Pharmacology and Treatment of Substance Abuse

COUNSELING AND PSYCHOTHERAPY:
INVESTIGATING PRACTICE FROM SCIENTIFIC, HISTORICAL, AND CULTURAL PERSPECTIVES

A Routledge book series
Editor, Bruce E. Wampold, University of Wisconsin

This innovative new series is devoted to grasping the vast complexities of the practice of counseling and psychotherapy. As a set of healing practices delivered in a context shaped by health delivery systems and the attitudes and values of consumers, practitioners, and researchers, counseling and psychotherapy must be examined critically. By understanding the historical and cultural context of counseling and psychotherapy and by examining the extant research, these critical inquiries seek a deeper, richer understanding of what is a remarkably effective endeavor.

Published

Counseling and Therapy with Clients Who Abuse Alcohol or Other Drugs
Cynthia E. Glidden-Tracy

The Great Psychothearpy Debate
Bruce Wampold

The Psychology of Working: Implications for Career Development, Counseling, and Public Policy
David Blustein

Neuropsychotherapy: How the Neurosciences Inform Effective Psychotherapy
Klaus Grawe

Beyond Evidence-Based Psychotherapy: Fostering the Eight Sources of Change in Child and Adolescent Treatment
George Rosenfeld

Principles of Multicultural Counseling
Uwe P. Gielen, Juris G. Draguns, Jefferson M. Fish

Cognitive Behavioral Therapy for Deaf and Hearing Persons with Language and Learning Problems
Neil Glickman

Intersections of Multiple Identities: A Casebook of Evidence-Based Practices with Diverse Populations
Miguel E. Gallardo and Brian W. McNeill

The Pharmacology and Treatment of Substance Abuse: Evidence and Outcomes Based Perspective
Lee Cohen, Frank Collins, Alice Young, Dennis McChargue

Forthcoming

The Handbook of Therapeutic Assessment
Stephen E. Finn

IDM Supervision: An Integrated Developmental Model for Supervising Counselors and Therapists, Third Edition
Cal Stoltenberg and Brian McNeill

The Great Psychotherapy Debate, Revised Edition
Bruce Wampold

Culture and the Therapeutic Process: A Guide for Mental Health Professionals
Mark M. Leach and Jamie Aten

Pharmacology and Treatment of Substance Abuse

Evidence- and Outcome-Based Perspectives

Edited by

Lee M. Cohen ◆ Frank L. Collins, Jr.

Alice M. Young ◆ Dennis E. McChargue

Thad R. Leffingwell ◆ Katrina L. Cook

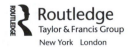
Routledge
Taylor & Francis Group
New York   London

Routledge
Taylor & Francis Group
270 Madison Avenue
New York, NY 10016

Routledge
Taylor & Francis Group
27 Church Road
Hove, East Sussex BN3 2FA

© 2009 by Taylor and Francis Group, LLC
Routledge is an imprint of Taylor & Francis Group, an Informa business

Printed in the United States of America on acid-free paper
10 9 8 7 6 5 4 3 2 1

International Standard Book Number: 978-0-8058-5968-3 (Hardback) 978-0-8058-5969-0 (Paperback)

Library of Congress Cataloging-in-Publication Data

Pharmacology and treatment of substance abuse : evidence- and outcome-based perspectives / Lee M. Cohen ... [et al.].
       p. ; cm. -- (Counseling and psychotherapy)
     Includes bibliographical references.
     ISBN 978-0-8058-5968-3 (hardback : alk. paper) -- ISBN 978-0-8058-5969-0 (pbk. : alk. paper)
     1. Substance abuse. I. Cohen, Lee M., Ph.D. II. Series: Counseling and psychotherapy.
     [DNLM: 1. Substance-Related Disorders--drug therapy. 2. Evidence-Based Medicine. 3. Treatment Outcome. WM 270 P5368 2009]

RC564.P484 2009
616.86--dc22
                                                                                          2008050336

Visit the Taylor & Francis Web site at
http://www.taylorandfrancis.com

and the Routledge Web site at
http://www.routledgementalhealth.com

This book is dedicated to the individuals struggling with addictions and the many professionals who have dedicated their careers to clinical research and the provision of services. We would also like to acknowledge the memory of three individuals who influenced our work:

Marian W. Fischman
Frank A. Holloway
Oscar A. Parsons

Contents

Part II
Conceptual Models and Principles of Substance Abuse Treatment

Part III
Assessment and Treatment of Substance Abuse

Part IV
Special Topics

Series Editor Preface

This innovative new series is devoted to grasping the vast complexities of the practice of counseling and psychotherapy. As a set of healing practices delivered in a context shaped by health delivery systems and the attitudes and values of consumers, practitioners, and researchers, counseling and psychotherapy must be examined critically. By understanding the historical and cultural contexts of counseling and psychotherapy and by examining the extant research, these critical inquiries seek a deeper, richer understanding of what is a remarkably effective endeavor.

Pharmacology and Treatment of Substance Abuse: Evidence- and Outcome-Based Perspectives, edited by Cohen, Collins, Young, McChargue, Leffingwell, and Cook, is everything that a comprehensive examination of the treatment of a mental disorder should be: evidence-based practice at its best. Cohen and colleagues use a transdisciplinary approach to bring together the best evidence from biology, neuroscience, psychology, and sociology in an understandable and integrated fashion. The first section offers a series of chapters that discuss from a variety of perspectives what is known about the biology of substance use and abuse. The second section describes the principles of substance use disorders, which form the basis for reviews of treatments for particular substances in the third section. The final section on special topics includes discussions of several important ancillary issues (e.g., drug testing in the workplace), particular intervention approaches, innovative perspectives (e.g., behavioral economics), and a view of the future. This volume does not take a perspective. Rather, it integrates the evidence from a variety of perspectives to provide a wonderfully rich understanding of substance abuse and its treatment.

Bruce E. Wampold
University of Wisconsin - Madison

Foreword

The Transdisciplinary Perspective

Mark S. Goldman

University of South Florida

It has long been noted that substance abuse is a biopsychosocial disorder, but for much of the time this term has been in use, it only has meant that one must acknowledge that separable biological, psychological, and social/cultural components all exert influence on outcomes of use. Only recently has the full meaning of this term, based on the truly interlocking and inseparable nature of these components, come into focus. Recent research has made it clear that the initiation, maintenance, and excessive use of psychoactive substances issue from a complex interplay of these components. In fact, these components operate so seamlessly that even the term "components" may represent unjustified separation. At times, what we call "components" instead may reflect that we are "shining the light" on different aspects of integrated and essentially unified processes. And in some instances, the "aspects" actually may just represent a different level of explanation of the very same process.

These components include genetically based individual differences in sensitivity, reactivity, and metabolism (pharmacokinetics and pharmacodynamics); individual differences in neurobiologically based learning and motivational pathways; individualized neuropsychological processes of self-regulation; varying family/social/peer influences; varying experiences and environmental exposures; and varying cultural norms. And, all these components of influence operate over developmental time. That is, as the individual grows and changes as they move through the different developmental phases of their lives, different aspects of these influences come to the fore and then recede.

This integrated perspective on substance abuse is emerging in the context of a revolution taking place in behavioral neuroscience that will allow us to move farther along on the path to a true multilevel, developmental perspective. Although examples of these revolutionary changes are far too extensive to recount here, I note a few that are critical in this domain.

Genetics

Because interest in genetics has become so ubiquitous in connection with substance abuse and dependence, it is perhaps appropriate to begin here. For many years, the approach to genetics involved the search for a gene, or genes, that served to increase risk, or sometimes to reduce (protect against) risk (e.g., Blum et al., 1990). Efforts to identify genes that confer risk have not ceased, of course, and one recent approach to drug development for addictions is to identify compounds that block the expression of certain gene products. At the same time, however, a more sophisticated understanding of gene operation has evolved, in which genes are understood to be active agents that interplay with successive environments over particular epochs in life to continuously adjust risk. Emphasized in the increased appreciation of genes as active agents is the concept of epigenesis, an increasingly popular and ever-evolving term in this age of genomics. Gottesman and Hanson (2005) report that the concept originated in embryology in reference to the emergence of complex organisms from undifferentiated cells, but broader definitions refer to gene expression profiles that include behavioral outcomes (Gottesman et al., 1982). The most expansive view of epigenetics best characterizes its meaning as it relates to substance abuse, however. In this sense of the term, Gottesman and Hanson (2005) relate epigenetics to "… the complexities of how multiple genetic factors and multiple environmental factors become integrated over time through dynamic, often nonlinear, sometimes nonreversible, processes to produce behaviorally relevant endophenotypes and phenotypes (p. 267)." The genetic factors are expressed as multilevel biological processes that range from those occurring within the nucleus of cells, to those that occur within single cells, to more complex processes that regulate the function of proximal groups of cells, and ultimately to distributed cell groupings that constitute brain "systems" (Breiter & Gasic, 2004). The environmental factors with which they interplay are diverse and may include familial influences, peer influences, community influences, and even historical influences that are operative within the lifespan of a single individual (e.g., prohibition in the early twentieth century in the United States).

The implications of this kind of thinking are far-reaching. Rather than directly conferring risk, genes may influence risk through an ongoing reciprocity with the environment that changes the very nature of the person as they develop. That is, gene/environment interactions generally do not operate in a simple manner (certain genes exposed to certain environments equal certain outcomes). Rather, genes that are activated by certain environments, at certain times in development, in certain sequences, may increase the likelihood of certain behavioral patterns that, when exposed to other environments, confer risk. And genes and environments do not just interact; genetically induced behavior patterns may influence individuals to seek environments that are consistent with the genetically induced pattern (gene/environment correlations) or may induce responses from the environment that then foster the original phenotype to become more extreme (gene/environment evocation).

Development

The role of development is so critical that it needs to be emphasized independently of its connection with genetics. An obvious aspect of development is sequencing; that is, behaviors and problem behaviors do not "pop up" instantly, but emerge over time as a consequence of sequences of events that occur in a particular order. In sequence, a recognizable pattern may emerge (e.g., the alcohol-dependence phenotype). Out of sequence, the same influences may not result in a recognizable pattern. But sequence is not enough; our biological substrate is primed to be receptive to event sequences at certain developmental epochs, and not at others. For substance abuse, a key example is the period that runs from what we might call peri-adolescence (the transition from childhood to adolescence) up to young adulthood. In the alcohol field, a recent report on underage drinking (Faden & Goldman, 2008) extensively reviews the multitude of influences that converge during this developmental phase to increase risk for adverse alcohol outcomes. And even within this time of life we commonly call adolescence, when events occur matters; early drinking is much more predictive of lifelong risk than is drinking later in this life period.

Decision Making and Incentive Valuation

Implied above is that risk in humans is not conferred through unyielding and automatic biological forces, but instead is usually conferred through tendencies (i.e., biases) built into the decision-making processes in some individuals. Humans are not robots, carrying out preset behaviors every time when triggered by a particular signal (context). Particular behaviors, even those that represent risk, occur probabilistically. Probabilities are adjusted by nuances of context, by temperaments and personality types, by social influences, and so on. Many advances in understanding how the brain renders decisions have been made in recent years, and these advances in understanding are increasingly being integrated with explanations of substance abuse. Most of these advances have been made in relation to normative tendencies in decision making (i.e., how the average person makes the decision). But even more recent work has revealed individual differences in decision-making tendencies especially when the decision needs to be made under conditions of uncertainty or risk; under these commonly occurring circumstances different individuals may interpret the same reinforcement in different ways (Cohen, 2008). Such individualized tendencies may be understood as one kind of behavioral phenotype in which the specific decision is not predetermined in any way, but instead the tendency to evaluate outcomes in particular ways influences choices.

When considering decision making, we first need to keep in mind that the occasion for making decisions is not just when we are presented with a conventional decision point, such as, do we want to buy a new car. In actuality, every moment of life represents a decision. Do we keep with the behavior sequence currently in play, or do we move to a new one? If we move to a new one, which one? These kinds of ongoing decisions require the capacity to place value on different behavioral choices, to compare these values "on-the-fly," and to successfully respond to contexts in which valued outcomes are, or are not, available. And ultimately, the goal of all choices is not just the conventional array of appetitive rewards, that is, food, water, sex, or money. Instead, it is what has been termed behavioral fitness, or the likelihood to have sufficient health and well-being, and sufficient social standing, to permit passing on of genes through procreation, and successful rearing of offspring until they can carry out an independent existence (to then procreate and pass on genes again; Glimcher, 2006). For this reason, we should consider the use of substances in this light; perhaps the goal of use is not just the influence of a consumed drug (or alcohol) on the user, but rather the effect of this use on behavioral patterns that lead to behavioral fitness. The point of getting intoxicated in late adolescence should not be seen as limited to the seeking of a pharmacological state (i.e., a direct effect of the drug on the brain); a better understanding of motivational influences may come from appreciating that such intoxication is occurring in a social context. Hence, that the behavioral state one achieves through substance use may serve to transiently increase bonding with your peers, or may increase the likelihood of a sexual encounter (in keeping with procreative urges), should not be dismissed as the actual penultimate goal. Certainly such patterns should be considered as operating prior to the end stage of use, when drug consumption may seem more autonomous.

Progress has been made in discerning the many kinds of decisions that human brains make, some of which involve different processing pathways in the brain (see Cardinal, 2006; Glimcher, Dorris, & Baker, 2005). So, for example, separate systems may evaluate delay of reward and effort necessary to obtain a reward (Rudebeck et al., 2006), and potential gains may be processed differently from potential losses (Weller et al., 2007). Extensive neural resources are devoted to social decision making, that is, cooperation or competition with an individual, or the decision to place trust in an individual (King-Casas, Tomlin, & Anen, 2005). Unlike other animals, humans can predict the hedonic consequences of events they have never experienced (Gilbert & Wilson, 2007). In the substance abuse field, considerable emphasis has been placed in recent years on the operation of dopamine pathways as a substrate for the evaluation of reward value (i.e., dopamine output as a signal for incentive salience or to note discrepancies between expected and actual rewards). It is, of course, these same dopamine pathways that have been linked to drugs of abuse, and are noted in many chapters in the present volume. Other neural pathways for decision making, possibly involving other neurotransmitters (e.g., norepinephrine, serotonin, glutamate), are being investigated for their involvement in substance use and abuse, with possible ramifications for new medication development.

Another aspect of reward valuation relates to immediate versus delayed reward. It is clear that drug abusers often opt for immediate as compared with delayed reward, and the mathematics of delay discounting has served as one base for the development of the emerging field of neuroeconomics (Loewenstein et al., 2008).

Social Behavior

As with any of the major themes discussed above, decision making transitions seamlessly into the next topic worth noting, that of social behavior. It is, of course, the social domain that is the primary zone of human decision making. Some theorists even suggest that the elaboration of the human brain beyond that of other species was based on the advantages for survival (evolutionary fitness) afforded by sophisticated social appraisal and decision making, and perhaps, most important, by pair bonding (Dunbar & Shultz, 2007). Social behavior relates to substance abuse in at least two important ways. First, it is becoming evident that for most people, the foundation for substance abuse at some point in a lifetime is established (as noted earlier) during adolescence, at a time when the importance of social development is paramount. And the use of substances (particularly alcohol) meshes perfectly with establishing social connections. Drug use is encouraged by social (peer) influences, typically begins and is maintained within social groupings, and has effects on social dynamics that are often facilitative. Particularly in adolescence and young adulthood, alcohol and drug use encourages more extreme social behavior, and a diminishment of responsibility for behavioral outputs while under the influence.

The significance of the social context for substance use and abuse cannot be sufficiently emphasized. More and more evidence is accruing that shows the human brain to be evolved for social functioning. As noted above, researchers who investigate decision making emphasize social decision making (competition, cooperation, trust) as the ultimate domain of choices we make. Other recent work shows that many brain cells are responsive to the actions of others (i.e., mirror neurons; Rizzolatti & Craighero, 2004), apparently as a device for understanding the intentions and goals of others in a social exchange. Even our ability to see the motions of others is built around the need to interpret the meaning of others' actions (Blake & Shiffrar, 2007). Once again, we must consider substance abuse as a social device for a species that is heavily invested at a fundamental level in emitting and interpreting social behavior.

Emotions

Perhaps it is unnecessary to point out that decision making, whether about appetitive or social goals, does not all (or even primarily) occur via thoughtful deliberation and calculation of payoffs. Although clearly such dispassionate consideration of options does occur, much of our decision making happens automatically, with the signal for the choice we are to follow coming in the form of an emotion: one that is positive and encouraging of a choice, or one that is aversive, discouraging a certain choice (Loewenstein et al., 2008). In this way, decision processes other than the one(s) mediated by dopaminergic pathways come to the fore. It is no great advance to recognize that drug use may alter emotion; perhaps the most common understanding of the motivation for drug use centers on the capacity of drugs to alter emotion. What is a newly emerging perspective is that cognition and emotion are intimately, perhaps inseparably, linked (Phelps, 2004). Hence, the influence of drugs may not just extend to emotional changes, but to actual changes in the way we think (process information). These kinds of alterations can lead an individual along different life pathways.

In particular, emotional reactions to stress can lead to long-term changes and perhaps differing life trajectories. It has been established (see Gunnar & Quevedo, 2007) that glucocorticoids, released in response to stress, influence gene expression in the nucleus of cells, leading to long-lasting effects of stress. Long-term recalibration of physiological set points has been deemed allostasis, and has been implicated in the etiology of substance abuse (Koob & Le Moal, 2008). Cycling us back to the inseparability of the themes we have addressed in this Preface, it is also established that environmental inputs, particularly maternal rearing practices, can alter these long-term stress response patterns, either by exacerbating them or by inducing resilience. Adolescent hyporesponsivity to some stress-inducing circumstances (Spear, 2000) can also be seen as a basis for the increases in risky behavior, including substance use, during this developmental phase.

Multiple Subsystems

One final point might be worth making in this discussion of etiological forces that influence substance use outcomes. The ongoing making of decisions about what behaviors in which we are to be engaged is not without internal conflict. I speak here not of the classic psychodynamic notions of competing motivations, but of the neural reality that our brains did not evolve in the way an engineer might have designed them with an efficient wiring scheme and program that converted a stimulus input into a desired output in the most direct and efficient fashion possible. Instead, our brains appear to be a collection of subsystems, each representing solutions to problems encountered at some point in our evolution. Some of these subsystems support deliberative processing, whereas others support automatic mechanisms of the kind described above (Kahneman, 2003). When presented with an environmental choice, these subsystems do not necessarily arrive at the same "best" solution. Which solution becomes preeminent in determining an output is not necessarily based on the optimal logic of the situation. It is these competing influences that result in what may appear to be suspect behavioral choices. On the whole, substance abuse may not seem to make much sense, but the processing logic of some subsystems may say otherwise in certain situations.

Implications for Prevention and Treatment

Given the multifaceted, and developmental, character of substance use and abuse noted above, it is no wonder that finding effective prevention and treatment approaches is a formidable task. It becomes clearer and clearer that what we are attempting to do is not to remove or replace a circumscribed biological process or behavioral characteristic, but instead to place our intervention into the flow of a multitude of forces, playing out over developmental time, that influence major pathways of life. Whatever we do to intervene, it is unlikely that we can influence all the unfolding processes that may play a role, or that we can set up new behavioral patterns that will not encounter new counterforces that emerge in response to our interventions. Whether we think we are carrying out prevention or treatment, what we are actually attempting is to alter life pathways in a reasonably permanent manner; because these pathways are multidetermined, they possess a kind of inertia, a resistance to change. Although treatment does not necessarily have to address the same processes that operate to produce a disorder (many upstream processes that eventually lead to a disorder no longer may be operative at the point that treatment is necessary, or may be irreversible), it may be the case that by thinking about more specific interventions as forays into these larger processes may offer some advantages. For example, by keeping in mind the sections on epigenesis and development, it becomes evident that some interventions might best be offered at certain times, or in certain sequences. When coming from the perspective of decision making, we might think of interventions, be they behavioral or pharmacological, as altering the "tipping point" in decision making about behaviors that are chosen for engagement. That is, they must alter relative valuations of outcomes, so that behavioral outputs are selected that have better long-term outcomes. And by invoking the essential social nature of humans, we can better understand why "common factors" often seem to have such influence, or why many interventions are easily offered in group settings.

And whether we think about them or not, the multifaceted forces are always operative, sometimes perhaps to thwart otherwise ideal plans. It is, of course, proper to ask how we can ever hope to make therapeutic inroads into these multifaceted, unfolding forces, Can an intervention ever be that broad? It is hoped the answer is that we do not have to influence all the forces. Instead, what we search for are what have been termed in different conceptual systems as nodes, attractors, or, more simply, points of leverage. A well-placed boulder can seriously alter the flow of a river, without needing to block all the water in play.

It is in this context that the chapters in this book are offered to present the best of current understanding about how to go about the change process. They represent the latest in creative approaches to change, along with the latest in empirical support for the methods offered. It is hoped they also represent points of leverage that will serve to influence the larger processes.

References

Blake, R., & Shiffrar, M. (2007). Perception of human motion. *Annual Review of Psychology, 58,* 47–73.

Blum, K., Noble, E. P., Sheridan, P. J., Montgomery, A., Ritchie, T., Jagadeeswaran, P., et al. (1990). Allelic association of human dopamine D2 receptor gene in alcoholism. *JAMA, 263,* 2055–2060.

Brieter, H., & Gasic, G. P. (2004). A general circuitry processing reward/aversion Information and its implication for neuropsychiatric illness. In M. Gazzaniga (Ed.), *The cognitive neurosciences* (3rd ed.). Boston: MIT Press.

Cardinal, R. N. (2006). Neural systems implicated in delayed and probabilistic reinforcement. *Neural Networks, 19,* 1277–1301.

Cohen, M. X. (2008). Neurocomputational mechanisms of reinforcement-guided learning in humans: A review. *Cognitive, Affective, and Behavioral Neuroscience, 8,* 113–125.

Dunbar, R. I. M., & Shultz, S. (2007). Evolution in the social brain. *Science, 317,* 1344–1347.

Faden, V., & Goldman, M. S. (2008). Underage drinking: Understanding and reducing risk in the context of human development, a supplement to *Pediatrics. Pediatrics, 121,* 231–354.

Gilbert, D. T., & Wilson, T. D. (2007). Prospection: Experiencing the future. *Science, 317,* 1351–1354.

Glimcher, P. W. (2005). Indeterminacy in brain and behavior. *Annual Review of Psychology, 56,* 25–56.

Glimcher, P. W., Dorris, M. C., & Bayer, H. M. (2005). Physiological utility theory and the neuroeconomics of choice. *Games & Economic Behavior, 52,* 213–256.

Gottesman, I. I., & Hanson, D. R. (2005). Human development: Biological and genetic processes. *Annual Review of Psychology,* 56, 263–286.

Gottesman, I. I., Shields, J., & Hanson, D. R. (1982). *Schizophrenia: The epigenetic puzzle.* London: Cambridge University Press.

Gunnar, M., & Quevedo, K. (2007). The neurobiology of stress and development. *Annual Review of Psychology, 58,* 145–173.

Kahneman, D. A. (2003). Perspective on judgment and choice: Mapping bounded rationality. *American Psychologist, 58,* 697–720.

King-Casas, B., Tomlin, D., & Anen, C. (2005). Getting to know you: Reputation and trust in a two-person economic exchange. *Science, 308,* 78–83.

Koob, G. F., & Le Moal, M. (2008). Addiction and the brain antireward system. *Annual Review of Psychology, 59,* 29–53.

Loewenstein, G., Rick, S., & Cohen, J. D. (2008). Neuroeconomics. *Annual Review of Psychology, 59,* 647–672.

Phelps, E. A. (2004). Human emotion and memory: Interactions of the amygdala and hippocampal complex. *Current Opinion in Neurobiology, 14,* 198–202.

Rizzolatti, G., & Craighero, L. (2004). The mirror-neuron system. *Annual Review of Neuroscience, 27,* 169–192.

Rudebeck, P. H., Walton, M. E., Smyth, A. N., Bannerman, D. M., & Rushworth, M. F. S. (2006). Separate neural pathways process different decision costs. *Nature Neuroscience, 9,* 1161–1168.

Spear, L. P. (2000). The adolescent brain and age-related behavioral manifestations. *Neuroscience and Biobehavioral Reviews, 24,* 417–463.

Weller, J. A., Levin, I. P., Shiv, B., & Bechara, A. (2007). Neural correlates of adaptive decision making for risky gains and losses. *Psychological Science, 18,* 958–964.

Part I

Psychopharmacology and Neurobiology of Substance Abuse

Alice M. Young
Texas Tech University
and Texas Tech University
Health Sciences Center

The chapters in this introductory section focus on conceptual models in pharmacology and psychopharmacology, and on how interactions among key behavioral, cellular, genetic, neuronal, and physiological processes contribute to substance use problems. The section begins with overviews of basic principles of drug action and of drug effects linked to substance abuse and dependence, and it finishes with discussions of the neurobiology and genetics of addiction. The breadth of these discussions illustrates that all drugs have multiple effects that can affect functions of multiple body systems and that are modified by the individual user's own particular biology, psychology, and experience.

All of the research knowledge described in this section relies on a framework of ethical, legal, research, and theoretical practices that protect vulnerable research participants. These chapters draw from in vitro studies of drug effects in cell cultures and brain tissues, from laboratory studies of behavioral and psychological effects of drugs in humans and other animals, and from clinical studies both in individuals who meet diagnostic criteria for substance use disorders and also in healthy research participants who have no history of substance abuse or misuse. By U.S. and international law, research with humans or animals is subject to rigorous review by Institutional Review Boards (for human participants) or Institutional Animal Care and Use Committees (for vertebrate animal subjects). Research involving administration of abused drugs is also subject to federal, state, and local controlled substance regulations. Ongoing development of our framework of ethical, legal, research, and theoretical practices will be critical to advancing research in this area and to translating research into clinical assessment and treatment.

Chapter 1 introduces key concepts of pharmacokinetics and pharmacodynamics. Paronis provides broad coverage of the principles of drug action, which in turn provide the foundations for the research strategies described in later chapters. Readers will quickly appreciate that drug effects are emergent effects, resulting from interactions of drugs and our normal biological processes, and that understanding the principles of drug actions will enable critical appreciation of theoretical and research approaches to treatment.

In Chapter 2, Cooper and Comer highlight the contributions that behavioral theory and research have made to development of potential pharmacotherapies for substance use disorders. They point out that the direct aim of a pharmacotherapy is to support and maintain abstinence from drug use, and argue that identification of such pharmacotherapies benefits from human laboratory studies that draw on the rich tradition of theory-based studies in animals. The chapter reviews the range of human laboratory models that do, or do not, provide predictive evidence of treatment effectiveness.

In Chapter 3, Vandrey and Mintzer address the clinical concern raised by impairments in cognitive functioning produced by abused drugs and drug abuse. They review what is known about which cognitive processes are affected by which drugs and under what conditions, about the impact of altered functioning on daily or specialized functioning, and about the relative severity of these effects across drug classes. In a discussion especially relevant to this volume, they discuss emerging evidence about whether drug effects on cognitive functioning may affect cognitive skills required by cognitive-behavioral or psychosocial treatment modalities.

Drug abuse and misuse can be accompanied by tolerance, sensitization, and/or physiological dependence. In Chapter 4, Allen draws upon research with animals and humans to guide the reader to a balanced understanding of these adaptive processes. As noted by Allen, brains and behaviors adapt in many ways to drug exposure, and an individual's specific learning opportunities play major roles in whether, when, and how tolerance and/or sensitization to effects of drugs occur. Moreover, the contributions of these processes to addiction are under vigorous scientific debate.

In Chapter 5, Koob provides a detailed conceptual model of how changes in biological and neurobiological processes mediate an individual's transition from occasional drug use to addiction. This evolving model begins with detailed information about how drug use engages normal brain circuits, learning processes, and neurochemical processes. The model then incorporates the critical feature that repeated use of addictive drugs changes how these processes operate, thereby creating a new trajectory that recruits new systems and motivational states.

The proposed stages of addiction and accompanying brain changes provide a theory-driven model to guide both basic and clinical research.

In Chapter 6, Ray and Hutchinson address another rapidly changing area, the genetics of addiction. They begin with an overview of basic principles of genetics and then review the complex work that will be required to unravel how a genetic variant acts to influence the risk and course of addiction in an individual. A major theme of this chapter is the likelihood that interactions among environments, genes, and behaviors are not unidirectional. A second theme is that genetic variation may either accelerate or slow changes in the neurobiological/psychological processes that shape or treat addiction.

Together, these chapters provide a conceptual review and background of biological and psychological processes that interact in addiction and substance abuse. Identification of potential substance use treatments builds upon the models and conceptualizations covered here. The evidence associated with substance use treatment is the focus of the remainder of this volume.

1

Principles of Drug Action: Pharmacokinetics and Pharmacodynamics

Carol A. Paronis

Northeastern University

Contents

Pharmacokinetics

Pharmacokinetic aspects of drug action concern the bioavailability of drugs, including how drugs are absorbed into, distributed throughout, and eventually metabolized and eliminated from the body. These processes are sometimes referred to in the aggregate by the acronym absorption, distribution, metabolism, excretion (ADME) and they establish the potency of drugs and the time course of the effects of drugs. Pharmacokinetic characteristics of drug action are determined in part by the physicochemical properties of the drug and in part by the physiology of the organism, which may be altered either intentionally or inadvertently. For example, a drug that has a fast onset and short duration of action may have its time course of activity altered by being chemically reformulated as a slow-release tablet. Alternatively, a drug that is expected to have effects that last eight hours based on studies in healthy individuals might last three days in someone suffering from liver failure. Despite these potential variations in pharmacokinetic properties, the principles introduced below generally apply in describing how drugs reach their site of action by being absorbed into, and distributed by, the circulatory system, and how drug action is terminated by metabolism to inactive products which are then eliminated from the body.

Administration

The administration of drugs refers to the process by which drugs are delivered to an organism. There are several different methods that can be used to deliver drugs, and the best route of administration varies according to the intended purpose for which the drugs are being administered. In humans, the most common routes of administration are oral (per os; PO), injection into the bloodstream (intravenous; IV), injection under the skin (subcutaneous; SC), injection into muscle (intramuscular; IM), or mucosal absorption, which occurs when a drug is taken by inhaled or buccal routes. A less common route of administration, but one that has application to substance abuse, is transdermal administration, in which a drug is slowly released from a patch and absorbed into the bloodstream through the skin. Each method of administering drugs has unique advantages and disadvantages, and all will differentially influence the rate at which drugs are absorbed into the bloodstream and the percentage of drug taken that ultimately enters the circulation, referred to as the bioavailability of the drug (see Figure 1.1).

Injection of drug by any of the routes mentioned above, IV, SC, or IM, is generally followed by a rapid and constant rate of absorption into the bloodstream. Of the common injection routes, IV administration results in the fastest onset to drug action with zero time to absorption as the drug is delivered directly to the bloodstream. IV administration also presents the best way to deliver precise doses of drugs; a drug administered by IV route is considered to be completely absorbed and therefore has 100% bioavailability (Levine, 1983). Injection of drugs by SC or IM routes also tends to result in relatively fast onset to action, although this can depend on the vehicle by which they are administered. "Vehicle," here, means the substances in which a drug is dissolved or otherwise formulated, serving the function of increasing the volume of the dose to be delivered. In most cases, drug vehicles are inert and do not influence direct effects of the drug; however, they can have physical properties that affect the drug absorption into the blood. Most drugs are dissolved in an aqueous solution and are rapidly absorbed, on the order of minutes. On occasion, however, drugs injected IM or SC may be formulated as suspensions which provide a slower absorption into the circulatory system. This slow absorption can allow drug effects that are sustained for days or even months. In addition to this ability to manipulate absorption by varying the vehicle, another advantage of administering drugs by injectable routes is the avoidance of "first-pass metabolism" in the liver. Disadvantages associated with drug injection include relatively high costs and the inherent risks of infection or other irritation occurring at the site of injection.

FIGURE 1.1

Theoretical plasma concentration of a drug following different routes of administration; IV (curve A), SC (curve B), IM (curve C), and PO (curve D). Drug administered IV is immediately and fully absorbed, yielding a large peak concentration that is cleared from the plasma relatively quickly. Oral administration produces the lowest peak concentration, but retains measurable concentrations for the longest period of time.

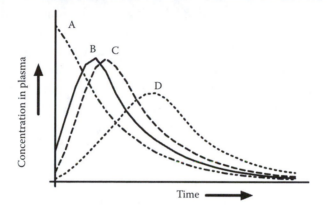

Oral administration is the most common method of taking drugs, either as therapeutics or as abused substances. Oral administration presents an easy and economical way to deliver drugs and virtually every drug can be taken orally. Despite its ease of use, however, oral drug administration has several disadvantages, including variable rates of absorption and low drug bioavailability. Drugs that are taken orally are sometimes absorbed into the bloodstream over minutes or sometimes hours, depending on the rate of gastric emptying, which, in turn, depends on a number of factors including the amount and type of food in the stomach, the gastric pH level, and the position and activity of the body. The rate of absorption can further vary as a function of the physicochemical properties of the drugs, especially their degree of ionization. Most drugs exist as weak acids or weak bases at a pH of 7.4, the normal pH of plasma, but in some organs, including the stomach and kidneys, the pH varies. In the stomach, the pH level decreases when food is eaten, changing the ionization of drugs, such that acids become less ionized and bases become more ionized at the lower pH. Hence, acids are more likely to diffuse into the blood and bases are less likely to enter the bloodstream after food is eaten (Levine, 1983). In addition to this variable absorption, bioavailability of drugs is almost always very low following oral administration because substances that enter the bloodstream from the alimentary canal must pass through the liver before being distributed to other tissues and organs in the body. Although drugs are metabolized throughout the body, the liver is the organ primarily associated with drug metabolism. Because orally delivered drugs enter the liver before the general circulation, it is often the case that a high percentage of the orally administered drug is metabolized to inactive products within the liver and eliminated from the body without ever producing a biological effect. This process, by which the drug is lost before entering the general circulation, is termed "first-pass metabolism."

Transmucosal administration is not a very common method for delivering therapeutics; however, it is the manner by which some drugs that are inhaled are absorbed into the circulation. Drugs that are available as vapors or aerosols, such as smoked nicotine, or as powders that are taken intranasally, are absorbed directly into the bloodstream from the mucosal membranes lining the mouth or nasal passages. Some drugs, for example nicotine gum, are administered buccally, that is they are taken by mouth but not swallowed, and these also are absorbed through mucosal linings. Because this route of administration avoids first-pass metabolism by entering the bloodstream at or near the site of administration, a drug that is administered by inhalation or buccally can be expected to have pharmacokinetic characteristics—high bioavailability and rapid onset to action—similar to those seen following injectable routes of administration.

In contrast to the rapid absorption seen with transmucosal administration, the slowest absorption of drugs occurs when a drug is administered using transdermal patches. Drug patches are comprised of multiple layers, including an impermeable outer layer, a drug reservoir, a porous membrane that controls the rate of release of the drug, and an adhesive to secure the patch to the skin. When the patch is affixed to the skin, the drug diffuses out of the reservoir, through the porous membrane, to the surface of the skin. The skin is nearly impermeable to all substances and so the movement of the drug particles across the skin and into the underlying blood vessels is very slow. One advantage of this method of drug delivery is that the steady release of the drug is excellent for maintaining consistent levels of the drug in blood for a period of weeks. However, in addition to the slow onset, other disadvantages of this route of administration are that patches must be formulated with very large quantities of drug and the dose cannot be easily adjusted for individuals. The transdermal route of administration has somewhat limited clinical utility, although it is an excellent way of delivering drugs for indications requiring constant blood levels of drugs for long periods of times, or when patient compliance is a concern. Patches originally were used to deliver scopolamine prophylactically for motion sickness; more recent indications for patch drug delivery systems are nicotine for smoking reduction, fentanyl for pain alleviation, and hormonal combinations for birth control (Gilman, Rall, Nies, & Taylor, 1993; Shiffman, Fant, Buchhalter, Gitchell, & Henningfield, 2005).

Absorption and Distribution

After a drug is administered, it is distributed throughout the body within the plasma, the liquid component of blood. Drugs enter or leave the plasma by diffusing across the biological membranes. The diffusion can be passive, by flowing from an area of high concentration to an area of low concentration without restriction, or it can be facilitated by coupling to other molecules in the body, called carrier proteins, that help transport substances across membranes that otherwise act as barriers to the substances due to their size, solubility, or ionization. The probability that a drug will diffuse across a membrane is determined not only by the concentrations of the drug on either side of the membrane, and of other molecules found in the blood or organ tissues, but also by the chemical structure of the drug, the composition of the membranes, and other physiological factors.

Most biological substances enter or leave the bloodstream within the capillaries, the smallest vessels of the circulatory system. The function of the capillaries is to allow the exchange of nutrients or other products between the circulating blood and the cells of other organs and so most solutes pass through the capillary walls easily. Both organic and inorganic substances, including drugs, can diffuse across the capillary membrane by going either through or between the capillary cells, depending on whether the substances are *hydrophilic* (water-loving) or *hydrophobic* (water-fearing). Like most cells in the body, the membranes of the capillary cells are comprised primarily of phospholipids, which are lipid molecules with charged head groups, oriented such that the lipids are internalized within the membrane and the charged head groups are found along the intracellular and extracellular surfaces of the cell. This arrangement results in a polar, or hydrophilic surface, and a nonpolar hydrophobic core within the membrane.

When drugs pass through the capillary walls, the size of the molecules and their lipid/water partition coefficient will influence the rate at which they diffuse across the capillary membranes. The lipid/water partition coefficient is essentially a measure of how hydrophilic or hydrophobic a substance is, and in living organisms the lipid/water partition coefficient of a drug can determine how rapidly it penetrates the capillary membrane (Levine, 1983). Hydrophobic drugs, such as heroin, will diffuse in and out of the blood very quickly, likely by going through the lipophilic membranes of the cells that form the capillary walls. In contrast, hydrophilic drugs, such as morphine, diffuse more slowly in and out of the blood, likely by passing through openings that occur between adjacent cells of the capillaries, which are lined by the hydrophilic headgroups of the phospholipids. For hydrophilic drugs, the size of the molecules may also directly influence their diffusion, as some molecules are simply too large to pass through the gaps and pores that form between cells. The rate at which hydrophilic drugs diffuse across membranes varies inversely with their molecular weight, up to a certain point, but very large molecules, for example, proteins, penetrate capillaries very poorly and are more likely to be transported across cell membranes by carrier molecules.

In addition to the physicochemical properties of the drug and the capillary membrane, several aspects of the physiology of the body will also influence the distribution of a drug either temporarily or permanently. For example, anything that increases blood flow, such as heat or exercise, will serve to also increase the distribution of drugs, or anything else, transported by the blood throughout the body. On the other hand, the volume of blood within an organism is not uniformly distributed throughout the body, but varies with the degree of vascularization in different tissues. The circulatory system is designed to deliver life-sustaining nutrients, remove waste, and transport hormones or other signaling molecules between organs. Because the needs of different tissues vary, the density of blood vessels in different tissues also varies, and a greater density of capillaries in well-vascularized tissues yields a large surface area available for the exchange of molecules across the capillary membranes. The most highly vascularized organ is the brain, which uses high amounts of energy and requires rapid delivery of nutrients to sustain its activities. As a result, drugs are delivered rapidly to brain tissue, although drugs that freely diffuse into brain tissue also will diffuse out of the brain and be rapidly redistributed by the plasma. Muscle and skin have a lower density of capillaries than does the brain, resulting in slower delivery of drugs to these tissues, although in terms of absorption this may facilitate the sustained absorption of drugs administered either IM or SC. Other tissues, such as fat, are poorly vascularized, and a drug that diffuses into fatty tissue will tend to stay there for a long time (Levine, 1983).

Some tissues have specialized structures that have developed to either facilitate or hinder transport across the cell membranes. In the liver and kidney, for example, capillary vessels contain large pores, which allow for easier exchange of large molecules. In contrast, the openings in the capillary walls within the central nervous system (CNS) are so small they are referred to tight junctions. In addition to decreased permeability as a function of the small openings, diffusion of many solutes into brain tissue is further hindered by a fatty sheath that surrounds the capillaries. Together, the tight junctions and the fatty sheath form what is called the blood–brain barrier, which counteracts the high vascularization of the brain by protecting the CNS from any large fluctuations in the constituents of the blood. However, although this barrier is impermeable to most charged or hydrophilic substances, drugs that are hydrophobic readily enter the CNS. For example, heroin is a hydrophobic drug that freely passes through the fatty barrier, whereas morphine is a hydrophilic drug that must achieve a higher concentration in plasma to create a diffusion gradient sufficient to support its crossing the blood–brain barrier. As a result, heroin is relatively potent, and morphine is relatively less potent. Interestingly, despite its potency, heroin itself is pharmacologically inert. After heroin enters the CNS, it is biotransformed to yield morphine, and it is only in this metabolized form that administered heroin is able to elicit a drug effect. This is not uncommon, and consideration of whether a drug must pass the blood–brain barrier is taken into account when new drugs are being developed. Psychoactive compounds must be able to penetrate the blood–brain barrier in order to produce their effects, and so ideally they should be small and hydrophobic. When a hydrophilic drug must be used to treat a disorder, it is sometimes possible to take advantage of mechanisms available for transport of other biological matter across the barrier. For example, levodopa, a precursor to dopamine that is used to treat Parkinson's disease, is transported across the blood–brain barrier via an amino acid carrier protein. Once in the brain, levodopa is converted to dopamine and becomes an effective treatment. Drugs developed for peripheral indications, such as hypertension or asthma, are designed specifically to remain in the periphery by incorporating molecules that are very large, or very polar, or both, and thus will have limited diffusion into the CNS.

Drug Reservoirs   The volume of distribution describes the total volume of fluid in which the drug is found in the body. Generally speaking, drugs distribute to three main water compartments within the body: the plasma, the extracellular fluid, and the intracellular fluid. Some drugs, however, accumulate at sites within the plasma or in tissues where they have no pharmacological actions but they happen to be more soluble in those environments or they bind to intracellular components of the tissue. These sites are known as reservoirs and when a drug is retained in a reservoir it may remain in the body for up to weeks or months. This is usually inconsequential as the compounds are released from the reservoir in quantities too small to have any effects. A potentially more deleterious effect of reservoirs is that a greater concentration of the drug exists in the tissue than in the plasma, reducing the potency of the drug and requiring that higher doses be administered.

Tissues such as fat or bone may store drug, but by far the most common reservoir for drugs are plasma proteins, which serve as carriers for different substances. One such carrier protein is hemoglobin, which transports iron in the blood; another plasma protein is albumin, which transports hydrophobic molecules in the blood. Albumin is the most abundant plasma protein, and it combines with a great variety of commonly used drugs including aspirin and some antibiotics. Similar to other reservoirs, binding of drug to plasma proteins greatly reduces the concentration of free drug and it is not unusual for more than 90% of a given drug to be bound to plasma proteins (Gilman et al., 1993). Because albumin serves to transport molecules through the blood, the binding of substances to albumin is necessarily reversible, allowing the transported compounds to come on and off easily. This binding process follows what is called the law of mass action, which simply states that when two reactants that bind in a reversible manner are at equilibrium, the rate of the formation of the product is equal to the rate of the dissociation of the product. The concentration of proteins in the plasma is relatively stable, so any amount of drug that exceeds the amount needed to saturate the protein is "free drug" are able to interact with its intended biological target. As free drug is eliminated from the body, the concentration in the plasma is reduced. This essentially triggers the drug–plasma protein complex to become unbound, releasing more free drug into the plasma.

Essentially the same relationship describes the movement of free drug in and out of all drug reservoirs, however, binding to plasma proteins is different from other tissue reservoirs because multiple drugs will bind to the same site on the protein. Thus, if another drug is added to the plasma, it will affect the equilibrium of the first drug. In other words, if drug A and drug B both bind albumin, then coadministration of drug A and drug B will result in competition for the albumin binding site, with the result that the protein will bind less than usual of both drugs, raising their free concentrations, and thus increasing their potency above normally expected levels.

Biotransformation

Biotransformation is often referred to as metabolism, although this is inaccurate as metabolism is the process of altering living material for the production of energy. In contrast, drugs are altered by the body, or biotransformed, to more water-soluble compounds to facilitate their elimination from the body. Biotransformation is most often a two-stage process of enzymatic reactions (Gilman et al., 1993; Levine, 1983). Phase I reactions are fast, resulting in compounds made more polar by the addition (oxidation) or removal (reduction) of oxygen, or cleavage of a compound by the addition of water (hydrolysis). Phase II reactions involve conjugations, or the chemical combination of the drug with a molecule present in the body, such as a carbohydrate or amino acid, yielding even more hydrophilic compounds. Biotransformation can occur anywhere in the body, although the liver is the primary organ associated with metabolic processes. Drug biotransformation usually results in inactive compounds that are readily eliminated by the body though sometimes active metabolites are formed, prolonging the duration of action of a drug instead of terminating it. Active compounds are more likely to result from Phase I than Phase II transformations. Codeine, aspirin, and diazepam are representative drugs that produce effects in their parent form and also following Phase I biotransformations. Other drugs represent another situation insofar as drugs are delivered in inactive forms, called prodrugs, which must be biotransformed to have a biological effect (Kenakin, 1993). Examples of prodrugs include heroin, which undergoes two hydrolysis reactions to become morphine before it can produce a biological effect, and levodopa, which is only active after decarboxylation (removal of a –COOH group) to become dopamine.

The rate at which drugs are biotransformed can follow either zero-order kinetics or first-order kinetics (see Figure 1.2). Zero-order kinetics describes a fixed or constant rate of removal of a set amount of drug per hour, independent of the concentration of the substrate. Very few

FIGURE 1.2

Rates of elimination following high and low doses of two drugs. Drug A is metabolized at a constant rate of 2 μg/ml per hour (zero-order kinetics); Drug B has a T1/2 of 90 min (first-order kinetics). Plasma concentration is shown on a linear scale (a) or a logarithmic scale (b and c); in c, the numbers indicate sequential half-lives for drug B.

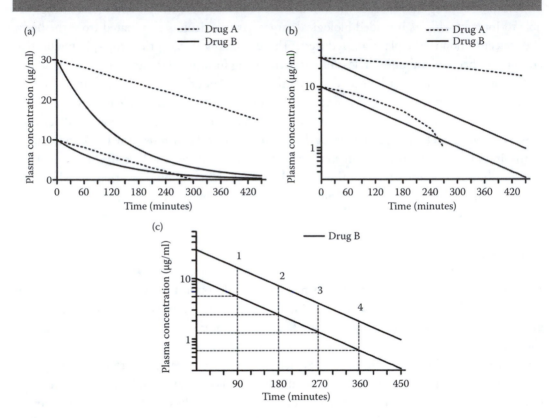

drugs are metabolized according to zero-order kinetics and those that are, such as aspirin and ethanol, tend to be administered in very large doses that are able to saturate the available enzyme. As an example, ethanol is oxidized by alcohol dehydrogenase, an enzyme that is quickly saturated. Once saturated, the alcohol dehydrogenase oxidizes ethanol at an average rate of 0.12 g/kg/hr regardless of how much alcohol is administered to the organism (Wilkinson, 1980). Most drugs, however, are transformed according to first-order kinetics, in which the rate of biotransformation varies directly with the concentration of the substrate (drug). In other words, the more drug that is available, the faster the enzymatic reaction and the more drug will be metabolized per unit time. Instead of describing this as a rate, the term half-life, or $T_{1/2}$, is applied. The half-life of a drug refers to the amount of time it takes to reduce the plasma concentration of the drug by 50% (Gilman et al., 1993). Knowing the $T_{1/2}$ of a drug can be of critical importance when determining dosage and dosing intervals for drugs that require more than a single administration. Drugs that are transformed according to first-order kinetics, when given at intervals that approximate their $T_{1/2}$, will yield a steady-state plasma concentration after approximately five half-lives (shown in Figure 1.3).

FIGURE 1.3
Schematic representation of the plasma concentrations of a drug, administered at one of two dosage levels and at intervals equal to the half-life of the drug (indicated by arrows). Hashed and dotted lines show fluctuations in plasma concentrations as each dose is absorbed and eliminated; solid lines represent the average plasma concentrations achieved by each dose.

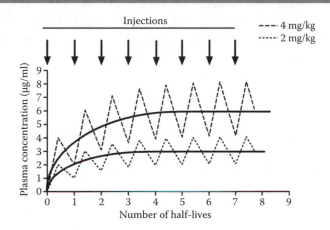

The term half-life is sometimes mistakenly used when discussing the time course of the effects of a drug. The $T_{1/2}$ of a drug is a constant measure of metabolism, calculated from plasma concentrations and independent of the dose administered, including whether single or multiple doses are given. In contrast, the time course of a drug effect varies directly with drug dose and applies only following a single administration of the drug. The time course of a drug effect takes into account the onset, duration, and offset of the drug action at the biological target, requiring distribution of the drug out of the plasma to the site of action. In order for there to be any measurable drug effect, first a certain threshold plasma concentration of drug must be gained. The drug effect then increases in intensity until the peak effect is obtained, and then the effect decreases as the drug is eliminated. Generally, the time course of action parallels the increases and decreases in plasma concentrations of the drug, but there is not always a one-to-one correspondence between the two measures. One might expect the plasma concentration needed for the onset and offset of drug effects to be the same, however, this is not necessarily the case and the effects of a drug may dissipate while plasma concentrations are relatively high (Maynert and Klingman, 1960). This phenomenon, sometimes referred to as the Mellanby phenomenon, cannot be fully explained, although redistribution from tissue to plasma, acute tolerance, or some other bioadaptation to the drug likely is involved.

Elimination

Most drugs are eliminated from the body by renal or hepatic clearance, although pulmonary, sweat, or other routes of elimination are also possible. As described above, biotransformation of many drugs occurs in the liver and the transformed products are then released from the liver through the bile duct into the small intestine. However, drugs tend to have low molecular weight, and their small size typically allows for passive diffusion of the compounds back into circulation, where they are then filtered through the kidney and excreted in urine (Levine, 1983). Untransformed drugs are rarely excreted from the body, and most urinalyses or other tests used to determine previous drug exposure assess levels of drug metabolites in addition to the parent compound. A very small fraction of an administered drug, instead of being eliminated, may become incorporated into the proteins of the body, for example, into hair or nails. This can occur when the drug or its metabolites, in the course of being distributed by the circulatory system, enters the hair glands or the matrix of the nail cuticle by passive diffusion (Scheidweiler, Cone, Moolchan, & Huestis, 2005). A drug also may be excreted by a sweat gland that happens to line a hair follicle, and from there become incorporated into the hair.

Pharmacokinetics Summary

Pharmacokinetics, or biodisposition, can determine the time course and the potency of drugs. Potency is determined largely by the route of administration and the hydrophilic or hydrophobic nature of the drug. The time course of action of drugs is determined by the route of administration, the drug distribution, and rate of biotransformation. Drugs are most potent when they are injected intravenously because there is no loss to first-pass metabolism before they enter the bloodstream. Drugs are least potent when they are given orally, as some drug is lost in each stage of the digestive process. In turn, drugs have the fastest onset when administered intravenously, and the slowest onset when taken orally. Hydrophobic drugs tend to be more potent than hydrophilic drugs as hydrophobic compounds more readily diffuse across biological membranes. Drug action is terminated by the biotransformation of the compound to an inactive form that is eliminated from the body. The time course, or duration of action of a drug, is not the same thing as the half-life, which is a measure of the metabolism of a drug. The duration of a drug's effect takes into account both onset and offset of the drug action, and where applicable can include the effects of active metabolites of the drug.

Pharmacodynamics

Pharmacodynamics is the study of the actions and effects drugs produce at the biochemical, cellular, tissue, or whole organism level. This is accomplished by establishing the relationship between doses or concentrations of drug and the responses they produce, and rests on the principle that increasing doses lead to increasing effects. The responses produced by most drugs result initially from their interactions with specific proteins, called receptors. The action of a drug binding to a receptor begins a cascade of events, and each subsequent event, from the subcellular to whole organism level can be considered a response.

The idea that drugs act at specific molecules within the body was based on the discovery of John Langley that nicotine elicits muscle contractions at the same site where curare blocks muscle contractions and, in fact, that nicotine and curare compete with each other for the site of action. Contemporaneous work of Paul Ehrlich suggested a relationship between the chemical structure of drugs and their recognition of biological substrates by demonstrating that, within a family of related compounds, some had biological activity, and others did not. This selectivity of action prompted Ehrlich to introduce the concept of "receptor," referring to a molecule within the body that was able to mediate the effects of drugs (Kenakin, 2006). Ehrlich further proposed that drugs and receptors work according to a lock and key model; that is, just as only some keys open particular locks, only some drugs activate particular receptors.

The contemporary view of receptors is that they may be any molecule that interacts with other substances and is able to transmit information to cells. To perform these actions, a receptor must have at least one binding site, for recognition of the drug or other stimuli (generically called ligands), and a functional site, able to elicit a biological response (Neubig, Spedding, Kenakin, & Christopoulos, 2003). For some membrane-bound receptors, the functional site is another binding site for a G-protein or other second messenger that is located intracellularly. Often, the term receptor is co-opted to specifically indicate such a membrane-bound protein; however, receptors comprise a diverse range of macromolecules that may be located on the cell surface or intracellularly. These different receptors subsume a variety of signaling functions by serving as enzymes, ion channels, genetic material, or transport proteins.

Hundreds of different molecules have been identified as serving as receptors for one or more substances, and these receptors have been grouped into dozens of receptor families, each consisting of one or more subtypes of receptors with varying degrees of overlap in terms of function, location, and structure. With this broad spectrum of available receptors, it is perhaps not surprising that many drugs and endogenous ligands are able to bind more than one receptor and, likewise, that receptors recognize more than one ligand. How then, is specificity of drug action determined? Historically, two pharmacological properties of a drug, affinity and efficacy, were believed to dictate the ability of the drug to elicit a response at a particular receptor. Contemporary theories of pharmacodynamic actions also recognize the role of the receptor and its microenvironment, which can dramatically modify drug effects. However, for illustrative purposes, this chapter focuses on the traditional view that responses to drugs vary as a function of the properties of the drug.

Drug–Receptor Interactions

Affinity The interactions between drugs and their receptors was originally described as being similar to enzymatic reactions, in which a substrate and an enzyme come together to form a substrate–enzyme complex, and this subsequently breaks down to form the enzyme and products. There is, however, a very important difference between drugs and receptors as compared to substrates and enzymes, and that is the interaction between drugs and receptors is fully reversible and neither is changed as a consequence of the process of the drug binding the receptor. In other words, the forward reaction of a drug and a receptor coming together to form a drug–receptor complex is counterbalanced by the reverse reaction, in which the drug–receptor complex become unbound, releasing free drug and receptor.

The affinity of a drug for a receptor is a measure of strength of the association between the drug and the receptor. Affinity can be directly determined from receptor binding studies or can be calculated from the ratio of the rates at which the drug binds to and dissociates from the receptor. The affinity of a drug is conventionally expressed by the term K_A, representing the concentration of drug necessary to bind 50% of the available receptors (Kenakin, 2006). A low K_A indicates a high affinity for a particular receptor, as a small concentration of drug is sufficient to bind half of the receptors. As mentioned above, very few drugs interact with only one receptor, however, drugs do tend to have different affinities for different receptors and receptor subtypes, and it is usually possible to identify a range of concentrations or doses in which a drug retains some selectivity of action at the receptor for which it has the highest affinity. In other words, a drug can be given at a dose that will occupy a certain proportion of one receptor, but does not occupy a noticeable fraction of another type of receptor. When administered at doses above this range, the drug will bind different receptors in addition to the one for which it has the highest affinity, conceivably resulting in a multitude of effects. When the dose range for selective actions is very small, the K_A values for a drug at different receptors are similar and the drug is considered to be nonselective.

Efficacy   Affinity is the measure of binding to a receptor but this does not bear any relation to the ability of the drug to elicit a change in the receptor, resulting in a response. Receptors are signaling molecules, and occupation of a receptor by a drug can initiate a cascade of cellular events that transmits the signal from the receptor to other cellular components. A response can be any event that occurs downstream as a consequence of the drug binding to the receptor. For example, the opening of an ion channel, a muscle contraction, or an increase in activity in a whole animal, might all be measurable responses related to receptor activation. The type and magnitude of response that a drug produces depends on its efficacy, or intrinsic activity. Intrinsic activity and efficacy are terms used to describe the ability of drugs to produce a change in the functional domain of the receptor, altering its interaction with other cellular molecules and initiating a response (Kenakin, 1993). For example, if a receptor is an ion channel, a drug that binds the receptor and has a high efficacy will produce a conformational change in the functional domain of the protein, such that the channel either opens or closes. The resulting flow of ions will change the intracellular and extracellular environment of the cell, potentially producing other changes, such as beginning an action potential, or contraction of the cell, or release of stored transmitter, which may then result in signaling between cells, initiating a change in the tissue or the whole animal.

Although every drug can produce a response, not all drugs have intrinsic activity. Drugs with intrinsic activity are able to produce a conformational change in the receptor, and are called agonists. Drugs that do not alter the receptor are antagonists. Another description of agonists is that they are substances able to either mimic or enhance the effects of the endogenous ligands at the receptor. This is a less specific description of drug action, but it is helpful in understanding the differences between agonists and antagonists, considering that the alternative definition of antagonists is that they are drugs that act solely by blocking the actions of endogenously or exogenously given substances. In other words, antagonists are ligands for receptors and are able to produce physiological effects, but only as a result of preventing the actions of another drug or ligand. Responses to antagonists, therefore, are best seen in receptor systems in which neurotransmitters, or other endogenous ligands, are constantly present. One example of such a receptor system is the dopamine system, in which an antagonist, such as haloperidol, can have profound effects by preventing dopamine from accessing the receptor.

It is hoped that the above descriptions of affinity and efficacy provide a useful platform for considering how drugs produce their effects; however, they represent a very simplified view of drug actions at the level of the receptor that does not incorporate physiological factors that necessarily impinge upon drug action. Another limitation of describing effects of drugs based solely on their immediate interactions with receptors is that many concepts of receptor theory consider only direct-acting ligands of membrane-bound receptors. However, many drugs produce significant physiological effects through indirect actions at these receptors (Neubig et al., 2003). Chief among these, as mentioned above, are antagonists that produce their effects only by blocking endogenous ligands. Haloperidol was one example cited; other antagonists with profound effects when given alone include the dissociative anesthetics, phencyclidine (PCP), and ketamine. In addition to antagonists, some agonists also act indirectly and are able to mimic or enhance the effects of the endogenous ligand without having an affinity for the receptor that directly mediates these actions. These indirect agonists produce their effects by increasing the concentration of the endogenous ligand by inhibiting its biotransformation, by acting as a precursor of the endogenous ligand, by increasing the release of the ligand from a cell, or by blocking removal of the ligand from the extracellular fluid. Notable indirect agonists include amphetamine and cocaine, which do not bind to dopamine receptors but produce their effects by increasing the concentration of extracellular dopamine.

Dose-Response Functions

Whether drugs act directly or indirectly to modify actions of a receptor, their responses are best quantified by evaluating dose-response functions, typically with the dose or concentration of drug plotted along the abscissa, and the response along the ordinate. The potency and efficacy, and in some circumstances the affinity, of drugs can be determined from dose-response functions (Kenakin, 2006). Drugs produce graded effects that increase with dose; when these effects are plotted according to the dose administered on a linear scale, the data yield a hyperbolic function. When the same data are plotted on a semi-logarithmic scale, the dose-effect function is sigmoidal, providing more detail in the effects of the lower doses and allowing effects of a greater range of doses to be depicted (shown in Figure 1.4). From such dose-effect functions, one can measure the relative potency of drugs, according to the position of the function along the x-axis, and the relative efficacy of the drug, according to the maximum effect produced. When the effect measured is simply the binding of the drug to the receptor, the point of the curve that crosses the 50% line is a measure of the affinity of the compound, defined as the concentration that occupies half of the available receptors. When the response measured is any effect downstream from binding at the receptor, the point on the dose-response function that passes through the 50% line is taken as the dose or concentration that produces 50% of the maximal response, designated the ED_{50} or EC_{50}, respectively. The ED_{50} value is a very commonly used measure of drug potency, but for different purposes, different points along the dose-effects function also may be used for comparisons, such as ED_{25} or ED_{80} representing, respectively, doses that produce 25% or 80% of the maximum possible effect.

Dose-response curves can be used to compare either the ability of a single drug to produce different responses, or the ability of several drugs to produce the same response. When different effects for a single drug are determined, comparing equieffective doses such as ED_{50} values

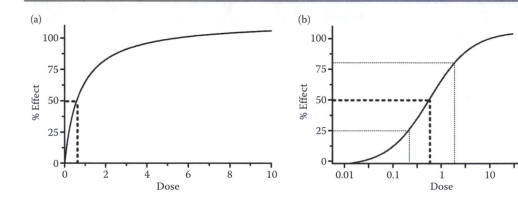

FIGURE 1.4

Comparison of the dose-effect functions of a drug graphed on an arithmetic scale and a semilogarithmic scale. The percentage of a maximal response is shown on the ordinate, and drug dose is shown along the abscissae on a linear scale (Panel a) or a logarithmic scale (Panel b). Dashed lines indicate the point at which 25, 50, or 80% of the maximum possible effect occurs, and the corresponding doses that result in these effects.

gives a measure of the selectivity of the drug in producing the effects. For example, if curves A, B, and C in Figure 1.5 represent different effects of drug X, one would surmise that a dose of X could be administered that would produce responses A and B, but would not produce measurable effects of response C. Such a separation of effects can be beneficial when some effects are desirable, and others are not desirable, provided, of course, that the undesirable effects are those that require the higher doses of drug. As a special case, if curve A represents a therapeutic effect of drug X, and curve C represents the lethal or toxic effects of drug X, the ratio of the ED_{50} values for A and C can provide a measure of the safety of the drug, termed the therapeutic index (Gilman et al., 1993). A caveat to this description is that although the simple ratio of the LD_{50}/ED_{50} is often used to introduce the concept of a therapeutic index, there is no universally accepted standard of what is considered to be a safe therapeutic index value, even when more conservative values are used. For instance, calculating an LD_1/ED_{90} ratio would compare a dose that is effective in 90% of the population to one that is lethal to 1% of the population. Although some would consider a dose that is lethal to 1% of the population to be unacceptably toxic, others might believe a dose effective in only 90% of the population to be inadequate.

When dose-response curves are used to compare the ability of several drugs to produce the same response, the relative potency of the different drugs can be determined. For example, if curves A, B, and C in Figure 1.5 represent the ability of drugs A, B, and C to produce effect X, drugs A and B would be considered approximately equipotent, whereas drug C is less potent. If a set of drugs is known to produce similar constellations of effects, comparing their order of potency across the different effects can give an indication of whether the same or different receptors mediate the responses to all drugs. A similar order of potency across effects indicates that the same, or similar, receptors mediate the different effects. When the drugs present a different order of potency across different effects, it can be assumed that different receptors

---

FIGURE 1.5
Comparison of the three dose-effect functions; the percentage of the maximal effect is shown on the ordinate, and drug dose is shown along the abscissae on a logarithmic scale. A, B, and C may represent either different effects of a single drug, or different drugs that produce the same response.

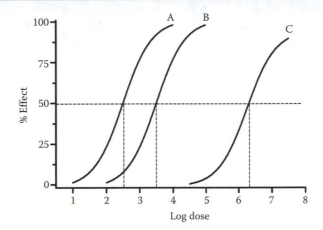

---

underlie the different responses. Thus, if the order of potency is A > B > C for effects X and Y, but is B > C > A for effect Z, one could assume that X and Y are mediated by similar receptors, and effect Z is mediated by a different receptor.

In addition to differences in potency, when effects of multiple drugs are compared, often it is apparent that not all drugs are able to produce the same maximum responses. This is most obvious when agonists and antagonists are compared, as the latter will yield flat dose-effect functions, yet even among agonists further distinctions can be made between full agonists, partial agonists, and in some cases, inverse agonists. The height of the dose-effect function for each drug is determined by the efficacy, or intrinsic activity of the drug, and this property defines the ability of each drug to produce a response. Drugs that produce maximum effects in a particular preparation or tissue are termed full agonists, and drugs that are not able to produce the maximal possible response in a preparation are partial agonists (Kenakin 1993; 2006). Drugs that are partial agonists are also sometimes referred to as mixed agonists/antagonists because their lower efficacy allows them also to function as antagonists under some circumstances. Drugs with different efficacy are shown in Figure 1.6a; here it can be seen that drugs A and B are full agonists, and drug C, although more potent than drug B, is a partial agonist that is not able to produce more than 50% of the maximum possible effect. In 1984, a new classification of efficacy, inverse agonism, was introduced to describe the effects of a new class of benzodiazepine ligands (Wood, Loo, Braunwalder, Yokoyama, & Cheney, 1984). These drugs produced physiological and biochemical effects opposite in nature to the effects of agonists. In Figure 1.6a, drug E represents anticipated responses to an inverse agonist. The term inverse agonist is used with increasing frequency based on effects of drugs in cell preparations although, excepting the benzodiazepines, often it is difficult to distinguish the effects of inverse agonists from antagonists in whole organisms.

FIGURE 1.6
Panel a. Theoretical functions comparing drugs that vary in intrinsic activity. Drugs A and B are able to produce maximal effects, drug C produces only 50% of the maximal response, drug D does not produce the response, and drug E results in a negative response. Panel b. Dose-effect function (response) and binding function (occupancy) for a single drug; the dashed lines indicate half-maximal effects and the corresponding concentrations that produce these effects.

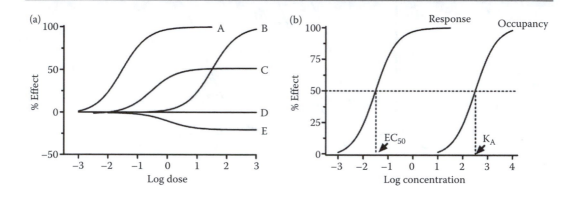

A corollary to drug efficacy is the concept of spare receptors, or a receptor reserve. By definition, any drug capable of producing a full effect is a full agonist, within this grouping, however, drugs may yet have varying degrees of efficacy, evidenced by the size of their receptor reserve. A receptor reserve exists when a drug with high efficacy is able to produce a maximal effect while occupying only a small fraction of the available receptors; the receptors not needed are considered the receptor reserve (Kenakin, 1993; Neubig et al., 2003). In Figure 1.6b, two dose-effect functions for drug X are compared. One function represents a response downstream from the receptor, and a maximum effect of this response occurs at the same concentration that produces 5% of the maximum of the second effect. If the second curve represents the binding of the drug to the receptor, it is clear that drug X is able to produce a maximal response at concentrations much lower than those needed to fully occupy the available receptors. For this response, the remaining 95% of the receptors are considered the receptor reserve for Drug X. The existence of a receptor reserve is important in formally distinguishing the concepts of intrinsic activity and efficacy. Heretofore, the two terms have been used interchangeably, and both relate to the ability of a drug to elicit a response at a receptor; however, they describe slightly different characteristics of agonists. As originally proposed by E. J. Ariens, intrinsic activity of a drug is measured according to the magnitude of effect it produces, on a scale that ranges from 0 to 1, which corresponds to a continuum that ranges from antagonists to full agonists. Efficacy is a more theoretical construct that defines the ability of a drug to produce a change in the receptor. Of the two descriptions of agonist actions, efficacy incorporates a role for receptor reserves, as a drug with a greater receptor reserve is considered to have a higher efficacy than a drug that must occupy all available receptors to produce a maximum effect. In contrast, any drug capable of producing a full effect, regardless of percentage receptor occupancy, can be considered to have an intrinsic activity equal to 1.

Despite being pharmacodynamic indices, both intrinsic activity and efficacy allow a role for physiology in modifying the responses produced by a particular drug by recognizing that a drug might produce a maximal effect in one preparation but have a submaximal effect in another preparation. Related to this are modern views of receptor theory, suggesting that different second messenger systems can interact with more than one receptor type and, furthermore, that different ligands might have the ability to direct the actions of these receptors by causing conformational changes that have greater or lesser affinity for either second messenger. The notion that the functional domain of a receptor might have multiple affinity states with different preferences for multiple second messenger systems is mirrored by similar theories that the binding domains of receptors also exist in multiple states that have different affinities for various ligands. From this standpoint, antagonists are described not as having zero efficacy, but instead as having a higher affinity for the receptor in the inactive state, whereas agonists have a higher affinity for receptors in an active state. Overall, improved technologies available for the study of drug action at the receptor level has led to the introduction of new terms to describe interactions between receptors and their ligands, including "functional selectivity," "protean agonism," and "receptor trafficking" among others (Urban et al., 2006). Nonetheless, for most purposes, traditional pharmacological principles still apply; that is, drugs produce graded responses that result from their ability to bind and activate receptors.

Drug–Drug Interactions

Everything discussed above considered the effects of a drug given alone, yet often one or more drugs are given in combination. Drugs administered simultaneously can modify the responses to each, such that effects of either drug are increased or diminished. Increased effects of direct acting agonists vary rarely occur at the level of the receptor, as few drugs act by increasing either the affinity or efficacy of other drugs. Instead, increasing the effects of a drug is often accomplished by giving another drug that produces the same response through a different mechanism. A very common example of this is the alleviation of pain by simultaneous administration of an opioid analgesic, such as morphine, and a nonsteroidal anti-inflammatory such as aspirin. Both morphine and aspirin reduce pain stimuli, but they do so through different mechanisms: morphine by activating mu-opioid receptors, and aspirin by inhibiting an enzyme required for the production of inflammatory compounds. The advantage of this approach is that the combination of the two drugs provides a greater measure of pain relief allowing lower doses of both drugs to be administered in combination than would be needed for either drug given alone. This, in turn, has the advantage of reducing undesirable effects of both drugs. Although the effects of morphine and aspirin combine in a positive manner in terms of pain relief, there is little interaction between the two drugs in other responses, such as gastric bleeding that can occur after high doses of aspirin, or respiratory depression that can occur with medium to high doses of opioids. Using low doses of both drug eliminates the need for high doses of either and their accompanying undesirable effects are avoided. Some drugs increase effects of each other inadvertently, as happens when drugs that bind plasma proteins are administered simultaneously. By competing for the same binding site on the albumin or other protein, the plasma concentration of free drug

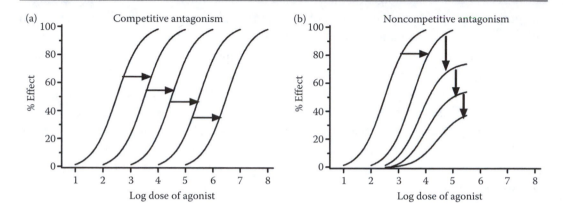

FIGURE 1.7

Graphic representation of competitive (Panel a) and noncompetitive (Panel b) antagonism. Increasing doses of a competitive antagonist produce progressive rightward shifts of the dose-response function of the agonist, but do not disrupt the ability of the agonist to produce a maximal response. A low dose of a noncompetitive antagonist shifts the dose-response function of the agonist to the right, higher doses decrease the maximal effect produced by the agonist.

is raised for both compounds. In this case, each drug literally increases the potency of the other drug, resulting in an increase in all of the effects produced by each drug.

An interaction between two drugs in which the resulting response is less than expected of either drug given alone is known as antagonism. Unlike increased drug effects, antagonism can be either pharmacological, by interfering with the binding of the other drug to the receptor, or physiological, which occurs when different drugs produce opposing effects. Pharmacological antagonism can be further described as competitive or noncompetitive (see Figure 1.7). When a drug acts as a competitive antagonist of another drug, it produces parallel rightward shifts of the dose-effect function for the other drug as the effects of competitive antagonism can be overcome with higher doses of the agonist, which effectively "competes" with the antagonist for access to the same binding site of the receptor (Kenakin, 2006). In contrast, a drug that acts noncompetitively will irreversibly bind the receptor, thus preventing the binding of the agonist (Neubig et al., 2003). Noncompetitive antagonism effectively removes receptors, reducing the ability of the agonist to bind and produce a response; this results in a downward shift of the dose-response function. A third type of antagonism, physiological or functional antagonism, results when drugs produce opposite effects on the same physiological function. For example, the sedative effects of pentobarbital, produced by actions at γ-aminobutyric acid (GABA) receptors may be antagonized by the simultaneous administration of amphetamine, a psychomotor stimulant that increases behavior by increasing the release of dopamine. It may seem counterintuitive to administer both a sedative and a stimulant, but consider the marketed drug, Tylenol No.3, which in some formulations contains acetaminophen and codeine and caffeine. The acetaminophen and codeine produce synergistic effects for pain relief, and the caffeine antagonizes the sedating effects of the codeine.

Tolerance and Dependence

Drug tolerance represents a special case of drug interaction, albeit sometimes it is a single drug that is given. The majority of pharmacological studies assess the effects of acute exposure to drugs, however, many drugs are taken on a long-term basis, and a drug given chronically sometimes produces a different constellation of effects than one sees following acute administration of the drug. This can include altering the responses to the same drug, given acutely, as well as responses to other drugs.

In many ways, tolerance is similar to pharmacological antagonism. Tolerance is defined as a rightward movement of the dose-effect function, resulting in a decreased response to a given dose, or the requirement of a higher dose to achieve a given response (Gilman et al., 1993). There are three types of tolerance: tachyphylaxis, metabolic tolerance, and pharmacodynamic tolerance. Tachyphylaxis is a rapid tolerance that can occur following a single exposure to a drug; relatively speaking, recovery from a tachyphylaxis tolerance is also rapid. Although underlying mechanisms of tachyphylaxis are not always understood, receptor internalization is one process that sometimes leads to rapid tolerance. In this case, a drug binding to a receptor is followed by movement of the receptor intracellularly. If a subsequent dose of drug is given before the receptor is reinserted in the cell membrane, there will be a reduced fraction of available receptors, and the drug will not be able to elicit a response. As soon as the receptor returns to the cell surface, drugs may again bind the receptor and function is restored. Metabolic tolerance is a pharmacokinetic tolerance that occurs when a drug given repeatedly causes an increase in the amount of circulating enzyme that metabolizes the drug. Most drug-metabolizing enzymes are able to biotransform multiple substances; therefore, metabolic tolerance is not specific to the drug that induces it. Instead, metabolic tolerance can result in decreases in the effects for many drugs that are not necessarily related by either function or physicochemical properties.

In contrast to metabolic tolerance, pharmacodynamic tolerance is a receptor-mediated event, in which a drug very selectively produces tolerance only to drugs that bind to the same receptor. Pharmacodynamic tolerance is sometimes, but not always, accompanied by drug dependence, a state in which chronic exposure to a given drug has altered the physiology of the organism, such that the drug must be administered in order to achieve a normative state (Gilman et al., 1993). In other words, drug dependence can only be seen in the absence of the drug (abstinence), and upon readministering the drug, dependence is no longer discernible. The mechanisms that underlie tolerance and dependence are largely unknown and vary in different receptor systems insofar as not every drug is able to produce either tolerance or dependence, nor does tolerance occur to all effects of a given drug. Although there is evidence that down-regulation of receptors and uncoupling of receptors from second messenger systems often play a role, other evidence indicates that nonpharmacological factors, such as environmental context, also may modify the development and expression of drug tolerance.

Pharmacodynamics Summary

Pharmacodynamic aspects of drug action revolve around the interactions of drugs with their receptors. All drugs are capable of interacting with more than one receptor type; however, the properties of affinity and efficacy impart selectivity in the effects drugs produce. Affinity is a measure of the strength of the association between a drug and a receptor; efficacy is a measure of the ability of a drug to activate the receptor. The effects of drugs, and drug interactions, are best analyzed by establishing the functional relationship between a range of doses and the effects they produce. So doing allows different drugs to be identified as agonists, antagonists, or partial agonists. All drugs produce their effects by interacting with receptors, yet receptors themselves encompass a wide assortment of macromolecules, inviting a great diversity of action. This allows drugs to interact with each other either directly, that is, by competing at the same receptor, or functionally, that is, by producing similar or dissimilar responses through separate mechanisms.

References

Gilman, A. G., Rall, T. W., Nies, A. S., & Taylor, P. (Eds.). (1993). *Goodman and Gilman: The pharmacological basis of therapeutics.* (8th ed.). New York: McGraw-Hill.

Kenakin, T. (1993). *Pharmacologic analysis of drug-receptor interaction.* (2nd ed.). New York: Raven Press.

Kenakin, T. (2006). *A pharmacology primer.* (2nd ed.). New York: Elsevier.

Levine, R. R. (1983). *Pharmacology: Drug actions and reactions.* (3rd ed.). Boston, MA: Little, Brown.

Maynert, E. W., & Klingman, G. I. (1960). Acute tolerance to intravenous anesthetics in dogs. *Journal of Pharmacology and Experimental Therapeutics, 128,* 192–200.

Neubig, R. R., Spedding, M., Kenakin, T., & Christopoulos, A. (2003). International Union of Pharmacology Committee on Receptor Nomenclature and Drug Classification. XXXVIII. Update on terms and symbols in quantitative pharmacology. *Pharmacological Reviews, 55,* 597–606.

Scheidweiler, K. B., Cone E. J., Moolchan, E. T., & Huestis, M. A. (2005). Dose-related distribution of codeine, cocaine, and metabolites into human hair following controlled oral codeine and subcutaneous cocaine administration. *Journal of Pharmacology and Experimental Therapeutics, 313,* 909–915.

Shiffman, S., Fant, R. V., Buchhalter, A. R., Gitchell, J. G., & Henningfield, J. E. (2005). Nicotine delivery systems. *Expert Opinion Drug Delivery, 2,* 563–577.

Urban, J. D., Clarke, W. P., von Zastrow, M., Nichols, D. E., Kobilka, B. K., Weinstein, H., et al. (2006). Functional selectivity and classical concepts of quantitative pharmacology. *Journal of Pharmacology and Experimental Therapeutics, 320,* 1–13.

Wilkinson, P. K. (1980). Pharmacokinetics of ethanol: A review. *Alcoholism, Clinical and Experimental Research, 4,* 6–21.

Wood, P. L., Loo, P., Braunwalder, A., Yokoyama, N., & Cheney, D. L. (1984). *In vitro* characterization of benzodiazepine receptor agonists, antagonists, inverse agonists, and agonist/antagonists. *Journal of Pharmacology and Experimental Therapeutics, 231,* 572–576.

2

Actions of Drugs Pertinent to Their Abuse: Targeting Subjective, Discriminative, and Reinforcing Effects for Evaluation of Potential Substance-Use Therapies

Ziva D. Cooper and Sandra D. Comer

Columbia University

Contents

Introduction to Drug Abuse and Dependence

Drugs that act on the central nervous system produce a variety of effects that directly or indirectly affect mood, behavior, and sensory perception. Many psychotropic therapeutic medications have little to no abuse potential, whereas others present a risk of abuse that is of concern to the medical community. Usually, psychotherapeutics that have little abuse potential are ones that either do not produce a perceptible change upon acute administration, or have only negative/aversive side effects. For instance, medications used to treat depression, such as selective serotonin reuptake inhibitors (SSRIs) do not produce immediate intoxicating effects, and therefore pose minimal abuse risk. Neuroleptics, a class of psychotherapeutics used to treat schizophrenia, are known for their negative side effects and therefore also pose no risk for abuse. In fact, patients prescribed neuroleptics typically have low rates of medication compliance due to the negative side effects. Therapeutics that produce positive subjective effects upon acute administration are more likely to have abuse potential. Examples of such drugs include opiates, which are used for pain relief, and stimulants, which are used for Attention Deficit Disorder (ADD). When taken as prescribed, the abuse liability of such medications is minimized, but taking larger amounts than prescribed can increase their abuse potential. In addition, the intoxicating effects of these medications depend in part upon the route by which they are administered. For example, oral use is generally associated with lower abuse potential than intranasal or intravenous use.

Drugs that have abuse potential, whether they have therapeutic indications (opiates and stimulants) or have little to no current therapeutic indications (alcohol and nicotine) can produce drug dependence when used repeatedly. People who use psychotropic medications for reasons other than their prescribed purposes may fit the *DSM–IV* criteria for drug abuse or drug dependence. Drug abuse, which can ultimately develop into drug dependence, can have severe detrimental effects on an individual's health and cognition, and therefore one's ability to function in his or her professional and personal lives (See Box 2.1 below). Drug dependence indicates use of a substance that has a more global impact on an individual's life (*DSM–IV*).

BOX 2.1   SUBSTANCE ABUSE AND DEPENDENCE AS DEFINED BY THE *DSM–IV*

Substance Abuse: Impairment or distress as manifested by any of the following points within a 12-month span:

- Recurrent substance use resulting in a failure to fulfill major role obligations at work, school, or home (such as repeated absences or poor work performance related to substance use; substance-related absences, suspensions, or expulsions from school; substance-related neglect of children or household).
- Recurrent substance use in situations in which it is physically hazardous (such as driving an automobile or operating a machine when impaired by substance use).
- Recurrent substance-related legal problems (such as arrests for substance related disorderly conduct).
- Continued substance use despite having persistent or recurrent social or interpersonal problems caused by the effects of the substance (for example, arguments with spouse about consequences of intoxication and physical fights).

Substance Dependence: A maladaptive pattern of substance use leading to clinically significant impairment or distress, as manifested by three (or more) of the following, occurring any time in the same 12-month period:

- Tolerance, as defined by either of the following: (a) A need for markedly increased amounts of the substance to achieve intoxication or the desired effect or (b) Markedly diminished effect with continued use of the same amount of the substance.
- Withdrawal, as manifested by either of the following: (a) The characteristic withdrawal syndrome from the substance or (b) The same (or closely related) substance is taken to relieve or avoid withdrawal symptoms.
- The substance is often taken in larger amounts or over a longer period of time than intended.
- There is a persistent desire or unsuccessful efforts to cut down or control substance use.
- A great deal of time is spent in activities necessary to obtain the substance, use the substance, or recover from its effects.
- Important social, occupational, or recreational activities are given up or reduced because of substance use.
- The substance use is continued despite knowledge of having a persistent physical or psychological problem that is likely to have been caused or exacerbated by the substance.

American Psychiatric Association (1994).

Commonly abused substances include a variety of drugs that act on a wide range of CNS targets. They therefore vary in their behavioral and subjective effects, and their abuse potential. Later chapters provide greater detail for each drug class and specific drugs that are popularly abused. Table 2.1 shows some commonly abused drugs listed according to their drug class, site of action, and typical route of administration.

Pharmacological Treatment Modalities

In addition to behavioral and cognitive-based therapies, a number of pharmacotherapies exist to assist with detoxification and maintenance of abstinence when an individual requests treatment for a substance use disorder. Typical pharmacotherapies include replacement therapy, antagonist treatment, and other therapies that directly or indirectly modify the actions of the abused drug. Regardless of modality, treatment for drug dependence and abuse is directly aimed at achieving and maintaining abstinence. Although many potential therapies have been reported to decrease drug craving, attenuation of drug craving has not been shown to be clinically predictive of sustained abstinence. Below is a brief description of the different pharmacological treatment approaches and examples of corresponding treatment options. It should be recognized that this is not a comprehensive list of possible treatment options.

TABLE 2.1
Some Commonly Abused Drugs

Drug Class	Commonly Used Drugs	Site of Action	Route of Administration
Depressants	Alcohol; Prescription benzodiazepines (Klonopin, Ambien, Valium, Ativan, Xanax)	GABA Benzodiazepine receptors	Oral Intranasal
Tobacco	Cigarettes, Cigars, Chewing tobacco	Nicotinic acetylcholine receptors	Oral Smoked
Opioids	Heroin; Prescription opioids (Vicodin, Percocet, Morphine, Codeine, OxyContin, Dilaudid, Demerol)	Mu-opiate receptor	Oral Intranasal, Intravenous
Stimulants	Cocaine and Crack-cocaine; Methamphetamine; Prescription Stimulants (Ritalin, Adderall, Dexedrin)	Dopamine, Norepinephrine	Oral Intranasal, Intravenous
Cannabis	Marijuana, Hashish, Sinsemilla	CB1 receptor	Oral Smoked
Hallucinogens and Dissociative Anesthetics	LSD; DMT; Peyote (mescaline); Mushrooms (psilocybin); MDMA ("Ecstasy"); Ketamine; PCP	Serotonin receptor NMDA receptor	Oral Intranasal

Agonist Replacement Therapy

The principle behind agonist replacement therapy is to introduce a medication that will act in place of the abused drug. The treatment generally has the same mechanism of action as the abused drug, but it produces a more sustained pharmacological effect with a slow onset of action, and thus does not afford the feeling of a "rush" or euphoria that is produced by a drug with a more rapid onset of action. The pharmacokinetic effects of the treatment are a fundamental component of its treatment efficacy. Tampering with the drug and administering it by routes other than the prescribed route of administration will alter the pharmacokinetic profile of the drug. The treatment can itself become a drug-abuse risk if not taken as prescribed. To prevent drug tampering, and in some cases, diversion, these medications are sometimes heavily federally regulated.

For opioid dependence, the most common form of agonist replacement pharmacotherapy is methadone. Methadone is administered orally, has a relatively slow onset of action, and a long half-life. The half-life of a drug describes how long it takes for half of the drug to be metabolized. One advantage of medications with long half-lives is that abrupt discontinuation of the medication results in milder withdrawal symptoms than drugs with shorter half-lives, such as heroin or oxycodone. Varying doses of methadone are prescribed depending on the therapeutic needs of the individual. Patients who report heavy heroin use prior to treatment usually will be maintained on a higher dose of methadone than those who report lighter use. One risk of methadone, however, is that it accumulates over several days, so that caution is needed when patients are initiated onto the medication. If the doses of methadone are increased too rapidly, significant toxicity, including death, can occur. A second type of replacement therapy for opioid dependence is buprenorphine. Buprenorphine is not effective orally because of significant first-pass metabolism, so it is prescribed for sublingual use in the treatment of opioid dependence. Like methadone, buprenorphine, when taken as prescribed, has a relatively slow onset of action and a long half-life. Unlike methadone, buprenorphine is a partial mu opioid agonist (and a kappa opioid antagonist) and therefore has a wide margin of safety and theoretically a lower abuse potential than methadone. However, a buprenorphine induction phase is required during which time the patient has to be carefully monitored when introduced onto the medication. If the patient is currently maintained on methadone or has recently taken another full opioid mu agonist, high doses of buprenorphine can precipitate opioid withdrawal symptoms. In these situations, the patient can experience abrupt severe opioid withdrawal. Therefore, buprenorphine has to be introduced carefully in opioid-dependent individuals.

Replacement therapy for nicotine dependence consists of various routes of nicotine administration. The transdermal patch adheres to the skin, which absorbs a relatively continuous level of nicotine for the lifetime of the patch. Depending upon the amount of cigarettes smoked prior to abstinence, the patient will begin with a patch that delivers a high dose of nicotine and subsequently patches with lower doses of nicotine are used. Nicotine delivered by a gum, lozenge, inhaler, or nasal spray have also been shown to help people who are trying to quit smoking. Unlike the patch, these methods produce sharp increases in plasma nicotine levels that are not sustained for very long and can induce a drug "rush" and are therefore a less favored pharmacotherapy for nicotine dependence. However, these increases in nicotine plasma levels are thought to better alleviate nicotine withdrawal in people who are trying to abstain from smoking. Varenicline is a partial agonist for the nicotinic acetylcholine receptor that has been shown to decrease nicotine withdrawal and craving and clinical efficacy for smoking cessation has been demonstrated in large clinical trials (Nides, 2008).

Marijuana dependence is a less well-known and recognized phenomenon. In the last 10 years, the number of people reporting difficulty quitting marijuana smoking has increased, and recent laboratory studies have demonstrated a marijuana-withdrawal syndrome when chronic marijuana users abstain from smoking (Haney, Ward, Comer, Foltin, & Fischman, 1999). Because this is a relatively newly recognized phenomenon, treatment options are currently being evaluated. One promising pharmacotherapy is oral THC, which provides sustained plasma THC levels, resulting in decreases in the marijuana withdrawal syndrome (Haney et al., 2004).

Although controversial as a treatment approach, there has been some success in demonstrating the clinical efficacy of agonist replacement therapy for cocaine dependence (for a recent review, see Karila et al., 2008). For example, laboratory studies and clinical trials investigating the use of modafinil as a potential replacement therapy show that it has some efficacy for the treatment of cocaine dependence (Dackis, Kampman, Lynch, Pettinati, & O'Brien, 2005; Hart, Haney, Vosburg, Rubin, & Foltin, 2008). Maintenance on oral amphetamine also showed efficacy in reducing cocaine use in both preclinical and clinical studies (Grabowski, Shearer, Merrill, & Negus, 2004).

Antagonist Therapy

An alternative approach to agonist replacement therapy is the use of antagonist treatments. An antagonist is a drug that blocks a specific receptor to which it binds from being activated by an agonist. The most successful antagonist treatment available is naltrexone, a drug that acts as an antagonist at the mu-opioid receptor. When administered, it blocks the effects of opiate agonists. Naltrexone can be used for rapid heroin detoxification or as a maintenance pharmacotherapy to increase abstinence from heroin. Medication compliance has been the biggest obstacle to widespread treatment success with naltrexone, but the development of newer, sustained-release formulations of naltrexone show great promise (Comer, Sullivan, & Hulse, 2007). Bupropion (Zyban and Wellbutrin), a medication that is used as an antidepressant, blocks the uptake of the neurotransmitters norepinephrine and dopamine and also has been shown to be a nicotinic receptor antagonist (Fryer and Lukas, 1999). Bupropion has been used successfully for nicotine dependence and somewhat less successfully for cocaine dependence.

Other Pharmacotherapy Modalities

There is a variety of other treatment modalities that do not interact directly with the receptor system at which the abused drug acts. Disulfiram, also called Antabuse is a drug that interferes with alcohol metabolism and leads to the build-up of acetaldehyde, the chemical that is implicated in the negative effects of alcohol, including nausea, vomiting, and headache. Naltrexone, a mu-opioid antagonist that was discussed above as a treatment for opioid dependence, has also been shown to have some clinical efficacy for alcohol abuse, but the mechanism for this effect is somewhat unclear. It has been suggested that naltrexone acts to improve rates of alcohol abstinence by blocking the effects of alcohol-induced release of endogenous opioids (Racz et al., 2008). Topiramate, acomprosate, and baclofen, drugs that enhance GABAergic activity have also been shown to be somewhat effective for alcohol dependence. Medications prescribed for mood disorders, such as depression, have shown some clinical efficacy for drug dependence, primarily when depression co-occurs with substance abuse.

Methods for Determining Effective Pharmacotherapies for Substance Abuse

The clinical efficacy of the above treatment options was determined based upon a number of methodological principles that focus on measuring modifications in behaviors relevant to drug abuse and dependence. These behaviors can range from verbal reports of how the potential treatment affects the subjective effects of the abused drug, including craving for the abused drug, behavior allocated to obtain the abused drug, and actual consumption of the abused drug. The basic principle of investigating a potential medication for the treatment of drug dependence is that ultimately it should decrease consumption of the abused drug. The mechanism of action, or neurobiological target (receptor system, neurotransmitter, etc.), of the abused drug of interest is frequently used as the rationale for choosing to test a potential medication. In some cases, treatments are geared more toward the alleviation of the withdrawal symptoms, and not the mechanism of action of the abused drug. This is especially true with benzodiaz-epine and alcohol dependence, when abrupt withdrawal from the drug can sometime produce serious physiological responses including seizures and disruption of cardiac function. Opiate withdrawal largely produces flu-like symptoms, but can also produce physiological disruptions including changes in thermoregulatory mechanisms and increases in heart rate and blood pres-sure. During abrupt withdrawal from these drugs, patients frequently are given medications to correct these physiological disturbances. These types of treatments are used during drug detoxification and do not have clinical efficacy for prolonged abstinence.

Prior to testing the efficacy of a certain medication for the treatment of drug dependence in a large clinical trial, smaller studies often are conducted in human laboratories where several doses of the proposed medication are tested in order to assess how the test drug dose depend-ently affects the behavioral effects of the abused substance. Behavioral studies with rodents (mice and rats) and nonhuman primates usually provide information regarding potential can-didates for medications that are assessed in preclinical human studies. Many methodological models used to study potential anti-addiction agents in animals have been translated into human laboratory models, some of which are described below.

Subjective Measures and Discrimination Procedures

The first method for investigating if a potential medication is effective as an agent to treat drug dependence is to evaluate its ability to alter the subjective responses produced by the abused drug. The subjective effect of an abused drug is called an *interoceptive stimulus*. The interocep-tive effects of a drug sometimes do not constitute any kind of observable behavior. Therefore, the challenge for the investigator is to develop a series of questions that will target those effects. If the appropriate questions are not asked, then the effects of the potential treatment medica-tion may be missed. This may be especially true if the abused drug produces a combination of effects that are shared by drugs from more than one class (e.g., 3,4-methylenedioxymetham-phetamine, also known as MDMA or "Ecstasy"). To determine if a test medication directly modifies the subjective effects of the abused drug, an investigator administers the abused drug to a study participant who is familiar with the effects of that drug. The participant then answers a series of questions regarding drug effects. Some of these questionnaires ask the par-ticipant to mark how they feel at that precise time on a 100 mm line anchored at one end with the words "not at all" and the other end "extremely." Other scales may require the participant to respond to true–false items, whereas others use a scale of 1–5, 1 being "not at all" and 5 being "very much so" to identify subjective drug effects. Examples of questions pertaining to subjective drug effects include items relevant to the quality of drug ("Good Drug Effect"; "Drug Liking"; "Strength of Drug Effect"), whereas others ask the participant to report the drug-elicited feelings ("Stimulated"; "Anxious"; "Irritable"). Once the subjective effects of the abused drug are established, a test medication is administered as a pretreatment to the abused drug. The effects of the test medication on the subjective effects of the abused drug should be reflected by a difference between the subjective ratings in the presence and absence of the test medication. Measurements of the subjective effects of the abused drug are essential to any assessment of potential medications for the treatment of substance abuse. However, difficulties in interpretation of the therapeutic utility of a potential medication may arise if the medica-tion reduces only some of the subjective effects produced by the abused drug.

The drug discrimination procedure is a method to directly assess the interoceptive stimulus effects of a given drug. A strength of the drug discrimination procedure is that it is a measure of the interoceptive effects of the abused drug that does not rely on a series of questions that may or may not comprehensively target the subjective effects of the abused drug. Examination of the effects of the treatment medication on both subjective responses and on discriminative responses may provide a more comprehensive assessment of a medication's therapeutic utility. When undergoing discrimination training, the participant usually is administered one of two drugs, the abused drug of interest and placebo. The administration of each drug is associated with external cues, such as a color, letter, number, and so on. The drugs are paired several times with the cues so that the participant learns to associate the interoceptive cues of the drug with the external cues (i.e., the assigned letter or color). Next, the participant is given one of the drugs and asked to choose the appropriate external cue that corresponds to the interoceptive stimulus of the administered drug. Usually, the participant is given a monetary reward upon correct discrimination of the administered drug. Once the discriminative stimuli of the two drugs are established over many sessions, the test medication is then given prior to the administration of the training drugs. A test medication that modifies the interoceptive cues of the training drug should also decrease the discriminative-stimulus effects of the training drug.

The following example is from a study that investigated the effects of aripiprazole, a drug that acts at the D2 subtype of dopamine receptor, on the interoceptive stimulus properties of amphetamine (Lile et al., 2005). The study rationale was supported by studies performed in animals, which demonstrated the therapeutic potential of drugs that act on the D2 receptors for stimulant abuse. In this study, participants were trained to discriminate 15 mg of *d*-amphetamine (training dose) from placebo. When discrimination of the training drug was achieved, participants received either the test medication (aripiprazole) or placebo before different doses of *d*-amphetamine were administered (2.5–15 mg). During each discrimination trial, participants provided subjective ratings of drug effects. Thus, in a single session, data pertaining to the effects of the study medication on both the subjective and discriminative-stimulus effects of *d*-amphetamine were collected. Figure 2.1 depicts participant ratings on a drug effects questionnaire. Subjective ratings of drug effect were measured on a scale of

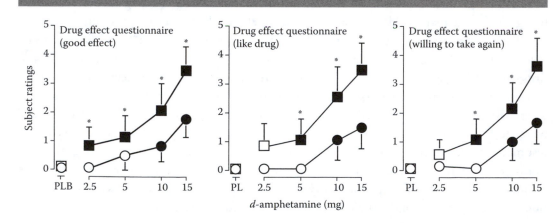

FIGURE 2.1
Aripiprizole decreases the subjective effects of d-amphetamine.

d-amphetamine (mg)

FIGURE 2.2
Aripiprizole decreases the discriminative-stimulus effects of d-amphetamine.

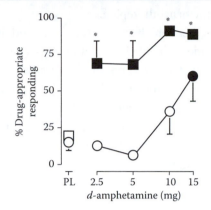

0–4 (0 = "Not at all"; 1 = "A little bit"; 2 = "Moderately"; 3 = "Quite a bit"; 4 = "Extremely"). Participants were asked several times after drug administration to report subjective ratings, which were analyzed according to the area under the curve. Placebo d-amphetamine (0 mg) did not produce ratings greater than 0 for subjective effects describing the positive qualities of the drug ("Good Effect") or drug liking ("Like Drug" and "Willing to Take Again"). In the absence of aripiprazole, ratings increased with increasing doses of d-amphetamine (squares, filled symbols indicate significant differences from placebo amphetamine), with peak ratings achieved with the highest dose of d-amphetamine tested (15 mg). Administration of aripiprazole (circles) prior to amphetamine decreased these subjective ratings for every dose of d-amphetamine tested (asterisks indicate significant differences in the presence and absence of aripiprazole for that dose of amphetamine).

Participants were then asked to identify if the drug received that day was the training drug. Drug-appropriate responding refers to the average percentage of times the participant identifies the test drug as the training drug. Figure 2.2 depicts the participants' ability to discriminate several doses of amphetamine in the presence and absence of the test medication. Placebo did not occasion drug-appropriate responding, meaning that placebo did not produce d-amphetamine-like interoceptive effects. All active doses of d-amphetamine occasioned drug-appropriate responding, indicating that all doses produced similar interoceptive effects as the training dose of d-amphetamine. When aripiprazole was administered prior to d-amphetamine, decreases in drug-appropriate responding were observed for all but the highest dose of d-amphetamine tested (Lile et al., 2005). Thus, this study demonstrated that the test medication decreased both the subjective and discriminative-stimulus effects of d-amphetamine, suggesting that the medication may be a good candidate for treating amphetamine dependence.

In addition to its utility in medications development for drug dependence, the drug discrimination procedure can also be used to determine whether two drugs share similar psychopharmacological profiles. If two drugs share similar mechanisms of action, the discriminative-stimulus effects of one should generalize to the other. In one study, participants were trained to discriminate the stimulant methylphenidate from placebo. When administered as a test drug, d-amphetamine dose-dependently increased methylphenidate-appropriate responding when it was substituted for methylphenidate. However, triazolam, a benzodiazepine, did not occasion methylphenidate-appropriate responding in these participants (Stoops, Lile, Glaser, & Rush, 2005). Although all three drugs increased reports of positive subjective drug effects, the discrimination paradigm was sensitive enough to detect differences in mechanism of action between the stimulants and the benzodiazepine.

Determining how a test-medication affects the subjective and discriminative-stimulus properties of an abused drug provides valuable information regarding the potential of the medication as an anti-addiction agent. However, one major disadvantage of discrimination studies is that they require multiple sessions for each phase (training and testing). Although it is premature to make definitive conclusions about the utility of drug discrimination procedures in humans, some studies suggest that these models may not necessarily provide predictive validity for efficacy in large clinical trials (Grabowski et al., 2000; Loebl et al., 2008; Rush, Stoops, Hays, Glaser, & Hays, 2003; Tiihonen et al., 2007).

Self-Administration Models

Assessing the effects of a test medication on the subjective and discriminative effects of the abused drug of interest addresses one aspect of a drug's effect. However, drug-taking behavior, the ultimate target of potential therapeutics, is not investigated using the above methods. Human self-administration studies have been modeled after animal self-administration models where access to drug is contingent upon some specified behavioral output. A drug serves as a reinforcer if the behavior upon which its presentation is contingent increases or is maintained over time. These models have proven to have good predictive validity for identifying medications for treating substance abuse (Comer et al., 2008; Haney & Spealman, 2008). As described above for the subjective effects and discrimination methods, the rationale behind choosing to investigate a potential therapeutic for drug dependence is guided by the mechanism of drug action and supportive findings from animal studies. Several different self-administration procedures are employed for the assessment of the reinforcing effects of a drug in a human laboratory setting.

Free Access and Verbal Choice Procedures

Under the free access paradigm, the drug's reinforcing effects are determined by allowing participants to have free access to the drug. In one inpatient study, caffeinated and decaffeinated coffee were made freely available on alternate days to coffee-drinking participants. The aim of the study was to determine if caffeinated coffee was more reinforcing than decaffeinated coffee. The results of the study demonstrated no difference in coffee consumption between the two types. However, when a choice was presented between the two types of coffee, participants chose caffeinated coffee more often than decaffeinated coffee (Griffiths, Bigelow, & Liebson, 1986). This study demonstrated that the choice procedure was sensitive to differences in the reinforcing effects of caffeinated and decaffeinated coffee. The verbal choice procedure has been extended to include choices between drug and placebo, drug and drug, and drug versus money. For these types of procedures, the operant response is a simple yes/no verbal choice. The essential premise of the verbal self-administration and choice procedures is that a potential therapeutic for drug abuse will decrease the reinforcing effects of the abused drug and will consequently lead to less drug self-administration and fewer choices made for drug when the choice is presented.

Nonverbal Self-Administration Procedures

Methods for nonverbal self-administration procedures arose from animal self-administration models developed in the 1960s to investigate the reinforcing effects of drugs in rats and monkeys (Deneau, Yanagita, & Seevers, 1969; Weeks & Collins, 1964). In these procedures, the animal is required to emit a response on a manipulandum, usually a lever, foot-pedal, or nose-poke and receives a dose of drug that is paired with an associated external cue (flashing light, noise, etc.). For human laboratory self-administration studies, the participant receives a drug during a preliminary sampling session. The identity of the drug is not disclosed but is associated with an external cue. Usually, the subjective effects of the drug are measured using questionnaires during the sampling session. During a subsequent session, the participant is given the option of working for the drug that was sampled earlier. This "work" can entail a simple behavior or response on a manipulandum such as a joystick, computer mouse, or bicycle. When the number of responses required to obtain drug is fixed, the participant is said to be working under a fixed-ratio schedule. The behavioral output can be increased or decreased in order to assess how hard the participant will work for the drug. The amount of behavior put forth to gain access to a drug is a way to measure the *reinforcing effects* of the drug. The simplest behavioral requirement would be a single response on a manipulandum to receive a dose of drug. A popular manipulation is to progressively increase the response requirement for each subsequent dose of drug (i.e., participants respond under a progressive ratio schedule). The *breakpoint* for a drug is the final behavioral requirement that the volunteer chooses to complete in order to gain access to the drug under this type of *schedule of reinforcement*. The breakpoint can thus be used to measure the reinforcing effects of the drug. Typically, the breakpoint when placebo is available is significantly lower than the breakpoint when active drug is available.

Determining how a potential therapeutic agent affects the breakpoint of an abused drug helps determine whether the test medication may have therapeutic utility. However, the face- and predictive-validity of the above-described self-administration paradigm can be improved by introducing an additional reinforcer and allowing the subject to choose between the two reinforcers. In animal studies, the subject is sometimes presented with a choice between the drug of interest and food. In human self-administration studies, participants typically are given the option to choose between drug and money or merchandise vouchers. The primary endpoints for the choice experiments are the (1) amount of behavior allocated to each reinforcer and (2) consumption (or money earned) in the presence or absence of the test medication.

The self-administration paradigm also can be used to investigate how the reinforcing effects of two drugs compare to each other. Similar to the choice procedure described above, the participant is given the opportunity to choose between two drugs. Volunteers are allowed to sample the drugs on separate occasions. To keep the participant blind to which drug he or she is receiving, each drug is associated with distinct external cues. After sampling both drugs, the participant is asked to choose between the two drugs during subsequent self-administration sessions. This experimental paradigm provides a good method of comparing the relative abuse liability of two drugs.

Human laboratory self-administration paradigms have been used to investigate potential therapeutics for heroin dependence. The therapeutic efficacy of buprenorphine for heroin dependence was measured in a choice procedure where heroin-dependent volunteers participated in an inpatient study during which they were maintained on sublingual buprenorphine. During the sampling session, the subjective effects of the various doses of heroin were also monitored. Thus, similar to the discrimination study discussed above, the current study was able to measure two relevant endpoints, the reinforcing and subjective effects of heroin during maintenance on buprenorphine (8 and 16 mg). Participants first sampled the dose of heroin that would be available for self-administration during a subsequent session. Again, the volunteer was blind to the drug and dose condition. Several hours after the sampling session, the volunteer was asked to choose between the dose of drug sampled earlier or money. The participant was presented with 10 choices, and was thus able to earn 1/10 of the sample dose or 1/10 of the available money for each choice. The ratio requirement increased with subsequent choice for a given reinforcer (drug or money). At the end of the choice session, the drug that was earned during the session was administered. Money earned during these sessions was given upon discharge from the inpatient study. This procedure allowed for the effects of buprenorphine on the relative reinforcing effects of heroin versus money to be measured. Figure 2.3 depicts the behavior allocated to either earn an infusion of heroin or money under a low dose of buprenorphine (8 mg, open circles) or a high dose of buprenorphine (16 mg, black circles). The y-axis depicts the breakpoint value supported by heroin (left panel) or money (right panel) when various doses of heroin were made available (0, 6.25, 12.5, and 25 mg, as depicted on the x-axis). As the dose of heroin increased across the choice session, participants allocated more behavior to gain access to heroin and less to earn money. The higher dose of buprenorphine (16 mg) decreased the number of choices made for heroin and increased the number of choices made for money when the two highest doses of heroin were made available (12.5 and 25 mg), thus the high dose of buprenorphine reduced the reinforcing efficacy of heroin.

Buprenorphine also dose-dependently decreased the positive subjective effects of heroin. Figure 2.4 illustrates four different subjective effects measured with visual analogue scales

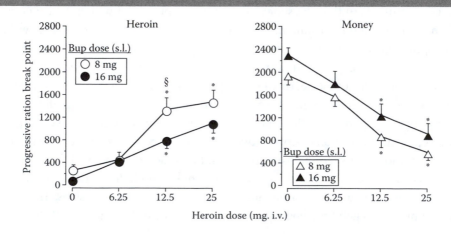

FIGURE 2.3
Sublingual buprenorphine decreases heroin self-administration.

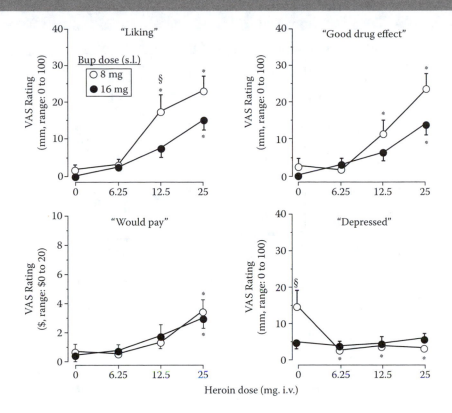

FIGURE 2.4
Effects of sublingual buprenorphine on subjective ratings of heroin.

(on the *y*-axis) as a function of heroin dose (on the *x*-axis) and maintenance dose of buprenorphine. Placebo did not produce any ratings of positive subjective effects, whereas heroin dose-dependently increased the positive subjective ratings of drug

"Liking" and "Good Drug Effect"   Participants also reported higher ratings of "Would Pay" for increasing doses of heroin. The higher dose relative to the low dose of buprenorphine decreased the subjective ratings of "Liking" and "Good Drug Effect" produced by heroin. Interestingly, reports of "Would Pay" did not differ between the two buprenorphine doses (Comer, Collins, & Fischman, 2001).

Recently, the effectiveness of a depot form of naltrexone for the treatment of heroin dependence was explored. The depot form of naltrexone delivers a sustained level of the mu-opioid antagonist, naltrexone, for about a month. After a detoxification procedure, previously heroin-dependent volunteers were allowed to choose between the dose of heroin they received during a sampling session (0–25 mg, i.v.) or $20. Using the same procedures as described above, the relative reinforcing effect of heroin versus money was determined prior to naltrexone administration and for several weeks after naltrexone administration. During the baseline week prior to naltrexone administration, breakpoint for heroin increased with increasing doses of heroin (Figure 2.5). Additionally, ratings of "Good Drug Effect" and miosis (reduction in pupil diameter, a physiological marker of opioid intoxication) increased

FIGURE 2.5
Depot naltrexone on blunts the behavioral and physiological effects of intravenous heroin.

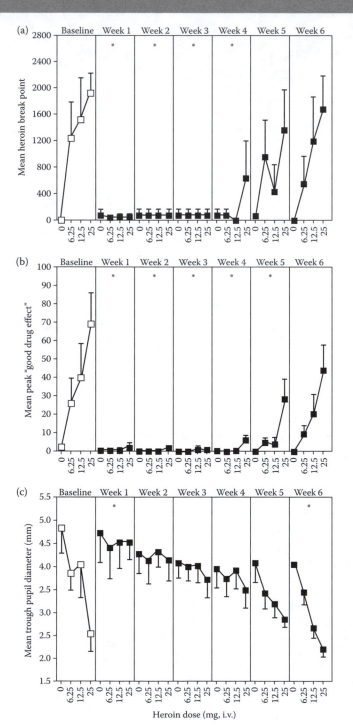

with increasing doses of heroin. After the depot form of naltrexone was given, the reinforcing, subjective, and physiological effects of heroin were antagonized for four weeks. These effects returned to baseline values six weeks after naltrexone administration, indicating that the effects observed during the first four weeks were due to mu-opioid blockade (Sullivan, Vosburg, & Comer, 2006). These findings provided substantial evidence for the potential clinical efficacy of depot naltrexone for heroin dependence, which was confirmed in a clinical trial (Comer et al., 2006).

Summary

A wide variety of drugs poses an abuse liability risk. There are several different psychotherapeutic modalities to assist individuals who struggle with drug dependence to achieve and maintain abstinence. Prior to large-scale clinical trials, determining the clinical efficacy of a novel therapeutic agent for drug dependence can be achieved in human laboratory studies. A medication is chosen as a potential therapeutic based upon its neurobiological mechanism and positive results in animal laboratory models of drug dependence. The methods used to assess a potential therapeutic agent are geared toward determining if the test medication decreases behaviors mediated by the drug of abuse. A potential therapeutic medication should ultimately promote long-term abstinence. Therefore, the self-administration model where the participant is given the option to take the abused drug, combined with measures of subjective responses, is thought to have the greatest predictive validity for clinical efficacy.

References

American Psychiatric Association. (1994). *Diagnostic and statistical manual of mental disorders* (4th ed., pp. 181–183). Washington, DC: American Psychiatric Press.

Comer, S. D., Ashworth, J. B., Foltin, R. W., Johanson, C. E., Zacny, J. P., & Walsh, S. L. (2008). The role of human drug self-administration procedures in the development of medications. *Drug and Alcohol Dependence, 96,* 1–15.

Comer, S. D., Collins, E. D., & Fischman, M. W. (2001). Buprenorphine sublingual tablets: Effects of IV heroin self-administration by humans. *Psychopharmacology, 154,* 28–37.

Comer, S. D., Sullivan, M. A., & Hulse, G. K. (2007). Sustained-release naltrexone: Novel treatment for opioid dependence. *Expert Opinion on Investigating Drugs, 16,* 1285–1294.

Comer, S. D., Sullivan, M. A., Yu, E., Rothenberg, J. L., Kleber, H. D., Kampman, K., et al. (2006). Injectable, sustained-release naltrexone for the treatment of opioid dependence: A randomized, placebo-controlled trial. *Archives of General Psychiatry, 63,* 210–218.

Dackis, C. A., Kampman, K. M., Lynch, K. G., Pettinati, H. M., & O'Brien, C. P. (2005). A double-blind, placebo-controlled trial of modafinil for cocaine dependence. *Neuropsychopharmacology, 30,* 205–211.

Deneau, G., Yanagita, T., & Seevers, M. H. (1969). Self-administration of psychoactive substances by the monkey. *Psychopharmacologia, 16,* 30–48.

Fryer, J. D., & Lukas, R. J. (1999). Noncompetitive functional inhibition at diverse, human nicotinic acetylcholine receptor subtypes by bupropion, phencyclidine, and ibogaine. *Journal of Pharmacology and Experimental Therapeutics, 288,* 88–92.

Galantar, M., & Kleber, H.D. (2004). Textbook of Substance Abuse Treatment (3rd ed.,). Washington, DC: American Psychiatric Press.

Grabowski, J., Rhoades, H., Silverman, P., Schmitz, J. M., Stotts, A., Creson, D., et al. (2000). Risperidone for the treatment of cocaine dependence: Randomized, double-blind trial. *Journal of Clinical Psychopharmacology, 20,* 305–1036.

Grabowski, J., Shearer, J., Merrill, J., & Negus, S. S. (2004). Agonist-like, replacement pharmacotherapy for stimulant abuse and dependence. *Addictive Behaviors, 29,* 1439–1464.

Griffiths, R. R., Bigelow, G. E., & Liebson, I. A. (1986). Human coffee drinking: Reinforcing and physical dependence producing effects of caffeine. *Journal of Pharmacology and Experimental Therapeutics, 239,* 416–425.

Haney, M., Hart, C. L., Vosburg, S. K., Nasser, J., Bennett, A., Zubaran, C., et al. (2004). Marijuana withdrawal in humans: Effects of oral THC or divalproex. *Neuropsychopharmacology, 29,* 158–170.

Haney, M., & Spealman, R. (2008). Controversies in translational research: Drug self-administration. *Psychopharmacology, 199,* 403–419.

Haney, M., Ward, A. S., Comer, S. D., Foltin, R. W., & Fischman, M. W. (1999). Abstinence symptoms following smoked marijuana in humans. *Psychopharmacology, 141,* 395–404.

Hart, C. L., Haney, M., Vosburg, S. K., Rubin, E., & Foltin, R. W. (2008). Smoked cocaine self-administration is decreased by modafinil. *Neuropsychopharmacology, 33,* 761–768.

Karila, L., Gorelick, D., Weinstein, A., Noble, F., Benyamina, A., Coscas, S., et al. (2008). New treatments for cocaine dependence: A focused review. *International Journal of Neuropsychopharmacology, 11,* 425–438.

Lile, J. A., Stoops, W. W., Vansickel, A. R., Glaser, P. E., Hays, L. R., & Rush, C. R. (2005). Aripiprazole attenuates the discriminative-stimulus and subject-rated effects of D-amphetamine in humans. *Neuropsychopharmacology, 30,* 2103–2114.

Loebl, T., Angarita, G. A., Pachas, G. N., Huang, K. L., Lee, S. H., Nino, J., et al. (2008). A randomized, double-blind, placebo-controlled trial of long-acting risperidone in cocaine-dependent men. *Journal of Clinical Psychiatry, 69,* 480–486.

Nides, M. (2008). Update on pharmacologic options for smoking cessation treatment. *American Journal of Medicine, 121,* S20–31.

Racz, I., Schürmann, B., Karpushova, A., Reuter, M., Cichon, S., Montag, C., et al. (2008). The opioid peptides enkephalin and beta-endorphin in alcohol dependence. *Biological Psychiatry, 64,* 989–997.

Rush, C. R., Stoops, W. W., Hays, L. R., Glaser, P. E., & Hays, L. S. (2003). Risperidone attenuates the discriminative-stimulus effects of d-amphetamine in humans. *Journal of Pharmacology and Experimental Therapeutics, 306,* 195–204.

Stoops, W. W., Lile, J. A., Glaser, P. E., & Rush, C. R. (2005). Discriminative stimulus and self-reported effects of methylphenidate, d-amphetamine, and triazolam in methylphenidate-trained humans. *Experimental and Clinical Psychopharmacology, 13,* 56–64.

Sullivan, M. A., Vosburg, S. K., & Comer, S. D. (2006). Depot naltrexone: Antagonism of the reinforcing, subjective, and physiological effects of heroin. *Psychopharmacology, 189,* 37–46.

Tiihonen, J., Kuoppasalmi, K., Fohr, J., Tuomola, P., Kuikanmaki, O., Vorma, H., et al. (2007). A comparison of aripiprazole, methylphenidate, and placebo for amphetamine dependence. *American Journal of Psychiatry, 164,* 160–162.

Weeks, J. R., & Collins, R. J. (1964). Factors affecting voluntary morphine intake in self-maintained addicted rats. *Psychopharmacologia, 6,* 267–279.

3

Performance and Cognitive Alterations

Ryan G. Vandrey and Miriam Z. Mintzer

Johns Hopkins University School of Medicine

Contents

Performance and Cognitive Alterations

Alteration of cognitive ability and function often accompanies the use and abuse of many psychoactive drugs. There is a particularly rich history of research on the cognitive consequences of drugs that are commonly abused (e.g., alcohol, opioids). This research includes the assessment of diverse levels of functioning, from basic sensory perception such as visual stimulus discrimination, to complex higher-order processes such as problem solving. Understanding the effects of drugs on cognitive performance has important clinical and social implications. For example, research has demonstrated that commonly abused drugs can significantly impair one's ability to drive a car, perform complex tasks required in the workplace, or even make one more prone to impulsive decision making.

The aim of this chapter is to provide an overview of the scientific research on the psychomotor and cognitive performance effects of commonly abused drugs. Particular attention is focused on the effects of benzodiazepines, alcohol, opioids, and cannabis because of the relative breadth of research conducted on these compounds and because they are generally associated with cognitive decrements of potential clinical importance. The cognitive effects of psychomotor stimulants (e.g., amphetamines, cocaine, nicotine), MDMA ("Ecstasy"), ketamine, and hallucinogens are also briefly reviewed.

In the interest of clarity, and to retain this text's focus on evidence-based, clinically relevant research, emphasis is placed on acute drug effects measured in controlled laboratory studies with healthy human volunteers. These qualities in research minimize the likelihood of invalid assumptions and ambiguity associated with generalizing effects across species. Also, although research on the long-term cognitive effects associated with chronic drug use (i.e., observational group comparison studies of substance abusers versus matched control participants) can provide clinically relevant information, and is discussed in brief, conclusions based on such studies are limited because they usually lack assessments of baseline function and rely on retrospective self-reports of drug use that are subject to error and recall bias. Furthermore, because substance abusers typically have histories of using more than one drug, comorbid psychiatric disorders, or central nervous system (CNS) injury, it is difficult to confidently attribute the cause of any observed cognitive deficits to use of a single drug. Last, by focusing on studies conducted with healthy (nondrug-dependent) participants, potential effects of drug withdrawal on baseline assessments are eliminated.

In addition to providing an overview of published data on the cognitive effects of abused drugs, brief comment is made regarding the relative severity of the acute effects observed for each drug class. Because the impairment caused by alcohol is generally considered significant (as evidenced by drinking and driving laws throughout the developed world), alcohol is used as a benchmark to provide comparative comment regarding the magnitude and clinical importance of the cognitive deficits described for other less familiar drugs (cf. Zacny, 1995).

Cognitive Functioning and Associated Measures

In the next section, the cognitive effects of abused drugs are presented grouped by drug class, and then within each drug class by distinct categories or types of cognitive function. In an effort to encompass a wide range of psychomotor and cognitive functions, the following categories were selected: (1) sensory acuity, (2) motor ability, (3) attention, and (4) memory. In some cases further distinction into subtypes was warranted. Higher-order cognitive functions such as problem solving, conceptual thinking, and decision making are not included here because they are not common in healthy volunteer studies and tend not to be conducive to the repeated measures designs typically used in acute drug effect studies. However, because these functions are clinically relevant and involve executive processes (control processes that serve to select, initiate, monitor, and schedule other cognitive activities) that have been linked to frontal lobe functioning and that are thought to play an important role in substance abuse, comment is made regarding the effects of chronic drug use on these functions.

In the interest of brevity and clarity, the data described for each type or subtype of cognitive functioning are limited to 1–3 measures that provide a relatively "pure" assessment of that function. An effort was also made to include the most commonly used of these measures to facilitate comparison across drug classes. Thus, measures for which outcome variables assess multiple types of functioning, or measures that have not been used across multiple drug classes were intentionally omitted. In this section, the selected measures are described in detail.

Sensory Acuity

The tasks selected provide measures of sensory acuity for the visual system, which is the sensory modality most commonly assessed in acute drug effect studies.

Flicker Fusion (Simonson & Brozek, 1952) Participants look through a viewing apparatus and see a light beam that is interrupted electronically at variable frequencies. At low frequencies the light beam appears to flash or flicker; at high frequencies the light beam appears to be uninterrupted. Participants use a toggle switch to indicate, on increasing and decreasing frequency curves, the points at which the beam appears, respectively, to stop and start flickering. The transition point on the ascending curve is called the threshold of fusion, and the transition point on the decreasing curve is called the threshold of flicker. The average of the thresholds of flicker and fusion is known as the critical flicker–fusion threshold (CFF), and is the primary outcome variable.

Maddox Wing (Hannington-Kiff, 1970) Participants look through a specially constructed apparatus that separates the visual field of each eye up to a central focal point. At that focal point, the left eye sees a horizontal scale, and the right eye sees a vertical arrow pointing at the scale. Participants are instructed to report the location on the scale at which the arrow appears to point. That location will shift depending on extraocular muscle balance. The focal point is centered if the muscles in both eyes are balanced. If the muscles in the eyes are unbalanced, the focal point will either shift to the left, indicating exophoria (eye divergence) or to the right indicating esophoria (eye convergence). Increased severity of exophoria or esophoria is associated with decreased visual perception (blurred or doubled vision).

Motor Ability

The tasks selected reflect relatively simple measures of motor ability. Performance changes on these tasks usually reflect gross alterations (excitation or depression) in CNS functioning.

Simple Tracking Participants are asked to track a randomly moving target (e.g., a circle) on a computer screen using a computer mouse (Nuotto & Korttila, 1991), or to track randomly illuminated lights on a panel of circularly arranged lights by pressing the button associated with each sequentially illuminated light as quickly as possible (Circular Lights; McLeod,

Griffiths, Bigelow, & Yingling, 1982). The outcome measure for a 1 min trial is either the number of errors (i.e., times the cursor deviates significantly from the moving target) or percent time on target for computer-based applications, and the number of correct button presses for the manual task.

Standing Steadiness   In the body sway task (Letz & Gerr, 1995), participants are asked to stand barefoot on a mechanized platform while anterior–posterior and medial–lateral body movements are measured in response to changes in the platform angle relative to baseline movements made when the platform is in a stable horizontal position. In the balance task, participants are asked to stand on one leg with eyes closed for as long as possible up to a maximum time interval (e.g., 30 seconds). If the participants touch the floor with the raised foot or open their eyes, the time expired is the score for that leg. The outcome measure is the total time balanced on both legs.

Finger Tapping (Reitan & Wolfson, 1985)   Participants are instructed to tap a panel or key as fast as possible for a fixed interval of time (e.g., 10 seconds). The outcome measure is the finger-tapping rate (i.e., the interval between taps).

Attention

Focused Attention   Focused attention refers to the ability to perceive and respond to a target stimulus of any type. To distinguish focused attention from sustained attention, only tasks lasting less than a total of 5 minutes are included.

Simple Reaction Time (RT)   Participants receive a series of discrete presentations of an auditory or visual stimulus and must respond by performing a simple motor behavior (e.g., button press) each time the stimulus is presented. The delay from presentation of the stimulus to the behavioral response, (RT), is the primary outcome variable.

Sustained Attention   Sustained attention refers to the ability to remain focused on a single task for an extended period of time without getting distracted or fatigued. Sustained attention is an important component of many work-related tasks, driving, and other daily activities. To distinguish from focused attention, only tasks lasting at least 10 minutes are included.

Rapid-visual Information Processing (RVIP; Wesnes & Warburton, 1983) or Continuous Performance Task (CPT; Riccio, Waldrop, Reynolds, & Lowe, 2001)   Similar to simple RT, participants must continuously attend to auditory or visual stimuli presented sequentially and perform a behavior (e.g., button press) each time a target stimulus or string of stimuli (e.g., 3 odd numbers in a row) occurs. Outcome variables are the number of correct and incorrect responses and RT for correct responses.

Selective Attention   Selective attention refers to the ability to direct your attention and respond selectively to one object or event that is directly relevant to a current goal, while ignoring other objects or events that are not relevant. For example, if you were interested in what a billboard said, you would want to focus on reading the text and not how many trees were beside it or how fast you were driving at the moment.

Stroop Task (Stroop, 1935)   Participants are presented with a series of color-word (e.g., the word "green") stimuli and either noncolor word (e.g., the word "mask") or nonword (e.g., a string of 0s) stimuli printed in different colors, and are instructed to speak the color of the stimulus as quickly as possible. The primary outcome measure is called the Stroop interference effect and refers to an increase in RT to name the color in which a stimulus is printed when the stimulus is a color-word printed in an incongruent color (e.g., the word "green" printed in the color red), relative to when the stimulus is a noncolor word or nonword stimulus.

Divided Attention   Divided attention is a critical aspect of performance for many daily activities. For example, when driving a car you must constantly monitor your speed, lane position, and distance from other cars, and also be attentive to peripheral objects such as traffic lights or debris that may appear or change unexpectedly.

Divided Attention Tasks   Participants must simultaneously attend to multiple stimuli and respond to them. These tasks come in many flavors, but generally involve performing one task at a central focal point (e.g., tracking an object in the middle of a computer screen with the mouse), while also attending and responding to peripheral stimuli (e.g., clicking the mouse button each time a target number appears in one corner of the computer screen). Outcome measures include separate scores for the central and peripheral tasks.

Memory

Short-Term/Working Memory   This type of memory enables one to hold onto and manipulate small amounts of information for short periods of time, and is critical to many daily tasks, such as holding in mind the beginning of a sentence until the end of the sentence in conversation or reading, retaining a phone number until it is dialed, or performing mental arithmetic.

Digit Span (Wechsler, 1981)   Digits are presented in successive trials and participants are asked to immediately recall the digits in the order of presentation (forward digit span) or in the reverse order (backward digit span). On each successive trial, the number of digits presented is increased by one and the outcome measure is the number of trials completed before an error occurred.

Sternberg Task (Sternberg, 1969)   Small sets of letters (typically 4–7) are presented briefly, immediately after which participants are presented with a probe letter and asked to indicate whether the probe letter was included in the presentation set. Outcome measures are the number of correct responses and RT.

Episodic Memory   Episodic memory refers to conscious long-term memory for a personally experienced event that occurred at a specific time and place (e.g., what you had for dinner last night).

Free Recall   Participants are presented with a list of words, which they are asked to recall following a delay (at least 10 min). The outcome measure is the number of words correctly remembered.

Recognition Memory   Participants are presented with a list of words. Following a delay, the participants are presented with words from the presentation list (old) as well as words that were not on the list (new) and are asked to distinguish between old and new words. Outcome measures are the proportion of old words identified as "old" (hit rate), proportion of new words identified as "old" (false alarm rate), and a measure of sensitivity in distinguishing between old and new words (d').

Semantic Memory   Semantic memory refers to conscious long-term memory for conceptual and factual knowledge, not associated with a specific time and place (e.g., Washington, DC is the capital of the United States; a dog is an animal).

Fluency   Participants are asked to produce as many items as possible from a specified category (e.g., fruits, words beginning with the letter "A") within a given period of time. The outcome measure is the number of correct items produced.

Implicit Memory   Implicit memory refers to long-term memory for a previous experience expressed unintentionally or without conscious recollection of the experience.

Word Stem Completion   Participants are presented with a list of words. Following a delay, the participants are presented with word stems (e.g., STR _ _ _) and instructed to complete each stem with the first word that comes to mind (e.g., STREAM). Implicit memory is manifested by the degree of priming, which refers to increased rates of completing stems with words from the presentation list, relative to words that had not been presented.

Effects of Drugs on Cognitive Functioning

This section provides an overview of the acute effects of most abused drugs on cognitive performance based on published placebo-controlled laboratory studies (studies in which a nondrug condition is included for comparison) in healthy, nondrug-dependent volunteers. For each drug class, the typical observed peak drug effects relative to placebo within each category of cognitive functioning are summarized and sample publications cited. For further information, the reader is referred to relevant recent reviews for each drug class. The effects of different doses are not considered separately; higher doses are associated with larger effects unless otherwise noted. As discussed earlier, in addition to summarizing the findings, comment is made regarding the relative severity of the observed effects. Last, the cognitive effects associated with chronic drug use and the long-term residual effects following drug discontinuation are discussed briefly. In the context of chronic effects, brief reference is made to epidemiological (traffic accident rates) and neuroimaging (brain changes) data, although in-depth discussion of these data is beyond the scope of this chapter.

Benzodiazepines

There is a vast literature on the acute effects of benzodiazepines on cognitive performance in healthy volunteers, with particular focus on memory-related effects (for reviews, see Curran, 2000; Ghoneim, 2004; Kunsman, Manno, Manno, Kunsman, & Przekop, 1992). The most commonly studied benzodiazepines in this area are lorazepam, midazolam, diazepam, alprazolam, and triazolam, and the most common route of administration is oral. The effects of different benzodiazepines and routes of administration are not considered separately; these variables generally only affect the time course of effects but are not associated with qualitatively different patterns of effects.

Sensory Acuity Benzodiazepines typically decrease CFF threshold (Curran & Birch, 1991; Curran, Pooviboonsuk, Dalton, & Lader, 1998; Hindmarch, Trick, & Ridout, 2005) and increase exophoria (Giersch, Boucart, Speeg-Schatz, Muller-Kauffmann, & Danion, 1996; Mattila, Aranko, & Kuitunen, 1993).

Motor Ability Benzodiazepines impair motor ability as evidenced by a decrease in tracking performance (Kirk, Roache, & Griffiths, 1990; Mintzer, Frey, Yingling, & Griffiths, 1997), impaired body sway (Bond, Silveira, & Lader, 1991) and balance (Kirk et al., 1990; Mintzer et al., 1997), and a decrease in finger-tapping rate (Bond et al., 1991; Curran & Birch, 1991; Curran et al., 1998).

Attention Benzodiazepines impair focused attention (File, 1992; Zacny, 2003), divided attention (Hindmarch et al., 2005; Moskowitz & Smiley, 1982), and sustained attention (Hindmarch et al., 2005). Findings for selective attention are mixed; three studies showed no benzodiazepine effect (Griffiths, Jones, & Richens, 1986; Mintzer & Griffiths, 2003; Preston et al., 1988) whereas one study (Kunsman et al., 1992) showed an increase in the Stroop interference effect.

Memory Benzodiazepines typically do not impair digit span performance (Bishop, Curran, & Lader, 1996; Kirkby, Montgomery, Badcock, & Daniels, 1995) but have been shown to impair short-term/working memory performance when task demands are greater (e.g., on versions of the Sternberg task; Mintzer & Griffiths, 2007; Verster, Volkerts, & Verbaten, 2002). Benzodiazepines impair episodic memory both on free recall and recognition memory tasks (Danion, Zimmermann, Willard-Schroeder, Grange, & Singer, 1989; Weingartner, Hommer, Lister, Thompson, & Wolkowitz, 1992). Benzodiazepines typically do not impair performance on fluency tasks (Danion et al., 1989; Krystal et al., 1998) but have been shown to impair semantic memory on more complex tasks, suggesting that some semantic memory processes may be disrupted (Bacon et al., 1998; Izaute, Paire-Ficout, & Bacon, 2004). For the most part, benzodiazepines do not impair priming on implicit memory tasks, although there is some evidence that lorazepam in particular may impair implicit memory (Bishop et al., 1996; Danion et al., 1989; Martin et al., 2002; Weingartner et al., 1992).

Comment Results of acute effect studies indicate that benzodiazepines reliably impair sensory acuity, motor ability, attention (focused, sustained, divided), and memory (short-term/working, episodic). Laboratory studies that have directly compared benzodiazepines to alcohol suggest that moderate doses of benzodiazepines produce psychomotor impairment comparable to that produced by alcohol doses that have been associated with driving impairment (Mintzer & Griffiths, 2002; Roache, Cherek, Bennett, Schenkler, & Cowan, 1993). Interestingly, in a recent study (Mintzer & Griffiths, 2002), the episodic memory impairment produced by a therapeutic dose of triazolam (0.25 mg/70 kg) was greater than that produced by a dose of alcohol resulting in breath alcohol concentrations (BAC) above the legal driving limit in most countries (mean BAC = 0.13%). This finding suggests that the acute amnestic effects of benzodiazepines are of a relatively large magnitude and would be expected to cause real-world functional impairment.

Supporting the clinical significance of the impairment associated with benzodiazepines, there is epidemiological evidence that patients prescribed benzodiazepines for anxiety disorders are at a significantly increased risk of involvement in a road traffic accident (Barbone et al., 1998). Likewise, results of a recent meta-analysis of observational studies (Barker, Greenwood, Jackson, & Crow, 2004a) suggest that long-term benzodiazepine users are significantly impaired relative to controls in all the cognitive domains tested (sensory processing, psychomotor speed, nonverbal memory, visuospatial skills, speed of processing, problem solving, attention/concentration, verbal memory, general intelligence, motor control/performance, working memory, and verbal reasoning). Results of a second meta-analysis by the same authors that examined residual effects of long-term benzodiazepine use following discontinuation suggest that although there is improvement postcessation in all cognitive domains tested, performance is still impaired relative to controls 6 months after discontinuation (Barker, Greenwood, Jackson, & Crowe, 2004b). Results of a recent neuroimaging study, however, did not find evidence that long-term benzodiazepine use is associated with brain abnormalities (Busto, Bremner, Knight, terBrugge, & Sellers, 2000).

Alcohol

As with benzodiazepines, extensive research has been conducted on the acute cognitive effects of alcohol in healthy volunteers (for reviews, see Finnigan & Hammerslay, 1992; Koelega, 1995), due in part to alcohol's widespread use in society and its association with traffic accidents.

Sensory Acuity   Alcohol has been shown to increase exophoria (Thapar, Zacny, Choi, & Apfelbaum, 1995a; Thapar, Zacny, Thompson, & Apfelbaum, 1995b) and to decrease CFF in some studies (Rammsayer, 1995; Yap, Mascord, Starmer, & Whitfield, 1993), but to have no effect on CFF in other studies (Liguori, D'Agostino, Dworkin, Edwards, & Robinson, 1999).

Motor Ability   Alcohol impairs motor ability as evidenced by a decrease in tracking performance (Heishman, Stitzer, & Bigelow, 1988; Mintzer & Griffiths, 2001), increase in body sway (Liguori et al., 1999; Yap et al., 1993), and a decrease in finger-tapping rate (Echeverria, Fine, Langolf, Schork, & Sampaio, 1991; Kennedy, Turnage, Wilkes, & Dunlap, 1993).

Attention   Alcohol typically impairs focused attention (Finnigan & Hammerslay, 1992; Maylor, Rabbitt, James, & Kerr, 1990), divided attention (Roehrs, Burduvali, Bonahoom, Drake, & Roth, 2003; Vermeeren et al., 2002; Yap et al., 1993), and sustained attention

(Linnoila et al., 1983; Tiplady et al., 2001). Alcohol appears not to affect selective attention as measured by the Stroop interference effect (Fillmore, Dixon, & Schweizer, 2000; Liguori & Robinson, 2001).

Memory Alcohol has been shown to impair short-term/working memory performance on the Sternberg task (Grattan-Miscio & Vogel-Sprott, 2005; Tiplady, Franklin, & Scholey, 2004). Alcohol-induced episodic memory impairment is observed both on free recall and recognition memory tasks, although the effect on recognition memory is less reliable (Hashtroudi, Parker, DeLisi, Wyatt, & Mutter, 1984; Mintzer & Griffiths, 2001; Soderlund, Parker, Schwartz, & Tulving, 2005). Alcohol has been shown to reduce the number of correct responses produced on the fluency task (Wendt & Risberg, 2001) and also to impair semantic memory on other tasks (Sayette, Martin, Perrott, & Wertz, 2001). Alcohol does not impair implicit memory performance (Hashtroudi et al., 1984; Lister, Gorenstein, Fisher-Flowers, Weingartner, & Eckardt, 1991; Soderlund et al., 2005).

Comment Results of acute effect studies indicate that alcohol reliably impairs sensory acuity (although effects on CFF are inconsistent), motor ability, attention (focused, sustained, divided), and memory (short-term/working, episodic, semantic). Consistent with alcohol's well-documented association with traffic accidents and driving impairment, the most profound deficits are in the areas of motor ability and attention. Alcohol is associated with as many fatal collisions as all other drugs combined, and a recent review concludes that significant impairment in functions relevant to driving performance can occur at BAC (< 0.02%), well below the legal intoxication limit in most countries (Ogden & Moskowitz, 2004).

Results of observational studies (for reviews, see Bates, Bowden, & Barry, 2002; Harper & Matsumoto, 2005) suggest that chronic alcohol abusers are impaired relative to controls in motor ability, memory, concept formation, abstraction, problem solving, and executive functions, and are prone to impulsive decision making (Dom, D'haene, Hulstijn, & Sabbe, 2006). Consistent with the observed deficits in motor ability, memory, and executive functions, brain changes have been observed, respectively, in the cerebellum, temporal cortex, and frontal cortex. There is evidence of recovered cognitive performance and brain functioning following sustained abstinence, although deficits have been observed even after years of abstinence and there is controversy regarding the rate of recovery for different cognitive functions. It also should be noted that a minority of chronic alcohol abusers develop Wernicke–Korsakoff syndrome, which is a persistent amnestic syndrome associated with thiamin deficiency.

Opioids

The acute cognitive effects of opioids that are used medically (e.g., morphine, fentanyl, oxycodone) have been studied fairly extensively in healthy volunteers (for a review, see Zacny, 1995). In controlled laboratory studies, acute doses are most commonly administered via intravenous or oral routes. There is evidence that some opioids may be associated with relatively more impairment than others. For this review, however, the typical effects observed across opioids are summarized and distinctions are not made based on route of administration.

Sensory Acuity   Opioids typically decrease CFF (Manner, Kanto, & Salonen, 1987; Saarialho-Kere, Mattila, & Seppala, 1989) and increase exophoria (Saarialho-Kere et al., 1989; Zacny, Conley, & Galinkin, 1997).

Motor Ability   Studies assessing the effects of opioids on motor ability have yielded mixed results. Opioids typically do not affect finger-tapping rate (Saarialho-Kere et al., 1989), and have been shown to impair tracking and body sway in some studies but not others (Hill & Zacny, 2000; Posner, Telekes, Crowley, Phillipson, & Peck, 1985; Saarialho-Kere, Mattila, & Seppala, 1986; Zacny et al., 1997).

Attention   Opioids have been shown to impair focused attention in some studies but not others (Hill, Black, & Sadeghi, 1998; Zacny, Lichtor, Flemming, Coalson, & Thompson, 1994; Zacny et al., 1993, 1997; Zacny). In the one study to our knowledge that examined effects of an opioid on selective attention, an increase in the Stroop interference effect was observed (Richens, Allen, Jones, Griffiths, & Marshall, 1983). Opioids do not appear to impair sustained attention (Rothenberg, Schottenfeld, Meyer, Krauss, & Gross, 1977) or divided attention (Saarialho-Kere et al., 1989), although few studies have examined opioid effects on these functions.

Memory   For the most part, opioids do not impair short-term/working memory (O'Neill, Hanks, White, Simpson, & Wesnes, 1995; Zacny, Lichtor, Klafta, Alessi, & Apfelbaum, 1996), episodic memory (Hill & Zacny, 2000; Zacny & Gutierrez, 2003), or semantic memory (Smith, Semke, & Beecher, 1962). To our knowledge, acute effects of single opioid doses on implicit memory have not been tested in laboratory studies with healthy volunteers.

Comment   Results of acute effect studies indicate that opioids can impair sensory acuity, motor ability, and focused attention, but the effects on motor ability and focused attention are not consistently observed. Opioids do not appear to significantly impair memory. Results of the one laboratory study to our knowledge that directly compared a single acute opioid dose to alcohol suggest that the acute cognitive effects of opioids are mild relative to an impairing dose of alcohol (Thapar et al., 1995b). Supporting the relatively low severity of acute opioid effects, opioids also produce less cognitive impairment than impairing doses of benzodiazepines (Hanks, O'Neill, Simpson, & Wesnes, 1995; O'Neill et al., 1995, 2000; Veselis, Reinsel, Feshchenko, & Wronski, 1997; Zacny, 2003). Consistent with the suggestion of minimal motor impairment, opioid users do not appear to have higher rates of traffic accidents or serious motor vehicle violations relative to nonusers (cf. Mintzer & Johnson, 2007).

The results of observational studies comparing chronic opioid abusers (mostly methadone maintenance patients) to nondrug abusers or abstinent former opioid abusers are inconsistent. Some studies suggest impairment in a wide range of functions (motor ability, attention, memory, problem solving, decision making) whereas others provide no evidence for impairment (for a review, see Mintzer & Johnson, 2007). However, evidence from several studies suggests that opioid abusers exhibit impairment in information processing at high speeds and decision making (i.e., tend to make more risky or impulsive decisions). Findings of impaired decision making (and memory in some studies) are consistent with observations in neuroimaging studies of altered brain function in the frontal and temporal areas in chronic opioid users compared with matched controls (cf. Mintzer & Johnson, 2007). Observational studies in abstinent opioid abusers suggest that recovery of brain functioning occurs during abstinence and that residual performance impairment is minimal (cf. Mintzer & Johnson, 2007).

Cannabis (Marijuana)

The acute cognitive effects of cannabis have been well studied, with particular attention paid to effects on tasks related to driving performance and memory (for reviews, see Beardsley & Kelly, 1999; Ramaekers, Berghaus, van Laar, & Drummer, 2004; Ranganathan & D'Souza, 2006). Most research has been conducted with smoked cannabis, although oral administration of delta-9-tetrahydracannbinol (THC), the primary psychoactive compound in cannabis, has also been used. Because the cognitive effects of oral THC are similar to those of smoked cannabis, these compounds are not differentiated below.

Sensory Acuity Mixed results have been observed with regard to the effects of cannabinoids on sensory acuity. In one study, CFF was increased, suggesting a stimulant-like effect (Hill, Goodwin, Schwin, & Powell, 1974), whereas no effect was observed in a second study (Liguori, Gatto, & Robinson, 1998). To our knowledge, no published studies have assessed the acute effects of cannabis on the Maddox Wing.

Motor Ability Cannabis has been shown to impair motor ability in some studies, but not others. Impaired tracking (Cone, Johnson, Moore, & Roache, 1986; Heishman, Huestis, Henningfield, & Cone, 1990) and body sway (Belgrave et al., 1979; Liguori, Gatto, & Jarrett, 2002; Liguori, Gatto, & Robinson, 1998) have been observed; however, the impaired tracking performance in the Heishman et al. (1990) study was described as "slight." In similar studies, effects on tracking (Heishman et al., 1988) and balance (Chait & Perry, 1994) were not observed. To our knowledge, finger tapping has not been assessed following acute administration of cannabis or THC in controlled studies.

Attention Cannabis typically impairs focused attention (Belgrave et al., 1979; Curran, Brignell, Fletcher, Middleton, & Henry, 2002). There is no evidence that cannabis impairs sustained attention (Curran et al., 2002). With regard to selective attention, an increase in the Stroop interference effect was found in one study (Hooker & Jones, 1987), but no effect was observed in another (Miller, Drew, & Kiplinger, 1972). Cannabis has been shown to reliably impair performance on divided attention tasks (Chait & Perry, 1994; Marks & MacAvoy, 1989).

Memory Cannabis did not impair digit span performance in two controlled studies (Chait & Perry, 1994; Hooker & Jones, 1987), but did in a third (Heishman, Stitzer, & Yingling, 1989). No effect was observed in the only study of Sternberg performance (Roth, Tinklenberg, & Kopell, 1977); however, that study used relatively short digit strings (1–4). The effects of cannabis on episodic memory have also been inconsistent, both on free recall and recognition memory tasks (Abel, 1971a, 1971b; Chait & Perry, 1994; Curran et al., 2002; Heishman, Arasteh, & Stitzer, 1997; Hooker & Jones, 1987). Cannabis has not been demonstrated to affect performance on semantic or implicit memory tasks (Curran et al., 2002).

Comment   Results of acute effect studies indicate that cannabis reliably impairs attention (focused, divided). There is some evidence that cannabis impairs motor ability and memory (short-term/working, episodic), but these effects do not appear to be very robust and are not observed consistently across studies. The acute effects of moderate doses of cannabis on motor ability and attention appear comparable to moderate doses of alcohol (BAC approximately 0.05%; Liguori et al., 1998; Ramaekers et al., 2004). In another study, impairment of episodic memory by multiple doses of alcohol and cannabis was shown to be dose-dependent and of comparable severity at parallel points in the dose-response curve (Heishman et al., 1997). With regard to the effects of cannabis on driving, research suggests that cannabis impairs driving ability and increases the risk of getting into an accident; however, under the influence of cannabis, drivers tend to go slower and be more cautious, and as a result are no more likely than drug-free drivers to get into an accident that results in serious or fatal injuries (for reviews, see Ramaekers et al., 2004; Smiley, 1999).

Results of observational studies suggest that chronic cannabis users are impaired relative to controls with respect to attention, memory, and some aspects of higher-order cognition including problem solving and mental flexibility (Kalant, 2004; Solowij et al., 2002). Consistent with these observed impairments in cognitive functioning, neuroimaging studies have shown that chronic cannabis users have altered brain function in the prefrontal cortex, cerebellum, and hippocampus compared with drug-free controls (Lundqvist, 2005). There is also evidence that chronic cannabis users perform significantly worse than matched controls on measures of risky decision making (Bolla, Eldreth, Matochik, & Cadet, 2005; Whitlow et al., 2004). Most research suggests that impairments associated with chronic cannabis use are reversed following extended abstinence (Fried & Gray, 2005; Pope, Gruber, Hudson, Huestis, & Yurgelun-Todd, 2001).

Stimulants

Summarizing the acute effects of drugs traditionally categorized as stimulants (amphetamines, caffeine, cocaine, methylphenidate, nicotine) in healthy volunteers is more challenging than for the drugs covered earlier in this chapter. Controlled studies of the cognitive effects of stimulants are largely inconsistent. One reason for this inconsistency is that the acute performance effects of stimulants tend to change relative to the magnitude of dose administered in what is called an "inverted U-shaped" function. What this means is that stimulants tend to improve performance at low doses and impair performance at high doses. Another issue is that a majority of the cognitive research on stimulants has been conducted either with chronic users or in combination with another variable (e.g., sleep deprivation or another drug) leaving relatively few studies that meet our criteria. Because of these issues, our overview of stimulant effects is more general and abbreviated compared with previous sections.

Acute administration of stimulants to healthy volunteers tends to result in improved sensory acuity, motor ability, focused attention, and sustained attention (for reviews, see Foltin & Evans, 1993; Heishman, Taylor, & Henningfield, 1994; Koelega, 1993). Stimulants tend not to have significant effects on selective or divided attention, or memory following acute drug administration. In other studies, the acute effects of stimulants have been shown to reliably counteract the performance impairments associated with fatigue (Lorist & Tops, 2003;

Newhouse et al., 1989). We were unable to find any evidence that strongly supported an association between use of stimulant drugs alone and increased risk for motor vehicle accidents.

Following chronic administration, stimulants have been reliably demonstrated to improve sensory acuity, attention, memory, and planning/cognitive flexibility in participants diagnosed with Attention Deficit–Hyperactivity Disorder (ADHD; Pietrzak, Mollica, Maruff, & Snyder, 2006). On the other hand, chronic abuse of illicit stimulant drugs (e.g., cocaine or methamphetamine) has been associated with impairment of focused and selective attention, short-term/working, episodic, and semantic memory, and higher-order functioning (cognitive flexibility, problem solving, and reasoning; Ersche, Clark, London, Robbins, & Sahakian, 2006; Jovanovski, Erb, & Zakzanis, 2005; Ornstein et al., 2000). Chronic abuse of cocaine and amphetamines is also associated with impaired decision making and increased impulsivity (Bornovalova, Daughters, Hernandez, Richards, & Lejuez, 2005; Coffey, Gudleski, Saladin, & Brady, 2003). Neuroimaging studies have demonstrated that chronic illicit stimulant use alters functioning in frontal, temporal, and subcortical brain areas (Lundqvist, 2005). Research suggests that impairment associated with chronic stimulant abuse is greater than that observed in chronic opiate abusers and can persist for up to one year of abstinence (Ersche et al., 2006; Verdejo-Garcia & Perez-Garcia, 2007).

Miscellaneous Other Drugs

This section provides brief summaries of the cognitive effects of drugs that were not covered in the major drug classes reviewed above, but which have been shown to be associated with some degree of impairment.

3,4-methylenedioxy-N-methamphetamine (MDMA, "Ecstasy")   Relatively few controlled studies have been conducted on the acute cognitive effects of MDMA. In these studies, MDMA impaired sensory acuity, attention (focused, sustained, divided), and free recall, but did not affect recognition memory (Cami et al., 2000; Farre et al., 2004; Hart, 2007; Kuypers & Ramaekers, 2005). In a study of driving ability, MDMA improved road-tracking performance, but reduced the accuracy of speed adaptation during a car-following task (Ramaekers, Kuypers, & Samyn, 2006). Far more studies have been conducted on the cognitive consequences of chronic MDMA use. Heavy MDMA users tend to have impaired motor ability, attention, memory, and reasoning compared with matched non-MDMA using controls (for a review, see Kalechstein, De La Garza II, Mahoney, Fantegrossi, & Newton, 2007). MDMA users have also been shown to have increased impulsivity and impaired decision making compared with controls (Quednow et al., 2007).

Hallucinogens   Studies conducted in the 1950s and 1960s suggest that acute administration of LSD results in impaired auditory RT and episodic and working memory, but has no effect on motor ability or visual RT (Abramson, Jarvik, & Hirsch, 1955a, 1955b; Jarvik, Abramson, & Hirsch, 1955; Silverstein & Klee, 1960). There is no clear evidence of impaired cognitive functioning following chronic use of hallucinogens. Some studies have reported slight decrements in visuospatial and memory abilities in heavy hallucinogen users compared with controls, but these effects were not replicated in other studies (for a review, see Halpern & Pope, 1999).

Ketamine   Research on the acute and chronic effects of the N-methyl-D-aspartic acid (NMDA) antagonist ketamine on cognitive performance has increased in recent years. In healthy volunteers, acute doses of ketamine typically produce dose-related impairment of motor ability (Lofwall, Griffiths, & Mintzer, 2006), focused attention, episodic memory, and some semantic and short-term/working memory processes, but do not appear to impair selective attention, implicit memory priming, or problem solving (Morgan & Curran, 2006). Acute effects on sustained attention have been inconsistent. Chronic ketamine users tend to be particularly impaired relative to controls with respect to episodic and semantic memory (Morgan & Curran, 2006).

Limitations

Some limitations of the overview of cognitive effects of abused drugs provided above warrant mention. As previously noted, causality cannot be inferred from observational studies in chronic users due to a lack of baseline performance assessment and the co-occurrence of other substance use or other factors that could contribute to performance impairment. Conclusions based on observational studies are also limited by methodological issues including small sample sizes, use of a limited range of performance measures, variability between studies in performance measures, and failure in some cases to appropriately match the chronic drug use and control groups on factors that may affect performance (e.g., IQ, years of education).

Our summary of acute drug administration studies in healthy volunteers also has limitations. First, despite our effort to select "pure" measures for each type of functioning, there is overlap across measures. For example, short-term/working memory is needed to remember what the target stimulus is in sustained attention tasks, and focused attention is needed to perform well on most memory tasks. Second, although measures are often collected at multiple time points, it is possible that the results reported do not reflect peak effects of acute dosing. Third, conclusions based on between-drug comparisons are constrained by dose selection issues. Likewise, some of the observed inconsistencies between studies within drug classes may be related to dose-selection issues.

Conclusions

Drugs of abuse can affect cognitive ability in many areas of functioning. Following acute administration, benzodiazepines, alcohol, opioids, cannabis, MDMA, and ketamine are generally associated with impaired performance, whereas stimulant drugs such as amphetamine and nicotine are generally associated with improved performance. The relative magnitude and clinical importance of the acute performance-impairing effects in different areas of functioning remain difficult to discern. Overall it appears that benzodiazepines and alcohol produce the greatest functional impairment, whereas opioids and cannabis produce relatively less impairment. Chronic drug abuse in general is associated with some degree of cognitive impairment, although in most cases the impairment is at least partially reversed following extended abstinence. Chronic drug abusers also tend to exhibit impairment in executive functions and to be more prone to impulsive decision-making or risk-taking behavior. The specific variables (e.g., genetic differences, drug use patterns) that mediate the development of long-term cognitive impairment following use of these drugs is not clear, but in most studies the magnitude of impairment was correlated with measures of drug use severity.

Significant clinical concerns arise related to these impairments in cognitive functioning. First, it is important to appropriately inform patients being prescribed medications or abusing the drugs described in this chapter about potential cognitive effects. This includes obvious recommendations about driving and operating dangerous machinery, but should also include information about the possibility of impaired visual perception and memory that can significantly interfere with daily functioning. Another clinical concern is that cognitive impairment can affect the ability to participate in and benefit from cognitive/psychosocial aspects of substance abuse treatment. Knowledge of the specific patterns of deficits associated with particular drugs of abuse can be used to tailor treatment interventions to individual cognitive capabilities and enhance treatment outcomes. In fact, there is evidence suggesting that success in substance abuse treatment is correlated with cognitive functioning (Teichner, Horner, & Harvey, 2001), and that certain treatment interventions are more effective than others for cognitively impaired substance abusers (Cooney, Kadden, Litt, & Getter, 1991; Higgins, Alessi, & Dantona, 2002; Teichner, Horner, Roitzsch, Herron, & Thevos, 2002). There is also the potential to enhance treatment outcomes by using cognitive rehabilitation/training techniques during treatment to directly target cognitive deficits that may be associated with continued drug use and relapse (e.g., impulsive decision making). For example, self-control training has been shown to reduce impulsive choices in children (Schweitzer & Sulzer-Azaroll, 1988).

The emergence of new technologies, such as functional magnetic resonance imaging (fMRI), should enable researchers to more clearly understand the neurobiological mechanisms that mediate the effects of abused drugs on cognitive performance and to measure the effects of these drugs on specific brain areas in real-time. Adding assessments of cognitive functioning to large-scale longitudinal studies could also assist in interpretation of the chronic effects of abused drugs by providing baseline (predrug use) measures of functioning. Further behavioral, neuroimaging, and longitudinal research is essential to developing a more complete understanding of the acute and long-term effects of drug use, and may be applied to improve treatment approaches and affect social policy.

References

Abel, E. L. (1971a). Marihuana and memory: Acquisition or retrieval? *Science, 173,* 1038–1040.

Abel, E. L. (1971b). Retrieval of information after use of marihuana. *Nature, 231,* 58.

Abramson, H. A., Jarvik, M. E., & Hirsch, M. W. (1955a). Lysergic acid diethylamide (LSD-25): VII. Effect upon two measures of motor performance. *The Journal of Psychology, 39,* 455–464.

Abramson, H. A., Jarvik, M. E., & Hirsch, M. W. (1955b). Lysergic acid diethylamide (LSD-25): X. Effect on reaction time to auditory and visual stimuli. *The Journal of Psychology, 40,* 39–52.

Bacon, E., Danion, J. M., Kauffmann-Muller, F., Schelstraete, M. A., Bruant, A., Sellal, F., et al. (1998). Confidence level and feeling of knowing for episodic and semantic memory: An investigation of lorazepam effects on metamemory. *Psychopharmacology, 138,* 318–325.

Barbone, F., McMahon, A. D., Davey, P. G., Morris, A. D., Reid, I. C., McDevitt, D. G., et al. (1998). Association of road-traffic accidents with benzodiazepine use. *Lancet, 352,* 1331–1336.

Barker, M. J., Greenwood, K. M., Jackson, M., & Crowe, S. F. (2004a). Cognitive effects of long-term benzodiazepine use: A meta-analysis. *CNS Drugs, 18*, 37–48.

Barker, M. J., Greenwood, K. M., Jackson, M., & Crowe, S. F. (2004b). Persistence of cognitive effects after withdrawal from long-term benzodiazepine use: A meta-analysis. *Archives of Clinical Neuropsychology : The official journal of the National Academy of Neuropsychologists, 19*, 437–454.

Bates, M. E., Bowden, S. C., & Barry, D. (2002). Neurocognitive impairment associated with alcohol use disorders: Implications for treatment. *Experimental and Clinical Psychopharmacology, 10*, 193–212.

Beardsley, P. M., & Kelly, T. H. (1999). Acute effects of cannabis on human behavior and central nervous system functions. In H. Kalant, W. A. Corrigall, W. Hall, & R. G. Smart (Eds.), *The health effects of cannabis* (pp. 127–170). Toronto: Centre for Addiction and Mental Health.

Belgrave, B. E., Bird, K. D., Chesher, G. B., Jackson, D. M., Lubbe, K. E., Starmer, G. A., et al. (1979). The effect of delta-9-tetrahydrocannabinol, alone and in combination with ethanol, on human performance. *Psychopharmacology, 62*, 53–60.

Bishop, K. I., Curran, H. V., & Lader, M. (1996). Do scopolamine and lorazepam have dissociable effects on human memory systems? A dose-response study with normal volunteers. *Experimental and Clinical Psychopharmacology, 4*, 292–299.

Bolla, K. I., Eldreth, D. A., Matochik, J. A., & Cadet, J. L. (2005). Neural substrates of faulty decision-making in abstinent marijuana users. *Neuroimage, 26*, 480–492.

Bond, A., Silveira, J. C., & Lader, M. (1991). Effects of single doses of alprazolam and alcohol alone and in combination on psychological performance. *Human Psychopharmacology, 6*, 219–228.

Bornovalova, M. A., Daughters, S. B., Hernandez, G. D., Richards, J. B., & Lejuez, C. W. (2005). Differences in impulsivity and risk-taking propensity between primary users of crack cocaine and primary users of heroin in a residential substance-use program. *Experimental and Clinical Psychopharmacology, 13*, 311–318.

Busto, U. E., Bremner, K. E., Knight, K., terBrugge, K., & Sellers, E. M. (2000). Long-term benzodiazepine therapy does not result in brain abnormalities. *Journal of Clinical Psychopharmacology, 20*, 2–6.

Cami, J., Farre, M., Mas, M., Roset, P. N., Poudevida, S., Mas, A., et al. (2000). Human psychopharmacology of 3,4-methylenedioxymeth-amphetamine (Ecstasy): Psychomotor performance and subjective effects. *Journal of Clinical Psychopharmacology, 20*, 455–466.

Chait, L. D., & Perry, J. L. (1994). Acute and residual effects of alcohol and marijuana, alone and in combination, on mood and performance. *Psychopharmacology, 15*, 340–349.

Coffey, S. F., Gudleski, G. D., Saladin, M. E., & Brady, K. T. (2003). Impulsivity and rapid discounting of delayed hypothetical rewards in cocaine-dependent individuals. *Experimental and Clinical Psychpharmacology, 11*, 18–25.

Cone, E. J., Johnson, R. E., Moore, J. D., & Roache, J. D. (1986). Acute effects of smoking marijuana on hormones subjective effects and performance in male human subjects. *Pharmacology, Biochemistry and Behavior, 24*, 1749–1754.

Cooney, N. L., Kadden, R. M., Litt, M. D., & Getter, H. (1991). Matching alcoholics to coping skills or interactional therapies: Two-year follow-up results. *Journal of Consulting and Clinical Psychology, 59*, 598–601.

Curran, H. V. (2000). Psychopharmacological approaches to human memory. In: M.S. Gazzaniga (Ed.), *The new cognitive neurosciences* (2nd ed., pp. 797–804). Boston: MIT Press.

Curran, H. V., & Birch, B. (1991). Differentiating the sedative, psychomotor and amnesic effects of benzodiazepines: A study with midazolam and the benzodiazepine antagonist, flumazenil. *Psychopharmacology, 103*, 519–523.

Curran, H. V., Brignell, C., Fletcher, S., Middleton, P., & Henry, J. (2002). Cognitive and subjective dose-response effects of acute oral delta-9-tetrahydrocannabinol (THC) in infrequent cannabis users. *Psychopharmacology, 164*, 61–70.

Curran, H. V., Pooviboonsuk, P., Dalton, J. A., & Lader, M. H. (1998). Differentiating the effects of centrally acting drugs on arousal and memory: An event-related potential study of scopolamine, lorazepam and diphenhydramine. *Psychopharmacology, 135*, 27–36.

Danion, J. M., Zimmermann, M. A., Willard-Schroeder, D., Grange, D., & Singer, L. (1989). Diazepam induces a dissociation between explicit and implicit memory. *Psychopharmacology, 99*, 238–243.

Dom, G., D'haene, P., Hulstijn, W., & Sabbe, B. (2006). Impulsivity in abstinent early- and late-onset alcoholics: Differences in self-report measures and a discounting task. *Addiction, 101*, 50–59.

Echeverria, D., Fine, L., Langolf, G., Schork, T., & Sampaio, C. (1991). Acute behavioural comparisons of toluene and ethanol in human subjects. *British Journal of Industrial Medicine, 48*, 750–761.

Ersche, K. D., Clark, L., London, M., Robbins, T. W., & Sahakian, B. J. (2006). Profile of executive and memory function associated with amphetamine and opiate dependence. *Neuropsychopharmacology, 31*, 1036–1047.

Farre, M., de la Torre, R., O Mathuna, B., Roset, P. N., Peiro, A. M., Torrens, M., et al. (2004). Repeated doses administration of MDMA in humans: Pharmacological effects and pharmacokinetics. *Psychopharmacology, 173*, 364–375.

File, S. E. (1992). Effects of lorazepam on psychomotor performance: A comparison of independent-groups and repeated-measures designs. *Pharmacology, Biochemistry, and Behavior, 42*, 761–764.

Fillmore, M. T., Dixon, M. J., & Schweizer, T. A. (2000). Alcohol affects processing of ignored stimuli in a negative priming paradigm. *Journal of Studies on Alcohol, 61*, 571–578.

Finnigan, F., & Hammersley, R. (1992). The effects of alcohol on performance. In D. M. Jones, & A. P. Smith (Eds.), *Handbook of human performance* (Vol. 2, pp. 73–126). London; San Diego: Academic Press.

Foltin, R. W., & Evans, S. M. (1993). Performance effects of drugs of abuse: A methodological survey. *Human Psychopharmacology, 8*, 9–19.

Fried, P. A., & Gray, W. R. (2005). Neurocognitive consequences of marihuana – A comparison with pre-drug performance. *Neurotoxicology and Teratology, 27*, 231–239.

Ghoneim, M. M. (2004). Drugs and human memory (part 2): Clinical, theoretical, and methodologic issues. *Anesthesiology, 100*, 1277–1297.

Giersch, A., Boucart, M., Speeg-Schatz, C., Muller-Kauffmann, F., & Danion, J. M. (1996). Lorazepam impairs perceptual integration of visual forms: A central effect. *Psychopharmacology, 126*, 260–270.

Grattan-Miscio, K. E., & Vogel-Sprott, M. (2005). Effects of alcohol and performance incentives on immediate working memory. *Psychopharmacology, 181*, 188–196.

Griffiths, A. N., Jones, D. M., & Richens, A. (1986). Zopiclone produces effects on human performance similar to flurazepam, lormetazepam and triazolam. *British Journal of Clinical Pharmacology, 21*, 647–653.

Halpern, J. H., & Pope, H. G. (1999). Do hallucinogens cause residual neuropsychological toxicity? *Drug and Alcohol Dependence, 53*, 247–256.

Hanks, G. W., O'Neill, W. M., Simpson, P., & Wesnes, K. (1995). The cognitive and psychomotor effects of opioid analgesics. II. A randomized controlled trial of single doses of morphine, lorazepam and placebo in healthy subjects. *European Journal of Clinical Pharmacology, 48*, 455–460.

Hannington-Kiff, J. G. (1970). Measurement of recovery from outpatient general anesthesia with a simple ocular test. *British Medical Journal, 18*, 132–135.

Harper, C., & Matsumoto, I. (2005). Ethanol and brain damage. *Current Opinion in Pharmacology, 5*, 73–78.

Hart, C. L. (2007). Personal Communication.

Hashtroudi, S., Parker, E. S., DeLisi, L. E., Wyatt, R. J., & Mutter, S. A. (1984). Intact retention in acute alcohol amnesia. *Journal of Experimental Psychology. Learning, Memory, and Cognition, 10*, 156–163.

Heishman, S. J., Arasteh, K., & Stitzer, M. L. (1997). Comparative effects of alcohol and marijuana on mood memory and performance. *Pharmacology, Biochemistry and Behavior, 58*, 93–101.

Heishman, S. J., Huestis, M. A., Henningfield, J. E., & Cone, E. J. (1990). Acute and residual effects of marijuana: Profiles of plasma THC levels, physiological, subjective, and performance measures. *Pharmacology, Biochemistry & Behavior, 37*, 561–565.

Heishman, S. J., Stitzer, M. L., & Bigelow, G. E. (1988). Alcohol and marijuana: Comparative dose effect profiles in humans. *Pharmacology, Biochemistry, and Behavior, 31*, 649–655.

Heishman, S. J., Stitzer, M. L., & Yingling, J. E. (1989). Effects of tetrahydrocannabinol content on marijuana smoking behavior subjective reports and performance. *Pharmacology, Biochemistry and Behavior, 34*, 173–179.

Heishman, S. J., Taylor, R. C., & Henningfield, J. E. (1994). Nicotine and smoking: A review of effects on human performance. *Experimental and Clinical Psychopharmacology, 2,* 345–395.

Higgins, S. T., Alessi, S. M., & Dantona, R. L. (2002). Voucher-based incentives. A substance abuse treatment innovation. *Addictive Behaviors, 27,* 887–910.

Hill, J. L., & Zacny, J. P. (2000). Comparing the subjective, psychomotor, and physiological effects of intravenous hydromorphone and morphine in healthy volunteers. *Psychopharmacology, 152,* 31–39.

Hill, S. Y., Goodwin, D. W., Schwin, R., & Powell, B. (1974). Marijuana: CNS depressant or excitant? *American Journal of Psychiatry, 131,* 313–315.

Hindmarch, I., Trick, L., & Ridout, F. (2005). A double-blind, placebo- and positive-internal-controlled (alprazolam) investigation of the cognitive and psychomotor profile of pregabalin in healthy volunteers. *Psychopharmacology, 183,* 133–143.

Hooker, W. D., & Jones, R. T. (1987). Increased susceptibility to memory intrusions and the Stroop interference effect during acute marijuana intoxication. *Psychophamacologia, 91,* 20–24.

Izaute, M., Paire-Ficout, L., & Bacon, E. (2004). Benzodiazepines and semantic memory: Effects of lorazepam on the moses illusion. *Psychopharmacology, 172,* 309–315.

Jarvik, M. E., Abramson, H. A., & Hirsch, M. W. (1955). Lysergic acid diethylamide (LSD-25): VI. Effect upon recall and recognition of various stimuli. *Journal of Psychology, 39,* 433–454.

Jovanovski, D., Erb, S., & Zakzanis, K. K. (2005). Neurocognitive deficits in cocaine users: A quantitative review of the evidence. *Journal of Clinical and Experimental Neuropsychology, 27,* 189–204.

Kalant, H. (2004). Adverse effects of cannabis on health: An update of the literature since 1996. *Progress in Neuro-Psychopharmacology & Biological Psychiatry, 28,* 849–863.

Kalechstein, A. D., De La Garza II, R., Mahoney, J. J., Fantegrossi, W. E., & Newton, T. F. (2007). MDMA use and neurocognition: A meta-analytic review. *Psychopharmacology, 189,* 531–537.

Kennedy, R. S., Turnage, J. J., Wilkes, R. L., & Dunlap, W. P. (1993). Effects of graded dosages of alcohol on nine computerized repeated-measures tests. *Ergonomics, 36,* 1195–1222.

Kirk, T., Roache, J. D., & Griffiths, R. R. (1990). Dose-response evaluation of the amnestic effects of triazolam and pentobarbital in normal subjects. *Journal of Clinical Psychopharmacology, 10,* 160–167.

Kirkby, K. C., Montgomery, I. M., Badcock, R., & Daniels, B. A. (1995). A comparison of age-related deficits in memory and frontal lobe function following oral lorazepam administration. *Journal of Psychopharmacology, 9,* 319–325.

Koelega, H. S. (1993). Stimulant drugs and vigilance performance: A review. *Psychopharmacology, 111,* 1–16.

Koelega, H. S. (1995). Alcohol and vigilance performance: A review. *Psychopharmacology, 118,* 233–249.

Krystal, J. H., Karper, L. P., Bennett, A., D'Souza, D. C., Abi-Dargham, A., Morrissey, K., et al. (1998). Interactive effects of subanesthetic ketamine and subhypnotic lorazepam in humans. *Psychopharmacology, 135,* 213–229.

Kunsman, G. W., Manno, J. E., Manno, B. R., Kunsman, C. M., & Przekop, M. A. (1992). The use of microcomputer-based psychomotor tests for the evaluation of benzodiazepine effects on human performance: A review with emphasis on temazepam. *British Journal of Clinical Pharmacology, 34,* 289–301.

Kuypers, K. P. C., & Ramaekers, J. G. (2005). Transient memory impairment after acute dose of 75 mg 3,4-methylene-dioxymethamphetamine. *Journal of Psychopharmacology, 19,* 633–639.

Letz, R., & Gerr, F. (1995). Standing steadiness measurements: Empirical selection of testing protocol and outcome measures. *Neurotoxicology and Teratology, 1,* 611–616.

Liguori, A., D'Agostino, R. B., Jr., Dworkin, S. I., Edwards, D., & Robinson, J. H. (1999). Alcohol effects on mood, equilibrium, and simulated driving. *Alcoholism, Clinical and Experimental Research, 23,* 815–821.

Liguori, A., Gatto, C. P., & Jarrett, D. B. (2002). Separate and combined effects of marijuana and alcohol on mood, equilibrium and simulated driving. *Psychopharmacology, 163,* 399–405.

Liguori, A., Gatto, C. P., & Robinson, J. H. (1998). Effects of marijuana on equilibrium, psychomotor performance, and simulated driving. *Behavioral Pharmacology, 9,* 599–609.

Liguori, A., & Robinson, J. H. (2001). Caffeine antagonism of alcohol-induced driving impairment. *Drug and Alcohol Dependence, 63*, 123–129.

Linnoila, M., Johnson, J., Dubyoski, T., Ross, R., Buchsbaum, M., Potter, W. Z., et al. (1983). Effects of amitriptyline, desipramine and zimeldine, alone and in combination with ethanol, on information processing and memory in healthy volunteers. *Acta Psychiatrica Scandinavica. Supplementum, 308*, 175–181.

Lister, R. G., Gorenstein, C., Fisher-Flowers, D., Weingartner, H. J., & Eckardt, M. J. (1991). Dissociation of the acute effects of alcohol on implicit and explicit memory processes. *Neuropsychologia, 29*, 1205–1212.

Lofwall, M. L., Griffiths, R. R., & Mintzer, M. Z. (2006). Cognitive and subjective acute dose effects of intramuscular ketamine in healthy adults. *Experimental and Clinical Psychopharmacology, 14*, 439–449.

Lorist, M. M., & Tops, M. (2003). Caffeine, fatigue, and cognition. *Brain and Cognition, 53*, 82–94.

Lundqvist, T. (2005). Cognitive consequences of cannabis use: Comparison with abuse of stimulants and heroin with regard to attention, memory and executive functions. *Pharmacology, Biochemistry, and Behavior, 81*, 319–330.

Manner, T., Kanto, J., & Salonen, M. (1987). Simple devices in differentiating the effects of buprenorphine and fentanyl in healthy volunteers. *European Journal of Clinical Pharmacology, 31*, 673–676.

Marks, D. F., & MacAvoy, M. F. (1989). Divided attention performance in cannabis users and non-users following alcohol and cannabis separately and in combination. *Psychopharmacology, 99*, 397–401.

Martin, J., Matthews, A., Martin, F., Kirkby, K. C., Alexander, J., & Daniels, B. (2002). Effects of lorazepam and oxazepam on perceptual and procedural memory functions. *Psychopharmacology, 164*, 262–267.

Mattila, M. J., Aranko, K., & Kuitunen, T. (1993). Diazepam effects on the performance of healthy subjects are not enhanced by treatment with the antihistamine ebastine. *British Journal of Clinical Pharmacology, 35*, 272–277.

Maylor, E. A., Rabbitt, P. M. A., James, G. H., & Kerr, S. A. (1990). Effects of alcohol and extended practice on divided-attention performance. *Perception & Psychophysics, 48*, 445–452.

McLeod, D. R., Griffiths, R. R., Bigelow, G. E., & Yingling, J. (1982). An automated version of the digit symbol substitution test (DSST). *Behavior Research Methods and Instrumentation, 14*, 463–466.

Miller, L., Drew, W. G., & Kiplinger, G. F. (1972). Effects on marijuana on recall of narrative material and Stroop colour-word performance. *Nature, 237*, 172–173.

Mintzer, M. Z., Frey, J. M., Yingling, J. E., & Griffiths, R. R. (1997). Triazolam and zolpidem: A comparison of their psychomotor, cognitive, and subjective effects in healthy volunteers. *Behavioural Pharmacology, 8*, 561–574.

Mintzer, M. Z., & Griffiths, R. R. (2001). Alcohol and false recognition: A dose-effect study. *Psychopharmacology, 159*, 51–57.

Mintzer, M. Z., & Griffiths, R. R. (2002). Alcohol and triazolam: Differential effects on memory, psychomotor performance and subjective ratings of effects. *Behavioural Pharmacology, 13*, 653–658.

Mintzer, M. Z., & Griffiths, R. R. (2003). Lorazepam and scopolamine: A single-dose comparison of effects on human memory and attentional processes. *Experimental and Clinical Psychopharmacology, 11*, 56–72.

Mintzer, M. Z., & Griffiths, R. R. (2007). Differential effects of scopolamine and lorazepam on working memory maintenance versus manipulation processes. *Cognitive, Affective, and Behavioral Neurosciencem, 7*, 120–129.

Mintzer, M. Z., & Johnson, M W. (2007). Neuropsychological consequences of opioid abuse. In: A. Kalechstein, & I W. Van Gorp (Eds.), *The neuropsychological consequences of substance abuse* (pp. 263–319). New York, NY: Taylor & Francis.

Morgan, C. J., & Curran, H. V. (2006). Acute and chronic effects of ketamine upon human memory: A review. *Psychopharmacology, 188*, 408–424.

Moskowitz, H., & Smiley, A. (1982). Effects of chronically administered buspirone and diazepam on driving-related skills performance. *The Journal of Clinical Psychiatry, 43*, 45–55.

Newhouse, P. A., Belenky, G., Thomas, M., Thorne, D., Sing, H. C., & Fertig, J. (1989). The effects of d-amphetamine on arousal, cognition, and mood after prolonged total sleep deprivation. *Neuropsychopharmacology, 2*, 153–164.

Nuotto, E. J., & Korttila, K. T. (1991). Evaluation of a new computerized psychomotor test battery: Effects of alcohol. *Pharmacology & Toxicology, 68,* 360–365.

Ogden, E. J., & Moskowitz, H. (2004). Effects of alcohol and other drugs on driver performance. *Traffic Injury Prevention, 5,* 185–198.

O'Neill, W. M., Hanks, G. W., Simpson, P., Fallon, M. T., Jenkins, E., & Wesnes, K. (2000). The cognitive and psychomotor effects of morphine in healthy subjects: A randomized controlled trial of repeated (four) oral doses of dextropropoxyphene, morphine, lorazepam and placebo. *Pain, 85,* 209–215.

O'Neill, W. M., Hanks, G. W., White, L., Simpson, P., & Wesnes, K. (1995). The cognitive and psychomotor effects of opioid analgesics. I. A randomized controlled trial of single doses of dextropropoxyphene, lorazepam and placebo in healthy subjects. *European Journal of Clinical Pharmacology, 48,* 447–453.

Ornstein, T. J., Iddon, J. L., Baldacchino, A. M., Sahakian, B. J., London, M., Everitt, B. J., et al. (2000). Profiles of cognitive dysfunction in chronic amphetamine and heroin abusers. *Neuropsychopharmacology, 23,* 113–126.

Pietrzak, R. H., Mollica, C. M., Maruff, P., & Snyder, P. J. (2006). Cognitive effects of immediate-release methylphenidate in children with attention-deficit/hyperactivity disorder. *Neuroscience and Biobehavioral Reviews, 30,* 1225–1245.

Pope, H. G., Jr., Gruber, A. J., Hudson, J. I., Huestis, M. A., & Yurgelun-Todd, D. (2001). Neuropsychological performance in long-term cannabis users. *Archives of General Psychiatry, 58,* 909–915.

Posner, J., Telekes, A., Crowley, D., Phillipson, R., & Peck, A. W. (1985). Effects of an opiate on cold-induced pain and the CNS in healthy volunteers. *Pain, 23,* 73–82.

Preston, G. C., Broks, P., Traub, M., Ward, C., Poppleton, P., & Stahl, S. M. (1988). Effects of lorazepam on memory, attention and sedation in man. *Psychopharmacology, 95,* 208–215.

Quednow, B. B., Kuhn, K. U., Westheide, J., Maier, W., Daum, I., & Wagner, M. (2007). Elevated impulsivity and impaired decision-making cognition in heavy users of MDMA ("Ecstasy"). *Psychopharmacology, 189,* 517–530.

Ramaekers, J. G., Berghaus, G., van Laar, M., & Drummer, O. H. (2004). Dose related risk of motor vehicle crashes after cannabis use. *Drug and Alcohol Dependence, 73,* 109–119.

Ramaekers, J. G., Kuypers, K. P., & Samyn, N. (2006). Stimulant effects of 3,4-methylenedioxymethamphetamine (MDMA) 75 mg and methylphenidate 20 mg on actual driving during intoxication and withdrawal. *Addiction, 101,* 1614–1621.

Rammsayer, T. (1995). Extraversion and alcohol: Eysenck's drug postulate revisited. *Neuropsychobiology, 32,* 197–207.

Ranganathan, M., & D'Souza, D. C. (2006). The acute effects of cannabinoids on memory in humans: A review. *Psychopharmacology, 188,* 425–444.

Reitan, R. M., & Wolfson, E. (1985). *The Halstead-Reitan Neuropsychological Test Battery.* Tuscon: Neuropsychology Press.

Riccio, C. A., Waldrop, J. J. M., Reynolds, C. R., & Lowe, P. (2001). Effects of stimulants on the Continuous Performance Test (CPT): Implications for CPT use and interpretation. *Journal of Neuropsychiatry and Clinical Neurosciences, 13,* 326–335.

Richens, A., Allen, E., Jones, D., Griffiths, A., & Marshall, R. (1983). A comparison of intramuscular meptazinol (100 mg) and papaveretum (20 mg) on human performance studies in healthy male volunteers. *Postgraduate Medical Journal, 59* (Suppl. 1), 19–24.

Roache, J. D., Cherek, D. R., Bennett, R. H., Schenkler, J. C., & Cowan, K. A. (1993). Differential effects of triazolam and ethanol on awareness, memory, and psychomotor performance. *Journal of Clinical Psychopharmacology, 13,* 3–15.

Roehrs, T., Burduvali, E., Bonahoom, A., Drake, C., & Roth, T. (2003). Ethanol and sleep loss: A "dose" comparison of impairing effects. *Sleep, 26,* 981–985.

Roth, W. T., Tinklenberg, J. R., & Kopell, B. S. (1977). Ethanol and marijuana effects on event-related potentials in a memory retrieval paradigm. *Electroencephalography and Clinical Neurophysiology, 42,* 381–388.

Rothenberg, S., Schottenfeld, S., Meyer, R. E., Krauss, B., & Gross, K. (1977). Performance differences between addicts and non-addicts. *Psychopharmacology, 52,* 299–306.

Saarialho-Kere, U., Mattila, M. J., & Seppala, T. (1986). Pentazocine and codeine: Effects on human performance and mood and interactions with diazepam. *Medical Biology, 64,* 293–299.

Saarialho-Kere, U., Mattila, M. J., & Seppala, T. (1989). Psychomotor, respiratory and neuroendocrinological effects of a mu-opioid receptor agonist (oxycodone) in healthy volunteers. *Pharmacology & Toxicology, 65*, 252–257.

Sayette, M. A., Martin, C. S., Perrott, M. A., & Wertz, J. M. (2001). Parental alcoholism and the effects of alcohol on mediated semantic priming. *Experimental and Clinical Psychopharmacology, 9*, 409–417.

Schweitzer, J. B., & Sulzer-Azaroff, B. (1988). Self-control: Teaching tolerance for delay in impulsive children. *Journal of the Experimental Analysis of Behavior, 50*, 173–186.

Silverstein, A. B., & Klee, G. D. (1960). The effect of lysergic acid diethylamide on digit span. *Journal of Clinical and Experimental Psychopathology, 21*, 11–14.

Simonson, E., & Brozek, J. (1952). Flicker fusion frequency background and applications. *Physiological Reviews, 32*, 349–378.

Smiley, A. (1999). Marijuana: On-road and driving-simulator studies. In H. Kalant, W. A. Corrigall, W. Hall, & R. G. Smart (Eds.), *The health effects of cannabis* (pp. 171–194). Toronto: Centre for Addiction and Mental Health.

Smith, G. M., Semke, C. W., & Beecher, H. K. (1962). Objective evidence of mental effects of heroin, morphine and placebo in normal subjects. *The Journal of Pharmacology and Experimental Therapeutics, 136*, 53–58.

Soderlund, H., Parker, E. S., Schwartz, B. L., & Tulving, E. (2005). Memory encoding and retrieval on the ascending and descending limbs of the blood alcohol concentration curve. *Psychopharmacology, 182*, 305–317.

Solowij, N., Stephens, R. S., Roffman, R. A., Kadden, T., Miller, R., Christiansen, M., et al. (2002). Cognitive functioning of long-term heavy cannabis users seeking treatment. *Journal of American Medical Association, 287*, 1123–1131.

Sternberg, S. (1969). The discovery of processing stages: Extensions of Donder's method. *ACTA Psychologica, 30*, 276–315.

Stroop, J. R (1935). Studies of interference in serial verbal reactions. *Journal of Experimental Psychology, 18*, 643–662.

Teichner, G., Horner, M. D., & Harvey, R. T. (2001). Neuropsychological predictors of the attainment of treatment objectives in substance abuse patients. *International Journal of Neuroscience, 106*, 253–263.

Teichner, G., Horner, M. D., Roitzsch, J. C., Herron, J., & Thevos, A. (2002). Substance abuse treatment outcomes for cognitively impaired and intact outpatients. *Addictive Behaviors, 27*, 751–763.

Thapar, P., Zacny, J. P., Choi, M., & Apfelbaum, J. L. (1995a). Objective and subjective impairment from often-used sedative/analgesic combinations in ambulatory surgery, using alcohol as a benchmark. *Anesthesia and Analgesia, 80*, 1092–1098.

Thapar, P., Zacny, J. P., Thompson, W., & Apfelbaum, J. L. (1995b). Using alcohol as a standard to assess the degree of impairment induced by sedative and analgesic drugs used in ambulatory surgery. *Anesthesiology, 82*, 53–59.

Tiplady, B., Drummond, G. B., Cameron, E., Gray, E., Hendry, J., Sinclair, W., et al. (2001). Ethanol, errors, and the speed-accuracy trade-off. *Pharmacology, Biochemistry, and Behavior, 69*, 635–641.

Tiplady, B., Franklin, N., & Scholey, A. (2004). Effect of ethanol on judgments of performance. *British Journal of Psychology, 95*, 105–118.

Verdejo-Garcia, A., & Perez-Garcia, M. (2007). Profile of executive deficits in cocaine and heroin polysubstance users: Common and differential effects on separate executive components. *Psychopharmacology, 190*, 517–530.

Vermeeren, A., Riedel, W. J., van Boxtel, M. P., Darwish, M., Paty, I., & Patat, A. (2002). Differential residual effects of zaleplon and zopiclone on actual driving: A comparison with a low dose of alcohol. *Sleep, 25*, 224–231.

Verster, J. C., Volkerts, E. R., & Verbaten, M. N. (2002). Effects of alprazolam on driving ability, memory functioning and psychomotor performance: A randomized, placebo-controlled study. *Neuropsychopharmacology: Official publication of the American College of Neuropsychopharmacology, 27*, 260–269.

Veselis, R. A., Reinsel, R. A., Feshchenko, V. A., & Wronski, M. (1997). The comparative amnestic effects of midazolam, propofol, thiopental, and fentanyl at equisedative concentrations. *Anesthesiology, 87,* 749–764.

Wechsler, D. (1981). *Manual for the Wechsler adult intelligence scale, revised.* New York: Psychological Corporation.

Weingartner, H. J., Hommer, D., Lister, R. G., Thompson, K., & Wolkowitz, O. (1992). Selective effects of triazolam on memory. *Psychopharmacology, 106,* 341–345.

Wendt, P. E., & Risberg, J. (2001). Ethanol reduces rCFB activation of left dorsolateral prefrontal cortex during a verbal fluency task. *Brain and Language, 77,* 197–215.

Wesnes, K., & Warburton, D. M. (1983). Effects of smoking on rapid information processing performance. *Neuropsychobiology, 9,* 223–229.

Whitlow, C. T., Liguori, A., Livengood, L. B., Hart, S. L., Mussat-Whitlow, B. J., Lamborn, C. M., et al. (2004). Long-term heavy marijuana users make costly decisions on a gambling task. *Drug and Alcohol Dependence, 76,* 107–111.

Yap, M., Mascord, D. J., Starmer, G. A., & Whitfield, J. B. (1993). Studies on the chronopharmacology of ethanol. *Alcohol and Alcoholism, 28,* 17–24.

Zacny, J. P. (1995). A review of the effects of opioids on psychomotor and cognitive functioning in humans. *Experimental and Clinical Psychopharmacology, 3,* 432–466.

Zacny, J. P. (2003). Characterizing the subjective, psychomotor, and physiological effects of a hydrocodone combination product (hycodan) in non-drug-abusing volunteers. *Psychopharmacology, 165,* 146–156.

Zacny, J. P., Conley, K., & Galinkin, J. (1997). Comparing the subjective, psychomotor and physiological effects of intravenous buprenorphine and morphine in healthy volunteers. *The Journal of Pharmacology and Experimental Therapeutics, 282,* 1187–1197.

Zacny, J. P., & Gutierrez, S. (2003). Characterizing the subjective, psychomotor, and physiological effects of oral oxycodone in non-drug-abusing volunteers. *Psychopharmacology, 170,* 242–254.

Zacny, J. P., Hill, J. L., Black, M. L., & Sadeghi, P. (1998). Comparing the subjective, psychomotor and physiological effects of intravenous pentazocine and morphine in normal volunteers. *The Journal of Pharmacology and Experimental Therapeutics, 286,* 1197–1207.

Zacny, J. P., Lichtor, J. L., Binstock, W., Coalson, D. W., Cutter, T., Flemming, D. C., et al. (1993). Subjective, behavioral and physiological responses to intravenous meperidine in healthy volunteers. *Psychopharmacology, 111,* 306–314.

Zacny, J. P., Lichtor, J. L., Flemming, D., Coalson, D. W., & Thompson, W. K. (1994). A dose-response analysis of the subjective, psychomotor and physiological effects of intravenous morphine in healthy volunteers. *The Journal of Pharmacology and Experimental Therapeutics, 268,* 1–9.

Zacny, J. P., Lichtor, J. L., Klafta, J. M., Alessi, R., & Apfelbaum, J. L. (1996). The effects of transnasal butorphanol on mood and psychomotor functioning in healthy volunteers. *Anesthesia and Analgesia, 82,* 931–935.

4

Tolerance, Sensitization, and Physical Dependence

Richard M. Allen

University of Colorado Denver

Contents

Operational Definitions

Tolerance is operationally defined as a *decrease* in the effectiveness of a drug given previous exposure to the drug. As a result, higher doses of the drug are required to produce a particular behavioral or physiological effect and previously effective doses lose some of their effectiveness. When the ability of a range of doses of a drug to produce a particular effect is measured, both before and after some exposure regimen, tolerance can be revealed by a shift to the right in the dose-effect function (i.e., the drug becomes less potent). Conversely, *sensitization* is operationally defined as an increase in the effectiveness of a drug given previous exposure to the drug. Thus, the effects of a particular dose of a drug become larger, and now lower doses of the drug may be sufficient to produce the target behavioral or physiological effect. When the ability of a range of doses of a drug to produce a particular effect is measured, sensitization can be revealed as a shift to the left in the dose-effect function (i.e., the drug becomes more potent). So, tolerance and sensitization are phenomena most often revealed by a change in drug potency that is attributable to previous exposure to the drug.

Physical dependence is a different animal. It shares with tolerance and sensitization the fact that it is a consequence of previous exposure to a drug. However, unlike tolerance and sensitization, it is not revealed by a change in the potency of a drug to produce a particular behavioral or physiological effect. Instead, physical dependence is said to have developed when, after exposure to a substance, removal of that substance from the body or abrupt termination of its pharmacological action reveals compensatory responses. The constellation of effects that emerge in a physically dependent person during drug abstinence or abrupt termination of the drug's action in the body is called a withdrawal syndrome. Thus, whereas drug effects develop tolerance and/or sensitization, measured in the presence of the drug, individuals develop physical dependence revealed by a withdrawal syndrome measured in the drug's absence.

Although tolerance, sensitization, and physical dependence have all been observed in humans, both anecdotally and in experimental and clinical situations, the use of animal models has been invaluable in establishing the principles and mechanisms by which tolerance, sensitization, and physical dependence develop. Indeed, such studies require careful control of individual differences in biology and drug history, and maintenance in a facility where drug can be repeatedly administered over days, weeks, or sometimes months. Much of our understanding of the neurobiological mechanisms that underlie these phenomena come from studies that require extracting central nervous system tissue. In experiments with animals, the behaviors measured are sometimes relatively simple (e.g., cocaine-induced locomotor activation, morphine-induced analgesia) and/or the drugs used may differ from those most commonly abused (e.g., morphine rather than heroin). This chapter describes the results of careful parametric experiments using animal subjects but also discusses the evidence from anecdote or empirical investigation in humans that often confirms or extends these findings.

Tolerance

Acute Tolerance and Chronic Tolerance

Both anecdote and experimental evidence reveal that tolerance to the effects of a drug can develop soon after a single drug administration, a phenomenon known as *acute tolerance* or *within-session* tolerance to distinguish it from the tolerance that develops across multiple drug exposures (i.e., *chronic* or *between-session* tolerance, discussed below). Because these studies typically require only one or two drug exposure(s), there are several clear examples of acute tolerance developing in human research participants.

One way acute tolerance is revealed is by comparing the effectiveness of a single administration of drug at a similar blood plasma concentration as concentration rises (during drug absorption) and falls (due to drug metabolism and elimination). Blood plasma concentrations are measured relatively easily in human research participants at various time points after drug administration, and these blood plasma levels can be compared with the behavioral and physiological effects produced by the drug at the various time points. In one such study with human participants, plasma cocaine concentration peaked approximately 18 minutes after participants smoked or were given an intravenous infusion of cocaine (Foltin & Fischman, 1991). Cocaine plasma concentration was of similar magnitude (i.e., lower than peak) at both 4 and 44 minutes postadministration (i.e., during the rising and falling phase of blood plasma concentration). Although plasma levels of cocaine were similar at these two time points, cocaine-elicited cardiovascular effects (increased heart rate and blood pressure) and some subjective effects (feeling "stimulated" and "high") were lower when measured 44 minutes (compared with 4 minutes) after administration; indeed, these subjective and physiological effects of cocaine had returned to near baseline levels by 44 minutes postadministration despite the significant measurable plasma cocaine levels at this time point. This specific form of acute tolerance is also called *tachyphylaxis*.

Another way to reveal acute tolerance is to administer a second dosing of a drug before the first dose has been completely eliminated, and compare the magnitude of effect produced by the first and second administration. Because the first dose of drug has not yet been completely eliminated, blood plasma levels measured after administration of the second dose will reach higher levels than after the first administration. Within the effective dose range, higher blood plasma concentrations of a drug are typically associated with larger behavioral effects, until plateau is reached at the maximum possible effect. However, Foltin and Haney (2004) demonstrated that increases in human participants' ratings of "positive drug effect", heart rate, and blood pressure produced by a first intranasal dose of cocaine were not produced by the same dose administered again 40 min later, even though the second administration nearly doubled participants' cocaine plasma concentrations.

Both acute (within-session) and chronic (between-session) tolerance can be measured in the same individual, suggesting that, under some conditions, these phenomena are controlled by distinct mechanisms. For example, Perkins et al. (1994) measured the effects of two administrations of nicotine during each experimental session in both nonsmokers and smokers. In both groups, some effects of the second dose of nicotine were lower than the first administration (acute tolerance). In this and similar studies, smaller behavioral and physiological effects were measured in smokers compared with the nonsmoker controls, and this was interpreted as evidence of chronic tolerance in smokers (Perkins et al., 1993, 1994). Although pre-existing differences in nicotine responsiveness between people who become smokers and nonsmokers cannot be ruled out, the experimental evidence from animal studies is clear that chronic nicotine exposure can produce tolerance to some effects of the drug. For example, mice that received 12 days of thrice-daily nicotine injections showed reduced nicotine effects on four behavioral and physiological measures relative to nicotine-naïve mice (Pauly, Grun, & Collins, 1992).

Tolerance Magnitude Increases with Level of Exposure

Just as the acute behavioral and physiological effects produced by a drug are dose-dependent, so too is the development of tolerance to those effects. In general, higher doses and/or more administrations, either in frequency or overall length of treatment, tend to lead to greater degrees of tolerance in both animals and humans.

Dose

The role of maintenance dose in the magnitude of tolerance has been demonstrated for many behavioral effects of many drugs of abuse, including (but not limited to) alcohol, THC, nicotine, cocaine and the amphetamines, and opiates, and only a couple of examples are discussed here. The effect of dose has been revealed for both acute and chronic tolerance, also. For example, in the Perkins et al. (1994) study discussed above, the second nicotine dose administered was always 20 μg/kg, but the first dose administered varied (0–20 μg/kg); the degree of acute tolerance that developed to nicotine's effects was greater when the first nicotine dose was higher. In the context of chronic tolerance, higher nicotine maintenance doses lead to greater degrees of tolerance; in mice, 200 μg/ml nicotine in drinking water produced greater tolerance to nicotine's analgesic, locomotor depressant, and hypothermic effects than 50 μg/ml in water (Sparks & Pauly, 1999; Grabus et al., 2005), and dose-related development of tolerance has been reported after continuous intravenous infusion of nicotine in mice (Marks, Stitzel, & Collins, 1986).

The relationship between maintenance dose and magnitude of tolerance has been very well characterized in animals administered opioid agonists, such as morphine. Many animal studies show that higher maintenance doses of morphine produce greater degrees of tolerance to morphine's antinociceptive (i.e., pain-relieving) effects. In these studies, the pain-relieving effects of a drug like morphine are measured both before and after some chronic regimen of morphine exposure. When these animals are administered larger doses of morphine, they develop more tolerance (Fernandes, Kluwe, & Coper, 1977, 1982; Mucha et al., 1979). For example, we have shown that dose-response functions for morphine antinociception were shifted approximately 3-, 6-, and 12-fold to the right when rats were administered 20, 40, and 80 mg/kg morphine, respectively, daily for seven days (Allen & Dykstra, 2000a).

A similar relationship was demonstrated for the discriminative stimulus effects of morphine in rats (Young et al., 1990). In the drug discrimination procedure, animals are trained to emit a specific response for a food reward (i.e., lever presses on a particular lever) when injected with a training drug and another response (i.e., lever presses on a second, distinct lever) when injected with saline control. During training, animals become quite good at pressing the drug-appropriate lever to earn their food reward only when they are injected with the training dose of the training drug (typically, > 80% accuracy). It is the internal stimulus effects of the drug (roughly equivalent to the "subjective" effects of the drug) that engenders drug-lever appropriate responding. Tolerance can be induced by introducing a regimen of daily drug administration either during continued training or when training is suspended for the chronic dosing regimen. Tolerance development in this procedure essentially means that higher doses of the training drug were needed after the chronic dosing regimen than were needed before the chronic dosing regimen in order for the animal to identify the drug injection as "training drug like." In a series of elegant and careful parametric analyses, Young et al. (1990) showed that chronic treatment with 3.2 mg/kg/day morphine did not alter the discriminative stimulus effects of morphine in rats. However, daily treatment with 10, 20, and 35.6 mg/kg day morphine produced dose-dependent shifts to the right in the function representing morphine discrimination.

Consistent with the animal literature, maintenance dose is directly related to the magnitude of tolerance that develops to the subjective effects people feel when administered morphine (Schuh, Walsh, Bigelow, Preston, & Stitzer, 1996). In this methodologically demanding study, six opioid-dependent human research participants were admitted to a research facility for nine weeks, during which time they were administered daily doses of morphine. Participants were administered 15 mg/day morphine during weeks 1–3, 30 mg/day during weeks 4 and 5, 60 mg/day during weeks 6 and 7, and 120 mg/day during weeks 8 and 9 (drug administered intramuscularly in four equal doses throughout the day, 7 AM to 10 PM). Thereafter, participants were transitioned to a methadone maintenance program. During weeks 3, 5, 7, and 9 of the study, participants were administered four tests, one each with morphine (30 mg), buprenorphine (6 mg; a low efficacy opioid agonist and a potential agonist maintenance therapy), naloxone (0.3 mg; an opioid receptor antagonist, to precipitate withdrawal), and placebo control, after which physiological (e.g., pupil constriction) and subjective effects (e.g., euphoria) were assessed. In total, each participant was tested 16 times in addition to their daily morphine maintenance. In this carefully controlled experimental study with people, the effect of morphine measured on the test days was reduced more by higher maintenance doses, to the point that the test dose of morphine (30 mg) produced no physiological or subjective effects when participants were maintained on the highest morphine maintenance dose (120 mg/day).

Frequency or Duration of Exposure

In addition to the influence of the chronically administered dose of a drug, under some circumstances tolerance magnitude is directly related to the frequency and/or duration of drug administration. This can be revealed by measuring the progressive decrement in effectiveness of a particular drug dose administered over days. For example, when 10 mg/kg morphine is administered daily to rats, and the effectiveness of that dose of morphine to produce pain relief is measured every other day, a progressive decrease in effectiveness is revealed across the days of the study (e.g., Trujillo & Akil, 1991). Thus, tolerance develops over time, and may reach some plateau for any particular dose of a drug. This can also be revealed by measuring the rightward shift in a drug dose-response curve before and after some chronic drug regimen (i.e., pre- and posttreatment effectiveness). For example, we have shown that chronic administration of 20 mg/kg/day morphine for 7 days shifts the morphine dose-response curve (for the pain relieving effects of morphine) ~3-fold to the right; an additional 7 days results in a total of ~5-fold shift to the right relative to control. This has also been demonstrated for the discriminative stimulus effects of morphine, where more frequent (once versus twice daily; Young et al., 1990) or longer exposure (one to three days; Young, Steigerwald, Makhay, & Kapitsopoulos, 1991) to 10 mg/kg morphine produced greater degrees of tolerance.

Adaptations are not Equal across Drug Effects

One important caveat to these findings is that, given the same chronic dosing regimen, tolerance can develop at different rates to the different behavioral effects produced by a drug. Indeed, under some conditions that produce tolerance to one behavioral effect, little or no tolerance (or even sensitization) may develop to other effects. In one report, Fernandes, Kluwe, and Coper (1977) administered morphine chronically to rats and measured changes in the antinociceptive, hyperthermic, and lethal effects of the drug. Despite an equivalent chronic exposure to morphine, the most tolerance developed to morphine's lethal effects and the least tolerance developed to morphine's hypothermic effects. In other studies with rodents, morphine produces time-dependent locomotor suppressant and stimulating effects, where an initial suppression of locomotor activity is followed by a delayed enhancement of locomotor activity after a single drug administration. Whereas tolerance can develop to the early suppressant effects of morphine, sensitization can develop to the delayed locomotor stimulating effects of morphine (Schnur, 1985).

Adaptations are not Equal across Drugs

There is good evidence that tolerance develops at different rates to drugs within the same pharmacological class. Again, the case can be made with the opioid analgesics. Research with opioids reveals that the amount of tolerance that develops to a particular drug effect (e.g., antinociception) varies with the chronically administered treatment drug (i.e., the toleragen). Thus, repeated treatment with equi-effective doses of the mu-opioid receptor agonists etorphine, morphine, and dezocine produce different degrees of tolerance, with no tolerance developing to the pain-relieving effects of etorphine, some tolerance developing to morphine (i.e., a 2.2-fold shift in the dose-response curve), and the greatest tolerance developing to dezocine (i.e., a 3.4-fold shift in the dose-response curve). However, although no tolerance was revealed when etorphine was both the chronic treatment drug (the toleragen) and the test compound, *cross-tolerance* (see below) was revealed after etorphine treatment when the lower-efficacy opioids morphine and dezocine were tested, suggesting that the etorphine treatment did alter the system in some way (Allen & Dykstra, 2000b).

Cross Tolerance Develops to Drugs with Similar Mechanisms of Action

Another interesting finding is that tolerance produced by repeated administration of one drug in a chemical class may confer tolerance to other chemicals in that class. This phenomenon is known as cross-tolerance. Again, this has been elegantly demonstrated for the opioid analgesics. In opioid cross-tolerance studies, the chronic opioid treatment is the same (e.g., 10 mg/kg morphine twice daily for seven days), but the effectiveness of a different drug is measured before and after the chronic drug treatment (e.g., the effects of the opioid agonist burprenorphine are measured before and after chronic morphine treatment). Studies with opioid agonists have repeatedly demonstrated that the magnitude of cross-tolerance conferred to test agonists differs, and is related to the intrinsic efficacy of the test agonist. In general, high-efficacy agonists (i.e., drugs that are very "efficient" when bound) show less cross-tolerance than low-efficacy agonists (i.e., drugs that are less "efficient" when bound) given a common chronic drug treatment (Allen & Dykstra, 2000b; Barrett, Cook, Terner, Craft, & Picker, 2001; Paronis & Holtzman, 1992; Walker & Young, 2001).

Some Mechanisms for Tolerance

There is an enormous literature describing potential mechanisms for the development of tolerance to the behavioral and physiological effects of psychoactive drugs. The specific mechanisms can vary across drug classes and even across effects for a particular drug. It appears that nervous systems adapt in many ways to drug exposure. Even for a specific drug effect, multiple neurobiological and behavioral mechanisms may mediate the development of tolerance. Thus, there is not a single mechanism that describes how the tolerance develops. This section presents some of the ways in which these adaptations are typically categorized, and describes some examples of each.

Livers Adapt

Tolerance is operationally defined as a decrease in drug effectiveness given previous drug exposure. Many of these adaptations involve a decrease in the effectiveness of the drug at its site of action in the central nervous system, either directly at the drug's receptor or at a cellular or systems level. However, one adaptation that can contribute to a decrease in drug effectiveness does not involve the central nervous system. Any change in the body that alters how much of a drug dose gets to its site of action is an example of pharmacokinetic tolerance. One example of this is *dispositional* or *metabolic tolerance,* which describes the condition whereby the metabolic activity of hepatic (liver) enzymes is up-regulated such that these enzymes now metabolize a drug at a faster rate. Thus, when the same dose of a drug is taken again, less of it is available to the central nervous system and the drug appears less effective, whether or not the effectiveness of the drug to interact with the central nervous system has changed. For example, up-regulation of the liver enzyme CYP2E1 can be induced by both ethanol and nicotine in rats (Howard, Micu, Sellers, & Tyndale, 2001). Such a mechanism could contribute to the doubling in the rate of alcohol metabolism observed in heavy drinkers (Lieber, 1994), and may contribute to the cross-tolerance observed between ethanol and nicotine, drugs with distinct primary mechanisms of action, under some circumstances (Collins, Wilkins, Slobe, Cao, & Bullock, 1996).

Neurons Adapt

When presented with psychoactive drugs, neurons show both immediate biological responses and can show different kinds of adaptations in the face of these drug interactions. Some of these adaptations appear to underlie drug tolerance; that is, the adaptation creates a situation where the drug's action on the neuron is diminished, and the subsequent cellular, systems-level, and behavioral or physiological responses that result from drug stimulation are reduced. This form of tolerance is often called *pharmacodynamic, cellular,* or *cellular-adaptive* tolerance to distinguish it from the tolerance that develops when a drug is metabolized at a faster rate (i.e., *pharmacokinetic or dispositional* tolerance) or that may be the result of learning (i.e., *conditioned* and *behavioral* tolerance, see below). In these latter cases, there may be no change in the ability of the drug to produce effects at its primary mechanism of action (i.e., no *pharmacokinetic* or *pharmacodynamic* tolerance) and this can be revealed under appropriate testing conditions.

Perhaps the most intuitive pharmacodynamic mechanism for tolerance, there is considerable evidence that the proteins that comprise the primary pharmacological sites of action for psychoactive drugs (e.g., pre- and postsynaptic neurotransmitter receptors, transporter proteins) can themselves adapt to the presence of a drug such that the drug becomes less effective at producing changes at the level of the receptor. This itself can occur in a number of ways, including alterations in receptor number expressed on the cell surface (i.e., up- or down-regulation of receptor number) or changes in the sensitivity of the receptor to drug stimulation (e.g., receptor sensitization or desensitization). For example, some receptors can rapidly desensitize and be removed from the neural cell surface (i.e., internalized for possible subsequent down-regulation) when stimulated with an agonist drug. For postsynaptic receptors, a decrease in the number of functional receptors available at the cell surface can lead to a decrease in the effectiveness of a given dose of drug. Furthermore, receptors can change in subunit composition, their interaction with other receptor types as heterodimers, or their functional connectivity to intracellular mechanisms in a manner that reduces the impact of activation. In this case, a drug may find a similar number of receptors available, but fewer of them will be functional. Chronic treatment with μ-opioid agonists such as morphine has been shown to produce such alterations in receptor number (Díaz et al., 1995; Yoburn, Billings, & Duttaroy, 1993), alterations in the functional state of the receptor (Sadée & Wang, 1995), and changes in the ratio of opioid receptor binding to inhibitory and stimulatory G-proteins (Wu et al., 1998). All of these phenomena may play some role in the reduced potency of opioid agonists to produce behavioral effects under some conditions.

The development of pharmacodynamic or cellular tolerance has also been revealed in effects further "downstream" from a drug's primary mechanisms of action and the most immediate intracellular consequences of those actions. One ultimate effect of a drug's interaction with a neurotransmitter receptor is to alter the firing rate of the neuron upon which that receptor is located. This in turn leads to increases or decreases in neurotransmitter release from those neurons, and tolerance (and sensitization) can develop to these effects. For example, morphine causes an increase in the neurotransmitter dopamine measured in the nucleus accumbens of rats. Repeated treatment with morphine can result in tolerance to this effect; that is, morphine produces less increase in nucleus accumbens dopamine. However, this effect may vary with time. Whereas tolerance to effects on dopamine release were observed early in withdrawal (within a day or two), morphine produced increases in dopamine release that were greater than control (i.e., led to sensitization of nucleus accumbens dopamine release) when the withdrawal period was longer (i.e., three to seven days withdrawal; Acquas & Di Chiara, 1992).

Organisms Learn

...About the Environment in which they Experience Drug Effects   Learning mechanisms can also explain the development of tolerance under some conditions. In now classic studies by Siegel (1975), rats were administered opiates (e.g., morphine or heroin) by daily injection, and the effectiveness of the drug was assessed either in the same environment where the daily injections were administered or in a novel environment. When tested in an environment in which the animals regularly experienced the drug effects, a profound degree of tolerance was revealed to the antinociceptive effects. Moreover, the effectiveness of the opiate was restored simply by testing these rats in a novel environment, suggesting that the development of tolerance was dependent on environmental conditions and little if any pharmacodynamic tolerance developed to the opiate.

Among the most striking examples of this form of tolerance came from studies in which the lethal effects of high doses of heroin were assessed in groups of rats that had been administered heroin in the same or a different environment as the final test dose (Siegel, Hinson, Krank, & McCully, 1982). This high dose was lethal in 64% of the rats that received the high dose in a different environment from the one in which they received their daily heroin injections. However, despite receiving equivalent amounts of heroin during the chronic dosing procedure (and thus, presumably, developing similar amounts of pharmacodynamic tolerance), this same high dose of heroin was lethal in only 32% of rats that received the test dose in the same environment in which they received their daily heroin injections. Just as with conditioned tolerance to the analgesic effects, greater tolerance was revealed when the test dose was administered in the same environment as the daily dose and more lethality was observed when the high test dose was administered in a novel environment. It is possible that some instances of overdose death in experienced users of heroin may be due to a similar mechanism.

...To Compensate for the Effects of Drugs on Behavior   A final form of drug tolerance involves learning to compensate for the (typically suppressing or deleterious) effects of a drug on ongoing behavior. For example, a person may learn to maintain balance or perform a task while intoxicated. As with conditioned tolerance, this can occur independently of or with a greater magnitude than the development of functional tolerance given the same drug treatment. Thus, the opportunity to perform a behavior under the influence of a drug (i.e., "intoxicated practice") may result in motor behaviors that compensate for the drug effect. Experimentally, such "behavioral tolerance" or "contingent tolerance" can be revealed by administering drug treatments, either prior to performance of some target behavior (a pre-exposure group) or after the performance of the behavior (a postexposure group), and comparing the magnitude

of tolerance that develops in the two groups. Because both groups received the same drug treatment, functional tolerance should be of the same magnitude. However, under some conditions, the amount of tolerance that develops in the pre-exposure group (the group that "practices" the behavior under the influence of the drug) is greater than that observed in the postexposure group (e.g., Fowler, Bowen, & Kallman, 1993; Holloway, Michaelis, Harland, Criado, & Gauvin, 1992).

The role of tolerance in drug addiction is discussed in more detail later in the chapter. However, it is important to note that tolerance is its own unique phenomenon and its occurrence may or may not be functionally related to the process of addiction in any given situation. To note, a person receiving repeated treatment with morphine in a medical setting, such as during hospitalization, may develop a degree of tolerance to the pain-relieving effects of morphine and may even develop some degree of physical dependence. However, it is unlikely that such individuals will engage in the compulsive, drug-seeking behavior that is characteristic of drug addiction or would classify them for a substance-related disorder once they leave the facility.

It is clear, however, that individuals who engage in repeated drug-taking behavior can develop tolerance to the effects of those drugs. Indeed, the most striking examples occur with alcohol and other sedative hypnotics, such as the benzodiazepines (e.g., Valium or diazepam, Xanax or alprazolam), the opiates (e.g., heroin and morphine), but also with drugs such as nicotine, cocaine, and methamphetamine. Studies conducted in the Netherlands in which heroin is prescribed to individuals as a maintenance therapy reveal that participant/patients in these trials administered individual doses of heroin intravenously that ranged from 66 to 450 mg (Rook, Huitema, van den Brink, van Ree, & Beijnen, 2006). Considering that the analgesic dose of heroin is approximately 1 mg or less, this represents an extraordinary degree of tolerance. Indeed, these doses would be lethal to drug-naïve individuals or even people with a limited drug-taking history (i.e., "recreational users").

Sensitization

Sensitization can be considered the opposite of tolerance, in that the effect of a drug becomes larger with repeated exposure. Many of the same principles that describe tolerance development also apply to sensitization. For example, the development of sensitization is dose-dependent, sensitization develops to some (but not all) effects of a drug given repeated exposure, and cross-sensitization is conferred to drugs with similar mechanisms of action. Under some conditions, sensitization may be mediated by mechanisms converse to those that underlie tolerance (e.g., receptor up-regulation) and in other cases may involve similar basic mechanisms (e.g., NMDA receptor activation). Just as is the case with tolerance, there is no single mechanism thought to underlie sensitization development, even for a specific drug and drug effect. Thus, this section covers some mechanisms for some effects of some drugs, noting that there are many ways that organisms adapt to repeated drug exposure. Although there are many similarities between tolerance and sensitization, there are some findings unique to, or at least more commonly studied with, sensitization and so, to avoid duplication, more focus is paid here to those findings.

Rate of Drug Administration and the Development of Sensitization

Several recent studies demonstrate that the rate at which a single drug dose is administered can affect the development of behavioral sensitization. Some recent studies show that psycho-motor sensitization, inhibition of dopamine uptake, and expression of immediate early genes in the corticomesolimbic system are greater with more rapid experimenter-administered IV cocaine infusions (e.g., 5 vs. 25 sec: Samaha, Li, & Robinson, 2002). When rats self-administer cocaine, rapid infusion rates are more likely to lead to sensitization to cocaine's reinforcing effects, although rapid infusion rates are not required for cocaine to function as a reinforcer (Liu, Roberts, & Morgan, 2005). These authors have argued that both the acute reinforcing effects of cocaine and the development of cocaine sensitization are factors that contribute to addiction and that both should be incorporated into models that study this process.

Evidence for Sensitization in Humans

Sensitization to the effects of drugs of abuse is most often studied by measuring increases in the locomotor stimulating effects of drugs in rodents (i.e., locomotor sensitization), a mea-sure that is not practical to measure in human research participants. There is considerable debate about the development of sensitization in humans (Bradberry, 2007) and its role in drug-taking behavior (Zernig et al., 2007), however, some researchers have demonstrated this phenomenon. Boileau et al. (2006) demonstrated sensitization to some, but not all effects of amphetamine measured in human subjects. In this study, men were administered three oral doses of amphetamine, once every other day, and then again 14 days (dose 4) and approximately one year later (dose 5), all during PET imaging sessions with the dopamine D_2/D_3 receptor agonist, raclopride (dose 1, 4, and 5), or a sham PET imaging session during which raclopride was not administered (dose 2 and 3). Compared with the first amphetamine administration, subjects showed an increase in eye blinking rate and reported greater alertness, energy, clear-headedness, and positive mood when readministered amphetamine up to 14 days withdrawal (i.e., dose 4); only the increase in energy was significantly greater after 1 year withdrawal (dose 5). A concomitant decrease in raclopride binding (suggesting an increase in the release of brain dopamine) was also measured. In contrast, there were no observed changes in heart rate or on measures of euphoria, high, rush, anxiety, or drug-wanting across the experiment. Sensitization may also develop to psychotomimetic effects of stimulants (Bartlett, Hallin, Chapman, & Angrist, 1997).

Sensitization may occur only in the earliest phases of drug taking, making it difficult to measure in human research participants who typically present after an extended history of drug taking. However, in addition to the above and other positive findings of sensitization in humans (Strakowski, Sax, Setters, & Keck, Jr., 1996), some authors report no obvious sensi-tization in human participants (Rothman et al., 1994) including stimulant-naïve participants (Wachtel & deWit, 1999). Alternatively, sensitization may play a role in behaviors that are typically difficult to measure empirically in human subjects, such as the "work" an individual is willing to do to procure and use their drug of abuse.

Another reason sensitization may be difficult to assess in humans is that human users typically increase their consumption over time. Although there are theories that attribute this escalation in part to a process that involves sensitization (e.g., incentive sensitization), some have argued that repeated high-dose drug exposure is more likely to lead to tolerance. Thus, increasing the frequency and amount of drug consumption might begin to engender more and more tolerance to effects that contribute to escalation and the early facilitation of drug taking due to sensitization of some drug effects is masked and inhibited.

Physical Dependence

The appearance of withdrawal symptoms upon discontinuation of a daily drug regimen is not limited to drugs of abuse. Indeed, withdrawal symptoms have been reported by some users upon discontinuation of several psychotropic medications with no apparent abuse liability (e.g., the SSRIs fluoxetine, flovoxamine, paroxetine, and sertraline; Price, Waller, Wood, & MacKay, 1996). However, under these conditions, these "withdrawal reactions" are typically less "intense" and reported in only a small portion of the drug-taking population. The basic principles that describe the likelihood and extent to which physical dependence will develop are discussed here. It is worth repeating that whereas tolerance and sensitization are phenomena that develop to drug effects, individuals develop physical dependence, revealed by a clear withdrawal syndrome upon discontinuation of drug use. In research studies, administration of a pharmacological "antagonist" to the treatment compound can immediately precipitate a withdrawal syndrome in dependent individuals.

Withdrawal Effects are Typically Opposite the Direct Effects of a Drug

Opiates such as heroin produce a range of physiological, subjective, and behavioral effects, including (but not limited to) pupil constriction, respiratory suppression, decreased body temperature (hypothermia), constipation, analgesia, and feelings of well-being or euphoria. The withdrawal syndrome that emerges upon drug abstinence in a dependent individual consists of a host of responses typically opposite to the direct effects of the drug, including (but again, not limited to) pupil dilation; increased respiration (panting/yawning); increased body temperature (hyperthermia); diarrhea; aching pain, and an increased sensitivity to painful stimuli (hyperalgesia); and dysphoria and other depressive symptoms. Thus, the withdrawal syndromes associated with different drugs of abuse differ from one another, and are typically characterized by effects opposite those produced by the drug of abuse.

Although the withdrawal syndrome is uncomfortable for many drugs, the withdrawal symptoms themselves appear to be life threatening only for alcohol and some CNS depressants. In either case, drugs within similar neurobiological/pharmacological mechanisms of action confer cross-dependence to one another just as cross-tolerance or cross-sensitization is observed to the direct effects of a drug. This cross-dependence provides the opportunity to transfer an individual to a compound similar to the drug of abuse (e.g., a benzodiazepine in place of alcohol, methadone in place of heroin) in order to begin the process of detoxification. Thus, administration of the medicinal compound prevents withdrawal, and dose can be tapered in an effort to reduce the unpleasantness (and, with alcohol, potential lethality) associated with abstinence. In the case of methadone, drug dose may not be tapered but rather increased to a dose that is effective at preventing illicit drug administration. In this case, methadone maintains opioid physical dependence throughout extended treatment.

A Drug's Half-Life Predicts the Onset and Duration of Acute Withdrawal Syndrome

In general, the appearance of a withdrawal syndrome is related to the half-life of the maintenance drug. Thus, withdrawal from heroin with a plasma half-life approximately < 1 hour will begin to appear within 8–12 hours and become severe within 2 days. In contrast, methadone-maintained patients are consuming a drug with a plasma half-life on the order of 15–40 hours, and typically readminister their medication once daily. Withdrawal effects generally do not appear during this time, consistent with methadone's longer duration of action and elimination rate. More recently approved maintenance medications, such as the opioid agonists LAAM and burprenorphine have even longer half-lives and may contribute to better compliance and easier management.

The long half-life of a drug and relatively mild withdrawal symptoms (i.e., relative to high-maintenance dose heroin withdrawal) could contribute to the notion that physical dependence is uncommon even with regular use of some psychoactive substances. A good case is point in marijuana (delta-9-THC) consumption in humans. Both delta-9-THC and some of its active metabolites have a very long half-life (up to 50 hours for some active metabolites). Given normal variations in rates of metabolism, it is can be methodologically difficult to assess a naturally occurring withdrawal syndrome, even in animal experiments. However, a withdrawal syndrome is demonstrated when compensatory responses are revealed in the absence of the pharmacological action of the maintenance drug. This can occur naturally, during abstinence and the half-life time-dependent clearance of the drug from the body, or it can be precipitated by administration of a pharmacological antagonist. Precipitated withdrawal following chronic THC exposure was first demonstrated in rats (Aceto, Scates, Lowe, & Martin, 1995; Tsou, Patrick, & Walker, 1995). Rats were administered THC via injection for 4 days. Subsequently, rats were injected with the cannabinoid receptor antagonist, SR141716A (Rimonabant), and behavioral changes noted. Within 10 minutes of the injection, animals displayed wet-dog shakes and facial rubbing, two classic signs of withdrawal in rodents, and, to a lesser extent, head shakes, biting, drooping eyelids, retropulsion (backing away), ear twitching, chewing, licking, and arching the back. In humans, increased anxiety and irritability, decreased food consumption, and difficulty sleeping are common effects measured in heavy users of marijuana upon abstinence (Haney, Ward, Comer, Foltin, & Fischman, 1999; Hart, Haney, Ward, Fischman, & Foltin, 2002). The emergence of these effects is time-dependent, typically beginning within a day or two after abstinence. The cannabis withdrawal syndrome has recently been reviewed by Budney and Hughes (1995).

Dose Exposure can Predict the Severity of Withdrawal Symptoms for a Particular Drug

As with tolerance and sensitization, higher maintenance doses can lead to more severe withdrawal symptoms. That said, acute dependence (i.e., dependence developing after a single drug administration) can occur. For example, June, Stitzer, and Cone (1995) revealed opiate withdrawal effects precipitated by an injection of nalxone at various time points (1–36 hours) after administration of a single dose of heroin (18 mg/70 kg, intramuscularly) to nondependent human participants. In rats administered chronic morphine and left to experience natural withdrawal through discontinuation of treatment, the magnitude of abstinence-induced weight loss was directly related to the amount of morphine upon which rats were chronically maintained (Yoburn, Chen, Huang, & Inturrisi, 1985). Similarly, in the Schuh et al. (1996) study discussed above (see Tolerance section), greater withdrawal effects were precipitated by naloxone during weeks in which the morphine maintenance dose was higher.

Glutamate and Drug Tolerance, Sensitization, and Physical Dependence

The neurotransmitter glutamate is one of the most ubiquitous neurotransmitters in the central nervous system. Among its many roles in central nervous system processes, glutamate has been shown to be involved in learning and neuroplasticity, and appears to play a critical role in the neural and behavioral adaptations related to drug tolerance, sensitization, and physical dependence. The N-methyl-D-aspartate (NMDA) subtype of the glutamate receptor plays a particularly important role in these adaptations. NMDA receptor antagonists have been shown to prevent the development of drug tolerance, sensitization, and/or the appearance of withdrawal symptoms that typically develop after repeated exposure to numerous psychoactive drugs, including opioids, major stimulants (e.g., cocaine, amphetamines), nicotine, cannabinoids (e.g., THC), and even alcohol which, interestingly, also possesses NMDA antagonist properties. Thus, even though there are many different types of neurobiological adaptations reported for the different behavioral and physiological effects produced by psychoactive drugs across drug classes, scores of studies now present data that suggest that activation of glutamatergic systems is a common adapation that underlies the change in these situations. This may in part be due to the near ubiquitous nature of glutatmate in the central nervous system, versus the relatively more restricted localization of other neurotransmitter systems.

A role for glutamate in drug tolerance is revealed in studies in which glutamate activity through the NMDA subtype of glutamate receptor is blocked by repeated or continuous treatment with an NMDA receptor antagonist during the chronic drug treatment. For example, noncompetitive NMDA receptor antagonists (Elliott, Hynanski, & Inturrisi, 1994; Trujillo & Akil, 1991), competitive NMDA receptor antagonists (Tiseo & Inturrisi 1993; Allen & Dykstra, 1999), and many other functional classes of NMDA receptor antagonist all prevent the development of tolerance to morphine's antinociceptive effects when coadministered with the drug during chronic treatment. NMDA receptor antagonists also prevent the development of tolerance to the discriminative stimulus effects of morphine (Bespalov, Balster, & Beardsley, 1999), some signs of opioid physical dependence (Trujillo & Akil, 1991), and motivational aspects of withdrawal (Medvedev, Dravolina, & Bespalov, 1998; Popik & Danysz, 1997). Worth noting are data that show both tolerance and sensitization develop to time-related locomotor effects of morphine: NMDA receptor antagonists prevent both of these behavioral adaptations (Trujillo, 2000).

Similarly, glutamate antagonists can block both the behavioral sensitization and neurochemical consequences of repeated cocaine administration in animal models. Again, the findings and caveats described in this literature have been thoroughly reviewed (e.g., Wolf, 1998; Vanderschuren & Kalivas, 2000); such a review is not reproduced here. However, it is important to highlight several key findings from this long and elegant line of research. Behavioral sensitization does not develop to a repeated cocaine regimen if rats are coadministered a glutamate antagonist along with each cocaine injection (e.g., Karler, Calder, Chaudhry, & Turkanis, 1989). Glutamate antagonists also prevent several neurobiological changes that accompany behavioral sensitization in these experiments, such as dopamine autoreceptor subsensitivity in the VTA, dopamine D1 receptor supersensitivity in the nucleus accumbens, and increases in tyrosine hydroxylase activity in the VTA (Li et al., 1999; Masserano, Baker, Natsukari, & Wyatt, 1996).

There are many other documented interactions between cocaine administration and glutamate function. Microdialysis studies show that single, experimenter-administered injections of cocaine elicit dose-dependent elevations in glutamate brain areas such as the prefrontal cortex (PFC), nucleus accumbens, and VTA of rats (e.g., Kalivas & Duffy, 1998). The elevation of glutamate elicited by cocaine is augmented (i.e., sensitized) in rats that receive repeated, experimenter-administered injections of cocaine, and this neurobiological adaptation is associated with the development of behavioral (locomotor) sensitization. Electrophysiological recordings of VTA neurons from rats that received repeated experimenter-administered injections of cocaine show a robust but transient increased responsiveness to locally administered glutamate (White, Hu, Zhang, & Wolf, 1995).

Glutamatergic mechanisms of learning and memory have been described in the experimental literature for quite some time. The basic finding that blockading glutamate function could prevent some forms of drug sensitization (and tolerance and physical dependence) suggested that the drug-related adaptations might also involve the same basic cellular mechanism thought to underlie learning and memory, namely long-term potentiation (LTP). There is some experimental evidence for this, but the story is not conclusive. For example, experimenter-administered injections of cocaine induce LTP in the corticomesolimbic system. Neurons in the nucleus accumbens and midbrain undergo NMDA-dependent and independent forms of LTP and long-term depression (LTD) in response to standard electrical stimulation (Bonci & Malenka, 1999; Pennartz, Ameerun, Groenewegen, & Lopes da Silva, 1993). Evidence for the formation of LTP in the nucleus accumbens and VTA following a single in vivo injection of cocaine has also been published, and this plasticity is blocked by coadministration of an NMDA receptor antagonist (Ungless, Whistler, Malenka, & Bonci, 2001). However, data from one study revealed that whereas behavioral sensitization developed over several exposures to cocaine, the synaptic modifications induced by repeated exposure to cocaine were no greater than those produced by a single injection of cocaine (Borgland, Malenka, & Bonci, 2004).

Role of Tolerance, Sensitization, and Withdrawal in Drug Addiction

Drug addiction has been defined as a chronic disorder characterized by compulsive use of a substance resulting in physical, psychological, or social harm to the user and continued use despite that harm (Rinaldi, Steindler, Wilford, & Goodwin, 1988). The development of drug tolerance, sensitization, and physical dependence are often invoked to explain the increase in the frequency or amount of drug consumed under these conditions (hereafter, "dose escalation"). Although dose escalation may be mediated by these phenomena, dose escalation is not synonymous with any one of them. The purpose of this final section of the chapter is to discuss the ways in which tolerance, sensitization, and physical dependence may play a role in addiction and, particularly, in dose escalation.

Psychoactive drugs elicit various behavioral and physiological effects through their direct actions on signaling proteins. Repeated exposure to a drug can change the effectiveness of the drug to produce these changes in physiology and behavior, through a variety of mechanisms resulting in tolerance and/or sensitization. It is changes in the magnitude of these elicited drug effects to which tolerance and sensitization should be restricted as descriptive constructs. In contrast, people emit behavior to acquire and ingest psychoactive substances. An increase in the frequency or amount of drug consumed does not directly imply tolerance to its effects have developed. Indeed, drug-taking behavior itself is not an elicited response (i.e., a "reflex" resulting from direct stimulation of receptors). Of interest, then, is to what degree tolerance or sensitization to particular drug effects influences the behavioral transition from occasional use of a psychoactive substance to drug dependence. Similarly, in what ways does the development of physical dependence alter drug-taking behavior?

A recent and very thorough review of the experimental and clinical literature on escalation of drug consumption reveals that this is not an easy question to answer. In their review, Zernig et al. (2007) describe six different models currently proposed to underlie escalation of drug consumption. These include (1) tolerance to the apparent reinforcing effects of a drug, (2) sensitization to the apparent reinforcing effects of a drug, (3) reward allostasis, (4) sensitization to the incentive salience of drug associated stimuli, (5) choice (changes in the relative reinforcing effectiveness of the drug versus other nondrug reinforcers, and (6) habit formation. Furthermore these authors describe 17 factors that can contribute to apparent drug reinforcement, all of which should be carefully monitored when assessing changes in apparent drug reinforcement that might lead to escalation of drug consumption. Only some of these theories are presented here.

To assert a role for tolerance in drug addiction, one must first ask to which effects does an individual become tolerant and then determine how those effects may contribute to the drug-taking behavior of the individual. Thus, we return to the idea that tolerance develops to drug effects, to the effects elicited by the action of the drug in the body. In the above example with heroin, it is presumably tolerance to the effects produced by the individual doses (perhaps the subjective effects) that leads to the profound increase in the amount of drug consumed at each administration, but such "escalation" of consumption probably involves other factors as well. For example, such individuals are consuming heroin multiple times each day, and these additional administrations (i.e., more than the once-a-day or lesser frequency that likely characterized initial drug use) account for some of the escalation as well. Zernig et al. (2007) argue that for some drugs, especially those with major or minor stimulant actions such as cocaine and nicotine, a larger portion of dose escalation is accounted for by an increase in the frequency of drug administrations, rather than the dose consumed at each administration. To note, a one or two pack a day smoker is consuming up to 40 cigarettes a day by smoking at more and more times throughout the day, rather than chain smoking every time he or she lights up a cigarette.

Under some conditions, tolerance and "addiction" can be temporally distinguished. For example, Perkins et al. (2001) argue that tolerance and dependence ("addiction") are not linearly related. They note that in their experiments, tolerance to the effects of nicotine appears to have developed at a similar magnitude in both dependent and nondependent smokers, and that tolerance appears to remain in former smokers who have been abstinent for many years. Thus, magnitude of tolerance to these effects was not related to the current amount of cigarette smoking. Tolerance may develop rapidly and early in a smoker's history. These and other nicotine researchers have also argued that tolerance may develop rapidly to the aversive effects of nicotine whereas sensitization may develop to the drug's positive effects. Solid empirical evidence for this idea is needed.

Individuals who consume a drug with some regularity may begin to develop both acute tolerance, which may, together with other behavioral variables, contribute to more frequent drug administration, as well as chronic tolerance, which may, along with other behavioral mechanisms, lead to increases in the amount of drug consumed at each administration. Although such tolerance may be one component of addiction, and may be a mechanism for escalation of consumption, clearly addiction involves other changes as well. For one example, increases in the amount and frequency of drug administration would lead to greater degrees of physical dependence, which could certainly increase motivation to self-administer the drug (see below).

Sensitization and Self-Administration

A role for sensitization in drug addiction continues to gain popularity, although there is considerable debate about the specific role it may play in addiction. Based largely upon preclinical investigations in rodents that are trained to self-administer drugs of abuse, some authors argue that exposure during the initial self-administration of drugs may produce sensitization of effects important for drug reinforcement processes, and this may naturally facilitate the associative learning processes necessary for acquisition of drug self-administration behavior (e.g., Robinson & Berridge, 2000; Schenk & Partridge, 1997), although this idea is somewhat controversial. Interestingly, rats that are exposed to experimenter-administered injections of psychomotor stimulants prior to the start of cocaine self-administration sessions acquire self-administration of cocaine more rapidly and/or achieve higher breakpoints under a PR schedule of cocaine reinforcement (Horger, Giles, & Schenk, 1992; Mendrek, Blaha, & Phillips, 1998; Suto et al., 2002). This may reflect sensitization to the reinforcing effectiveness of cocaine because lower doses of cocaine now support the same behavior (i.e., rate of acquisition, break point) as higher doses under control conditions. Sensitization to the reinforcing effectiveness of cocaine has also been demonstrated in cocaine self-administering rats that are subsequently permitted daily exposure to cocaine under a PR schedule of reinforcement (as evidenced by an "escalation" of break point over time; Morgan, Liu, & Roberts, 2006).

Similarly, sensitization to incentive salience (i.e., incentive sensitization) has been proposed as a mechanism to explain differences in the motivational effects of cocaine and cocaine-paired cues and to explain compulsive drug-seeking behavior in human "addicts" (Robinson & Berridge, 1993, 2000). According to the incentive sensitization theory of addiction, sensitization to the incentive effects of drugs (and environmental stimuli associated with them) occurs as a result of repeated drug taking. These incentive effects, which are proposed to underlie drug wanting (as opposed to liking) grow and grow with repeated drug administrations. This is thought to be one mechanism that can lead to the excessive motivation to readminister drug in the addicted individual. It is important to note that the subjective state produced by the drugs (e.g., drug-elicited euphoria), or the drug *liking* is not thought to undergo sensitization and may in fact develop tolerance. Thus, according to this theory, drug liking develops tolerance and the power of the drug and drug-paired stimuli to motivate behavior (*wanting*) develops sensitization. There is evidence in humans that the subjective effects of a drug diminish with repeated exposure and that, despite this reduction, motivation to readminister increases (e.g., "chasing" the high during a cocaine binge, in which the profound effects of the first dose are not re-experienced with subsequent administrations during the binge).

Physical dependence/withdrawal can serve to evoke drug-seeking behavior, just as a state of food or water deprivation can evoke eating or drinking. Thus, the development of physical dependence (and subsequent experience of withdrawal) could evoke drug-seeking behavior even though physical dependence was not required for the initial development of that behavior. Furthermore, the alleviation of withdrawal symptoms by drug administration in a physically dependent person could provide an additional behavioral mechanism maintaining the reinforcing effects of the drug. There seems to be no question in clinical circles that avoidance of aversive withdrawal effects can be a powerful motivator of drug-taking behavior.

There is some good experimental evidence showing that withdrawal can increase the relative reinforcing effectiveness of drugs of abuse. Using a choice procedure with heroin-dependent rhesus monkeys, Negus (2006) demonstrated that, when experiencing withdrawal, monkeys would begin to select lower doses of heroin over food than they would when not experiencing withdrawal, confirming and extending the findings of others (e.g., Griffiths, Wurster, & Brady, 1975). Opiate-dependent animals will also work harder (i.e., emit more lever presses) to receive heroin injections than their nondependent counterparts under some conditions. (Carrera, Schulteis, & Koob, 1999).

Summary

Tolerance, sensitization, and physical dependence are examples of adaptations that occur in individuals that are exposed to psychoactive substances. These phenomena are not inevitable consequences of drug administration, but instead depend on a range of factors including dose, frequency of administration, abstinence period, learning history, and many other variables. Although there is no single biological mechanism that can describe all the ways in which tolerance, sensitization, and physical dependence develop, a role for glutamate in these phenomena is being established as a fairly ubiquitous mechanism for the adaptations. Finally, tolerance, sensitization, and physical dependence stand as phenomena in their own right, independent of addiction. There are many ways that these phenomena might contribute to certain aspects of addiction, such as dose escalation, but their specific role is undergoing vigorous debate.

References

Aceto, M. D., Scates, S. M., Lowe, J. A., & Martin, B. R. (1995). Cannabinoid precipitated withdrawal by the selective cannabinoid receptor antagonist, SR 141716A. *European Journal of Pharmacology, 282,* R1–2.

Acquas, E., & Di Chiara, G. (1992). Depression of mesolimbic dopamine transmission and sensitization to morphine during opiate abstinence. *Journal of Neurochemistry, 58,* 1620–1625

Allen, R. M., & Dykstra, L. A. (1999). The competitive NMDA receptor antagonist LY235959 modulates the progression of morphine tolerance in rats. *Psychopharmacology (Berl), 142,* 209–214.

Allen, R. M., & Dykstra, L. A. (2000a). Role of morphine maintenance dose in the development of tolerance and its attenuation by an NMDA receptor antagonist. *Psychopharmacology, (Berl), 148,* 59–65.

Allen, R. M., & Dykstra, L. A. (2000b). Attenuation of mu-opioid tolerance and cross-tolerance by the competitive N-methyl-D-aspartate receptor antagonist LY235959 is related to tolerance and cross-tolerance magnitude. *Journal of Pharmacology and Experimental Therapeutics, 295,* 1012–1021.

Barrett, A. C., Cook, C. D., Terner, J. M., Craft, R. M., & Picker, M. J. (2001). Importance of sex and relative efficacy at the mu opioid receptor in the development of tolerance and cross-tolerance to the antinociceptive effects of opioids. *Psychopharmacology (Berl), 158,* 154–164.

Bartlett, E., Hallin, A., Chapman, B., & Angrist, B. (1997). Selective sensitization to the psychosis-inducing effects of cocaine: A possible marker for addiction relapse vulnerability? *Neuropsychopharmacology, 16,* 77–82.

Bespalov, A. Y., Balster, R. L., & Beardsley, P. M. (1999). N-Methyl-D-aspartate receptor antagonists and the development of tolerance to the discriminative stimulus effects of morphine in rats. *Journal of Pharmacology and Experimental Therapeutics, 290,* 20–27.

Boileau, I., Dagher, A., Leyton, M., Gunn, R. N., Baker, G. B., Diksic, M., et al. (2006). Modeling sensitization to stimulants in humans: An [11C]raclopride/positron emission tomography study in healthy men. *Archives of General Psychiatry, 63,* 1386–1395.

Bonci, A., & Malenka, R. C. (1999). Properties and plasticity of excitatory synapses on dopaminergic and GABAergic cells in the ventral tegmental area. *Journal of Neuroscience, 19,* 3723–3730.

Borgland, S. L., Malenka, R. C., & Bonci, A. (2004). Acute and chronic cocaine-induced potentiation of synaptic strength in the ventral tegmental area: Electrophysiological and behavioral correlates in individual rats. *Journal of Neuroscience, 24,* 7482–7490.

Bradberry, C. W. (2007). Cocaine sensitization and dopamine mediation of cue effects in rodents, monkeys, and humans: Areas of agreement, disagreement, and implications for addiction. *Psychopharmacology (Berl), 191,* 705–717.

Carrera, M. R., Schulteis, G., & Koob, G. F. (1999). Heroin self-administration in dependent Wistar rats: increased sensitivity to naloxone. *Psychopharmacology (Berl), 144,* 111–120.

Collins, A. C., Wilkins, L. H., Slobe, B. S., Cao, J. Z., & Bullock, A. E. (1996). Long-term ethanol and nicotine treatment elicit tolerance to ethanol. *Alcoholism: Clinical and Experimental Research, 20,* 990–999.

Diaz, A., Ruiz, F., Flórez, J., Hurlé, M. A., & Pazos, A. (1995). Mu-opioid receptor regulation during opioid tolerance and supersensitivity in rat central nervous system. *Journal of Pharmacology and Experimental Therapeutics, 274,* 1545–1551.

Elliott, K., Hynansky, A., & Inturrisi, C. E. (1994). Dextromethorphan attenuates and reverses analgesic tolerance to morphine. *Pain, 59,* 361–368.

Fernandes, M., Kluwe, S., & Coper, H. (1977). The development of tolerance to morphine in the rat. *Psychopharmacology (Berl), 54,* 197–201.

Fernandes, M., Kluwe, S., & Coper, H. (1982). Development and loss of tolerance to morphine in the rat. *Psychopharmacology (Berl), 78,* 234–238.

Foltin, R. W., & Fischman, M. W. (1991). Smoked and intravenous cocaine in humans: Acute tolerance, cardiovascular and subjective effects. *Journal of Pharmacology and Experimental Therapeutics, 257,* 247–261.

Foltin, R. W., & Haney, M. (2004). Intranasal cocaine in humans: Acute tolerance, cardiovascular and subjective effects. *Pharmacology Biochemistry and Behavior, 78,* 93–101.

Fowler, S. C., Bowen, S. E., & Kallman, M. J. (1993). Practice-augmented tolerance to triazolam: Evidence from an analysis of operant response durations and interresponse times. *Behavioural Pharmacology, 4,* 147–157.

Grabus, S. D., Martin, B. R., Batman, A. M., Tyndale, R. F., Sellers, E., & Damaj, M. I. (2005). Nicotine physical dependence and tolerance in the mouse following chronic oral administration. *Psychopharmacology (Berl), 178,* 183–192.

Griffiths, R. R., Wurster, R. M., & Brady, J. V. (1975). Discrete-trial choice procedure: Effects of naloxone and methadone on choice between food and heroin. *Pharmacological Reviews, 27,* 357–365.

Haney, M., Ward, A. S., Comer, S. D., Foltin, R. W., & Fischman, M. W. (1999). Abstinence symptoms following smoked marijuana in humans. *Psychopharmacology (Berl), 141,* 395–404.

Hart, C. L., Haney, M., Ward, A. S., Fischman, M. W., & Foltin, R. W. (2002). Effects of oral THC maintenance on smoked marijuana self-administration. *Drug and Alcohol Dependence, 67,* 301–309.

Holloway, F. A., Michaelis, R. C., Harland, R. D., Criado, J. R., & Gauvin, D. V. (1992). Tolerance to ethanol's effects on operant performance in rats: Role of number and pattern of intoxicated practice opportunities. *Psychopharmacology (Berl), 109,* 112–120.

Horger, B. A., Giles, M. K., & Schenk, S. (1992). Preexposure to amphetamine and nicotine predisposes rats to self-administer a low dose of cocaine. *Psychopharmacology (Berl), 107,* 271–276.

Howard, L. A., Micu, A. L., Sellers, E. M., & Tyndale, R. F. (2001). Low doses of nicotine and ethanol induce CYP2E1 and chlorzoxazone metabolism in rat liver. *Journal of Pharmacology and Experimental Therapeutics, 299,* 542–550.

June, H. L., Stitzer, M. L., & Cone, E. (1995). Acute physical dependence: Time course and relation to human plasma morphine concentrations. *Clinical Pharmacology & Therapeutics, 57,* 270–280.

Kalivas, P. W., & Duffy, P. (1998). Repeated cocaine administration alters extracellular glutamate in the ventral tegmental area. *Journal of Neurochemistry, 70,* 1497–1502.

Karler, R., Calder, L. D., Chaudhry, I. A., & Turkanis, S. A. (1989). Blockade of "reverse tolerance" to cocaine and amphetamine by MK-801. *Life Sciences, 45,* 599–606.

Li, Y., Hu, X. T., Berney, T. G., Vartanian, A. J., Stine, C. D., Wolf, M. E., et al. (1999). Both glutamate receptor antagonists and prefrontal cortex lesions prevent induction of cocaine sensitization and associated neuroadaptations. *Synapse, 34,* 169–180.

Lieber, C. S. (1994). Hepatic and metabolic effects of ethanol: Pathogenesis and prevention. *Annals of Medicine, 26,* 325–330.

Liu, Y., Roberts, D. C., & Morgan, D. (2005). Sensitization of the reinforcing effects of self-administered cocaine in rats: Effects of dose and intravenous injection speed. *European Journal of Neuroscience, 22,* 195–200.

Marks, M. J., Stitzel, J. A., & Collins, A. C. (1986). Dose-response analysis of nicotine tolerance and receptor changes in two inbred mouse strains. *Journal of Pharmacology and Experimental Therapeutics, 239,* 358–364.

Masserano, J. M., Baker, I., Natsukari, N., & Wyatt, R. J. (1996). Chronic cocaine administration increases tyrosine hydroxylase activity in the ventral tegmental area through glutaminergic- and dopaminergic D2-receptor mechanisms. *Neuroscience Letters, 217,* 73–76.

Medvedev, I. O., Dravolina, O. A., & Bespalov, A. Y. (1998). Effects of N-methyl-D-aspartate receptor antagonists on discriminative stimulus effects of naloxone in morphine-dependent rats using the Y-maze drug discrimination paradigm. *Journal of Pharmacology and Experimental Therapeutics, 286,* 1260–1268.

Mendrek, A., Blaha, C. D., & Phillips, A. G. (1998). Pre-exposure of rats to amphetamine sensitizes self-administration of this drug under a progressive ratio schedule. *Psychopharmacology (Berl), 135,* 416–422.

Morgan, D., Liu, Y., & Roberts, D. C. (2006). Rapid and persistent sensitization to the reinforcing effects of cocaine. *Neuropsychopharmacology, 31,* 121–128.

Mucha, R. F., Kalant, H., & Linseman, M. A. (1979). Quantitative relationships among measures of morphine tolerance and physical dependence in the rat. *Pharmacology, Biochemistry, and Behavior, 10,* 397–405.

Negus, S. S. (2006). Choice between heroin and food in nondependent and heroin-dependent rhesus monkeys: Effects of naloxone, buprenorphine, and methadone. *Journal of Pharmacology and Experimental Therapeutics, 317,* 711–723.

Paronis, C. A., & Holtzman, S. G. (1992). Development of tolerance to the analgesic activity of mu agonists after continuous infusion of morphine, meperidine or fentanyl in rats. *Journal of Pharmacology and Experimental Therapeutics, 262,* 1–9.

Pauly, J. R., Grun, E. U., & Collins, A. C. (1992). Tolerance to nicotine following chronic treatment by injections: A potential role for corticosterone. *Psychopharmacology (Berl), 108,* 33–39.

Pennartz, C. M., Ameerun, R. F., Groenewegen, H. J., & Lopes da Silva, F. H. (1993). Synaptic plasticity in an in vitro slice preparation of the rat nucleus accumbens. *European Journal of Neuroscience, 5,* 107–117.

Perkins, K. A., Gerlach, D., Broge, M., Sanders, M., Grobe, J., Fonte, C., et al. (2001). Quitting cigarette smoking produces minimal loss of chronic tolerance to nicotine. *Psychopharmacology (Berl), 158,* 7–17.

Perkins, K. A., Grobe, J. E., Epstein, L. H., Caggiula, A., Stiller, R. L., & Jacob, R. G. (1993). Chronic and acute tolerance to subjective effects of nicotine. *Pharmacology Biochemistry and Behavior, 45,* 375–381.

Perkins, K. A., Grobe, J. E., Fonte, C., Goettler, J., Caggiula, A. R., Reynolds, W. A., et al. (1994). Chronic and acute tolerance to subjective, behavioral and cardiovascular effects of nicotine in humans. *Journal of Pharmacology and Experimental Therapeutics, 270,* 628–638.

Popik, P., & Danysz, W. (1997). Inhibition of reinforcing effects of morphine and motivational aspects of naloxone-precipitated opioid withdrawal by N-methyl-D-aspartate receptor antagonist, memantine. *Journal of Pharmacology and Experimental Therapies, 280,* 854–865.

Price, J. S., Waller, P. C., Wood, S. M., & MacKay, A. V. (1996). A comparison of the post-marketing safety of four selective serotonin re-uptake inhibitors including the investigation of symptoms occurring on withdrawal. *British Journal of Clinical Pharmacology, 42,* 757–763.

Rinaldi, R. C., Steindler, E. M., Wilford, B. B., & Goodwin, D. (1988). Clarification and standardization of substance abuse terminology. *Journal of the American Medical Association, 259,* 555–557.

Robinson, T. E., & Berridge, K. C. (1993). The neural basis of drug craving: An incentive-sensitization theory of addiction. *Brain Research Brain Research Reviews, 18,* 247–291.

Robinson, T. E., & Berridge, K. C. (2000). The psychology and neurobiology of addiction: An incentive-sensitization view. *Addiction, 95* (Suppl. 2) S91–117.

Rook, E. J., Huitema, A. D., van den Brink, W., van Ree, J. M., & Beijnen, J. H. (2006). Population pharmacokinetics of heroin and its major metabolites. *Clinical Pharmacokinetics, 45,* 401–417.

Rothman, R. B., Gorelick, D. A., Baumann, M. H., Guo, X. Y., Herning, R. I., Pickworth, W. B., et al. (1994). Lack of evidence for context-dependent cocaine-induced sensitization in humans: Preliminary studies. *Pharmacology Biochemistry and Behavior, 49,* 583–588.

Samaha, A. N., Li, Y., & Robinson, T. E. (2002). The rate of intravenous cocaine administration determines susceptibility to sensitization. *Journal of Neuroscience, 22,* 3244–3250.

Sadée, W., & Wang, Z. (1995). Agonist induced constitutive receptor activation as a novel regulatory mechanism. Mu receptor regulation. *Advances in Experimental Medicine and Biology, 373,* 85–90.

Schenk, S., & Partridge, B. (1997). Sensitization and tolerance in psychostimulant self-administration. *Pharmacology Biochemistry and Behavior, 57,* 543–550.

Schnur, P. (1985). Morphine tolerance and sensitization in the hamster. *Pharmacology Biochemistry and Behavior, 22,* 157–158.

Schuh, K. J., Walsh, S. L., Bigelow, G. E., Preston, K. L., & Stitzer, M. L. (1996). Buprenorphine, morphine and naloxone effects during ascending morphine maintenance in humans. *Journal of Pharmacology and Experimental Therapeutics, 278,* 836–846.

Siegel, S. (1975). Evidence from rats that morphine tolerance is a learned response. *Journal of Comparative Physiology and Psychology, 89,* 498–506.

Siegel, S., Hinson, R. E., Krank, M. D., & McCully, J. (1982). Heroin "overdose" death: Contribution of drug-associated environmental cues. *Science, 216,* 436–437.

Sparks, J. A., & Pauly, J. R. (1999). Effects of continuous oral nicotine administration on brain nicotinic receptors and responsiveness to nicotine in C57Bl/6 mice. *Psychopharmacology (Berl), 141,* 145–153.

Strakowski, S. M., Sax, K. W., Setters, M. J., & Keck, P. E. Jr. (1996). Enhanced response to repeated d-amphetamine challenge: Evidence for behavioral sensitization in humans. *Biological Psychiatry, 40,* 872–880.

Suto, N., Austin, J. D., Tanabe, L. M., Kramer, M. K., Wright, D. A., & Vezina, P. (2002). Previous exposure to VTA amphetamine enhances cocaine self-administration under a progressive ratio schedule in a D1 dopamine receptor dependent manner. *Neuropsychopharmacology, 27,* 970–979.

Tiseo, P. J., & Inturrisi, C. E. (1993). Attenuation and reversal of morphine tolerance by the competitive N-methyl-D-aspartate receptor antagonist, LY274614. *Journal of Pharmacology and Experimental Therapeutics, 264,* 1090–1096.

Trujillo, K. A. (2000). Are NMDA receptors involved in opiate-induced neural and behavioral plasticity? A review of preclinical studies. *Psychopharmacology (Berl), 151,* 121–141.

Trujillo, K. A., & Akil, H. (1991). Inhibition of morphine tolerance and dependence by the NMDA receptor antagonist MK-801. *Science, 251,* 85–87.

Tsou, K., Patrick, S. L., & Walker, J. M. (1995). Physical withdrawal in rats tolerant to delta 9-tetrahydrocannabinol precipitated by a cannabinoid receptor antagonist. *European Journal of Pharmacology, 280,* R13–15.

Ungless, M. A., Whistler, J. L., Malenka, R. C., & Bonci, A. (2001). Single cocaine exposure in vivo induces long-term potentiation in dopamine neurons. *Nature, 411,* 583–587.

Vanderschuren, L. J., & Kalivas, P. W. (2000). Alterations in dopaminergic and glutamatergic transmission in the induction and expression of behavioral sensitization: A critical review of preclinical studies. *Psychopharmacology (Berl), 151,* 99–120.

Wachtel, S. R., & de Wit, H. (1999). Subjective and behavioral effects of repeated d-amphetamine in humans. Behavioral Pharmacology, 10, 271–281.

Walker, E. A., & Young, A. M. (2001). Differential tolerance to antinociceptive effects of mu opioids during repeated treatment with etonitazene, morphine, or buprenorphine in rats. *Psychopharmacology (Berl), 154,* 131–142.

White, F. J., Hu, X. T., Zhang, X. F., & Wolf, M. E. (1995). Repeated administration of cocaine or amphetamine alters neuronal responses to glutamate in the mesoaccumbens dopamine system. *Journal of Pharmacology and Experimental Therapeutics, 273,* 445–454.

Wolf, M. E. (1998). The role of excitatory amino acids in behavioral sensitization to psychomotor stimulants. *Progress in Neurobiology, 54,* 679–720.

Wu, G., Lu, Z. H., Wei, T. J., Howells, R. D., Christoffers, K. & Ledeen, R. W. (1998). The role of GM1 ganglioside in regulating excitatory opioid effects. *Annals of the New York Academy of Sciences, 845,* 126–138.

Yoburn, B. C., Billings, B., & Duttaroy, A. (1993). Opioid receptor regulation in mice. *Journal of Pharmacology Experimental Therapeutics, 265,* 314–320.

Yoburn, B. C., Chen, J., Huang, T., & Inturrisi, C. E. (1985). Pharmacokinetics and pharmacodynamics of subcutaneous morphine pellets in the rat. *Journal of Pharmacology and Experimental Therapeutics, 235,* 282–286.

Young, A. M., Sannerud, C. A., Steigerwald, E. S., Doty, M. D., Lipinski, W. J., & Tetrick, L. E. (1990). Tolerance to morphine stimulus control: Role of morphine maintenance dose. *Psychopharmacology (Berl), 102,* 59–67.

Young, A. M., Steigerwald, E. S., Makhay, M. M., & Kapitsopoulos, G. (1991). Onset of tolerance to discriminative stimulus effects of morphine. *Pharmacology Biochemistry and Behavior, 39,* 487–493.

Zernig, G., Ahmed, S. H., Cardinal, R. N., Morgan, D., Acquas, E., Foltin, R. W., et al. (2007). Explaining the escalation of drug use in substance dependence: Models and appropriate animal laboratory tests. *Pharmacology, 80,* 65–119.

5

Neurobiology of Addiction

George F. Koob
The Scripps Research Institute

Contents

Introduction

What is Addiction? The Clinical Syndrome Relevant to the Neurobiology of Addiction

Drug addiction, also known as substance dependence, is a chronically relapsing disorder characterized by (1) compulsion to seek and take the drug, (2) loss of control in limiting intake, and (3) emergence of a negative emotional state (e.g., dysphoria, anxiety, irritability) when access to the drug is prevented (defined here as dependence; Koob & Le Moal, 1997).

Addiction and *Substance Dependence* (as currently defined by the *Diagnostic and Statistical Manual of Mental Disorders*, 4th edition [*DSM-IV*]; American Psychiatric Association, 1994) is used interchangeably throughout this chapter and refers to a final stage of a usage process that moves from drug use to addiction. Clinically, the occasional but limited use of a drug with the potential for abuse or dependence is distinct from the emergence of a chronic drug-dependent state, and this becomes an important element in the pursuit of the neurobiological mechanisms of addiction. An important goal of current neurobiological research is to understand the molecular, neuropharmacological, and neurocircuitry changes that mediate the transition from occasional, controlled drug use to the loss of behavioral control over drug-seeking and drug-taking that defines chronic addiction. The hypothesis elaborated here is that both excessive drug-taking and genetic vulnerability, separately or combined, engage similar mechanisms that mediate the vulnerability to addiction.

A useful psychiatric-motivational framework that integrates well with animal models of addiction is the conceptualization that drug addiction has aspects of both impulse control disorders and compulsive disorders (see Figure 5.1). Impulse control disorders are characterized by an increasing sense of tension or arousal before committing an impulsive act; pleasure, gratification, or relief at the time of committing the act; and there may or may not be regret, self reproach, or guilt following the act (American Psychiatric Association, 1994). A classic impulse control disorder is kleptomania where there is an increase in tension before stealing an object or objects that are not needed, relief after the act, but little or no regret or self-reproach. In contrast, compulsive disorders are characterized by anxiety and stress before committing a compulsive repetitive behavior and relief from the stress by performing the compulsive behavior. A classic compulsive disorder is obsessive-compulsive disorder where obsessions of contamination or harm drive anxiety, which then requires repetitive compulsive acts to reduce the anxiety. As an individual moves from an impulsive disorder to a compulsive disorder there is a shift from positive reinforcement to negative reinforcement driving the motivated behavior (Koob, 2004). Drug addiction has been conceptualized as a disorder that progresses from impulsivity to compulsivity in a collapsed cycle of addiction composed of three stages: *preoccupation/anticipation*, *binge/intoxication*, and *withdrawal/negative affect*.

Animal Models

Although no animal model of addiction fully emulates the human condition, they do permit investigation of specific elements of the process of drug addiction. Such elements can be defined by models of actual symptoms of addiction within different stages of the addiction cycle. Different animal models for the study of the neurobiology of addiction can be superimposed on these three stages which are conceptualized as feeding into each other, becoming more intense, and ultimately leading to the pathological state known as addiction (Koob & Le Moal, 1997).

Animal models for the *binge/intoxication* stage of the addiction cycle incorporate the construct of drug reinforcement. Animal models of drugs as reinforcers are extensive and well validated. Animals and humans will readily self-administer drugs in the nondependent state. Drugs of abuse have powerful reinforcing properties. Animals will perform many different tasks and procedures to obtain the drugs, even in the nondependent state. Drugs that are self-administered by animals correspond well with those that have high abuse potential in humans,

FIGURE 5.1

Diagram showing stages of impulse control disorder and compulsive disorder cycles related to the sources of reinforcement. In impulse control disorders, an increasing tension and arousal occurs before the impulsive act, with pleasure, gratification or relief during the act. Following the act, there may or may not be regret or guilt. In compulsive disorders, there are recurrent and persistent thoughts (obsessions) that cause marked anxiety and stress followed by repetitive behaviors (compulsions) that are aimed at preventing or reducing distress (American Psychiatric Association, 1994). Positive reinforcement (pleasure/gratification) is more closely associated with impulse control disorders. Negative reinforcement (relief of anxiety or relief of stress) is more closely associated with compulsive disorders.

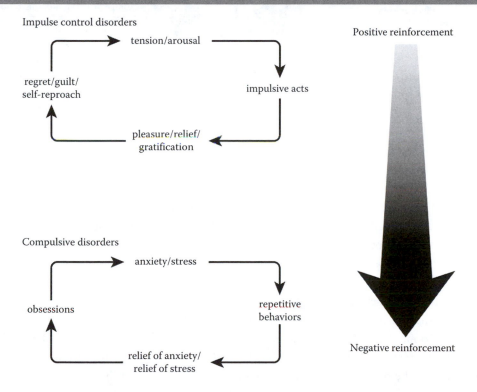

Source. Koob, G. F., Alcoholism: Allostasis and Beyond. *Alcoholism: Clinical and Experimental Research, 27,* 2003. Reproduced with permission.

and intravenous drug self-administration is considered an animal model that is predictive of abuse potential (Collins, Weeks, Cooper, Good, & Russell, 1984). Two other animal models have been used extensively to measure drug reward indirectly: conditioned place preference and brain stimulation reward (Figure 5.2). Conditioned place preference is a nonoperant procedure for assessing the reinforcing efficacy of drugs using a classical or Pavlovian conditioning procedure. Animals typically exhibit a conditioned place preference for an environment

FIGURE 5.2
Animal models associated with the three stages of the addiction cycle (preoccupation/anticipation, binge/intoxication, withdrawal/negative affect).

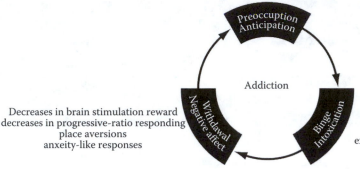

Drug-induced reinstatement
Cue-induced reinstatement
Stress-induced reinstatement
Protracted abstinence-stress responsivity incubation effect

Preoccuption Anticipation

Addiction

Withdrawal Negative affect

Binge Intoxication

Decreases in brain stimulation reward
decreases in progressive-ratio responding
place aversions
anxeity-like responses

Drug self-administration
conditioned place preference
brain stimulation reward
binge drug self-administration
extended access self-administration
self-administration with
aversive consequences

associated with drugs that are self-administered by humans and avoid environments that induce aversive states (i.e., conditioned place aversion). Lowering of brain stimulation reward thresholds also are reliable measures of drug reward. Drugs of abuse decrease thresholds for brain stimulation reward, and there is good correspondence between the ability of drugs to decrease brain reward thresholds and their abuse potential (Kornetsky & Bain, 1990).

Although a large focus in animal studies has been on the synaptic sites and molecular mechanisms in the central nervous system on which drugs of abuse act initially to produce their rewarding effects, animal models now have been designed to address elements of the *binge/intoxication* stage and the increased motivation to seek drugs. Such measures include binge drug-taking (Tornatzky & Miczek, 2000), increased drug intake produced by extended access to drugs (Ahmed & Koob, 1998), and drug-seeking despite negative or aversive consequences (Deroche-Gamonet, Belin, & Piazza, 2004; Vanderschuren & Everitt, 2004; Figure 5.2). Such increased self-administration in dependent animals has now been observed with cocaine, methamphetamine, nicotine, heroin, and alcohol (Ahmed & Koob, 1998; Ahmed, Walker, & Koob, 2000; Kitamura, Wee, Specio, Koob, & Pulvirenti, 2006; O'Dell & Koob, 2007; Roberts, Heyser, Cole, Griffin, & Koob, 2000). Equally compelling are studies showing drug-taking in the presence of aversive consequences in animals with extended access to the drug. Rats with extended access to cocaine do not suppress drug-seeking in the presence of an aversive conditioned stimulus which has face validity for the *DSM-IV* criterion of "continued substance use despite knowledge of having a persistent physical or psychological problem" (Vanderschuren & Everitt, 2004).

For the *withdrawal/negative affect* stage, animal models exist for the somatic signs of withdrawal for virtually all drugs of abuse. However, more relevant for addiction are the animal models of components of the negative reinforcing effects of dependence which are beginning to be used to explore how the nervous system involved in motivation adapts to drug use (Figure 5.2). These include conditioned place aversion, elevations in reward thresholds, and decreases in responding for nondrug rewards on a progressive-ratio schedule. Animal models of the negative reinforcing effects of dependence include the same models used for the rewarding effects of drugs of abuse (see above), but with changes in valence of the reward. Animals will show a conditioned place aversion to precipitated withdrawal from chronic administration of a drug. For example, in a conditioned place preference procedure, rodents avoid the compartment paired with an acute withdrawal syndrome precipitated by administration of an antagonist to the neurochemical system under study. Thus, rats will show a conditioned place aversion to precipitated opioid, cannabinoid, and nicotine withdrawal, each precipitated by opioid, cannabinoid, and nicotinic antagonists (Tzschentke, 1998). Similarly, precipitated or spontaneous withdrawal from all drugs of abuse raise, instead of lower, brain reward thresholds (Markou, Kosten, & Koob, 1998).

For the *preoccupation/anticipation* stage, there are models of craving involving drug-, cue-, and stress-induced reinstatement of drug-seeking behavior (Figure 5.2). Animal models of craving involve both the conditioned rewarding effects of drugs of abuse and measures of the conditioned aversive effects of dependence (Shippenberg & Koob, 2002). Resistance to extinction has been used to measure the residual motivational properties of drugs by assessing the persistence of drug-seeking behavior in the absence of response-contingent drug availability. Other measures of craving have examined the motivational properties of the drugs themselves or cues paired with the drugs after extinction. Drug-induced reinstatement first involves extinction then presentation of a priming injection of a drug. Latency to reinitiate responding, or the amount of responding on the previously extinguished lever, is hypothesized to reflect the motivation for drug-seeking behavior. Similarly, drug-paired or drug-associated stimuli can reinitiate drug-seeking behavior (cue-induced reinstatement). Other measures of craving include second-order schedules of reinforcement where animals can be trained to work for a previously neutral stimulus that predicts drug availability.

From the aversive side, acute stressors also can reinitiate drug-seeking behavior in animals that have been extinguished, and this is called stress-induced reinstatement. Increased brain reward thresholds and increases in anxiety-like behavior have been shown to persist after acute withdrawal in animal studies and have been hypothesized to reflect protracted abstinence. Finally, with opioids, conditioned withdrawal has been observed where previously neutral stimuli paired with precipitated opioid withdrawal have been shown not only to produce place aversions but also to have motivational properties in increasing self-administration of opioids (Kenny, Chen, Kitamura, Markou, & Koob, 2006).

Neurobiological Mechanisms—Binge/Intoxication Stage

The neurobiological mechanisms of addiction that are involved in various stages of the addiction cycle have a specific focus on certain brain circuits, and the neuroadaptational changes within those circuits, during the transition from drug-taking to drug addiction and how those changes persist in the vulnerability to relapse. In addition, an evolving hypothesis is that there are molecular changes within the brain circuits associated with addiction that form the basis for the circuitry changes. Whether the molecular changes are pre-existing, convey vulnerability, or are induced by the insult of heavy drug-taking (or both) remains to be determined. Insights to date argue for ultimately some common substrates upon which vulnerability to acquire addiction and sustain addiction can be linked. These common elements are the focus of the review that follows.

Brain Reward Systems

A long-hypothesized key element of drug addiction is that drugs of abuse activate brain reward systems, and understanding the neurobiological bases for acute drug reward is a key to how these systems change with the development of addiction (Koob & Le Moal, 1997; Koob, 2004). A principle focus of research on the neurobiology of the positive reinforcing effects of drugs with addiction potential has been the origins and terminal areas of the mesocorticolimbic dopamine system, and there is compelling evidence for the importance of this system in psychostimulant reward. However, the specific circuitry associated with drug reward in general has been broadened to include the many neural inputs and outputs that interact with the basal forebrain. More recently, specific components of the basal forebrain that have been identified with drug reward have focused on both the nucleus accumbens and amygdala (Koob, Sanna, & Bloom, 1998; Koob & Le Moal, 2001; Figure 5.3). As the neural circuits for the reinforcing effects of drugs with dependence potential have evolved, the role of neurotransmitters and neuromodulators within those circuits also has evolved, and five of those systems have been identified to have a role in the acute reinforcing effects of drugs: dopamine, opioid peptides, γ-aminobutyric acid (GABA), serotonin, and endocannabinoids (Table 5.1).

The nucleus accumbens and its projections became a focal point for drug reward with the discovery that this structure formed an interface between limbiclike structures and motor systems (Mogenson & Yang, 1991). Subsequent work showed that the nucleus accumbens received afferents from the medial prefrontal cortex, medial thalamus, hippocampus, and basolateral amygdala (Burns, Annett, Kelley, Everitt, & Robbins, 1996; Kelley & Domesick, 1982) and projected to the ventral pallidum (Groenwegen, Berendse, Wolters, & Lohman, 1990; Groenwegen, Berendse, & Haber, 1993). Substantive neuroanatomical and functional analyses showed that the core of the nucleus accumbens is a ventral extension of the cortical-pallidal-thalamic-cortical loops long hypothesized to mediate motor function in the extrapyramidal motor system (Heimer & Alheid, 1991; Groenewegen et al., 1993) but with a more allocortical rather than cortical input. Both stimulant and opioid drug reward were shown to involve the nucleus accumbens and the ventral pallidal connection from the nucleus accumbens, supporting the hypothesized role of this circuit in drug reward (Hubner & Koob, 1990).

Another basal forebrain structure implicated in drug reward is the *extended amygdala* (Heimer & Alheid, 1991). The extended amygdala is composed of the bed nucleus of the stria terminalis, the central nucleus of the amygdala, and a transition zone in the medial subregion of the nucleus accumbens (shell of the nucleus accumbens). Each of these regions has cytoarchitectural and circuitry similarities (Heimer & Alheid, 1991). The extended amygdala receives numerous afferents from limbic structures such as the basolateral amygdala and hippocampus and sends efferents to the medial part of the ventral pallidum and a large projection to the lateral hypothalamus, thus further defining the specific brain areas that

FIGURE 5.3

Sagittal section through a representative rodent brain illustrating the pathways and receptor systems implicated in the acute reinforcing actions of drugs of abuse. The arrows between N Acc, AMG, and BNST represent the interactions within the extended amygdala system hypothesized to have a key role in psychostimulant reinforcement. The arrows from N Acc to VP to DMT to FC to N Acc represent an hypothesized nucleus accumbens-ventral pallidum circuit. The nucleus accumbens forms an interface between limbic-like structures and motor systems. It projects to the ventral pallidum and receives afferents from the medial prefrontal cortex, medial thalamus, hippocampus, and basolateral amygdala. The core of the nucleus accumbens is a ventral extension of the cortical-pallidal-thalamic-cortical loops hypothesized to mediate motor function in the extrapyramidal motor system but with a more allocortical input rather than cortical input. Both stimulant and opioid drug reward involve the nucleus accumbens and the ventral pallidal connection from the nucleus accumbens supporting the hypothesized role of this circuit in drug reward. AC, anterior commissure; AMG, amygdala; ARC, arcuate nucleus; BNST, bed nucleus of the stria terminalis; Cer, cerebellum; C-P, caudate-putamen; DMT, dorsomedial thalamus; FC, frontal cortex; Hippo, hippocampus; IF, inferior colliculus; LC, locus coeruleus; LH, lateral hypothalamus; N Acc., nucleus accumbens; OT, olfactory tract; PAG, periaqueductal gray; RPn, reticular pontine nucleus; SC, superior colliculus; SNr, substantia nigra pars reticulata; VP, ventral pallidum; VTA, ventral tegmental area.

Neurochemical neurocircuits in drug reward

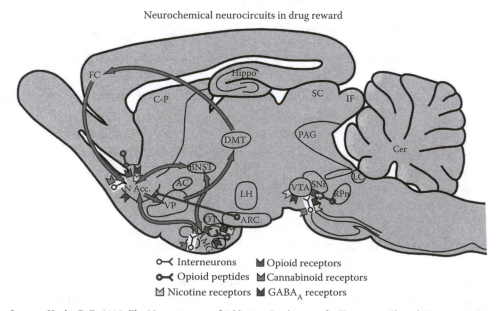

Source. Koob, G. F., 2005. The Neurocircuitry of Addiction: Implications for Treatment. *Clinical Neuroscience Research*, 5, p.92. Copyright 2005, Elsevier Inc. All rights reserved. Reprinted with permission.

TABLE 5.1
Neurobiological Substrates for the Acute Reinforcing Effects of Drug Abuse

Drug of Abuse	Neurotransmitter	Site
Cocaine and amphetamines	Dopamine	Nucleus accumbens
	γ-Aminobutyric acid	Amygdala
Opioids	Opioid peptides	Nucleus accumbens
	Dopamine	Ventral tegmental area
	Endocannabinoids	
Nicotine	Dopamine	Nucleus accumbens
	γ-Aminobutyric acid	Ventral tegmental area
	Opioid peptides	Amygdala
Δ^9-Tetrahydrocannabinol	Endocannabinoids	Nucleus accumbens
	Opioid peptides	Ventral tegmental area
	Dopamine	
Alcohol	Dopamine	Nucleus accumbens
	Opioid peptides	Ventral tegmental area
	γ-Aminobutyric acid	Amygdala
	Glutamate	
	Endocannabinoids	

interface classical limbic (emotional) structures with the extrapyramidal motor system (Alheid, De Olmos, & Beltramino, 1995). Neurochemical studies have implicated the shell of the nucleus accumbens as a sensitive site for dopamine release in response to acute administration of drugs of abuse (Di Chiara et al., 2004), but also the amygdala as a sensitive site for drug reward (Koob et al., 1998; see below).

Neurochemical Systems in Drug Reward

Dopamine released in the terminal structures of the mesolimbic dopamine system such as the nucleus accumbens is well established as having a critical role in the activating and reinforcing effects of indirect sympathomimetics such as cocaine, methamphetamine, and nicotine. However, although all drugs of abuse acutely activate the mesolimbic dopamine system, particularly in the medial shell region of the nucleus accumbens, the role of dopamine becomes less critical for the acute reinforcing effects of drugs of abuse as one moves to opioids, alcohol, and Δ^9-tetrahydrocannabinol (THC). Indeed, more recent theories have implicated dopamine in a more general associative function (Young, Ahier, Upton, Joseph, & Gray, 1998; Wise, 2004) or incentive salience (Robinson & Berridge, 2001). Other neurotransmitter systems such as opioid peptides, GABA, and endocannabinoids may play key roles in the acute reinforcing effects of drugs of abuse either in series or independent of activation of the mesolimbic dopamine system. For example, a particularly sensitive site for blockade of the acute reinforcing effects of alcohol with opioid and GABAergic antagonists appears to be the central nucleus of the amygdala (Koob, 2003). Opioid peptide antagonists also block the reinforcing effects of Δ^9-THC, a key active ingredient in marijuana.

Serotonin receptors at specific subtypes modulate psychostimulant and alcohol reward, and endocannabinoid mechanisms have been implicated in psychostimulant, opioid, alcohol, and cannabinoid reward. For example, serotonin 5-hydroxytryptamine-1B (5-HT$_{1B}$) receptor agonists facilitate cocaine reward (Parsons, Weiss, & Koob, 1998) and decrease alcohol reward (Tomkins & O'Neill, 2000). Cannabinoid CB$_1$ antagonists block opioid, alcohol, and cannabinoid reward (Justinova, Tanda, Munzar, & Goldberg, 2004; Justinova, Solinas, Tanda, Redhi, & Goldberg, 2005). In summary, multiple neurotransmitters are implicated in the acute reinforcing effects of drugs of abuse. Key players in the nucleus accumbens and amygdala are dopamine, opioid peptide, and GABA systems with modulation via serotonin and endocannabinoids.

Neurobiological Mechanisms—Withdrawal/Negative Affect Stage

The neural substrates and neuropharmacological mechanisms for the negative motivational effects of drug withdrawal may involve disruption of the same neural systems implicated in the positive reinforcing effects of drugs. Measures of brain reward function during acute abstinence from all major drugs with dependence potential have revealed increases in brain reward thresholds as measured by direct brain stimulation reward (Epping-Jordan, Watkins, Koob, & Markou, 1998; Gardner & Vorel, 1998; Markou & Koob, 1991; Paterson, Myers, & Markou, 2000; Schulteis, Markou, Cole, & Koob, 1995; Schulteis, Markou, Gold, Stinus, & Koob, 1994). These increases in reward thresholds may reflect decreases in the activity of reward neurotransmitter systems in the midbrain and forebrain implicated in the positive reinforcing effects of drugs of abuse.

Changes at the neurochemical level that reflect changes in the neurotransmitter systems implicated in acute drug reward have been hypothesized to be within-system neuroadaptations to chronic drug exposure. A within-system neuroadaptation that can be defined as "the primary cellular response element to the drug would itself adapt to neutralize the drug's effects; persistence of the opposing effects after the drug disappears would produce the withdrawal response" (Koob & Bloom, 1988). These changes include decreases in dopaminergic and serotonergic transmission in the nucleus accumbens during drug withdrawal as measured by in vivo microdialysis (Parsons & Justice, 1993; Weiss, Markou, Lorang, & Koob, 1992), increased sensitivity of opioid receptor transduction mechanisms in the nucleus accumbens during opioid withdrawal (Stinus, Le Moal, & Koob, 1990), decreased GABAergic and increased N-methyl-D-aspartate (NMDA) glutamatergic transmission during alcohol withdrawal (Davidson, Shanley, & Wilce, 1995; Morrisett, 1994; Roberts, Cole, & Koob, 1996; Weiss et al., 1996), and differential regional changes in nicotinic receptor function (Collins, Bhat, Pauly, & Marks, 1990; Dani & Heinemann, 1996). The decreases in reward neurotransmitters have been hypothesized to contribute significantly to the negative motivational state associated with acute drug abstinence. The decreased reward system function may persist in the form of long-term biochemical changes that contribute to the clinical syndrome of protracted abstinence and vulnerability to relapse.

The emotional dysregulation associated with the *withdrawal/negative affect* stage also may involve a between-system neuroadaptation where neurochemical systems other than those involved in positive rewarding effects of drugs of abuse are recruited or dysregulated by chronic activation of the reward system (Koob & Bloom, 1988) and have been termed "anti-reward" systems (see below). Brain neurochemical systems involved in stress modulation are engaged within the neurocircuitry of the brain stress systems, and the hypothesis is that this is an attempt to overcome the chronic presence of the perturbing drug and to restore normal function despite the presence of the drug (Koob & Le Moal, 2005). Both the hypothalamic-pituitary-adrenal axis and the brain stress system mediated by corticotropin-releasing factor (CRF) are dysregulated by chronic administration of all major drugs with dependence or abuse potential, with a common response of elevated adrenocorticotropic hormone, corticosterone, and amygdala CRF during acute withdrawal (Delfs, Zhu, Druhan, & Aston-Jones, 2000; Koob, Heinrichs, Menzaghi, Pich, & Britton, 1994; Merlo-Pich et al., 1995; Olive, Koenig, Nannini, & Hodge, 2002; Rasmussen et al., 2000; Rivier, Bruhn, & Vale, 1984). Acute withdrawal from drugs also may increase the release of norepinephrine in the bed nucleus of the stria terminalis and decrease levels of neuropeptide Y (NPY) in the central and medial nuclei of the amygdala (Roy & Pandey, 2002).

These results suggest that during the development of dependence a change occurs in the function of neurotransmitters associated with the acute reinforcing effects of drugs (dopamine, opioid peptides, serotonin, GABA, and endocannabinoids) together with recruitment of the brain stress system (CRF and norepinephrine) and dysregulation of the NPY brain anti-stress system (Koob & Le Moal, 2001; Table 5.2). Activation of the brain stress systems may not only contribute to the negative motivational state associated with acute abstinence but also may contribute to the vulnerability to stressors observed during protracted abstinence in humans.

The concept of an anti-reward system has been recently formulated to accommodate the significant changes in brain emotional systems associated with the development of dependence (Koob & Le Moal, 2005). The anti-reward concept is based on the hypothesis that there are brain systems in place to limit reward (Koob & Bloom, 1988), an opponent process

TABLE 5.2

Neurotransmitters Implicated in the Motivational Effects of Withdrawal from Drugs of Abuse

Neurotransmitter	Functional Effect
↓ Dopamine	"Dysphoria"
↓ Serotonin	"Dysphoria"
↓ γ-Aminobutyric acid	Anxiety, panic attacks
↓ Neuropeptide Y	Antistress
↑ Dynorphin	"Dysphoria"
↑ Corticotropin-releasing factor	Stress
↑ Norepinephrine	Stress

concept that forms a general feature of biological systems. The concept of an anti-reward system is derived from the hypothesis of between-system neuroadaptations to activation of the reward system at the neurocircuitry level. A between-system neuroadaptation is a circuitry change where circuit B (anti-reward circuit) is activated by circuit A (reward circuit). This concept has its origins in the theoretical pharmacology that predates opponent process theory (Martin, 1967). Thus, the activation of brain stress systems such as CRF, norepinephrine, and dynorphin with concomitant dysregulation of the NPY system may represent recruitment of an anti-reward system in the extended amygdala that produces the motivational components of drug withdrawal and provides a baseline hedonic shift that facilitates craving mechanisms (Koob & Le Moal, 2005; Figure 5.4).

Neurobiological Mechanisms—Preoccupation/Anticipation Stage

The *preoccupation/anticipation* stage, or "craving" stage, of the addiction cycle has long been hypothesized to be a key element of relapse in humans and defines addiction as a chronic relapsing disorder. Although often linked to the construct of craving, craving per se has been difficult to measure in human clinical studies (Tiffany, Carter, & Singleton, 2000) and often does not correlate well with relapse. Nevertheless, the stage of the addiction cycle where the individual reinstates drug-seeking behavior after abstinence remains a challenging focus for neurobiological mechanisms and medications development for treatment.

Animal models of craving can be divided into two domains: drug-seeking induced by stimuli paired with drug-taking, and drug-seeking induced by an acute stressor or a state of stress (Table 5.3). *Craving Type-1* animal models involve the use of drug-primed reinstatement and cue-induced reinstatement. *Craving Type-2* animal models involve stress-induced reinstatement in animals that have acquired drug self-administration and then have been subjected to extinction of responding for the drug (Shippenberg & Koob, 2002) and animal models of protracted abstinence.

Most evidence from animal studies suggests that drug-induced reinstatement is localized to the medial prefrontal cortex/nucleus accumbens/ventral pallidum circuit mediated by the neurotransmitter glutamate (McFarland & Kalivas, 2001). In contrast, neuropharmacological and neurobiological studies using animal models for cue-induced reinstatement involve the basolateral amygdala as a critical substrate with a possible feedforward mechanism through the prefrontal cortex system involved in drug-induced reinstatement (Everitt & Wolf, 2002; Weiss et al., 2001). The association of previously neutral stimuli paired with precipitated opioid withdrawal (conditioned withdrawal) also depends critically on the basolateral amygdala (Schulteis, Ahmed, Morse, Koob, & Everitt, 2000), and such stimuli may have motivational significance (Kenny et al., 2006). In contrast, stress-induced reinstatement of drug-related responding in animal models appears to depend on the activation of both CRF and norepinephrine in elements of the extended amygdala (central nucleus of the amygdala and bed nucleus of the stria terminalis; Shaham, Shalev, Lu, De Wit, & Stewart, 2003; Shalev, Grimm, & Shaham, 2002). Protracted abstinence, largely described in alcohol dependence

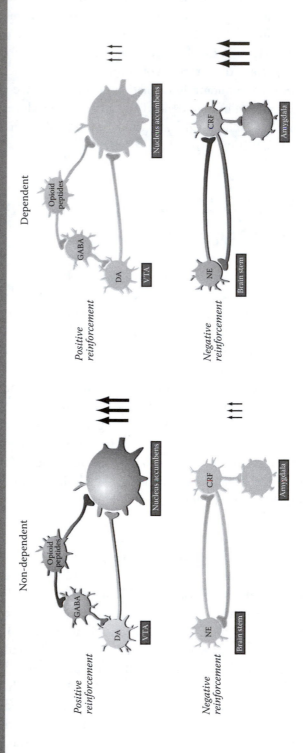

FIGURE 5.4

Neurocircuitry associated with the acute positive reinforcing effects of drugs of abuse and the negative reinforcement of dependence and how it changes in the transition from nondependent drug-taking to dependent drug-taking. Key elements of the reward circuit are dopamine and opioid peptide neurons that intersect at both the ventral tegmental area (VTA) and the nucleus accumbens and are activated during initial use and the early binge/intoxication stage. Key elements of the stress circuit are corticotropin-releasing factor (CRF) and noradrenergic neurons that converge on γ-aminobutyric acid (GABA) interneurons in the central nucleus of the amygdala and are activated during the development of dependence. DA, dopamine; NE, norepinephrine.

Source.   Nestler, E. J., Is There a Common Molecular Pathway for Addiction? *Nature Neuroscience,* 8, Macmillan Publishers Ltd. Copyright 2005. Reprinted with permission.

TABLE 5.3 Drug Craving	
Drug Craving	"Drug craving is the desire for the previously experienced effects of a psychoactive substance. This desire can become compelling and can increase in the presence of both internal and external cues, particularly with perceived substance availability. It is characterized by an increased likelihood of drug-seeking behavior and, in humans, drug-related thoughts" (Markou et al., 1992).
Craving Type 1	• Induced by stimuli that have been paired with drug self-administration, such as environmental cues. • Termed *conditioned positive reinforcement* in experimental psychology. • Animal model: Cue-induced reinstatement where a cue previously paired with access to a drug reinstates responding for a lever that has been extinguished.
Craving Type 2	State of protracted abstinence in drug-dependent individuals weeks after acute withdrawal. Conceptualized as a state change characterized by anxiety and dysphoria. Animal model: Residual hypersensitivity to states of stress and environmental stressors that lead to relapse to drug-seeking behavior.

models, appears to involve overactive glutamatergic and CRF systems (De Witte, Littleton, Parot, & Koob, 2005; Valdez et al., 2002).

Overall Neurocircuitry of Addiction

In summary, three neurobiological circuits have been identified that have heuristic value for the study of the neurobiological changes associated with the development and persistence of drug dependence (Figures 5.3 and 5.4). The acute reinforcing effects of drugs of abuse that comprise the *binge/intoxication* stage most likely involve actions with an emphasis on the ventral striatum and extended amygdala reward system and inputs from the ventral tegmental area and arcuate nucleus of the hypothalamus. In contrast, the symptoms of acute withdrawal important for addiction, such as negative affect and increased anxiety associated with the *withdrawal/negative affect* stage, most likely involve decreases in function of the extended amygdala reward system but also recruitment of brain stress neurocircuitry. The *preoccupation/anticipation* (craving) stage involves key afferent projections to the extended amygdala and nucleus accumbens, specifically the prefrontal cortex (for drug-induced reinstatement) and basolateral amygdala (for cue-induced reinstatement). Compulsive drug-seeking behavior is hypothesized to engage ventral striatal-ventral pallidal-thalamic-cortical loops which may subsequently engage dorsal striatal-pallidal-thalamic-cortical loops (Vanderschuren & Everitt, 2004, 2005), both systems driven by substantive reward deficits in the extended amygdala (Koob & Le Moal, 2005).

Molecular and Cellular Targets Within the Brain Circuits Associated with Addiction

An exciting area of pursuit in the neurobiology of addiction is which genetic and environmental factors produce the vulnerability to addiction. One hypothesis is that molecular changes at the gene or gene transcription level will provide the key to understanding such vulnerability.

The search at the molecular level has shown how repeated perturbation of intracellular signal transduction pathways by drugs of abuse leads to changes in nuclear function and altered rates of transcription of particular target genes (Nairn et al., 2004; Nestler, Barrot, & Self, 2001). Altered expression of such genes would lead to altered activity of the neurons where such changes occur, and ultimately to changes in the function of neural circuits in which those neurons operate.

Two transcription factors in particular have been implicated in the plasticity associated with addiction: cyclic adenosine monophosphate (cAMP) response element binding protein (CREB) and ΔFosB (Carlezon, Duman, & Nestler, 2005; Nestler, 2001, 2005). CREB regulates the transcription of genes that contain a CRE site (cAMP response element) within the regulatory regions and can be found ubiquitously in genes expressed in the central nervous system such as those encoding neuropeptides, synthetic enzymes for neurotransmitters, signaling proteins, and other transcription factors. CREB can be phosphorylated by protein kinase A and by protein kinases regulated by growth factors, putting it at a point of convergence for several intracellular messenger pathways that can regulate the expression of genes.

Much work in the addiction field has shown activation of CREB in the nucleus accumbens as a consequence of chronic exposure to opiates, cocaine, and alcohol, and deactivation of CREB in the central nucleus of the amygdala with alcohol and nicotine. The activation of CREB is linked to the activation of the "dysphoria"-inducing κ opioid receptor binding the opioid peptide dynorphin and has led to the hypothesis that up-regulation of the cAMP pathway and CREB in the nucleus accumbens represents a mechanism of "motivational tolerance and dependence." More specifically, these molecular adaptations may decrease an individual's sensitivity to the rewarding effects of subsequent drug exposures (tolerance) and impair the reward pathway (dependence) such that after removal of the drug the individual is left in an amotivational, dysphoric, or depressed-like state (Nestler, 2004). Thus, at the molecular level, these changes may be the basis of another source of a between-system, opponent process-like anti-reward system (i.e., recruitment of the dynorphin system; Carlezon et al., 1998; McLaughlin, Land, Li, Pintar, & Chavkin, 2006; Newton et al., 2002; Spangler, Unterwald, & Kreek, 1993; Wagner, Terman, & Chavkin, 1993).

In contrast, decreased CREB phosphorylation has been observed in the central nucleus of the amygdala during alcohol withdrawal and has been linked to decreased NPY function and consequently the increased anxiety-like responses associated with acute alcohol (Pandey, 2004). Increased CREB in the nucleus accumbens and decreased CREB in the central nucleus of the amygdala are not necessarily mutually exclusive and point to transduction mechanisms that could produce neurochemical changes in the neurocircuits outlined above as important for breaks with reward homeostasis in addiction.

The molecular changes associated with long-term changes in brain function as a result of chronic exposure to drugs of abuse also have been linked to changes in transcription factors (i.e., factors that can change gene expression and produce long-term changes in protein expression and as a result neuronal function). Although acute administration of drugs of abuse can cause a rapid (hours) activation of members of the Fos family, such as c-*fos*, FosB, Fra-1, and Fra-2 in the nucleus accumbens, other transcription factors (i.e., isoforms of ΔFosB) accumulate over longer periods of time (days) with repeated drug administration (Nestler, 2004). Animals with activated ΔFosB have exaggerated sensitivity to the rewarding effects of drugs of abuse, and thus ΔFosB may be a sustained molecular trigger that helps to initiate and maintain a state of addiction. How changes in ΔFosB that can last for days can translate into vulnerability to relapse remains a challenge for future work (Nestler, 2004).

Genetic and molecular genetic animal models have provided a molecular basis to support the neuropharmacological substrates identified in neurocircuitry studies. High alcohol-preferring rats have been bred that show high voluntary consumption of alcohol, increased anxiety-like responses, and numerous neuropharmacological phenotypes such as decreased dopaminergic and NPY activity (McBride, Murphy, Lumeng, & Li, 1990; Murphy et al., 2002). In an alcohol-preferring and nonpreferring cross, a quantitative trait locus was identified on chromosome 4, a region to which the gene for NPY has been mapped. Follow-up studies with expression profiling in congenic strains of inbred-preferring (iP) and inbred-nonpreferring (iNP) rat strains confirmed a decrease in NPY expression in iNP animals and changes in regulation of the protein kinase C pathway (Carr et al., 1998, 2007). Quantitative trait loci analyses of the high alcohol-preferring (HAP) and low alcohol-preferring (LAP) mouse lines confirmed specific regions on chromosomes 9, 2, and 5, with possible candidate genes *Drd2* and GABA$_A$ receptors (Bice et al., 2006).

Advances in molecular biology have led to the ability to systematically inactivate the genes that control the expression of proteins that make up receptors or neurotransmitter/neuromodulators in the central nervous system using the gene knockout approach. Knockout mice have a gene inactivated by homologous recombination. A knockout mouse deficient in both alleles of a gene is homozygous for the deletion and is termed a null mutation (–/–). A mouse that is deficient in only one of the two alleles for the gene is termed a heterozygote (+/–). Transgenic mice may also have an extra gene introduced into their germ line. An additional copy of a normal gene is inserted into the genome of the mouse to examine the effects of overexpression of the product of that gene. Alternatively, a new gene not normally found in the mouse can be added, such as a gene associated with a specific pathology in humans. Wildtype controls are animals bred through the same breeding strategies involving mice that received the transgene injected into the fertilized egg (transgenics) or a targeted gene construct injected into the genome via embryonic stem cells (knockout) but lacking the mutation on either allele of the gene in question. Although such an approach does not guarantee that these genes are the ones that are vulnerable in the human population, they provide viable candidates for exploring the genetic basis of endophenotypes associated with addiction (Koob, Bartfai, & Roberts, 2001).

Notable positive results with gene knockout studies in mice have focused on knockout of the μ-opioid receptor, which eliminates opioid, nicotine, and cannabinoid reward and alcohol drinking in mice (Contet, Kieffer, & Befort, 2004). Opioid (morphine) reinforcement as measured by conditioned place preference or self-administration is absent in μ knockout mice, and there is no development of somatic signs of dependence to morphine in these mice. Indeed, to date all morphine effects tested, including analgesia, hyperlocomotion, respiratory depression, and inhibition of gastrointestinal transit, are abolished in μ knockout mice (Gaveriaux-Ruff & Kieffer, 2002).

Selective deletion of the genes for expression of different dopamine receptor subtypes and the dopamine transporter has revealed significant effects to challenges with psychomotor stimulants. Dopamine D_1 receptor knockout mice show no response to D_1 agonists or antagonists and show a blunted response to the locomotor-activating and rewarding effects of cocaine and amphetamine (Caine et al., 2007; Smith et al., 1998; Xu, Gue, Vorhees, & Zhang, 2000; Xu et al., 1994). D_1 knockout mice also are impaired in their acquisition of intravenous cocaine self-administration compared to wildtype mice (Caine et al., 2007). D_2 knockout mice have severe motor deficits and blunted psychostimulant responses to psychostimulants and opiates, but the effects on psychostimulant reward are less consistent. Dopamine transporter knockout mice are dramatically hyperactive but also show a blunted response to psychostimulants. Although developmental factors must be taken into account for the compensatory effect of deleting any one or a combination of genes, it is clear that D_1 and D_2 receptors and the dopamine transporter play important roles in the actions of psychomotor stimulants (Caine et al., 2002).

Brain Imaging Circuits Involved in Human Addiction

Brain imaging studies using positron emission tomography with ligands for measuring oxygen utilization or glucose metabolism or using magnetic resonance imaging techniques are providing dramatic insights into the neurocircuitry changes in the human brain associated with the development, maintenance, and vulnerability to addiction. These imaging results overall show a striking resemblance to the neurocircuitry identified by animal studies. During acute intoxication with alcohol, morphine, nicotine, and cocaine, there is an activation of the orbitofrontal cortex, prefrontal cortex, anterior cingulate, extended amygdala, and ventral striatum (Becerra, Harter, Gonzalez, & Borsook, 2006; Breiter et al., 1997; Childress et al., 1999; Grant et al., 1996; Montgomery, Lingford-Hughes, Egerton, Nutt, & Grasby, 2007; Volkow & Fowler, 2000; Volkow et al., 1992, 1993, 1999; Yoder et al., 2007). This activation often is accompanied by an increase in availability of the neurotransmitter dopamine in the nucleus accumbens with psychostimulant challenge (Volkow et al., 1997; Martinez et al., 2005). During acute and chronic withdrawal there is a reversal of these changes with decreases in metabolic activity, particularly in the orbitofrontal cortex, prefrontal cortex, and anterior cingulate, and decreases in basal dopamine activity as measured by decreased D_2 receptors in the ventral striatum and prefrontal cortex (Martinez et al., 2005; Volkow et al., 1993, 1996, 2001; Wang et al., 1997). Similar results have been observed in rhesus macaques with decreases in D_2 dopamine receptor binding persisting for up to 1 year postexposure (Nader et al., 2006). This decrease in D_2 receptors has been hypothesized to reflect a hypodopaminergic state (Volkow & Fowler, 2000). Cue-induced reinstatement appears to involve a reactivation of these circuits much like acute intoxication (Bonson et al., 2002; Breiter, Aharon, Kahneman, Dale, & Shizgal, 2001; Childress et al., 1999). Craving or cues associated with heroin, cocaine, and nicotine produce activation of the prefrontal cortex and anterior cingulate gyrus (Lee, Lim, Wiederhold, & Graham, 2005; Risinger et al., 2005; Xiao et al., 2006). Imaging studies also show evidence that cues associated with cocaine craving increase dopamine release in the striatum as well as opioid peptides in the anterior cingulate and frontal cortex (Hermann et al., 2006; Gorelick et al., 2005; Volkow et al., 2006; Wong et al.,

FIGURE 5.5

Key common neurocircuitry elements in drug-seeking behavior associated with drug addiction. Three major circuits that underlie addiction can be distilled from the literature. A drug reinforcement circuit ("reward" and "stress") is composed of the extended amygdala including the central nucleus of the amygdala, the bed nucleus of the stria terminalis, and a transition zone in the shell of the nucleus accumbens. A drug- and cue-induced reinstatement ("craving") neurocircuit based on animal studies is composed of the prefrontal (anterior cingulate, prelimbic, orbitofrontal) cortex and basolateral amygdala with a primary role hypothesized for the basolateral amygdala in cue-induced craving and a primary role for the medial prefrontal cortex in drug-induced craving. The striatal-pallidal-thalamic loops reciprocally move from the prefrontal cortex to orbitofrontal cortex to motor cortex, ultimately leading to drug-seeking behavior.

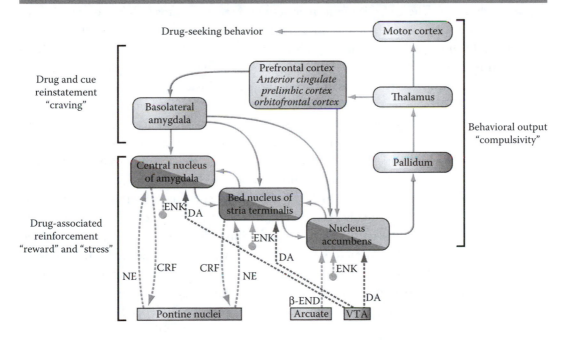

Source. Koob G. F., & Le Moal, M., *Neurobiology of Addiction*, p. 415. London: Academic Press, Copyright 2006. Elsevier Inc. All rights reserved. Reprinted with permission.

2006). Craving in alcoholics appears to be correlated with higher opioid peptide activity in the striatum but lower dopaminergic activity (Heinz et al., 2004, 2005). Thus, imaging studies to date reveal baseline decreases in orbitofrontal function and dopamine function during dependence but a reactivation of dopamine and reward system function during acute craving episodes consistent with the early formulation of different neural substrates for *Craving Type-1* and *Type-2* (see above).

Summary and Conclusions

Much progress in neurobiology has provided a useful neurocircuitry framework with which to identify the neurobiological mechanisms involved in the development of drug addiction (See Figure 5.5 above). A conceptual framework has evolved with a focus on dysregulation of brain reward systems as a function of the different stages of the addiction process that affect aspects of positive reinforcement, negative reinforcement, and conditioned reinforcement. The brain reward system implicated in the development of addiction is composed of key elements of the basal forebrain with a focus on the nucleus accumbens (nucleus accumbens-ventral pallidum-thalamic-cortical loops) and central nucleus of the amygdala (extended amygdala). Neuropharmacological studies in animal models of addiction have provided evidence for the activation of specific neurochemical mechanisms in specific brain reward neurochemical systems in the basal forebrain (dopamine, opioid peptides, GABA, serotonin, and endocannabinoids) during the *binge/intoxication* stage. During the *withdrawal/negative affect* stage, there is a dysregulation of the same brain reward neurochemical systems in the basal forebrain (dopamine, opioid peptides, GABA, serotonin, and endocannabinoids). There also is recruitment of brain stress systems (CRF and norepinephrine) and dysregulation of brain anti-stress systems (NPY) that contribute to the negative motivational state associated with drug abstinence. During the *preoccupation/anticipation* stage, neurobiological circuits that engage the frontal cortex glutamatergic projections to the nucleus accumbens are critical for drug-induced reinstatement, whereas basolateral amygdala and ventral subiculum glutamatergic projections to the nucleus accumbens are involved in cue-induced reinstatement. Stress-induced reinstatement appears to be mediated by recruitment of sensitivity in the anti-reward systems of the extended amygdala. The changes in craving and anti-reward (stress) systems are hypothesized to remain outside a homeostatic state, and as such convey the vulnerability for development of dependence and relapse in addiction. Genetic studies to date in animals suggest roles for the genes encoding the neurochemical elements involved in the brain reward (dopamine, opioid peptide) and stress (NPY) systems in the vulnerability to addiction. Molecular studies have identified transduction and transcription factors that may mediate the dependence-induced reward dysregulation (CREB) and chronic-vulnerability changes (ΔFosB) in neurocircuitry associated with the development and maintenance of addiction. Human imaging studies reveal similar neurocircuits involved in acute intoxication, chronic drug dependence, and vulnerability to relapse.

Imaging studies reveal that two salient changes in established and unrecovered substance-dependent individuals that cut across different drugs are decreases in orbitofrontal/prefrontal cortex function and decreases in brain dopamine D_2 receptors. No molecular markers are sufficiently specific yet to predict vulnerability to addiction, but changes in certain intermediate early genes with chronic drug exposure in animal models show promise of long-term changes in specific brain circuits that may be common to all drugs of abuse. The continually evolving knowledge base of biological and neurobiological aspects of substance use disorders provides a heuristic framework to better develop the diagnoses, prevention, and treatment of substance abuse disorders.

Acknowledgments

This is publication number 20007 from The Scripps Research Institute. Research was supported by the Pearson Centre for Alcoholism and Addiction Research and National Institutes of Health grants AA06420 and AA08459 from the National Institute on Alcohol Abuse and Alcoholism, DA04043 and DA04398 from the National Institute on Drug Abuse, and DK26741 from the National Institute of Diabetes and Digestive and Kidney Diseases. The authors would like to thank Michael Arends for his assistance with manuscript preparation.

References

Ahmed, S. H., & Koob, G. F. (1998). Transition from moderate to excessive drug intake: Change in hedonic set point. *Science, 282*, 298–300.

Ahmed, S. H., Walker, J. R., & Koob, G.F. (2000). Persistent increase in the motivation to take heroin in rats with a history of drug escalation. *Neuropsychopharmacology, 22*, 413–421.

Alheid, G. F., De Olmos, J. S., & Beltramino, C. A. (1995). Amygdala and extended amygdala. In: G. Paxinos (Ed.), *The rat nervous system* (pp. 495–578). San Diego, CA: Academic Press.

American Psychiatric Association. (1994). *Diagnostic and statistical manual of mental disorders* (4th ed.). Washington DC: American Psychiatric Press.

Becerra, L., Harter, K., Gonzalez, R. G., & Borsook, D. (2006). Functional magnetic resonance imaging measures of the effects of morphine on central nervous system circuitry in opioid-naive healthy volunteers. *Anesthesia and Analgesia, 103*, 208–216.

Bice, P. J., Foroud, T., Carr, L. G., Zhang, L., Liu, L., Grahame, N. J., et al. (2006). Identification of QTLs influencing alcohol preference in the High Alcohol Preferring (HAP) and Low Alcohol Preferring (LAP) mouse lines. *Behavior Genetics, 36*, 248–260.

Bonson, K. R., Grant, S. J., Contoreggi, C. S., Links, J. M., Metcalfe, J., Weyl, H. L., et al. (2002). Neural systems and cue-induced cocaine craving. *Neuropsychopharmacology, 26*, 376–386.

Breiter, H. C., Aharon, I., Kahneman, D., Dale, A., & Shizgal, P. (2001). Functional imaging of neural responses to expectancy and experience of monetary gains and losses. *Neuron, 30*, 619–639.

Breiter, H. C., Gollub, R. L., Weisskoff, R. M., Kennedy, D. N., Makris, N., Berke, J. D., et al. (1997). Acute effects of cocaine on human brain activity and emotion. *Neuron, 19*, 591–611.

Burns, L. H., Annett, L., Kelley, A. E., Everitt, B. J., & Robbins, T. W. (1996). Effects of lesions to amygdala, ventral subiculum, medial prefrontal cortex, and nucleus accumbens on the reaction to novelty: Implication for limbic-striatal interactions. *Behavioral Neuroscience, 110*, 60–73.

Caine, S. B., Negus, S. S., Mello, N. K., Patel, S., Bristow, L., Kulagowski, J., et al. (2002). Role of dopamine D2-like receptors in cocaine self-administration: Studies with D2 receptor mutant mice and novel D2 receptor antagonists. *Journal of Neuroscience, 22*, 2977–2988.

Caine, S. B., Thomsen, M., Gabriel, K. I., Berkowitz, J. S., Gold, L. H., Koob, G. F., et al. (2007). Lack of self-administration of cocaine in dopamine D1 receptor knockout mice. *Journal of Neuroscience, 27*, 13140–13150.

Carlezon, W. A., Jr., Duman, R. S., & Nestler, E. J. (2005). The many faces of CREB. *Trends in Neurosciences, 28*, 436–445.

Carlezon, W. A. Jr., Thome, J., Olson, V. G., Lane-Ladd, S. B., Brodkin, E. S., Hiroi, N., et al. (1998). Regulation of cocaine reward by CREB. *Science, 282*, 2272–2275.

Carr, L. G., Foroud, T., Bice, P., Gobbett, T., Ivashina, J., Edenberg, H., et al. (1998). A quantitative trait locus for alcohol consumption in selectively bred rat lines. *Alcoholism: Clinical and Experimental Research, 22*, 884–887.

Carr, L. G., Kimpel, M. W., Liang, T., McClintick, J. N., McCall, K., Morse, M., et al. (2007). Identification of candidate genes for alcohol preference by expression profiling of congenic rat strains. *Alcoholism: Clinical and Experimental Research, 31*, 1089–1098.

Childress, A. R., Mozley, P. D., McElgin, W., Fitzgerald, J., Reivich, M., & O'Brien, C. P. (1999). Limbic activation during cue-induced cocaine craving. *American Journal of Psychiatry, 156,* 11–18.

Collins, A. C., Bhat, R. V., Pauly, J. R., & Marks, M. J. (1990). Modulation of nicotine receptors by chronic exposure to nicotinic agonists and antagonists. In G. Bock & J. Marsh (Eds.), *The biology of nicotine dependence,* series title: Ciba Foundation Symposium (Vol. 152, pp. 87–105). New York: John Wiley.

Collins, R. J., Weeks, J. R., Cooper, M. M., Good, P. I., & Russell, R. R. (1984). Prediction of abuse liability of drugs using IV self-administration by rats. *Psychopharmacology, 82,* 6–13.

Contet, C., Kieffer, B. L., & Befort, K. (2004). Mu opioid receptor: A gateway to drug addiction. *Currrent Opinion in Neurobiology, 14,* 370–378.

Dani, J. A., & Heinemann, S. (1996). Molecular and cellular aspects of nicotine abuse. *Neuron, 16,* 905–908.

Davidson, M., Shanley, B., & Wilce, P. (1995). Increased NMDA-induced excitability during ethanol withdrawal: A behavioural and histological study. *Brain Research, 674,* 91–96.

De Witte, P., Littleton, J., Parot, P., & Koob, G. F. (2005). Neuroprotective and abstinence-promoting effects of acamprosate: Elucidating the mechanism of action. *CNS Drugs, 19,* 517–537.

Delfs, J. M., Zhu, Y., Druhan, J. P., & Aston-Jones, G. (2000). Noradrenaline in the ventral forebrain is critical for opiate withdrawal-induced aversion. *Nature, 403,* 430–434.

Deroche-Gamonet, V., Belin, D., & Piazza, P. V. (2004). Evidence for addiction-like behavior in the rat. *Science, 305,* 1014–1017.

Di Chiara, G., Bassareo, V., Fenu, S., De Luca, M. A., Spina, L., Cadoni, C., et al. (2004). Dopamine and drug addiction: The nucleus accumbens shell connection. *Neuropharmacology, 47* (Suppl. 1), 227–241.

Epping-Jordan, M. P., Watkins, S. S., Koob, G. F., & Markou, A. (1998). Dramatic decreases in brain reward function during nicotine withdrawal. *Nature, 393,* 76–79.

Everitt, B. J., & Wolf, M. E. (2002). Psychomotor stimulant addiction: A neural systems perspective. *Journal of Neuroscience, 22,* 3312–3320.

Gardner, E. L., & Vorel, S. R. (1998). Cannabinoid transmission and reward-related events. *Neurobiology of Disease, 5,* 502–533.

Gaveriaux-Ruff, C., & Kieffer, B. L. (2002). Opioid receptor genes inactivated in mice: The highlights. *Neuropeptides, 36,* 62–71.

Gorelick, D. A., Kim, Y. K., Bencherif, B., Boyd, S. J., Nelson, R., Copersino, M., et al. (2005). Imaging brain mu-opioid receptors in abstinent cocaine users: Time course and relation to cocaine craving. *Biological Psychiatry, 57,* 1573–1582.

Grant, S., London, E. D., Newlin, D. B., Villemagne, V. L., Liu, X., Contoreggi, C., et al. (1996). Activation of memory circuits during cue-elicited cocaine craving. *Proceedings of the National Academy of Sciences USA, 93,* 12040–12045.

Groenewegen, H. J., Berendse, H. W., & Haber, S. N. (1993). Organization of the output of the ventral striatopallidal system in the rat: Ventral pallidal efferents. *Neuroscience, 57,* 113–142.

Groenewegen, H. J., Berendse, H. W., Wolters, J. G., & Lohman, A. H. (1990). The anatomical relationship of the prefrontal cortex with the striatopallidal system, the thalamus and the amygdala: Evidence for a parallel organization. In H. B. M. Uylings, C. G. van Eden, J. P. C. de Bruin, M. A. Corner & M. G. P. Feenstra (Eds.), *The prefrontal cortex: Its structure, function, and pathology,* series title: *Progress in brain research* (Vol. 85 pp. 95–116). New York: Elsevier.

Heimer, L., & Alheid, G. (1991). Piecing together the puzzle of basal forebrain anatomy. In T. C. Napier, P. W. Kalivas & I. Hanin (Eds.), *The basal forebrain: Anatomy to function,* series title: *Advances in experimental medicine and biology* (Vol. 295 pp. 1–42). New York: Plenum Press.

Heinz, A., Reimold, M., Wrase, J., Hermann, D., Croissant, B., Mundle, G., et al. (2005). Correlation of stable elevations in striatal mu-opioid receptor availability in detoxified alcoholic patients with alcohol craving: A positron emission tomography study using carbon 11-labeled carfentanil. *Archives of General Psychiatry, 62,* 57–64.

Heinz, A., Siessmeier, T., Wrase, J., Hermann, D., Klein, S., Grusser, S. M., et al. (2004). Correlation between dopamine D(2) receptors in the ventral striatum and central processing of alcohol cues and craving. *American Journal of Psychiatry, 161,* 1783–1789.

Hermann, D., Smolka, M. N., Wrase, J., Klein, S., Nikitopoulos, J., Georgi, A., et al. (2006). Blockade of cue-induced brain activation of abstinent alcoholics by a single administration of amisulpride as measured with fMRI. *Alcoholism: Clinical and Experimental Research, 30,* 1349–1354.

Hubner, C. B., & Koob, G. F. (1990). The ventral pallidum plays a role in mediating cocaine and heroin self-administration in the rat. *Brain Research, 508,* 20–29.

Justinova, Z., Solinas, M., Tanda, G., Redhi, G. H., & Goldberg, S. R. (2005). The endogenous cannabinoid anandamide and its synthetic analog R(+)-methanandamide are intravenously self-administered by squirrel monkeys. *Journal of Neuroscience, 25,* 5645–5650.

Justinova, Z., Tanda, G., Munzar, P., & Goldberg, S. R. (2004). The opioid antagonist naltrexone reduces the reinforcing effects of delta 9 tetrahydrocannabinol (THC) in squirrel monkeys. *Psychopharmacology, 173,* 186–194.

Kelley, A. E., & Domesick, V. B. (1982). The distribution of the projection from the hippocampal formation to the nucleus accumbens in the rat: An anterograde- and retrograde-horseradish peroxidase study. *Neuroscience, 7,* 2321–2335.

Kenny, P. J., Chen, S. A., Kitamura, O., Markou, A., & Koob, G. F. (2006). Conditioned withdrawal drives heroin consumption and decreases reward sensitivity. *Journal of Neuroscience, 26,* 5894–5900.

Kitamura, O., Wee, S., Specio, S. E., Koob, G. F., & Pulvirenti, L. (2006). Escalation of methamphetamine self-administration in rats: A dose-effect function. *Psychopharmacology, 186,* 48–53.

Koob, G. F. (2003). Alcoholism: Allostasis and beyond. *Alcoholism: Clinical and Experimental Research, 27,* 232–243.

Koob, G. F. (2004). Allostatic view of motivation: Implications for psychopathology. In. R. A. Bevins & M. T. Bardo (Eds.), *Motivational factors in the etiology of drug abuse,* series title: *Nebraska symposium on motivation* (Vol. 50 pp. 1–18). Lincoln, NE: University of Nebraska Press.

Koob, G. F. (2005). The neurocircuitry of addiction: Implications for treatment. *Clinical Neuroscience Research, 5,* 89–101.

Koob, G. F., Bartfai, T., & Roberts, A. J. (2001). The use of molecular genetic approaches in the neuropharmacology of corticotropin-releasing factor. *International Journal of Comparative Psychology, 14,* 90–110.

Koob, G. F., & Bloom, F. E. (1988). Cellular and molecular mechanisms of drug dependence. *Science, 242,* 715–723.

Koob, G. F., Heinrichs, S. C., Menzaghi, F., Pich, E. M., & Britton, K. T. (1994). Corticotropin releasing factor, stress and behavior. *Seminars in the Neurosciences, 6,* 221–229.

Koob, G. F., & Le Moal, M. (1997). Drug abuse: Hedonic homeostatic dysregulation. *Science, 278,* 52–58.

Koob, G. F., & Le Moal, M. (2001). Drug addiction, dysregulation of reward, and allostasis. *Neuropsychopharmacology, 24,* 97–129.

Koob, G. F., & Le Moal, M. (2005). Plasticity of reward neurocircuitry and the 'dark side' of drug addiction. *Nature Neuroscience, 8,* 1442–1444.

Koob, G. F., & Le Moal, M. (2006). *Neurobiology of addiction.* London: Academic Press.

Koob, G. F., Sanna, P. P., & Bloom, F. E. (1998). Neuroscience of addiction. *Neuron, 21,* 467–476.

Kornetsky, C., & Bain, G. (1990). Brain–stimulation reward: A model for drug induced euphoria. In M. W. Adler & A. Cowan (Eds.), *Testing and evaluation of drugs of abuse,* series title: *Modern methods in pharmacology* (Vol. 6 pp. 211–231). New York: Wiley-Liss.

Lee, J. H., Lim, Y., Wiederhold, B. K., & Graham, S. J. (2005). A functional magnetic resonance imaging (FMRI) study of cue-induced smoking craving in virtual environments. *Applied Psychophysiology and Biofeedback, 30,* 195–204.

Markou, A., & Koob, G. F. (1991). Post-cocaine anhedonia: An animal model of cocaine withdrawal. *Neuropsychopharmacology, 4,* 17–26.

Markou, A., Kosten, T. R., & Koob, G. F. (1998). Neurobiological similarities in depression and drug dependence: A self-medication hypothesis. *Neuropsychopharmacology, 18,* 135–174.

Martin, W. R. (1967). Opioid antagonists. *Pharmacological Reviews, 19,* 463–521.

Martinez, D., Gil, R., Slifstein, M., Hwang, D. R., Huang, Y., Perez, A., et al. (2005). Alcohol dependence is associated with blunted dopamine transmission in the ventral striatum. *Biological Psychiatry, 58,* 779–786.

McBride, W. J., Murphy, J. M., Lumeng, L., & Li, T. K. (1990). Serotonin, dopamine and GABA involvement in alcohol drinking of selectively bred rats. *Alcohol, 7,* 199–205.

McFarland, K., & Kalivas, P. W. (2001). The circuitry mediating cocaine-induced reinstatement of drug-seeking behavior. *Journal of Neuroscience, 21,* 8655–8663.

McLaughlin, J. P., Land, B. B., Li, S., Pintar, J. E., & Chavkin, C. (2006). Prior activation of kappa opioid receptors by U50,488 mimics repeated forced swim stress to potentiate cocaine place preference conditioning. *Neuropsychopharmacology, 31*, 787–794.

Merlo-Pich, E., Lorang, M., Yeganeh, M., Rodriguez de Fonseca, F., Raber, J., Koob, G. F., et al. (1995). Increase of extracellular corticotropin-releasing factor-like immunoreactivity levels in the amygdala of awake rats during restraint stress and ethanol withdrawal as measured by microdialysis. *Journal of Neuroscience, 15*, 5439–5447.

Mogenson, G. J., & Yang, C. R. (1991). The contribution of basal forebrain to limbic-motor integration and the mediation of motivation to action. *Advances in Experimental Medicine and Biology, 295*, 267–290.

Montgomery, A. J., Lingford-Hughes, A. R., Egerton, A., Nutt, D. J., & Grasby, P. M. (2007). The effect of nicotine on striatal dopamine release in man: A [11C]raclopride PET study. *Synapse, 61*, 637–645.

Morrisett, R. A. (1994). Potentiation of N-methyl-D-aspartate receptor-dependent afterdischarges in rat dentate gyrus following in vitro ethanol withdrawal. *Neuroscience Letters, 167*, 175–178.

Murphy, J. M., Stewart, R. B., Bell, R. L., Badia-Elder, N. E., Carr, L. G., McBride, W. J., et al. (2002). Phenotypic and genotypic characterization of the Indiana University rat lines selectively bred for high and low alcohol preference. *Behavior Genetics, 32*, 363–388.

Nader, M. A., Morgan, D., Gage, H. D., Nader, S. H., Calhoun, T. L., Buchheimer, N., et al. (2006). PET imaging of dopamine D2 receptors during chronic cocaine self-administration in monkeys. *Nature Neuroscience, 9*, 1050–1056.

Nairn, A. C., Svenningsson, P., Nishi, A., Fisone, G., Girault, J. A., & Greengard, P. (2004). The role of DARPP-32 in the actions of drugs of abuse. *Neuropharmacology, 47*(Suppl. 1), 14–23.

Nestler, E. J. (2001). Molecular neurobiology of addiction. *American Journal on Addictions, 10*, 201–217.

Nestler, E. J. (2004). Historical review: Molecular and cellular mechanisms of opiate and cocaine addiction. *Trends in Pharmacological Sciences, 25*, 210–218.

Nestler, E. J. (2005). Is there a common molecular pathway for addiction? *Nature Neuroscience, 8*, 1445–1449.

Nestler, E. J., Barrot, M., & Self, D. W. (2001). DeltaFosB: A sustained molecular switch for addiction. *Proceedings of the National Academy of Sciences USA, 98*, 11042–11046.

Newton, S. S., Thome, J., Wallace, T. L., Shirayama, Y., Schlesinger, L., Sakai, N., et al. (2002). Inhibition of cAMP response element-binding protein or dynorphin in the nucleus accumbens produces an antidepressant-like effect. *Journal of Neuroscience, 22*, 10883–10890.

O'Dell, L. E., & Koob, G. F. (2007). "Nicotine deprivation effect" in rats with intermittent 23-hour access to intravenous nocotine self-administration. *Pharmacology Biochemistry and Behavior, 86*, 346–353.

Olive, M. F., Koenig, H. N., Nannini, M. A., & Hodge, C. W. (2002). Elevated extracellular CRF levels in the bed nucleus of the stria terminalis during ethanol withdrawal and reduction by subsequent ethanol intake. *Pharmacology Biochemistry and Behavior, 72*, 213–220.

Pandey, S. C. (2004). The gene transcription factor cyclic AMP-responsive element binding protein: Role in positive and negative affective states of alcohol addiction. *Pharmacology and Therapeutics, 104*, 47–58.

Parsons, L. H., & Justice, J. B. Jr. (1993). Perfusate serotonin increases extracellular dopamine in the nucleus accumbens as measured by in vivo microdialysis. *Brain Research, 606*, 195–199.

Parsons, L. H., Weiss, F., & Koob, G. F. (1998). Serotonin-1B receptor stimulation enhances cocaine reinforcement. *Journal of Neuroscience, 18*, 10078–10089.

Paterson, N. E., Myers, C., & Markou, A. (2000). Effects of repeated withdrawal from continuous amphetamine administration on brain reward function in rats. *Psychopharmacology, 152*, 440–446.

Rasmussen, D. D., Boldt, B. M., Bryant, C. A., Mitton, D. R., Larsen, S. A., & Wilkinson, C. W. (2000). Chronic daily ethanol and withdrawal: 1. Long-term changes in the hypothalamo-pituitary-adrenal axis. *Alcoholism: Clinical and Experimental Research, 24*, 1836–1849.

Risinger, R. C., Salmeron, B. J., Ross, T. J., Amen, S. L., Sanfilipo, M., Hoffmann, R. G., et al. (2005). Neural correlates of high and craving during cocaine self-administration using BOLD fMRI. *Neuroimage, 26*, 1097–1108.

Rivier, C., Bruhn, T., & Vale, W. (1984). Effect of ethanol on the hypothalamic-pituitary-adrenal axis in the rat: Role of corticotropin-releasing factor (CRF). *Journal of Pharmacology and Experimental Therapeutics, 229,* 127–131.

Roberts, A. J., Cole, M., & Koob, G. F. (1996). Intra-amygdala muscimol decreases operant ethanol self-administration in dependent rats. *Alcoholism: Clinical and Experimental Research, 20,* 1289–1298.

Roberts, A. J., Heyser, C. J., Cole, M., Griffin, P., & Koob, G. F. (2000). Excessive ethanol drinking following a history of dependence: Animal model of allostasis. *Neuropsychopharmacology, 22,* 581–594.

Robinson, T. E., & Berridge, K. C. (2001). Incentive-sensitization and addiction. *Addiction, 96,* 103–114.

Roy, A., & Pandey, S. C. (2002). The decreased cellular expression of neuropeptide Y protein in rat brain structures during ethanol withdrawal after chronic ethanol exposure. *Alcoholism: Clinical and Experimental Research, 26,* 796–803.

Schulteis, G., Ahmed, S. H., Morse, A. C., Koob, G. F., & Everitt, B. J. (2000). Conditioning and opiate withdrawal: The amygdala links neutral stimuli with the agony of overcoming drug addiction. *Nature, 405,* 1013–1014.

Schulteis, G., Markou, A., Cole, M., & Koob, G. F. (1995). Decreased brain reward produced by ethanol withdrawal. *Proceedings of the National Academy of Sciences USA, 92,* 5880–5884.

Schulteis, G., Markou, A., Gold, L. H., Stinus, L., & Koob, G. F. (1994). Relative sensitivity to naloxone of multiple indices of opiate withdrawal: A quantitative dose-response analysis. *Journal of Pharmacology and Experimental Therapeutics, 271,* 1391–1398.

Shaham, Y., Shalev, U., Lu, L., De Wit, H., & Stewart, J. (2003). The reinstatement model of drug relapse: History, methodology and major findings. *Psychopharmacology, 168,* 3–20.

Shalev, U., Grimm, J. W., & Shaham, Y. (2002). Neurobiology of relapse to heroin and cocaine seeking: A review. *Pharmacological Reviews, 54,* 1–42.

Shippenberg, T. S., & Koob, G. F. (2002). Recent advances in animal models of drug addiction and alcoholism. In K. L. Davis, D. Charney, J. T. Coyle & C. Nemcroff (Eds.), *Neuropsychopharmacology: The fifth generation of progress* (pp. 1381–1397). Philadelphia: Lippincott Williams and Wilkins.

Smith, D. R., Striplin, C. D., Geller, A. M., Mailman, R. B., Drago, J., Lawler, C. P., et al. (1998). Behavioural assessment of mice lacking D1A dopamine receptors. *Neuroscience, 86,* 135–146.

Spangler, R., Unterwald, E. M., & Kreek, M. J. (1993). 'Binge' cocaine administration induces a sustained increase of prodynorphin mRNA in rat caudate-putamen. *Molecular Brain Research, 19,* 323–327.

Stinus, L., Le Moal, M., & Koob, G. F. (1990). Nucleus accumbens and amygdala are possible substrates for the aversive stimulus effects of opiate withdrawal, *Neuroscience, 37,* 767–773.

Tiffany, S. T., Carter, B. L., & Singleton, E. G. (2000). Challenges in the manipulation, assessment and interpretation of craving relevant variables. *Addiction, 95*(Suppl. 2), s177–s187.

Tomkins, D. M., & O'Neill, M. F. (2000). Effect of 5-HT(1B) receptor ligands on self-administration of ethanol in an operant procedure in rats. *Pharmacology Biochemistry and Behavior, 66,* 129–136.

Tornatzky, W., & Miczek, K. A. (2000). Cocaine self-administration "binges": Transition from behavioral and autonomic regulation toward homeostatic dysregulation in rats. *Psychopharmacology, 148,* 289–298.

Tzschentke, T. M. (1998). Measuring reward with the conditioned place preference paradigm: A comprehensive review of drug effects, recent progress and new issues. *Progress in Neurobiology, 56,* 613–672.

Valdez, G. R., Roberts, A. J., Chan, K., Davis, H., Brennan, M., Zorrilla, E. P., et al. (2002). Increased ethanol self-administration and anxiety-like behavior during acute withdrawal and protracted abstinence: Regulation by corticotropin-releasing factor. *Alcoholism: Clinical and Experimental Research, 26,* 1494–1501.

Vanderschuren, L. J., & Everitt, B. J. (2004). Drug seeking becomes compulsive after prolonged cocaine self-administration. *Science, 305,* 1017–1019.

Vanderschuren, L. J., & Everitt, B. J. (2005). Behavioral and neural mechanisms of compulsive drug seeking. *European Journal of Pharmacology, 526,* 77–88.

Volkow, N. D., Chang, L., Wang, G. J., Fowler, J. S., Ding, Y. S., Sedler, M., et al. (2001). Low level of brain dopamine D2 receptors in methamphetamine abusers: Association with metabolism in the orbitofrontal cortex. *American Journal of Psychiatry, 158,* 2015–2021.

Volkow, N. D., & Fowler, J. S. (2000). Addiction, a disease of compulsion and drive: Involvement of the orbitofrontal cortex. *Cerebral Cortex, 10,* 318–325.

Volkow, N. D., Fowler, J. S., Wang, G. J., Hitzemann, R., Logan, J., Schlyer, D. J., et al. (1993). Decreased dopamine D2 receptor availability is associated with reduced frontal metabolism in cocaine abusers. *Synapse, 14,* 169–177.

Volkow, N. D., Hitzemann, R., Wang, G. J., Fowler, J. S., Wolf, A. P., Dewey, S. L., et al. (1992). Long-term frontal brain metabolic changes in cocaine abusers. *Synapse, 11,* 184–190.

Volkow, N. D., Wang, G. J., Fowler, J. S., Logan, J., Gatley, S. J., Gifford, A., et al. (1999). Prediction of reinforcing responses to psychostimulants in humans by brain dopamine D2 receptor levels. *American Journal of Psychiatry, 156,* 1440–1443.

Volkow, N. D., Wang, G. J., Fowler, J. S., Logan, J., Gatley, S. J., Hitzemann, R., et al. (1997). Decreased striatal dopaminergic responsiveness in detoxified cocaine-dependent subjects. *Nature, 386,* 830–833.

Volkow, N. D., Wang, G. J., Fowler, J. S., Logan, J., Hitzemann, R., Ding, Y. S., et al. (1996). Decreases in dopamine receptors but not in dopamine transporters in alcoholics. *Alcoholism: Clinical and Experimental Research, 20,* 1594–1598.

Volkow, N. D., Wang, G. J., Telang, F., Fowler, J. S., Logan, J., Childress, A. R., et al. (2006). Cocaine cues and dopamine in dorsal striatum: Mechanism of craving in cocaine addiction. *Journal of Neuroscience, 26,* 6583–6588.

Wagner, J. J., Terman, G. W., & Chavkin, C. (1993). Endogenous dynorphins inhibit excitatory neurotransmission and block LTP induction in the hippocampus. *Nature, 363,* 451–454.

Wang, G. J., Volkow, N. D., Fowler, J. S., Logan, J., Abumrad, N. N., Hitzemann, R. J., et al. (1997). Dopamine D2 receptor availability in opiate-dependent subjects before and after naloxone-precipitated withdrawal. *Neuropsychopharmacology, 16,* 174–182.

Weiss, F., Ciccocioppo, R., Parsons, L. H., Katner, S., Liu, X., Zorrilla, E. P., et al. (2001). Compulsive drug-seeking behavior and relapse: Neuroadaptation, stress, and conditioning factors. In V. Quinones-Jenab (Ed.), *The biological basis of cocaine addiction,* series title: *Annals of the New York Academy of Sciences* (Vol. 937 pp. 1–26). New York: New York Academy of Sciences.

Weiss, F., Markou, A., Lorang, M. T., & Koob, G. F. (1992). Basal extracellular dopamine levels in the nucleus accumbens are decreased during cocaine withdrawal after unlimited-access self-administration. *Brain Research, 593,* 314–318.

Weiss, F., Parsons, L. H., Schulteis, G., Hyytia, P., Lorang, M. T., Bloom, F. E., et al. (1996). Ethanol self-administration restores withdrawal-associated deficiencies in accumbal dopamine and 5-hydroxytryptamine release in dependent rats. *Journal of Neuroscience, 16,* 3474–3485.

Wise, R. A. (2004). Dopamine, learning and motivation. *Nature Reviews Neuroscience, 5,* 483–494.

Wong, D. F., Kuwabara, H., Schretlen, D. J., Bonson, K. R., Zhou, Y., Nandi, A., et al. (2006). Increased occupancy of dopamine receptors in human striatum during cue-elicited cocaine craving. *Neuropsychopharmacology, 31,* 2716–2727.

Xiao, Z., Lee, T., Zhang, J. X., Wu, Q., Wu, R., Weng, X., et al. (2006). Thirsty heroin addicts show different fMRI activations when exposed to water-related and drug-related cues. *Drug and Alcohol Dependence, 83,* 157–162.

Xu, M., Guo, Y., Vorhees, C. V., & Zhang, J. (2000). Behavioral responses to cocaine and amphetamine administration in mice lacking the dopamine D1 receptor. *Brain Research, 852,* 198–207.

Xu, M., Hu, X. -T., Cooper, D. C., Moratalla, R., Graybiel, A. M., White, F. J., et al. (1994). Elimination of cocaine-induced hyperactivity and dopamine-mediated neurophysiological effects in dopamine D1 receptor mutant mice. *Cell, 79,* 945–955.

Yoder, K. K., Constantinescu, C. C., Kareken, D. A., Normandin, M. D., Cheng, T. E., O'Connor, S. J., et al. (2007). Heterogeneous effects of alcohol on dopamine release in the striatum: A PET study. *Alcoholism: Clinical and Experimental Research, 31,* 965–973.

Young, A., M., Ahier, R., G., Upton, R. L., Joseph, M. H., & Gray, J. A. (1998). Increased extracellular dopamine in the nucleus accumbens of the rat during associative learning of neutral stimuli. *Neuroscience, 83,* 1175–1183.

6

Genetics of Addiction

Lara A. Ray

University of California

Kent E. Hutchison

University of New Mexico and Mind Research Network

Contents

Behavioral Genetics of Addiction

Behavioral genetics is the field of study that seeks to understand both the genetic and environmental contributions to individual variation in human behavior. In order to accomplish such a challenging task, a number of research strategies are often employed, such as family, twin, and adoption studies designed to parse out the biological from environmental influences on a given behavior. More recently, genetic linkage and association studies have been used to identify location for genes associated with a given disorder and specific genes underlying the disorder, respectively. Genetics and molecular biology methods have developed rapidly and have provided important insight into the mechanisms by which genes may come to influence human behavior. The first step in studying behavioral genetics is to determine that the behavior, or in this case, psychiatric disorder of interest, is indeed substantially influenced by genetics. In order to determine the relative contribution of genetic and environmental factors to a given psychiatric disorder, behavioral geneticists traditionally rely on three basic strategies: family, twin, and adoption studies.

Family Studies

Family studies are designed to address the following question: "Does this disorder run in families?" The study design consists of comparing relatives of affected individuals (usually termed "probands," as the individuals who brought the family into the study) to relatives of unaffected individuals or controls. The presence of a control group is critical to drawing inferences in family studies. In short, if the prevalence of the disorder of interest is significantly higher among relatives of affected individuals (i.e., cases) compared to relatives of controls, we may infer that the disorder of interest runs in families. Additionally, family studies generally assume that first-degree relatives should be at greater risk for developing the disorder than second-degree relatives, which in turn should be at greater risk than third-degree relatives. This is because first-degree relatives share, on average, half their genes identical by descent, in common with the proband, whereas second-degree relatives share only one fourth of their genes with the proband, and third-degree relatives share one eighth of their genes with the proband, on average.

Family studies of addictions have generally supported the notion that addictive behaviors such as alcoholism (e.g., Cotton, 1979), marijuana use (Hopfer, Stallings, Hewitt, & Crowley, 2003), and tobacco use (i.e., "ever smoking;" Cheng, Swan, & Carmelli, 2000) tend to run in families. A study comparing probands dependent on alcohol, opioids, cocaine, or cannabis, versus controls found that the rate of drug dependence among relatives of controls was 3.5%, compared to 20.5% among relatives of opioid-dependent probands, 14.9% among relatives of cocaine-dependent probands, and 21.3% among relatives of cannabis-dependent probands (Merikangas et al., 1998). The aforementioned study estimated an eightfold increase risk for a substance use disorder among relatives of probands affected by an addictive disorder and supported the notion that addiction runs in families, although this study could not disentangle the method of familial transmission, namely genetic or environmental. Family study designs are also useful in identifying location for genes associated with a given disorder using linkage analyses (discussed in detail below).

Twin Studies

Demonstrating that a disorder runs in families does not conclusively establish that genes contribute to the etiology of the disorder given that environmental mechanisms of familial transmission may also take place. Twin and adoption studies are used to parse out the relative contribution of genetic and environmental factors to a given disorder. Twin studies capitalize on the occurrence of twinning, which provides a powerful natural experiment in human genetics. Specifically, monozygotic (MZ), or identical, twins share 100% of their genes with each other, such that any differences between MZ twins must be due to environmental effects. Dizygotic (DZ), or fraternal, twins share only 50% of their genes with each other, which is the same genetic similarity observed among full siblings. Therefore, if genetic factors influence a given disorder then the disorder should co-occur more frequently among MZ twins than among DZ twins and full siblings. For example, a twin study of alcoholism (McGue, Pickens, & Svikis, 1992) indicated that the concordance rate for male MZ twin pairs was 77%, as compared to 54% for male DZ twins. This study estimated the heritability of alcoholism at 54%, such that 54% of the variability in risk for alcoholism was estimated to be due to genetic factors and 46% of the variability in risk was attributed to environmental factors. Results of twin studies of alcoholism among females are more equivocal and generally provide weaker support for the role of genetic factors underlying the risk for alcoholism in women (Heath, Slutske, & Madden, 1997).

Twin methodology allows researchers to mathematically partition the cause of disorders into three sources, namely heritability, shared environment, and unique environment. Heritability refers to the degree to which the vulnerability to develop a disorder is due to genes. Environmental factors are divided into common, or shared, environment, and unique environment. Shared environment refers to environmental factors shared by the twins, such as social economic status, for example. Unique environment refers to environmental factors not shared by twins, such as exposure to peer group, for example. Shared environmental factors are thought to make twins more similar to each other whereas unique environmental factors are likely to make them less similar to each other. Although the methods for computing the genetic and environmental estimates of contribution to a given disorder are beyond the scope of this chapter, clinicians should be familiar with the basic model of heritability which partitions the vulnerability for a given disorder into what is known in behavioral genetics as the ACE model, where A represents additive genetic effects, C stands for shared environmental effects, and E represents unique environmental effects. The estimate of heritability is referred to as h^2. See Figure 6.1.

Adoption Studies

Adoption studies provide another method for parsing out the genetic and environmental contributions to the familial aggregation of a given psychiatric disorder. Specifically, children adopted at an early age have a genetic relationship with their biological parents and an environmental relationship with their adoptive parents. If genes are primarily responsible for the familial transmission of the disorder, one would expect that the offspring would be more similar to their biological parents than to their adoptive parents. Statistical methods allow us

FIGURE 6.1

ACE model for partitioning the cause of mental disorders into three sources: heritability (A), common environment (C), and unique environment (E).

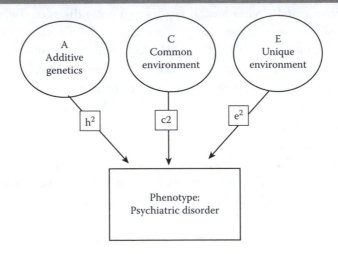

to quantify those genetic and environmental contributions to the etiology of a disorder using adoption data.

Adoption studies have shown that the rate of alcoholism in adopted (i.e., reared away) male offspring of alcohol-dependent probands ranged between 18 and 63%, as compared to generally smaller rates for adopted offspring of nonalcohol-dependent parents, ranging between 5 and 24% (McGue, 1999). These studies generally concluded that adopted sons of alcohol-dependent probands were 1.7 to 6.5 times more likely to develop alcoholism, as compared to adopted sons of controls. Studies of adopted daughters of alcohol-dependent probands indicated odds ratios between 0.5 and 8.9 (McGue, 1999). Adoption studies have also shown that drug abuse and dependence in adoptees was related to drug abuse/dependence and deviant behavior in the biological parents (Cadoret, Troughton, O'Gorman, & Heywood, 1986).

Summary of Twin and Adoption Findings

In review, twin and adoption studies have indicated that approximately 50% of the variance in risk for developing substance abuse and dependence can be explained by genetic factors (Gordis, 2000; Heath & Phil, 1995; Kendler, Neale, Heath, Kessler, & Eaves, 1994; Lumeng, Murphy, McBride, & Li, 1995). Recent studies have demonstrated that genetic factors account for a significant portion of variance in drug use, abuse, and dependence (e.g., see Bierut et al., 1998; Grove et al., 1990; Gynther, Carey, Gottesman, & Vogler, 1995; Kendler, Thornton, & Pedersen, 2000; Kendler, Prescott, Meyers, & Neale, 2003; Tsuang et al., 1996, 1998). In addition, the progression from initial use to abuse or dependence for marijuana and cocaine also appears to be largely due to genetic factors (Kendler & Prescott, 1998a, 1998b).

It is important to note that behavioral genetics research has shown that the effect of genetic factors on behavior can vary significantly across development. For example, a study of Finish twins found that genetics accounted for only 18% of the variance in drinking initiation at age 14. However, at age 16 genetic factors accounted for one third of the variability in drinking patterns, and by age 18 genetic factors accounted for half of the variability in drinking behavior (Rose, Dick, Viken, Pulkkinen, & Kaprio, 2001). These findings highlight the importance of considering developmental factors when studying genetic and environmental factors underlying substance use and abuse.

Common and Specific Genetic Risk

A number of genetic studies have examined common genetic and environmental factors influencing the vulnerability to substance use disorders. For example, a large population-based study of male twins found that the genetic and shared environmental effects on risk for the use and misuse of six classes of illicit substances (i.e., cannabis, cocaine, hallucinogens, sedatives, stimulants, and opiates) were largely or entirely nonspecific to any particular drug class. Unique environmental experiences were found to largely determine whether predisposed individuals will use or misuse one class of drugs or another (Kendler et al., 2003). A large twin study found support for a common genetic vulnerability model, influenced by both genetic and environmental factors, that cuts across various classes of illicit drugs. Specifically, results from the Harvard Twin Study of Substance Abuse revealed that between 50 and 85% of the vulnerability to drug use is common across different categories of illicit drugs (Tsuang, Bar, Harley, & Lyons, 2001).

Twin studies have also shown that common genetic factors may underlie the vulnerability to alcohol and drug dependence. The genetic correlation between alcohol and drug dependence was partially explained by the genetic risk both disorders share with adolescent conduct disorder (Button et al., 2007). An alternative conceptualization of this covariation is that conduct disorder represents an early, adolescent, manifestation of the same genetic loading that influences adult alcohol dependence later in life (Dick, Rose, & Kaprio, 2006). Genetic factors underlying alcohol and nicotine dependence were also found to overlap substantially (True et al., 1999). A large twin study investigating genetic and environmental risk factors underlying the comorbidity among 10 lifetime psychiatric disorders, including alcohol and drug dependence, concluded that the pattern of comorbidity between substance use disorders and other highly prevalent psychiatric disorders, such as mood and anxiety disorders, are largely due to common genetic risk factors (Kendler et al., 2003).

These results are generally consistent with clinical observations of high levels of comorbidity between alcohol and drug use disorders, addictions and conduct disorder in adolescence, and substance use disorders and mood/anxiety disorders in adulthood. Common genetic factors underlying the vulnerability to frequently comorbid disorders suggests that disorders that are correlated at the phenotypic level may be correlated at the genotypic level as well. It should be noted that studies have also identified genetic risk factors that are specific to a given addictive disorder, alcoholism being the most notable example (e.g., Edenberg & Foroud, 2006). Taken together, family, twin, and adoption study findings highlight the central role of environmental factors, such as drug availability, which are often required before any genetic and biological vulnerability can be phenotypically expressed. They also underscore something that clinicians are well aware of: the importance of environmental factors as determinants of human behavior.

Molecular Genetics of Addiction

After determining that genes play a substantial role in the etiology of addictive disorders through multiple family, twin, and adoption studies, the next step in genetics research often consists of identifying specific genes that contribute to the etiology of these disorders. In many ways, research on genetics of addiction has already transitioned from establishing that genetic variables contribute to the variance in a disorder to identifying the specific genetic variables that actually contribute to the disorder. Recent advances in technology have also driven this transition as scientists have unprecedented access to genetic data. It is only a matter of time before scientists will have information about the entire genome, or roughly 3 billion pieces of genetic code for any given individual.

Polygenetic and Multifactorial Genetic Transmission

When considering genetic factors underlying the vulnerability to addictions, it is important to consider the complexity of these behavioral phenotypes and reconsider traditional notions regarding modes of genetic transmission. Specifically, the single-gene inheritance mode of transmission does not apply to addictive disorders, or more broadly, to psychiatric disorders. To date, scientists have succeeded in unraveling the genetic basis of several disorders and examples of diseases with known genetic loci including cystic fibrosis, fragile-X syndrome, ocular albinisms, Huntington disease, and retinoblastoma. Over 5000 human conditions are known to be inherited in a single gene, Mendelian fashion. Understanding the concepts of Mendelian inheritance is certainly invaluable for grasping how scientists go about finding genes and provides a foundation for recognizing more complex modes of inheritance.

Despite the intuitive appeal and simplicity of the single-gene mode of inheritance, most psychiatric disorders, including addictions, are not caused by a single aberrant gene. Instead, complex disorders such as addictions are thought to be transmitted through a multifactorial polygenic model of inheritance, which proposes that a large, unspecified number of genes and environmental factors combine in an additive fashion to cause the disease. Importantly, these genetic and environmental factors can combine in an interactive or epistatic manner, which can complicate matters further. In short, addictive disorders clearly constitute disorders of complex genetics likely caused by multiple genetic factors, environmental factors, and their interactions, including gene × gene interactions, referred to as epistasis.

Phenotypes and Endophenotypes

Behavioral and clinical scientists are largely interested in the behavioral manifestation of a given disorder, namely a phenotype. The behavioral phenotypes used in many of the association studies (e.g., a diagnosis of drug abuse or dependence) are influenced by many different genetic, as well as environmental, components. Because there are so many different factors that influence whether an individual has a diagnosis of dependence, it is important to identify a specific and narrowly defined behavioral phenotype (i.e., intermediate phenotype or endophenotype) that is related to the larger disorder. A narrowly defined phenotype increases power to detect significant associations and facilitates the interpretation of the findings.

An ideal behavioral phenotype is one that is narrowly defined, readily identifiable, empirically related to the clinical manifestation of the disorder, related to an underlying biological mechanism, and theoretically related to a candidate gene.

Linkage and Association: An Overview

Two methodological approaches are commonly used in efforts to identify specific genes underlying vulnerability for psychiatric disorders: linkage and association studies. Linkage analysis consists of examining family pedigrees of affected individuals (i.e., probands) in order to find chromosomal regions that tend to be shared among affected relatives but not shared among unaffected relatives. In other words, linkage analysis finds genetic locations in the chromosome by showing that a genetic marker of known genetic location tends to be transmitted along with the disease within families. It is important to note that the transmission of the marker among affected relatives needs to be significantly greater than the transmission of the marker that is expected by chance. In genetics research "lod scores" are commonly used as a quantitative index of linkage such that higher scores indicate greater evidence of linkage. The classical critical lod score is 3 or higher.

Following linkage studies, which help identify chromosomal regions that may be involved in the disorder of interest, genetic association studies are often used to identify specific genes underlying the disorder or a disorder-related phenotype. Association studies take a "candidate gene" approach by examining the frequency of specific genotypes among cases (i.e., affected individuals) versus controls (i.e., unaffected individuals). Association studies seek to demonstrate that the frequency of the candidate gene of interest is higher among cases relative to controls, thereby supporting the hypothesis that the candidate gene may be associated with the disorder of interest. Association studies can be conducted in population-based samples as well as in family-based samples. Family-based association studies are thought to be less biased by potential ethnic differences between cases and controls, commonly referred to as "population stratification" effects. However, the relative impact of population stratification effects in association studies may not be as detrimental as initially thought (Hutchison, Stallings, McGeary, & Bryan, 2004). Recently, high-throughput methods have become available through "gene chip" technology, such that multiple markers can be examined concomitantly in a single association study, rather than testing one genetic marker at a time. There are now a number of centers that utilize high-throughput tools to genotype vast numbers of genetic markers in the hopes of establishing links between markers and behavioral disorders such as addictions. These methods are certainly promising and their main drawback is the lack of theoretical rationale for why and how certain genes may be associated with psychiatric disorders using high-throughput methods. In short, linkage and association studies are two of the most common genetic methods for identifying specific genes underlying the vulnerability for psychiatric disorders.

Linkage and Association: Brief Review of Findings

Studies to date have largely failed to identify specific genetic factors that contribute a large amount of variance in the risk for alcohol and drug dependence. There are several reasons why research to date has not identified specific genetic factors that contribute to the etiology of addictions. For example, in the alcohol field, despite the evidence for a strong genetic contribution to drinking behavior, it is highly unlikely that any one specific gene accounts for the development of alcohol dependence (e.g., Gordis, 2000; Kendler, Prescott, Neale, & Pedersen, 1997; Li, 2000; Reich et al., 1998; Schuckit, 1998). As discussed above, the behavioral phenotypes used in many of the association studies (e.g., a diagnosis of alcohol dependence) are highly heterogeneous and, as a result, are likely influenced by a multitude of genes as well as a multitude of environmental factors. As a result, investigations often lack the statistical power necessary for detecting an association. Another methodological limitation is that many genetic studies lack a strong a priori theoretical framework that infers a causal connection among a particular genetic factor, a biological mechanism, and a behavioral outcome.

Large studies designed to uncover genetic variation linked to alcohol and drug dependence have been underway for some time. A great example is the Consortium on Genetics of Alcoholism (COGA). This project started in 1989 with the primary goal of identifying specific genes underlying the vulnerability to alcohol dependence. The COGA project uses a family study design in which pedigrees from over 300 extended families densely affected by alcoholism were extensively assessed resulting in a rich dataset of clinical, neuropsychological, electrophysiological, biochemical, and genetic data (Begleiter et al., 1995). The COGA research group has published various papers linking genetic variation to alcohol dependence. Specifically, results from COGA have advanced the knowledge about genetics of alcoholism in many ways, including linkage and association findings.

Linkage analyses from the COGA project revealed that two of the most consistent loci for alcohol phenotypes were in chromosomes 4 and 7 (Dick, Jones, et al., 2006). Additionally, within these loci, important candidate genes have emerged. Some of the most notable genes associated with alcoholism and alcohol endophenotypes include the cluster of γ-aminobutric acid (GABA$_A$) receptors on chromosome 4q with specific genes including: GABRG1, GABRA2, GABRA4, and GABRB1 (Edenberg et al., 2004). One of the most consistent findings of this cluster is that of an association between polymorphisms within the GABRA2 gene and alcohol dependence, which has been replicated in independent samples (Covault, Gelernter, Hesselbrock, Nellissery, & Kranzler, 2004; Kranzler, Covault, Gelernter, & Nellissery, 2004; Xu et al., 2004).

Additionally, within chromosome 7, there was a linkage peak located directly at a muscarinic cholinergic receptor gene (CHRM2) thought to be involved in processes such as cognition and memory. Follow-up association studies found a significant relationship between multiple single nucleotide polymorphisms (SNPs) in the CHRM2 gene and both alcohol dependence and major depression (Wang et al., 2004). However, the risk alleles differed for each disorder suggesting evidence of common and specific genetic effects on both disorders. It is only a matter of time before the COGA group has examined all of the genetic variation. To many, it might seem that uncovering genetic variation linked to alcohol dependence is the endgame. In truth, it is only the beginning. Once genetic variants that are associated with addiction are identified, the focus of research will shift to unraveling how the variation influences the course of addiction and scientists will also need to consider how this information might be used. Several molecular studies are currently underway to unravel the functional significance of genetic variation in many of the candidate genes identified by the COGA group (e.g., GABRA2) in order to understand how specific genetic variation may be involved in the predisposition to alcohol dependence and related alcohol endophenotypes (Dick, Jones et al., 2006).

Large studies of the genetics of drug abuse are also currently in place, including the National Institute on Drug Abuse (NIDA) Genetics Consortium. There are also many smaller studies that have examined specific genetic markers that might be involved in addiction. For example, in a review of the literature on candidate genes for nicotine dependence, there was considerable focus on genes involved in the dopaminergic reward pathway, such as genes involved in dopamine synthesis (e.g., tyrosine hydroxylase; TH), receptor activation (e.g., dopamine receptors DRD1-DRD5), dopamine reuptake (dopamine transporter; DAT1), and dopamine metabolism (e.g., Catechol-o-methultransferase COMT; dopamine β-hydroxylase DBH) (see Rossing, 1998).

There is considerable overlap in candidate genes for various substance use disorders. For example, similar polymorphisms such as those of the dopamine receptor genes, and COMT have been examined for their association with opioid dependence, and the DBH gene and dopamine receptor genes have been extensively examined as genetic determinants of cocaine dependence (see Saxon, Oreskovich, & Brkanac, 2005). Likewise, a functional polymorphism of the μ-opioid receptor (OPRM1) gene coding for an amino acid change from asparagine to aspartic acid (A118G SNP) has received considerable attention as a candidate gene for addictive disorders such as opioid and cocaine dependence (Schinka et al., 2002; Tan, Tan, Karupathivan, & Yap, 2003), alcoholism (e.g., Kranzler, Gelernter, O'Malley, Hernandez-Avila, & Kaufman, 1998; Schinka et al., 2002; Town et al., 1999), and alcohol sensitivity (Ray & Hutchison, 2004), an alcohol endophenotype. This polymorphism has been shown to affect receptor activity for endogenous ligand β-endorphin, such that the Asp40 variant binds β-endorphin three times stronger than the Asn40 allele (Bond et al., 1998); however, a more recent study suggested that this polymorphism may have deleterious effects on mRNA and protein yield (Zhang, Wang, Johnson, Papp, & Sadée, 2005). In short, molecular studies have shown that this polymorphism is functional, which strengthens its rationale as a possible candidate gene for addictive behaviors.

In summary, association studies examining the significance of individual genes to the diagnostic phenotypes of substance use disorders and/or endophenotypes for those disorders have generally examined candidate genes thought to underlie the pathophysiology of addictions. Although there are too many association studies to be reviewed in this chapter, the present findings describe the general approach taken in genetic association studies of addictions. It is important to note that the findings of association studies to date are largely inconclusive and marked by multiple failures to replicate reported associations, especially associations with diagnostic phenotypes. As recently articulated by Dick, Jones, and colleagues (2006), endophenotypes have led to more successful gene identification for alcoholism in the COGA study and offer a promising approach to candidate gene studies on addictions.

Elucidating the Pathways Between Genes and Behavior

As noted previously, the focus of research is likely to shift from identifying which genetic variables contribute to addiction to how those variants contribute to addiction. A change in the genetic code does not lead directly to a change in behavior. In fact, a change in the genetic

FIGURE 6.2
Translational model for how genetic variability may influence human behavior.

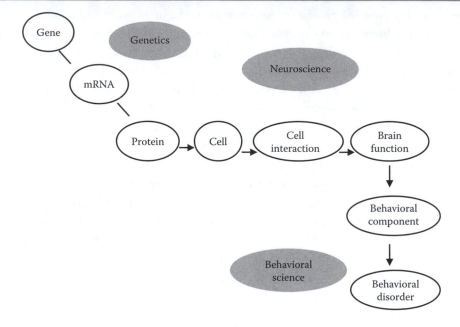

code leads to a molecular change in mRNA, or the protein for which it codes, or a change in the amount of protein that is produced. In turn, these molecular changes lead to changes in the function of cells, and changes in how cells interact. Further downstream, these changes alter brain function and specific behavioral components that then contribute to the overall risk for addiction (Figure 6.2). The neurobiology of addiction is further complicated by the fact that it is likely that the interaction of genetic variation and repeated exposure to psychoactive drugs is responsible for altering the neurobiological factors, such as the interaction of cells and brain function which in turn may contribute to addiction. Thus, it is not a simple unidirectional model.

For example, genetic variation might accelerate the process by which drugs of abuse hijack the reward and craving circuitry in the brain. Specifically, the incentive salience and craving model of addiction posit that activation along mesolimbic dopamine substrates is critical to the development of the motivational and appetitive properties of tobacco, alcohol, and other drugs (e.g., Berridge & Robinson, 2003; Robinson & Berridge, 1993, 2001). Thus, incentive salience (i.e., craving) for substances of abuse is produced by repeated drug/alcohol ingestion and the associated release of dopamine. Genetic factors may operate in conjunction with repeated alcohol or drug exposure leading to differential incentive salience or craving among individuals with certain genetic predispositions. As an example, variation in a dopamine receptor (DRD4) gene has been associated with differential craving response to alcohol and nicotine in previous laboratory studies (Hutchison, LaChance, Niaura, Bryan, & Smolen, 2002; Hutchison, McGeary, Smolen, Bryan, & Swift, 2002; MacKillop, Mengen, McGeary, & Lisman, 2007).

It also seems likely that genetic variation may accelerate, or alternatively, protect against the changes that are posited to underlie allostatic processes in the brain's stress pathways that result from alcohol use and withdrawal and ultimately contribute to alcohol dependence. In the allostatic model of dependence (Koob, 2003; Koob & LeMoal, 2001, 2005), the development of alcohol dependence is characterized as an allostatic process that involves changes in reward and stress circuits that become dysregulated with repeated exposure to alcohol. This process putatively involves alterations of corticotrophin-releasing factor (CRF) and neuropeptide Y (NPY) in the central nucleus of the amygdala and bed nucleus of the stria terminalis. In turn, these changes confer vulnerability to relapse among alcohol-dependent patients. Interestingly, polymorphisms in the neuropeptide Y (NPY) gene have been associated with alcohol dependence in humans (e.g., Mottagui-Tabar et al., 2005) and in multiple animal models of alcohol addiction. In short, this is a demonstration of how genetic markers may be involved in specific neurobiological processes relevant to addictions. It is important to note that integrating genetic findings into such models may elucidate the specific mechanisms by which genetic variation ultimately influences one's vulnerability to addiction.

There are certainly many different possibilities for how genetic variation may underlie the risk of addiction at a behavioral level. As another example, genetic variation that contributes to variability in behavioral expressions of impulsivity, risk-taking, and stress responsivity may lead to early experimentation with drugs. As articulated by Kreek, Nielsen, Butelman, and LaForge (2005), physiological and personality factors may have differential effects on the various stages of addiction. To that end, understanding genetic variation leading to individual differences in personality constructs may be relevant to unravel the genetic risk for addiction. In summary, there are many pathways through which genetic variation may contribute to addiction processes. The studies reviewed herein provide an overview of how research on genetics of addiction seeks to understand the specific pathways by which genetic variation may come to influence complex behaviors such as substance use and abuse.

Gene × Environment Interactions

An important conceptual issue that only recently began to materialize in genetics research of addictions is that of gene by environment interactions. Twin and adoption models consider genes and environment as latent constructs (i.e., not measured constructs) whereas molecular studies examine genes as observed or measured constructs. However, few studies operationalize the environment and examine how specific environmental factors may come to interact with genetic polymorphisms to produce a given clinical outcome or behavior. For example, marital status and religiosity have been found to attenuate the effects of additive genetics on alcohol use (Heath, Eaves, & Martin, 1998; Koopmans, Slutske, van Baal, & Boomsma, 1999). Likewise, recent results from the COGA project revealed that marital status moderates the effects of the GABRA2 genotype on alcohol dependence, such that the effects of genotype were magnified among individuals who were married (Dick, Agrawal et al., 2006). The authors hypothesize that genetic risk for alcoholism may become more salient among individuals in a lower risk environment (i.e., those stably married). In short, research on gene by environment interactions is in its initial stages and much work has yet to be done in order to translate the elusive, and most often latent, construct of "environment" into meaningful operational definitions that can in turn elucidate specific risk mechanisms and hence treatment alternatives for addictive disorders.

Addiction Treatment and Genetics

Basic research on the human genome is progressing at a rapid pace and investigations of genetic factors that influence the development, expression, and treatment of alcohol and drug dependence is one of the most promising areas of research in addictions. This is a significant development in the field of addictions because many believe that genetic information will eventually be used to "individualize" or "personalize" treatment. It is only a matter of time (albeit, perhaps, a long time) before most of the genes that contribute to the risk for addiction are uncovered, and likewise, only a matter of time before clinicians begin to utilize genetic information to match individuals with the treatment that is most likely to benefit them.

Pharmacogenetics: An Overview

Pharmacogenetics is a field of research that seeks to understand individual differences in the metabolism and efficacy of drugs. Specifically, pharmacogenetics research focuses on identifying genetic factors that account for variability in pharmacotherapy effects, both in terms of pharmacodymamic and efficacy (Evans & Johnson, 2001). The field of pharmacogenetics has grown rapidly and has greatly benefited from advancements in molecular genetic tools for identifying gene polymorphisms, developments in bioinformatics and functional genomics, and new findings from the human genome project (Evans & Johnson, 2001). The foremost goal of this line of research is to optimize drug therapy by identifying genetic factors that predict who is more likely to respond to certain pharmacotherapies and who will not respond, therefore matching patients to medications on the basis of genetic factors.

Genetic factors can account for individual differences in drug toxicity and response in many ways. Genetic polymorphisms may lead to functional differences in drug metabolism and disposition, such as functional differences in enzyme activity or drug transporters. Alternatively, genetic polymorphisms may affect the target of a drug, such as a particular receptor. An example of the first case is a polymorphism of the CYP2D6 gene, which is involved in the availability of specific drug-metabolizing enzymes associated with one's response to opioid pain killers, such as codeine or morphine. Individuals who are homozygous for the nonfunctional CYP2D6 alleles have been found to be resistant to the analgesic effects of opioid pain killers (e.g., Poulsen et al., 1996). On the other hand, genetic polymorphisms involved in the drug target may also affect one's response to pharmacotherapy. For example, polymorphisms of the dopamine receptor gene (DRD4) have been associated with differential response to antipsychotic medications (e.g., Cohen et al., 1999).

Pharmacogenetics of Addictions

A few studies to date have investigated genetic polymorphisms in the context of pharmacotherapies for alcohol and cocaine dependence. One of such studies has found that a polymorphism of the OPRM1 was associated with clinical response to naltrexone among alcohol-dependent patients (Oslin et al., 2003). The relationship was such that individuals with at least one copy of the variant allele that codes for more potent μ-opioid receptors (the A to G substitution) showed lower relapse rates and longer time to return to heavy drinking when treated with naltrexone, an opioid antagonist (Oslin et al., 2003). More recently, a double-blind placebo-controlled laboratory trial of naltrexone (50 mg) suggested that individuals who were carriers of the G allele of the OPRM1 gene showed significantly greater naltrexone-induced blunting of alcohol "high," as compared to individuals who were homozygous for the A allele (Ray & Hutchison, 2007). These findings suggest that the differential clinical response to naltrexone may be due to differential blunting of alcohol-induced reward as a function of genotype and propose a mechanism for this important pharmacogenetic relationship.

A series of pharmacogenetic studies have tested the association between olanzapine, a medication that targets dopamine receptors, alcohol craving, and a polymorphism of the dopamine D4 receptor (DRD4 VNTR; Hutchison, McGeary et al., 2002; Hutchison et al., 2003, 2006). One study has found an association between the long allele of the DRD4 VNTR polymorphism with increased craving for alcohol after a priming dose of alcohol (Hutchison, McGeary et al., 2002). Another study has found that olanzapine decreases craving after a priming dose of alcohol in a nonclinical sample of college drinkers (Hutchison et al., 2003). Finally, results from a recent clinical trial revealed that the efficacy of olanzapine in the treatment of alcohol dependence was moderated by the DRD4 VNTR SNP, such that individuals with at least one copy of the long allele showed greater reductions in cue-elicited craving and greater decreases in alcohol consumption during the 12-week clinical trial, as compared to individuals who were homozygous for the short allele (Hutchison et al., 2006). Taken together, these series of laboratory and clinical trials have established a relationship among a polymorphism of the D4 receptor gene (DRD4), craving for alcohol in the laboratory, and response to a medication that targets dopamine receptors. More recently, animal research has suggested that genetic variation in the dopamine beta-hydroxylase (DBH) gene was associated with differential response to disulfiran (Antabuse®), a DBH inhibitor (Bordelat-Parks et al., 2005; Schank et al., 2006). This is especially relevant given that disulfiran has shown promise as a pharmacoptherapy for cocaine dependence and these findings are consistent with the putative role of the dopaminergic system in addictions.

Translational approaches such as these have the potential to inform clinical practice by identifying individuals who are more likely to benefit from a given pharmacotherapy on the basis of genetic factors. At present, efforts at optimizing pharmacotherapy on the basis of genetic factors, often referred to as personalized medicine, are in their initial stages and considerable research is required before these findings can be translated into clinical practice. Important issues such as the differential frequency of certain gene variants among various ethnic groups and the clinical significance of these differential treatment responses must be evaluated carefully in future pharmacogenetic trials and before translating these findings to clinical practice. Nevertheless, research efforts such as these hold considerable promise for optimizing treatment for a host of disorders, including addictions.

Clinical Implications

There are a number of implications for clinical practice that can be drawn from the current knowledge of genetics of addictions. As clinicians we can learn a lot about the psychiatric conditions of our patients by knowing which disorders affect their family members. As articulated by Faraone, Tsuang, and Tsuang (1999), family-based diagnosis can be useful especially in terms of answering complex diagnostic questions. For example, when making a differential diagnosis, knowledge of a family history may be informative, particularly when diagnostic data are scarce. A clear diagnosis in a family member may provide clues to the nature of an ambiguous or atypical disorder presentation in a relative. This approach may be particularly useful when making diagnostic decisions regarding substance-induced psychiatric disorders and when disentangling comorbidity issues between substance use disorders and other *DSM–IV* axis I disorders. Using valid and reliable measures for assessing family history of psychiatric problems may be especially useful in such endeavors. Some of the empirically supported assessments for family history include semistructured interviews such as (1) the Family History Assessment Module (FHAM; Bucholz et al., 1994) used by the COGA; (2) the Family History Research Diagnostic Criteria (FHRDC; Andreasen, Endicott, Spitzer, & Winokur, 1977); and (3) the National Institute of Mental Health (NIMH) Genetics Initiative's Family Interview for Genetic Studies (Nurnberger et al., 1994).

In addition to the assessment issues discussed above, clinicians who are informed in psychiatric genetics are in a unique position to provide patients with psychoeducation about the role of genes and environment and the etiology of addictive disorders. This knowledge can be used to affect the therapeutic process of change and to help patients make sense of genetic information as it becomes available in the media, which can often lead patients and families to develop misconceptions about the role of genetics in the etiology of addictions. Perhaps one of the most powerful of such misconceptions is what Paul Meehl called "therapeutic nihilism," which is the notion that only biological treatments can help individuals affected by a biological or genetic disorder. Psychoeducation represents an important clinical tool for addressing those issues, which often inhibit psychosocial treatment engagement and recovery. Specifically, clinicians can engage patients in a discussion of levels of vulnerability, the role of the environment, the patient's role in treatment and recovery, and the polygenic multifactorial model of inheritance thought to explain the transmission of complex disorders such as substance abuse and dependence.

Lastly, patients presenting for addictions treatment often believe they have "an addictive personality" or "the addictive gene." Such beliefs may inhibit the patient's ability to develop a sense of self-efficacy for coping with high-risk situations, and more broadly, for recovering from an addiction. Clinicians who are familiar with evidence-based psychiatric genetics are well positioned to educate patients on the complex nature of their disorder and may integrate knowledge of genetics of addiction into their case conceptualization, particularly in the context of the biopsychosocial model of psychiatric disorders.

Limitations and Future Directions

The field of genetics of addiction has certainly progressed rapidly over the past decade, largely fueled by advances in the understanding of the human genome. However, a number of challenges remain for researchers in psychiatric genetics. One of the largest challenges is to start to put together the pieces of the puzzle and to more clearly delineate the specific risk associated with particular genes in conjunction with the environment and developmental considerations

(Dick, Rose, et al., 2006). Otherwise, we may end up with a series of genotypes that are associated with intermediate phenotypes which cannot be tied to the development or treatment of addictions. The issue of developmental and environmental considerations is hugely important as it may explain some of the inconsistencies in association findings and gene identification for specific disorders. Gene × environment and gene × gene interactions continue to challenge researchers to integrate large amounts of information in order to capture the full and complex picture of substance use disorders. The field of psychiatric genetics has certainly come a long way, and yet has a long road ahead. Ultimately, research on genetics of addiction holds tremendous promise to significantly enhance our understanding of the development, maintenance, and treatment of addictive disorders.

References

Andreasen, N., Endicott, J., Spitzer, R., & Winokur, G. (1977). The family history method using diagnostic criteria. *Archives General Psychiatry, 34,* 1229–1235.

Begleiter, H., Reich, T., Hesselbrock, V., Projesz, B., Li, T. K., Schuckit, M., et al. (1995). The collaborative study on the genetics of alcoholism. *Alcohol Health and Research World, 19,* 228–236.

Berridge, K. C., & Robinson, T. E. (2003). Parsing reward. *Trends in Neuroscience, 26,* 507–513.

Bierut, L. J., Dinwiddie, S. H., Begleiter, H., Crowe, R., Hesselbrock, V., Nurnberger, J. I., et al. (1998). Familial transmission of substance dependence: Alcohol, marijuana, cocaine, and habitual smoking. *Archives of General Psychiatry, 55,* 982–988.

Bond, C., LaForge, K. S., Tian, M., Melia, D., Zhang, S., Borg, L., et al. (1998). Single-nucleotide polymorphism in the human mu opioid receptor gene alters β-endorphin binding and activity: Possible implications for opiate addiction. *Neurobiology, 95,* 9608–9613.

Bourdelat-Parks, B. N., Anderson, G. M., Donaldson, Z. R., Weiss, J. M., Bonsall, R. W., Emery, M. S., et al. (2005). Effects of dopamine beta-hydroxylase genotype and disulfiram inhibition on catecholamine homeostasis in mice. *Psychopharmacology, 183,* 72–80.

Bucholz, K. K., Cadoret, R., Cloninger, C. R., Dinwiddie, S. H., Hesselbrock, V. M., Nurnberger, J. I., Jr, et al., (1994). A new, semi-structured psychiatric interview for use in genetic linkage studies: A report on the reliability of the SSAGA. *Journal of Studies on Alcohol, 55,* 149–158.

Button, T. M., Rhee, S. H., Hewitt, J. K., Young, S. E., Corley, R. P., & Stallings, M. C. (2007). The role of conduct disorder in explaining the comorbidity between alcohol and illicit drug dependence in adolescence. *Drug and Alcohol Dependence, 87,* 46–53.

Cadoret, R. J., Troughton, E., O'Gorman, T. W., & Heywood, E. (1986). An adoption study of genetic and environmental factors in drug abuse. *Archives of General Psychiatry, 43,* 1131–1136.

Cheng, L. S., Swan, G. E., & Carmelli, D. (2000). A genetic analysis of smoking behavior in family members of older adult males. *Addiction, 95,* 427–435.

Cohen, B. M., Ennulat, D. J., Centorrino, F., Matthysse, S., Konieczna, H., Chu, H. M., et al. (1999). Polymorphisms of the dopamine D4 receptor and response to antipsychotic drugs. *Psychopharmacology, 141,* 6–10.

Cotton, N. S. (1979). The familial incidence of alcoholism: A review. *Journal of Studies on Alcohol, 40,* 89–116.

Covault, J., Gelernter, J., Hesselbrock, V., Nellissery, M., & Kranzler, H. R. (2004). Allelic and haplotypic association of GABRA2 with alcohol dependence. *American Journal of Medical Genetics, 129B,* 104–109.

Dick, D. M., Agrawal, A., Schuckit, M., Bierut, L., Fox, L., Mullaney, J., et al. (2006). Marital status, alcohol dependence, and GABRA2: Evidence for gene-environment correlation and interaction. *Journal of Studies on Alcohol, 67,* 185–194.

Dick, D. M., Jones, K., Saccone, N., Hinrichs, A., Wang, J. C., Goate, A., et al. (2006). Endophenotypes successfully lead to gene identification: Results from the Collaborative Study on the Genetics of Alcoholism. *Behavior Genetics, 36,* 112–126.

Dick, D. M., Rose, R. J., & Kaprio, J. (2006). The next challenge for psychiatric genetics: Characterizing the risk associated with identified genes. *Annals of Clinical Psychiatry, 18,* 223–231.

Edenberg, H. J., Dick, D. M., Xuei, X., Tian, H., Almasy, L., Bauer, L. O., et al. (2004). Variations in GABRA2, encoding the alpha 2 subunit of the GABA(A) receptor, are associated with alcohol dependence and with brain oscillations. *American Journal of Human Genetics, 74,* 705–714.

Edenberg, H. J., & Foroud, T. (2006). The genetics of alcoholism: Identifying specific genes through family studies. *Addiction Biology, 11,* 386–396.

Evans, W. E. & Johnson, J. A. (2001). Pharmacogenomics: The inherited basis for interindividual differences in drug response. *Annual Review of Genomics and Human Genetics, 2,* 9–39.

Faraone, S. V., Tsuang, M. T., & Tsuang, D. W. (1999). *Genetics of mental disorders: What practitioners and students need to know.* New York: Guildford Press.

Gordis, E. (2000). Contributions of behavioral science to alcohol research: Understanding who is at risk and why. *Experimental and Clinical Psychopharmacology, 8,* 264–270.

Grove, W. M., Eckert, E. D., Heston, L., Bouchard, T. J., Segal, N., & Lykken, D. T. (1990). Heritability of substance abuse and antisocial behavior: A study of monozygotic twins reared apart. *Biological Psychiatry, 27,* 1293–1304.

Gynther, L. M., Carey, G., Gottesman, I. I., & Vogler, G. P. (1995). A twin study of non-alcohol substance abuse. *Psychiatry Research, 56,* 213–220.

Heath, A. C., Eaves, L. J., & Martin, N. G. (1998). Interaction of marital status and genetic risk for symptoms of depression. *Twin Research, 1,* 119–122.

Heath, A. C., & Phil, D. (1995). Genetic influences on alcoholism risk: A review of adoption and twin studies. *Alcohol Health & Research World, 19,* 166–171.

Heath, A. C., Slutske, W. S., & Madden, P. A. F. (1997). Gender differences in the genetic contribution to alcoholism risk and to alcohol consumption patterns. In R. W. Wilsnack & S. C. Wilsnack (Eds.), *Gender and Alcohol: Vol. 3. Alcohol, culture, and social control monograph series* (pp. 114–119). New Brunswick, NJ: Rutgers University Press.

Hopfer, C. J., Stallings, M. C., Hewitt, J. K., & Crowley, T. J. (2003). Family transmission of marijuana use, abuse, and dependence. *Journal of the American Academy of Child and Adolescent Psychiatry, 42,* 834–841.

Hutchison, K. E., LaChance, H., Niaura, R., Bryan, A. D., & Smolen, A. (2002). The DRD4 VNTR polymorphism influences reactivity to smoking cues. *Journal of Abnormal Psychology, 111,* 134–143.

Hutchison, K. E., McGeary, J., Smolen, A., Bryan, A., & Swift, R. M. (2002). The DRD4 VNTR polymorphism moderates craving after alcohol consumption. *Health Psychology, 21,* 139–146.

Hutchison, K. E., Ray, L. A., Sandman, E., Rutter, M. C., Peters, A., & Swift, R. (2006). The effect of olanzapine on craving and alcohol consumption. *Neuropsychopharmacology, 31,* 1310–1317.

Hutchison, K. E., Stallings, M., McGeary, J., & Bryan, A. (2004). Population stratification in the candidate gene study: Fatal threat or red herring? *Psychological Bulletin, 130,* 66–79.

Hutchison, K. E., Wooden, A., Swift, R. M., Smolen, A., McGeary, J., & Adler, L. (2003). Olanzapine reduces craving for alcohol: A DRD4 VNTR polymorphism by pharmacotherapy interaction. *Neuropsychopharmacology, 28,* 1882–1888.

Kendler, K. S., Neale, M. C., Heath, A. C., Kessler, R. C., & Eaves, L. J. (1994). A twin-family study of alcoholism in women. *American Journal of Psychiatry, 151,* 707–715.

Kendler, K. S., & Prescott, C. A. (1998a). Cannabis use, abuse, and dependence in a population-based sample of female twins. *American Journal of Psychiatry, 155,* 1016–22.

Kendler, K. S., & Prescott, C. A. (1998b). Cocaine use, abuse and dependence in a population-based sample of female twins. *The British Journal of Psychiatry: The Journal of Mental Science, 173,* 345–350.

Kendler, K. S., Prescott, C. A., Meyers, J., & Neale, M. C. (2003). The structure of genetic and environmental risk factors for common psychiatric and substance use disorders in men and women. *Archives of General Psychiatry, 60,* 929–937.

Kendler, K. S., Prescott, C. A., Neale, M. C., & Pedersen, N. L. (1997). Temperance board registration for alcohol abuse in a national sample of Swedish male twins, born 1902 to 1949. *Archives of General Psychiatry, 54,* 178–184.

Kendler, K. S., Thornton, L. M., & Pedersen, N. L. (2000). Tobacco consumption in Swedish twins reared apart and reared together. *Archives of General Psychiatry, 57,* 886–892.

Koob, G. F. (2003). Neuroadaptive mechanisms of addiction: Studies on the extended amygdale [Special issue: Neuropsychopharmacology of Addiction]. *European Neuropsychopharmacology, 13,* 442–452.

Koob, G. F., & LeMoal, M. (2001). Drug addiction, dysregulation of reward, and allostasis. *Neuropsychopharmacology, 24,* 97–129.

Koob, G. F., & LeMoal, M. (2005). Plasticity of reward neurocircuitry and the 'dark side' of drug addiction. *Nature Neuroscience, 8,* 1442–1444.

Koopmans, J. R., Slutske, W. S., van Baal, G. C. M., & Boomsma, D. I. (1999). The influence of religion on alcohol use initiation: Evidence for genotype x environment interaction. *Behavior Genetics, 29,* 445–453.

Kranzler, H. R., Covault, J., Gelernter, J., & Nellissery, M. (2004). Allelic and haplotypic association of GABA alpha-2 gene with alcohol dependence. *Alcoholism: Clinical and Experimental Research, 28,* 49A.

Kranzler, H. R., Gelernter, J., O'Malley, S., Hernandez-Avila, C. A., & Kaufman, D. (1998). Association of alcohol or other drug dependence with alleles of the μ opioid receptor gene (OPRM1). *Alcoholism: Clinical and Experimental Research, 22*(6), 1359–1362.

Kreek, M. J., Nielsen, D. A., Butelman, E. R., & LaForge, K. S. (2005). Genetic influences on impulsivity, risk taking, stress responsivity and vulnerability to drug abuse and addiction. *Nature Neuroscience, 8,* 1450–1457.

Li, T. K. (2000). Pharmacogenetics of responses to alcohol and genes that influence alcohol drinking. *Journal of Studies on Alcohol, 61,* 5–12.

Lumeng, L., Murphy, J. M., McBride, W. J., & Li, T. K. (1995). Genetic influences on alcohol preference in animals. In H. Begleiter & B. Kissin (Eds.), *The genetics of alcoholism* (pp. 165–201). New York: Oxford University Press.

MacKillop, J., Menges, D. P., McGeary, J. E., & Lisman, S. A. (2007). Effects of craving and DRD4 VNTR genotype on the relative value of alcohol: An initial human laboratory study. *Behavioral and Brain Functions, 3,* 11.

McGue, M. (1999). Behavioral genetic models of alcoholism and drinking. In K. E. Leonard & H. T. Blane (Eds.), *Psychological theories of drinking and alcoholism* (pp. 372–421). New York: Guildford Press.

McGue, M., Pickens, R. W., & Svikis, D. S. (1992). Sex and age effects on the inheritance of alcohol problems: A twin study. *Journal of Abnormal Psychology, 101,* 3–17.

Merikangas, K. R., Stolar, M., Stevens, D. E., Goulet, J., Preisig, M., Fenton, B., et al. (1998). Familial transmission of substance use disorders. *Archives of General Psychiatry, 55,* 973–979.

Mottagui-Tabar, S., Prince, J. A., Wahlestedt, C., Zhu, G., Goldman, D., & Heilig, M. (2005). A novel single nucleotide polymorphism of the neuropeptide Y (NPY) gene associated with alcohol dependence. *Alcoholism: Clinical and Experimental Research, 29,* 702–707.

Nurnberger, J. I., Jr, Blehar, M. C., Kaufmann, C. A., York-Cooler, C., Simpson, S. G., Harkavy-Friedman J., et al. (1994). Diagnostic interview for genetic studies. Rationale, unique features, and training. NIMH Genetics Initiative. *Archives of General Psychiatry 51,* 849–859.

Oslin, D. W., Berrettini, W., Kranzler, H. R., Pettinati, H., Gelernter, J., Volpicelli, J. R., et al. (2003). A functional polymorphism of the mu-opioid receptor gene is associated with naltrexone response in alcohol-dependent patients. *Neuropsychopharmacology, 28,* 1546–1552.

Poulsen, L., Brosen, K., Arendt-Nielsen, L., Gram, L. F., Elbaek, K., & Sindrup, S. H. (1996). Codeine and morphine in extensive and poor metabolizers of sparteine: Pharmacokinetics, analgesic effect and side effects. *European Journal of Clinical Pharmacology, 51,* 289–295.

Ray, L., & Hutchison, K. E. (2004). A polymorphism of the μ-opioid receptor gene (OPRM1) and sensitivity to the effects of alcohol in humans. *Alcoholism Clinical and Experimental Research, 28,* 1789–1795.

Ray, L. A., & Hutchison, K. E. (2007). A double-blind placebo-controlled study of the effects of naltrexone on alcohol sensitivity and genetic moderators of medication response. *Archives of General Psychiatry, 64,* 1069–1077.

Reich, T., Edenberg, H. J., Goate, A., Williams, J. T., Rice, J. P., Van Eerdewegh, P., et al. (1998). Genome-wide search for genes affecting the risk for alcohol dependence. *American Journal of Medical Genetic, 81,* 207–215.

Robinson, T. E., & Berridge, K. C. (1993). The neural basis of drug craving: An incentive sensitization theory of addiction. *Brain Research. Brain Research Reviews, 18,* 247–291.

Robinson, T. E., & Berridge, K. C. (2001). Incentive-sensitization and addiction. *Addiction, 96,* 103–114.

Rose, R. J., Dick, D. M., Viken, R. J., Pulkkinen, L., & Kaprio, J. (2001). Drinking or abstaining at age 14: A genetic epidemiological study. *Alcoholism: Clinical and Experimental Research, 25,* 637–643.

Rossing, M. A. (1998). Genetic influences on smoking: Candidate genes. *Environmental Health Perspectives, 106,* 231–238.

Saxon, A. J., Oreskovich, M. R., & Brkanac, Z. (2005). Genetic determinants of addictions to opioids and cocaine. *Harvard Review of Psychiatry, 13,* 218–232.

Schank, J. R., Ventura, R., Puglisi-Allegra, S., Alcaro, A., Cole, C. D., Liles, L. C., et al. (2006). Dopamine beta-hydroxylase knockout mice have alterations in dopamine signaling and are hypersensitive to cocaine. *Neuropsychopharmacology, 31,* 2221–2230.

Schinka, J. A., Town, T., Abdullah, L., Crawford, F. C., Ordorica, P. I., Francis, E., et al. (2002). A functional polymporphism within the μ-opioid receptor gene and risk for abuse of alcohol and other substances. *Molecular Psychiatry, 7,* 224–228.

Schuckit, M. A. (1998). Biological, psychological and environmental predictors of the alcoholism risk: A longitudinal study. *Journal of Studies on Alcohol, 59,* 485–494.

Tan, E., Tan, C., Karupathivan, U., & Yap, E. P. H. (2003). Mu opioid receptor gene polymorphisms and heroin dependence in Asian populations. *Neuroreport, 14,* 569–572.

Town, T., Abdullah, L., Crawford, F., Schinka, J., Ordorica, P. I., Francis, E., et al. (1999). Association of a functional μ-opioid receptor allele (+ 118A) with alcohol dependency. *American Journal of Medical Genetics, 88,* 458–461.

True, W. R., Xian, H., Scherrer, J. F., Madden, P. A. F., Bucholz, K. K., Heath, A. C., et al. (1999). Common genetic vulnerability for nicotine and alcohol dependence in men. *Archives of General Psychiatry, 56,* 655–661.

Tsuang, M. T., Bar, J. L., Harley, R. M., & Lyons, M. J. (2001). The Harvard twin study of substance abuse: What we have learned. *Harvard Review of Psychiatry, 9,* 267–279.

Tsuang, M. T., Lyons, M. J., Eisen, S. A., Goldberg, J., True, W., Lin, N., et al. (1996). Genetic influences on the DSM-III-R drug abuse and dependence: A study of 3,372 twin pairs. *American Journal of Medical Genetics, 67,* 473–477.

Tsuang, M. T., Lyons, M. J., Meyer, J. M., Doyle, T., Eisen, S. A., Goldberg, J., et al. (1998). Co-occurrence of abuse of different drugs in men: The role of drug-specific and shared vulnerabilities. *Archive of General Psychiatry, 55,* 967–972.

Wang, J. C., Hinrichs, A. L., Stock, H. l., Budde, J., Allen, R., Bertelsen, S., et al. (2004). Evidence of common and specific genetic effects: Association of the muscarinic acetylcholine receptor M2 (CHRM2) gene with alcohol dependence and major depressive syndrome. *Human Molecular Genetics, 13,* 1903–1922.

Xu, K., Westly, E., Aubman, J., Astor, W., Lipsky, R. H., & Goldman, D. (2004). Linkage disequilibrium relationships among GABRA cluster genes located on chromosome 4 with alcohol dependence in two populations. *Alcoholism: Clinical and Experimental Research, 28,* 48A.

Zhang, Y., Wang, D., Johnson, A. D., Papp, A. C., & Sadée, W. (2005). Allelic expression imbalance of human mu opioid receptor (OPRM1) caused by variant A118G. *The Journal of Biological Chemistry, 280,* 32618–32624.

Part II

Conceptual Models and Principles of Substance Abuse Treatment

Frank L. Collins
University of North Texas

Introduction

This section of the book focuses on broad conceptual models and how these models can be applied to the assessment and treatment of substance use problems. It begins with an overview of current perspectives on evidence-based practice and includes chapters on individual and group treatment, community reinforcement models and prevention.

Chapter 7 emphasizes the critical components of evidence-based practice. Collins, Leffingwell, Callahan, and Cohen point out that evidence-based practice involves the integration of the best available research evidence with clinical expertise and patient values. This chapter provides a cautionary note to readers who mistakenly link evidence-based practice to empirically supported procedures and provides a strong rationale as to why the other components are critical for understanding the best assessment and treatment approaches.

Peirce, King, and Brooner highlight the need for individualized treatment in Chapter 8. They point out the disconnect between treatment of most mental health problems and the treatment of individuals with substance use disorders. This chapter highlights the effectiveness of individualized treatments as well as providing much needed information about factors commonly used for treating other mental health problems that may need to be modified for effective treatment of individuals with substance use disorders. They provide a detailed discussion of adaptive treatment strategies as the "next wave" of therapy for substance use disorders.

Chapter 9 (Morrell and Myers) focuses on group therapy, which is the most frequently used form of psychotherapy for treating individuals with substance use disorders. The chapter provides an introduction to group treatment by highlighting many of the factors which influence the manner in which groups are formed and the methods used. Finally, the authors provide a review of the treatment effectiveness literature for group therapy.

In Chapter 10, Gianini, Lundy, and Smith provide a detailed conceptual model based on the community reinforcement approach (CRA) to the assessment and treatment of substance use disorders. This form of therapy is discussed in terms of the conceptual background and methods used for implementing community reinforcement. One of the most unique aspects of this approach is the focus on the family members of individuals with substance use disorders. This approach (Community Reinforcement and Family Training, CRAFT) emphasizes the need to include other members of the client's community in treatment. Outcome studies for both CRA and CRAFT are presented to highlight the effectiveness of these approaches.

Finally, in Chapter 11, Steiker, Goldbach, Sagun, Hopson, and Laird focus on the need for prevention of substance use disorders. As the authors note, much of the prevention literature has focused on children and adolescents because these are the individuals most vulnerable to initiation of substance use. The chapter provides definitions of incidence and prevalence, a history of prevention programs in the United States and an overview of different prevention strategies. The chapter provides an overview of issues related to harm reduction and the debate regarding the need for abstinence. The authors also discuss the importance of culturally grounded prevention efforts and efforts at prevention across the lifespan.

Together, these chapters provide a conceptual review and background for the assessment and treatment of substance use disorders. Although not always specifically mentioned in the chapters in Part III, these models form the basis for the assessment and treatment of each of the drug categories addressed in Part III, thus helping the reader with a greater understanding of the broad issues involved.

7

Evidence-Based Practice

Frank L. Collins
University of North Texas

Thad R. Leffingwell
Oklahoma State University

Jennifer L. Callahan
University of North Texas

Lee M. Cohen
Texas Tech University

Contents

What is Evidence-Based Treatment?

The most widely used definition of EBP has its foundation in the definition of evidence-based medicine articulated by Sackett and colleagues: "… the conscientious, explicit, and judicious use of current best evidence in making decisions about the care of individual patients … integrating individual clinical expertise with the best available external clinical evidence from systematic research" (Sackett, Rosenberg, Gray, Haynes, & Richardson, 1996, p. 71).

This definition was adapted and expanded upon in an influential report by the Institute of Medicine (IOM, 2001), and more recently forms the basis for the American Psychological Association's (APA) landmark policy statement regarding EBP in psychology, "[EBP is] the integration of the best available research with clinical expertise in the context of patient characteristics, culture, and preferences" (APA, 2005, p. 1).

Thus, EBP for substance use disorders must focus on the integration of the best available research evidence with clinical expertise and patient values. Integration is highlighted in this definition to stress the importance of all three components of this definition. Although integration of these components is critical, identification of the core components is likewise important.

What is Research Evidence?

What is research evidence? What counts as research evidence? Where does one find research evidence? How does one apply research evidence to answer clinical questions? In general, research evidence refers to knowledge obtained through careful and controlled observations applying the scientific method and methodologies generally accepted by a professional field. Sackett et al. (1996) define "best available clinical evidence" as "clinically relevant research, often from the basic sciences of medicine, but especially from patient-centered clinical research… (p. 71)." The IOM (2001) uses essentially the same definitions. The APA (2005) policy statement similarly defines "best research evidence" as "scientific results related to intervention strategies, assessment, clinical problems, and patient populations in laboratory and field settings as well as to clinically relevant results of basic research in psychology and related fields (p. 1)." Notably, all three definitions cast a wide net to include as evidence not only the results of randomized clinical trials (RCTs) of specific treatments with defined populations or problems, but also research involving assessment (reliability, validity, clinical utility, etc.), psychopathology (including description, etiology, and prognosis), treatment process, fundamental psychological processes (e.g., learning, cognition, or emotion), and a host of other relevant areas of scientific knowledge.

Quality of the Evidence

When trying to define the boundaries of research evidence, however, it becomes easy for reasonable professionals to disagree. Rather than approaching the issue in search of an arbitrary boundary of what is or is not research evidence, we favor an approach that treats all evidence as existing on a continuum (McCabe, 2004). Simply put, some research evidence is stronger and more trustworthy than others. For example, research evidence from a single unreplicated experiment is less trustworthy than research evidence supported by a number of replicated experiments. Similarly, research evidence from a cross-sectional correlation study is not as trustworthy as research evidence from a carefully controlled longitudinal study in terms of the independent variable's strength of inference. Thus, we find it more useful to consider all possible research evidence as existing on a continuum that takes into account the strength of the evidence, including the validity and reliability of the finding, the strength of inference offered by the research design, the generalizability to a population of interest, and the size of the effect in both statistical and clinical terms. An example of a continuum-based hierarchical organization of sources of scientific evidence can be found in Table 7.1.

TABLE 7.1
Hierarchical Levels of Evidence

Level I: Evidence from true experimental designs.
1. Evidence derived from rigorous reviews of several experimental studies, including meta-analyses.
2. Evidence from one or more well-controlled randomized study.
3. Evidence from practice guidelines derived from rigorous reviews of scientific evidence.

Level II: Evidence from quasi-experimental designs.
1. Evidence derived from well-designed, controlled trials without randomization.
2. Evidence from multiple time series, cohort, or case-control studies.
3. Evidence from dramatic results in one uncontrolled study (sometimes seen in medicine or public health, but rare in behavioral science)

Level III: Evidence from expert consensus.
1. Evidence derived from the multiple opinions of respected authorities, based upon known clinical and/or research experience.

Level IV: Evidence from qualitative literature reviews and other publications.
1. Evidence derived from a qualitative review of published evidence without quantitative synthesis (as in meta-analysis).
2. Evidence derived from opinion essays, case reports, etc.
3. Evidence derived from opinions of influential individuals, if those opinions are based upon relevant personal clinical experience (e.g., authors of popular books).

Level V: "Someone once told me…" or "I once treated a case like this…"
1. Evidence based upon a single training experience (e.g., expert advice from a supervisor or course instructor).
2. Evidence based on recollection of single similar case in one's history without rigorous data and/or follow-up.

Source. McCabe, O. L. Crossing the quality chasm in behavioral health care: The role of evidence-based practice. *Professional Psychology: Research & Practice*, 35, 571 (2004), and American Psychiatric Association (2004).

Relevance of the Evidence

Evidence can come from a variety of types of research, from basic laboratory science to applied clinical science with clinical populations. Some evidence is more directly relevant to the clinical question than others. For example, when considering a decision about the ideal treatment for a Hispanic-American man with cocaine dependence, the following lines of research are increasingly relevant to the clinical question (although all may be useful): (a) basic research describing fundamental learning processes (e.g., modeling, operant, and classical conditioning); (b) laboratory research with animals studying learning processes relative to cocaine as a reinforcer; (c) laboratory research with humans studying behavioral economics of alternative reinforcers; (d) laboratory research with humans who are dependent on cocaine studying behavioral economics and behavioral choice; (e) correlational research with cocaine-dependent men studying deficiencies in alternative reinforcement; (f) a randomized controlled trial of a treatment featuring contingency management/community reinforcement as a treatment for alcohol dependence in men; (g) a randomized controlled trial of a treatment featuring contingency management/community reinforcement as treatment for cocaine dependence in Hispanic-American men; and (h) a randomized controlled trial for a treatment featuring contingency management/community reinforcement for cocaine dependence in Hispanic-American men.

Of course, one would be quick to observe that the "level" of each study is not independent; each incorporates and builds upon knowledge generated by the other. In fact, one might observe that in a well-developed field of scientific inquiry, each subsequent level explicitly and carefully builds upon the best available evidence from the previous levels. Nonetheless, the final study mentioned above is most closely related to the clinical question and would likely be considerably more useful in informing clinical decision making. Frequently, however, this type of evidence may not yet be available in the research literature, and the practitioner may have to integrate other levels of evidence, or extrapolate from evidence regarding similar problems or populations, with expertise and patient values to answer the clinical questions and derive a treatment plan.

Where does One Find Evidence?

Although debates continue about what constitutes evidence that should inform clinical practice, there is little disagreement that evidence exists in the scientific literature that can serve in this role. One issue however, is that the evidence available in the literature grows exponentially over time, and generally becomes more complex and sophisticated in regard to sampling, design, measurement, and analysis strategies as science progresses and the evidence base matures. To further complicate matters, the nature of scientific evidence is such that historic evidence will over time be superseded or replaced by new evidence, requiring all practitioners of EBP to remain abreast of new developments in the research. The abundance of evidence and the dynamic nature of evidence are such that relying upon primary sources is simply not feasible (Sackett, Straus, Richardson, Rosenbert, & Haynes, 2000) and other means of obtaining and utilizing evidence are necessary (referred to as "evidence management" by McCabe, 2004). Members of the practice community often lack the time and resources (e.g., access to database searches or full-text copies of literature) to make personal primary-source searches for evidence practical or even possible. Fortunately, a growing number of resources are available that provide credible reviews and summaries of the most current evidence available which are much more useful to practitioners. These resources generally represent Level I or Level II sources of evidence relative to the hierarchy depicted in Table 7.1.

Commissioned Reviews or Institute Reports   Given the importance of EBP to inform policy, governments may at times commission summaries of evidence to guide prudent use of our limited health care resources. One example of this type of report from the field of psychotherapy are the reports by Roth and Fonagy (2004) commissioned by the National Health Service of the United Kingdom. Examples from the addictions field include reports from the National Institute on Drug Abuse (NIDA) and the National Institute on Alcohol Abuse and Alcoholism (NIAAA) such as, *Principles of Drug Addiction Treatment* (National Institute of Drug Abuse, 1999) or the *Treatment Improvement Protocol Series* (TIPS; SAMHSA, 2008) that combine brief reviews of the research evidence with practical protocols for implementing empirically supported practices in real-world settings. Another example of commissioned reviews is the summary of empirically supported psychological treatments commissioned by David Barlow, then president of Division 12 (clinical psychology) of the APA (Task Force on Promotion and Dissemination of Psychological Procedures, 1995; Chambless et al., 1996, 1998).

Clinical Practice Guidelines and Consensus Statements   Clinical practice guidelines can be initiated and produced by a variety of sources. The Michigan Quality Improvement Consortium has developed an extensive list of health care practice guidelines (see http://www.mqic.org). The National Guideline Clearinghouse lists 39 clinical practice guidelines for "substance-related disorders" including the popular *Treating Tobacco Use and Dependence* clinical practice guideline issued by the U.S. Public Health Service (Fiore et al., 2000).

Cochrane Reviews   Since 1993, the Cochrane Collaboration has produced and distributed dozens of reviews of randomized controlled trials of treatments for health problems (see http://www.cochrane.org). Although the collaboration's primary focus is on medical health care, the Cochrane Library (see http://www.cochranelibrary.com) also includes a number of reviews on the prevention and treatment of drug and alcohol dependence (pharmacological and psychosocial).

Textbooks   Although there are a number of textbooks devoted to the assessment and treatment of substance abuse, including this text, Sackett and colleagues (2000) suggest caution in using texbooks as a sole source of evidence summaries because they may be biased editorially and become out of date quickly as the status of the evidence is always changing. In general, we would caution against placing trust in textbooks that offer little connection to research evidence or evidence-rich textbooks more than a few years old as authoritative guides for practice. The present text has attempted to provide the reader with guidelines regarding the current state of assessment and treatment at the time of publication, and encouragement for continued reading and life-long learning.

What is the Evidence Telling Us?

RCTs testing the efficacy of specific treatments to ameliorate specific problems are frequently considered the gold standard for informing EBP (Behar & Borkovec, 2003). When rigorously designed, these between-group experimental trials provide the strongest possible inference about the treatment by controlling for and ruling out several other rival hypotheses. For this reason, RCTs are widely used in medicine and remain the standard for approval of any new medicine or medical procedure. RCTs were also the primary design used by the Division 12 Task Force in determining whether to designate a certain treatment as "empirically supported."

The major concern about focusing too much on RCTs is that it is tempting to equate EBP with RCTs and to assume EBP is the implementation of Empirically Supported Treatments (Collins, Leffingwell, & Belar, 2007). Some have expressed fears that a movement towards EBP will result in a policy-driven prescription of certain treatments for some problems, a prohibition of some therapeutic activities, or an end to creative pursuit of new, innovative, and potentially more effective approaches. Such outcomes would indeed be unfortunate, but will only occur if the movement towards EBP is misunderstood or misrepresented. EBP, as defined by Sackett et al. (2000) and APA (2005) recognizes that current research evidence will always be inadequate to guide all (if not most) clinical decision making and treatment planning, and retains the professional clinician, in the context of each individual patient, to be the arbiter of decision making through the integration of evidence with clinical expertise and patient values.

If RCTs are not to be construed as the be-all-end-all standard of evidence, then what is to be gleaned from this evidence? Borkovec and colleagues (Behar & Borkovec, 2003; Borkovec & Castonguay, 1998) argue that what we learn primarily from well-designed RCTs is not an answer to the question, "Does this treatment work?" but rather we learn something fundamental about the nature of human problems and the processes by which change in those problems is most likely to occur. Perhaps the question best answered by RCTs, and the most useful answer for informing EBP, is "What is the nature of the disorder and its maintaining conditions such that this particular component or combination of components specifically leads to improvement?" (Behar & Borkovec, 2003, p. 218). Viewed in this manner, RCTs are easier to view as integrated with so-called "basic science" findings that contribute to a conceptual understanding of the disorder itself, which should in turn lead to more rapid scientific advances and the most efficient development of more powerful treatments (Miranda & Borkovec, 1999). The NIDA guide, *Principles of Drug Treatment* described earlier (National Institute of Drug Abuse, 1999) is an exemplar of a summary including research evidence that integrates both basic and applied research in order to extrapolate evidence-based principles of best practices (see Table 7.2).

What is Clinical Expertise?

The second component of EBP is clinical expertise. Although clinical expertise is recognized as an important aspect for effective EBP, it may well be the most misunderstood and controversial component. Clinical expertise incorporates therapist characteristics, skills, attitudes,

TABLE 7.2
Research-Based Principles of Substance Use Disorder Treatment

1. No single treatment is appropriate for all individuals.

2. Treatment needs to be readily available.

3. Effective treatment attends to multiple needs of the individual, not just his or her drug use.

4. An individual's treatment and services plan must be assessed continually and modified as necessary to ensure that the plan meets the person's changing needs.

5. Remaining in treatment for an adequate period of time is critical for treatment effectiveness.

6. Counseling (individual and/or group) and other behavioral therapies are critical components of effective treatment for addiction.

7. Medications are an important element of treatment for many patients, especially when combined with counseling and other behavioral therapies.

8. Addicted or drug-abusing individuals with coexisting mental disorders should have both disorders treated in an integrated way.

9. Medical detoxification is only the first stage of addiction treatment and by itself does little to change long-term drug use.

10. Treatment does not need to be voluntary to be effective.

11. Possible drug use during treatment must be monitored continuously.

12. Treatment programs should provide assessment for HIV/AIDS, hepatitis B and C, tuberculosis, and other infectious diseases, and counseling to help patients modify or change behaviors that place themselves or others at risk for infection.

13. Recovery from drug addiction can be a long-term process and frequently requires multiple episodes of treatment.

Source. National Institute of Drug Abuse, *Principles of Drug Addiction Treatment.* (NIH Publication No. 99–4180. Rockville, MD (1999). Reprinted with permission.

competencies, and experience. There is no single agreed-upon definition, nor is there a single measure that can be used to determine the presence or absence of clinical expertise.

In this section, we address this question by first identifying general components of clinical expertise that are important for EBP in the assessment and treatment of substance use disorders and to discuss methods for the identification of components thought to be important for effective clinical expertise. Although there are clear gaps in our knowledge, particularly agreement as to the best method(s) for assessment of these competencies, we focus on aspects of expertise that have been shown to be associated with positive outcomes. Finally, we provide a summary discussion of the importance of identifying aspects of clinical competence for substance abuse counseling. These aspects include level of professional training and draw heavily on competencies identified for professional practice in related disciplines. These competencies are the foundation upon which clinical expertise is based and it is critical for substance abuse practitioners to ensure that they have acquired these minimal practice competencies.

Although focusing on clinical expertise and the importance of expertise for influencing treatment outcome, it is not our intention to overemphasize the unique contribution of clinical expertise. Consistent with the definition of EBP, we fully believe that best practice is accomplished when therapy is based on the integration of the best research evidence with clinical expertise and patient characteristics, values, and context. Outcomes are influenced by treatments used (Barlow, 2004), individual patient characteristics, and other characteristics that are outside the therapeutic relationship such as social support or the presence of other Axis I disorders (Lambert & Barley, 2002). Thus, evidence-based treatment of substance use disorders involves the integration of a multitude of factors, with clinical expertise being one factor. However, the ability to effectively accomplish this integration is, in part, at the heart of clinical expertise and, as such, it is important that this aspect of EBP remain a central component of practice.

Components of Clinical Expertise

Recently, clinical expertise has been defined as "the ability to integrate knowledge, experience, technical and relational skill, critical thinking, prediction, decision-making, and self-assessment within a fluid situation that often is uncertain and ambiguous" (Goodheart, 2006). This definition implies a level of cognitive decision making that, although easy to conceptualize and affirm, is difficult to objectively observe and identify. As such, it may be most useful to identify components of expertise and use clinical outcomes as an indirect method for assessing expertise.

An alternative to this more cognitive conceptualization of clinical expertise is to focus on the components of expertise. Lambert and his colleagues (Lambert & Barley, 2002) have identified three major categories that comprise clinical expertise that are not mutually exclusive: Therapist Attributes, Facilitative Conditions, and Therapeutic Alliance. These categories are somewhat arbitrary and very interdependent upon one another, however, it seems to us to be useful to discuss these distinct components of clinical expertise using this framework.

Therapist Attributes and Facilitative Conditions   It has been well understood for some time that some therapists are more effective than others. Orlinsky and Howard (1978) reviewed the outcomes of 23 therapists for 143 female clients. Their review indicated significant variability between therapists. Clients of some therapists were more likely to have better outcomes than others and these differences were not obviously related to the type of treatment used. In fact, even for therapists who, on average, showed less effective client outcomes, some of their clients displayed positive outcomes. These findings have been supported in other studies (Luborsky, McLellan, Diguer, Woody, & Seligman, 1997), including focused manualized treatments (cf., Shapiro, Firth-Cozens, & Stiles, 1989).

Several factors have been identified that appear to characterize more effective therapists. More effective therapists have been described as sensitive, gentle, and honest (Lazarus, 1971), or as warm, attentive, interested, understanding, and respectful (Strupp, Fox, & Lessler, 1969). Orlinsky, Grawe, and Parks (1994) in a review of studies found several characteristics to be related to positive outcomes: (a) therapist credibility, (b) therapist skill, (c) empathic understanding, (d) affirmation of the patient, (e) ability to engage with the patient, (f) ability to focus on the patient's problems, and (g) ability to direct the patient's attention to the patient's affective experience.

The most frequently identified therapist variables appear to be characterized into three components: (a) empathic understanding, (b) nonpossessive warmth and positive regard, and (c) congruence. These components have been shown to be important for cognitive behavioral treatments (Ablon & Jones, 1999; Murphy, Cramer, & Lillie, 1984), interpersonal psychotherapy (Ablon & Jones, 1999), and behavioral treatment of alcohol consumption (Miller, Taylor & West, 1980).

Other therapist characteristics that have at times been shown to be related to specific treat-ment outcomes include gender, race, cultural attitudes, emotional well-being, and therapeutic style. It should also be noted that few studies have focused on these characteristics with sub-stance-using clients alone. It is possible that therapist characteristics that are associated with positive outcomes will be similar for most disorders, however, it is also possible that for some characteristics, the relationship between the characteristic and successful treatment outcome will be different for specific substance-using populations. Thus, we have encouraged all authors to address these issues where appropriate, even if the conclusion is that more research is needed to better understand these relationships.

Therapeutic Alliance   In addition to the therapist characteristics reviewed above, therapeutic alliance appears to be an important aspect of treatment effectiveness (Horvath & Greenberg, 1994). Therapeutic alliance is a conceptually derived, but empirically supported, construct that describes the relationship between a therapist and client. Most definitions of therapeutic alliance focus on three aspects of this construct: (a) a collaborative relationship, (b) an affective bond between the client and therapist, and (c) mutual agreement upon treatment goals and tasks (Martin, Garske, & Davis, 2000). Measurement of therapeutic alliance has grown from observer rating scales to self-report scales used by therapists and/or clients. Regardless of how it is measured though, the importance of the therapeutic alliance appears to be independent of treatment modality (Martin et al., 2000).

Research has consistently shown a moderate effect size (.22–.26) between alliance and therapy outcomes (Horath & Bedi, 2002; Horvath & Greenberg, 1994). Most studies reported in the literature measure alliance early in treatment (before session 5). It is interesting to note studies that measure alliance at different time points show small differences in the relationship between alliance to outcomes with the strongest relationships observed for measures made early and late in treatment. This pattern has been well replicated empirically and is underscored by theoretical explanations (for additional information, see Horvath & Bedi, 2002; Wampold, 2001).

In short, the measurement of alliance early in treatment is very important and the ability to develop a positive therapeutic alliance early in treatment should be viewed as a positive indica-tion of clinical expertise.

Enhancing Clinical Expertise

It may seem presumptuous to begin to talk about enhancing clinical expertise when there is no agreed-upon definition or method(s) for assessment of expertise (Keen & Freeston, 2008). However, to a large extent, clinical expertise represents the development of professional com-petencies that are tied to aspirational goals of professional training programs. In professional psychology, for example, core competencies for practice have already been identified (Kaslow et al., 2004). As practice competencies are developed for addiction counseling, it is likely that they will be modeled after related disciplines and focus on such broad areas as clini-cal intervention and assessment, as well as cross-cutting competencies such as multicultural competence, ethical and professional development, and consultation and interdisciplinary relationships.

In the chapters in Section III of this text, attention is given where available to specific competencies that have been shown to be related to positive outcomes. It is important to point out, however, that professional education and training are lifelong. One must maintain skills and competencies, and like research evidence, knowledge about effective clinical expertise is evolving and treatment providers must adapt to this knowledge base.

When is Clinical Expertise Present?

Although specific definitions and assessment methods do not exist, we believe that it is possible to identify the presence of clinical expertise by looking at client outcomes. Specifically, in a clinical setting with a number of treatment providers, there will be variability both between clinicians and between clients for a particular clinician. With respect to variability in outcomes between clinicians, it is important to develop local norms and it is critical that systematic outcome data be collected by all clinicians for all clients. Staff need to evaluate these data and identify those clinicians for whom clients have poor outcomes.

Having identified clinicians who are not successful with clients allows for retraining, continuing education, and/or self-exploration to determine why lower outcomes are present. Just as one would use those treatment strategies that produce superior outcomes, one must determine how to maximize outcomes for specific clinicians. To our knowledge, this is rare outside training clinics. However, EBP demands that not only does the clinician use those treatment strategies that have been shown to be more effective, clinicians must develop (and use) those clinical skills that are also more effective. This may require systemwide assessment.

Likewise, individual clinicians need to be aware of the characteristics of clients that they see who show differential outcomes. Specifically, clinicians need to understand the extent to which they are not as effective with particular client groups and through self-observation and supervision, understand the extent to which these differential outcomes are due to different therapist behaviors with different clients or whether the same therapist behaviors are differentially effective. From a system perspective, it is possible that an agency could use different clinicians for different types or clients, or clinicians could refer out the types of clients for whom they are less effective. All of these alternatives would be consistent with enhanced EBP.

New Competencies Required for EBP

In addition to the clinical competencies already described, the clinician must also develop new competencies specific to the practice of EBP. These competencies include skills for accessing relevant research evidence and integrating it into clinical decisions. Such skills include asking well-formulated questions, searching for and acquiring evidence, evaluating the evidence, and applying that evidence to the question at hand. Recognizing the need for training in these new skills, the Office of Behavioral and Social Sciences within the National Institutes of Health has funded the development of an Internet resource, EBBP.org, for disseminating and enhancing competencies related to EBP. This resource will include online training modules for each of the new competencies required for EBP.

Identification of Clinical Expertise for Substance Abuse Counseling

As noted previously, each of the chapters in Section III of this text provides information about what is currently known about the research on treatment effectiveness, clinical expertise, and patient values. The integration of research evidence, clinical expertise, and patient values is only possible if the clinician has sufficient clinical expertise to accomplish this integration. Although we believe that specific components of clinical expertise can be identified and trained, the whole is greater than the sum of the parts. By knowing that clients are improving, and fortunately in the area of substance abuse outcome measures can be quite specific (e.g., abstinence), one can identify effective practice.

This process of identification of competencies for substance abuse counseling must draw on the knowledge gained in the psychotherapy literature while at the same time being open to divergent perspectives. Just as treatment techniques are subjected to rigorous evaluation, we must rigorously evaluate competencies needed for effective practice, and when such competencies are shown to be critical for effective outcomes, ensure that all treatment providers master those critical competencies.

What are Patient Values?

We now turn to the third and final component of EBP, with a particular emphasis on the treatment of substance-related disorders. Patient values refers to "the unique preferences, concerns and expectations that each patient brings to a clinical encounter and that must be integrated into clinical decisions if they are to serve the patient" (IOM, 2001, p. 147). Despite the fact that this component is mentioned third, it is important to note that the definition addresses a true integration of all three components without indicating that one is more important than the next. Although the EBP movement has returned to prominence the idea that patient–treatment interactions are related to clinical outcomes, research reports from the past three decades have indicated that treatment outcomes can be enhanced by carefully matching individuals, based on personal characteristics, to specific treatment approaches.

We first review the normative data on what types of treatments work for whom, with a focus on the findings from Project Matching Alcoholism Treatments to Client Heterogeneity (MATCH), a multisite clinical trial for the treatment of alcohol-use problems. Next, we outline general client characteristics that have been shown to be related to outcome and retention in psychotherapy and follow with a discussion of patient characteristics that may be unique to substance use disorders. Finally, we provide a summary of how a clinician might incorporate the personal values of the client and his or her preferences into the available effective treatment interventions.

What Works for Whom: Findings from Project MATCH

During the 1980s, psychotherapy research began to study client characteristics with greater rigor and numerous small studies (e.g., de Jong, Treiber, & Henrich, 1986; Emmelkamp, Brilman, & Kuiper, 1986; McCrady, Noel, Abrans, & Stout, 1986) seemed to indicate that behaviorally oriented treatments might significantly interact with such characteristics.

The National Academy of Science's IOM consequently recommended a large-scale investigation of matching specific treatments to specific patients, with the idea that this would result in better outcomes, increased cost-effectiveness, and improved utilization of available treatment resources. The NIAAA responded to this challenge and, in 1989, launched an eight-year, multisite trial of "MATCH" (a.k.a. Project MATCH; 1993, 1997).

Three psychosocial treatments were selected for inclusion in the trial, each distinctive from the other, and all having demonstrated effectiveness in previous, well-controlled research trials. The three treatments were 12-step facilitation therapy, cognitive-behavioral therapy, and motivational enhancement therapy. An indeterminate number of patient characteristics could have been investigated, but to preserve power in analyses, Project MATCH focused on those supported by research evidence and/or widely believed theory, including a demographic variable (i.e., gender), alcohol-related variables (i.e., severity of alcohol involvement, typology of alcoholism, social support for drinking versus abstinence), and individual differences (i.e., cognitive impairment, sociopathy, level of conceptual reasoning, meaning-seeking, psychiatric severity, and motivational readiness to change). Response to treatment was operationalized as the average number of drinks per drinking day and the percentage of days abstinent during the year following the course of treatment provided through Project MATCH. A total of 64 potential interactions could have been examined, although only 16 relationships were formally proposed in hypotheses. During analyses, the only identified "match" that emerged was between patients with low psychiatric severity and 12-step facilitative treatment. Such individuals reported more days of abstinence than those individuals treated in the cognitive-behavioral condition. Notably, this relationship was not explicitly stated in the initial hypotheses. As a result of Project MATCH many researchers and clinicians concluded that matching of patients to treatment does not substantially alter outcomes and research investigations began to shift in emphasis to better elucidating the biophysical mechanisms of dependence.

Despite the enormous amount of time and money invested in this undertaking, Project MATCH was not without methodological weaknesses. Specifically, although the treatments provided were tightly controlled to ensure high quality and standard delivery, patients were not prohibited from pursuing parallel informal experiences that may have affected treatment. Most notably, many of the patients assigned to cognitive-behavioral or motivational enhancement therapy concurrently attended meetings of Alcoholics Anonymous. Although this was conceptualized by the researchers as more of a mutually supportive fellowship, rather than a formalized treatment, it is unclear how this may have manifested itself when the data were being analyzed.

Furthermore, and perhaps more relevant to this chapter, is that Project MATCH was not intended to examine client preferences, concerns, or expectations, which is inconsistent with our working definition of evidenced-based treatment. However, a closer examination of the project's findings may indeed reveal significant relationships reflecting patient values. For example, outpatient clients who were categorized as being more motivated for treatment evidenced better outcomes, suggesting that differing outcome expectancies may have been present. Similarly, social support for drinking was found to be predictive of poorer outcomes which may reflect differing individual preferences pertaining to ending or limiting those relationships. Additional information revealing the importance of client preferences is found in

Project MATCH's report of participant recruitment. Specifically, 459 potential participants declined to participate following the initial screening because they considered participation in the study to be too inconvenient or time consuming. Other possible participants were excluded because they evidenced concurrent drug dependencies, did not have stable housing, or reported legal or probation problems. It is quite likely that such individuals would report differing preferences, concerns, expectations, and values compared to those participants who were included in the study. Although the purpose of this chapter is predominantly one of exploring client values in the form of preferences, concerns, and expectations, these variables cannot be extricated from individual characteristics, including personality variables, and the familial and societal cultures pertaining to the individual.

Client Characteristics and Psychotherapy: What is Generally Known?

Age Psychotherapy studies generally indicate that age is not strongly related to treatment retention or treatment outcome (Dubrin & Zastowny, 1988; Sledge, Moras, Hartley, & Levine, 1990). Younger individuals, however, appear to be more likely to have a history of mental health service utilization and report stronger intentions of using such services in the future (Smith, Peck, & McGovern, 2004). However, in the case of the substance-related disorders, youth appears to be a specific risk factor for premature termination and poorer outcome (Agosti, Nunes, & Ocepeck-Welikson, 1996).

Gender Research examining the relationship of gender and psychotherapy outcome also generally reveals no differences (Garfield, 1994; Petry, Tennen, & Affleck, 2000), with the possible exception of those in treatment for depression (Thase, Frank, Kornstein, & Yonkers, 2000). However, the possibility exists that gender differences are exerting an influence in how treatment options are evaluated by clients, prior to actually initiating psychotherapy. For example, Smith et al. (2004) observed that women were more likely to possess positive attitudes about help-seeking behavior. They also reported that women were more likely to have a history of utilizing mental health services and to report an intention of utilizing mental health services in the future if needed.

Robertson and Fitzgerald (1992) provide further evidence suggesting the presence of gender differences with respect to the initiation of psychological services. In this study, men were asked to rate their preferences when presented with descriptions of mental health services. As a group, men reported greater preference for the more structured service options, considering them to be less emotionally involving. In a more recent study (Blazina & Marks, 2001), men who endorsed traditional masculine gender roles were more likely to report a negative reaction when presented with treatment options, with the most pronounced negativity directed at unstructured group services (i.e., a men's support group). Although both of these studies were conducted with non-help-seeking, male undergraduates, who may not be comparable to help-seeking populations, NIMH has acknowledged that gender may play a significant role in treatment initiation and selection given their development of the *Real Men, Real Depression* marketing campaign.

More specifically to substance-abusing populations, a study of adolescents suffering from sub-stance-abuse problems (Blood & Cornwall, 1994) found no significant predictors of treatment completion among female participants, but four distinct predictors among male participants: (1) severity of problems with alcohol; (2) greater use of drugs other than alcohol, cannabis, and tobacco; (3) lower self-esteem; and (4) more internalizing symptoms of emotional distress. The finding regarding the role of internalizing symptoms is unclear however, given that another study of adolescents (Rivers, Greenbaum, & Goldberg, 2001) revealed that males who reported more internalizing symptomatology reduced their drug use more compared to their low internalizing peers. With respect to female participants, those who initially reported experiencing more family problems became more self-efficacious about future drug avoidance.

Within adult substance-abusing populations, there also appear to be some gender-specific findings. In one study it was found that an alcohol-related diagnosis was predictive of treatment initiation in females (Green, Polen, Dickinson, Lynch, & Bennett, 2002). Completion of the course of treatment was predicted both by having a higher income and by being referred by an agency or legal entity. Length of treatment course was predicted by alcohol- or opiate-related diagnoses and also by legal/agency referral. In contrast, failure to initiate treatment was predicted by the presence of one or more mental health diagnoses and failure to complete treatment was predicted by greater impairment in employment and comorbid substance-dependence diagnoses. For men, initiation of treatment was predicted by being employed and by being married. Less education was predictive of a failure to initiate treatment, and treatment completion was predicted by older age. Fewer mental health diagnoses, higher education, domestic victim status, or prior 12-step attendance were all predictive of length of time in treatment. Failure to complete treatment was predicted by worse psychiatric status, receiving Medicaid, and motivation for entering treatment.

Ethnicity and Culture   Research into the relationship among ethnicity, culture, and psychotherapy outcome suggests that the client–therapist alliance is especially salient when working with ethnic minority populations (e.g., Gibbs, 1985; Griffith & Jones, 1979; Jenkins, 1997; Sue & Zane, 1987). For example, literature in this field indicates that egalitarian attitudes by therapists may be particularly useful when working with low-income, African-American clients (Ross, 1983). Some research indicates that the biases and/or discomfort of the therapist when working with members of a different ethnicity may adversely affect treatment outcome (Garb, 1997; Whaley, 1998). However, other research suggests that the impact of therapist attitude may actually be related to SES status, rather than ethnic status (Lerner, 1972).

Cultural variables and how they may influence treatment outcome has also been examined empirically. Specifically, judgments pertaining to satisfaction in life may be influenced by the individual's subjective determination of needs and goals which appear to be influenced by the individual's experience and understanding of culture and society (Diener & Lucus, 2000). A study examining Asian-American college students found that the level of self-reported cultural identity was a significant moderator of credibility ratings for treatment rationales of both time-limited psychotherapy as well as cognitive therapy (Wong, Kim, & Zane, 2003). Other studies have noted that common constructs of Western psychotherapy may inherently conflict with conventional expectations in non-Western cultures (e.g., Leong, 1986), particularly in terms of emphasis on individualism versus collectivism (Duan & Wang, 2000).

Cultural differences are also likely to play a significant role in cases of immigration. A large-scale study of disability levels and health utilization in Australia found that individuals from non-English-speaking backgrounds, particularly those born in Asia, Africa, or the Middle East, were less likely to utilize health services and, consequently, more likely to suffer from high levels of disability (Boufous, Silove, Bauman, & Steel, 2005). Thus, the importance of cultural differences should not be overlooked as their influence may be misinterpreted by clinicians as indicative of resistance (Reid, 1999) and, in turn, be linked to premature termination and unsuccessful courses of treatment.

A recent meta-analysis examining smoking cessation treatment programs concluded that although treatments appear to be effective across racial and ethnic groups, there are no studies that have examined the relative efficacy rates (Piper, Fox, Welsch, Fiore, & Baker, 2001). Nevertheless, evidence does suggest that use and dependence factors may vary across groups. Value systems may also vary significantly between groups in ways that are relevant to treatment. For example, Ortega and Alegría (2002) reported that an attitude of self-reliance was related to utilization of mental health services in low-income Puerto Ricans. Specifically, those with higher levels of self-reliant attitudes were less likely to access services, even when deemed to be in need of such services.

Intelligence   General intellectual abilities are not typically thought to relate significantly to therapy outcome (Haaga, DeRubeis, Stewart, & Beck, 1991). However, most studies reporting no differences include only a restricted range of cognitive abilities. As such, a comprehensive review of this area is beyond the scope of this chapter. For a more detailed review of psychotherapy involving persons with mental retardation, including suggestions of modifications that might be useful for each of the major schools of psychotherapy, see Nezu and Nezu (1994).

Psychiatric Comorbidity   The existing treatment outcome literature suggests that fewer comorbid mental health problems lead to a better prognosis (AuBuchon & Malatesta, 1994; McDermut & Zimmerman, 1998; Rossiter, Agras, Telch, & Schneider, 1993); however, this is overly simplistic. At present, a preponderance of psychotherapy research is centered on examining the efficacy of specific treatments in clinical populations with a singular diagnosis (for illustrative purposes, see Chambless et al., 1998). As such, a paucity of research is devoted to developing treatments for those with comorbid diagnoses. In general, it appears that the presence of one or more personality disorders is a specific risk for premature treatment discontinuation, with estimates ranging from 42 to 67% (Chiesa, Drahorad, & Longo, 2000; Gunderson et al., 1989; Shea et al., 1990; Skodol, Buckley, & Charles, 1983).

The examination of symptom severity is another way of investigating this issue, regardless of diagnoses. It has been widely and repeatedly demonstrated that higher levels of symptomatic distress are related to poorer treatment outcomes, and this finding holds true in substance abusing populations (McLellan, Luborsky, Woody, Druley, & O'Brien, 1983; McLellan et al., 1994).

Expectancies   Research on psychotherapy attrition (or "premature termination") has estimated that 30 to 60% of clients in outpatient settings discontinue treatment before the therapist considers termination appropriate (Sledge et al., 1990). In fact, in some urban mental health centers as many as 37–45% may not return after the first session (Fiester & Rudestam,

1975; Pekarik, 1983). One contributing factor that has been identified as predictive of which individuals may experience negative initial outcome is disconfirmed expectations (Garfield, 1994). Research examining expectancies has demonstrated that clients with more accurate expectations for treatment evidence better outcomes (e.g., Gaston, Marmar, Gallagher, & Thompson, 1989; Joyce & Piper, 1998). Conversely, clients who formulate a negative impression of their therapist, based on whatever subjective or idiosyncratic variables they consider salient, have been found to be more likely to drop out of treatment (Beckham, 1989), perhaps because these clients do not expect that such therapists will be able to help them effectively with their presenting concerns.

Preferences   Clients present with idiosyncratic preferences that may also influence treatment, including treatment selection and continuation, acceptance of treatment rationales, decision making, and delivery of feedback. For example, a large study examining preferences related to treatment options in Germany found that psychotherapy was the preferred treatment over medication (Riedel-Heller, Matschinger, & Angermeyer, 2005). What is also notable from this study, given the overall theme of this book, is that it appears that research evidence may not be well known, or perhaps as influential, in guiding clients when faced with making treatment-related decisions. Instead, clients appeared to rely more heavily on their beliefs, expectations, and preferences in making treatment decisions.

Agreement of treatment attrition predictors across treatment populations is not readily found in the literature, but several studies pose strong heuristic value and lay groundwork for the subsequent substance- and population-specific chapters. An excellent review of these factors is available in Ciraulo, Piechniczek-Buczek, and Iscan (2003).

Clients not only appear to differ in terms of the information they consider in decision making, they also vary in their preferences for how decisions are made during treatment. A recent population-based survey of a representative sample examining decision making in medical settings found that most individuals (96%) wanted to be offered treatment choices and have their opinion solicited in the decision-making process (Levinson, Kao, & Kuby, 2005). Nevertheless, 44% of the respondents reported that they preferred to rely on their providers for information and not seek that information themselves, illustrating the importance of providers being fully up to date on the research evidence for available practice options. This point is further confirmed by the finding that more than half (52%) of the respondents identified that their preference is to leave the final treatment decisions up to the provider.

Interestingly, this study also revealed group differences in preferences. Specifically, more active decision-making involvement was desired by females, people in good health, and those with more education. Up to the age of 45, a preference for greater involvement was evident, although this preference subsequently declined. Regardless of age, individuals identifying themselves as African-American or Hispanic were more likely to state a preference for their provider to make treatment-related decisions.

Clients also may have differing preferences for communication exchanges, including preferences for how they disclose information and how those disclosures are responded to by the provider. Floyd, Lang, and McCord (2005) examined this issue in a primary care setting and found that clients who reported they would most likely share their concerns by simply describing their symptoms preferred being asked biomedical questions by the provider in response.

In contrast, clients who indicated they would provide a "clue" to their underlying concern while sharing their symptoms noted no clear preference and were equally comfortable with the provider responding by posing biomedical questions, exploring the clue, or simply facilitating further disclosure. Finally, those clients who indicated they would explicitly state their concern to the provider preferred that the provider respond by, first, acknowledging the concern and, then, exploring the source of the concern.

Client differences in disclosure preferences indicate that previous treatment encounters with a provider may influence level of disclosure (Maguire, 1984; Passik et al., 2002). Unfortunately, some clients withhold information because they consider their provider to be too busy to be bothered by their concerns (Maguire, 1984). Client personality variables may also influence disclosure. For example, a fatalistic orientation in thinking style can moderate a client's willingness to disclose or solicit treatment-related information (Aitken-Swan & Paterson, 1955). Similarly, patterns of interpersonal control can influence how and when a client makes a disclosure to her provider (Street, Krupat, Kravitz, & Haidet, 2003). Factors specific to the nature of the disclosure are also salient. Clients may be reluctant to disclose information to their provider for fear of appearing foolish or mentally unstable (Cornford, Morgan, & Ridsdale, 1993) and some anticipate feeling shameful or humiliated by disclosure (Lazare, 1987).

Finally, it is important to consider that clients may have preferences for how negative feedback is provided. To our knowledge, there are no studies examining this issue in the mental health literature, but a recent study examining how patients prefer to be given bad news from physicians can be informative (Mast, Kindlimann, & Langewitz, 2005). In this study a patient-centered communication style produced higher ratings of perceived physician emotional expression, availability, and hopefulness. In addition, they were viewed as less domineering and more appropriate in conveying information. Overall, patients were more satisfied with the visit and reported less of an increase in negative emotions following being told the bad news. More specific to substance-related disorders, client preferences may vary widely. These preferences are considered in greater detail in later chapters, including preferences related to moderation approaches versus abstinence models, inpatient versus outpatient settings, and individual versus family modalities. In brief, Patkar and colleagues (2004) noted that when making predictions of treatment outcome, one should be very cautious when such predictions are based on the primary drug of abuse, but client demographics and preferences may be useful. Future research in this area is likely to include novel, Web-based approaches, with early indications being that hazardous drinkers may prefer such interventions (Kypri, Saunders, & Gallagher, 2003).

We encourage practitioners to balance client preferences and characteristics, such as those just listed, with available effective treatments. A study by Thornton et al. (2003) may provide an illustrative example. In this study it was found that clients who displayed a more "helpless" demeanor achieved better outcomes in behaviorally oriented, structured treatments. In contrast, a less-structured, facilitative treatment milieu was found to be more efficacious for those deemed less "helpless."

Values The overview of client preferences thus far may lead a practitioner to conclude that adopting a patient-centered communication style will ensure the best outcomes. Alas, research in this area illustrates that patient-centered care is more complicated than simply using patient-centered communication. Patient-centered care requires the care to center on the patient, which includes appreciating their value systems. Somewhat ironically this means that, for some clients, patient-centered communication may conflict with the values of a particular individual client (Aita, McIlvain, & Backer, 2005). Nevertheless, the IOM's (2001) definition of EBP requires that the individual's unique values be integrated into clinical decision making.

Although it is heavily encouraged that practitioners discuss client values in session rather than make assumptions about personal values, an unusually large ($N = 77,528$) multinational ($N = 70$) study examining gender differences is worth keeping in mind (Schwartz & Rubel, 2005). In this study, 10 basic values were examined, and small, but significant effect sizes ($d = .15-.32$) were found suggesting that men more highly value power, stimulation, hedonism, achievement, and self-direction. In contrast, women were shown to value benevolence and universalism more highly. No gender differences were found for values of tradition and conformity and differences in valuing security were inconsistent. Although the study focused on gender differences, the authors also noted that culture moderated all gender differences. In all, research examining the relationship of values in psychotherapy has demonstrated that some values may be more (e.g., Jensen & Bergin, 1988; Strupp, 1980), or less (e.g., Furnham & Bochner, 1986), facilitative of patients' subjective well-being. Subjective well-being, in turn, is thought to contribute to positive psychotherapy outcome (Barkham et al., 1996; Callahan, Swift, & Hynan, 2006).

Clinical lore has long held that individuals may expect to feel worse before they begin feeling better in psychotherapy. Although the preceding studies offer strong evidence that such lore is unfounded (Barkham et al., 1996; Callahan et al., 2006; Howard, Lueger, Maling, & Martinovich, 1993), there is some evidence to suggest that when an individual's values are incompatible with those of an environment they may experience internal conflict (Schwartz, 1992; Tetlock, 1986) and a decline in subjective well-being (Oles, 1991; Sagiv & Schwartz, 2000). Given the demonstrated importance of subjective well-being to successful psychotherapy, it is important for practitioners to be mindful of client values and their congruence with the treatment environment.

Implementing EBP for Substance Abuse Assessment and Treatment

Effective assessment and treatment of substance abuse disorders requires attention to each of the three components of EBP and continued integration of each of these components. Thus, one must remain current on the most recent evidence in assessment and treatment. Developing strategies for life-long learning are essential as well as developing habits that allow for easy access to the most current research literature. The field needs to develop better methods for access to current research, but more work is needed to ensure that access will result in inclusion of research findings into practice (cf., Hardisty & Haaga, 2008, for a discussion of these issues).

Each of the chapters in Section III of this text addresses EBP for specific disorders. We hope that each chapter provides a foundation and that this foundation serves to encourage you to learn more about assessment and treatment. Continued training, through workshops, supervised experiences, and self-exploration is critical. What we know today will be replaced by new and more effective strategies.

References

Ablon, J. S., & Jones, E. E. (1999). Psychotherapy process in the national institute of mental health treatment of depression collaborative research program. *Journal of Consulting and Clinical Psychology, 67,* 64–75.

Agosti, V., Nunes, E., & Ocepeck-Welikson, K. (1996). Client factors related to early attrition from an outpatient cocaine research clinic. *American Journal of Drug and Alcohol Abuse, 22,* 29–39.

Aita, V., McIlvain, H., & Backer, E. (2005). Patient-centered care and communication in primary care practice: What is involved? *Patient Education and Counseling, 58,* 296–304.

Aitken-Swan, J., & Paterson, R. (1955). The cancer patient: Delay in seeking advice. *British Medical Journal, 12,* 623–627.

American Psychological Association (2005). Policy statement on evidence-based practice in psychology. Retrieved July 4, 2008, from http://www2.apa.org/practice/ebpstatement.pdf

AuBuchon, P. G., & Malatesta, V. J. (1994). Obsessive compulsive patients with comorbid personality disorder: Associated problems and response to a comprehensive behavior therapy. *Journal of Clinical Psychiatry, 55,* 448–453.

Ball, S. A., Carroll, K. M., Canning-Ball, M., & Rounsaville, B. J. (2006). Reasons for dropout from drug abuse treatment: Symptoms, personality, and motivation. *Addictive Behaviors, 31,* 320–330.

Barkham, M., Rees, A., Stiles, W. B., Shapiro, D. A., Hardy, G. E., & Reynolds, S. (1996). Dose-effect relations in time-limited psychotherapy for depression. *Journal of Consulting and Clinical Psychology, 64,* 927–935.

Barlow, D. H. (2004). Psychological treatments. *American Psychologists, 59,* 869–878.

Beckham, E. E. (1989). Improvement after evaluation in psychotherapy of depression: Evidence of a placebo effect? *Journal of Clinical Psychology, 45,* 945–950.

Behar, E., & Borkovec, T. D. (2003). Between-group psychotherapy outcome research. In J. A. Schinka & W. Velicer (Eds.), *Comprehensive handbook of psychology: Research Methods* (Vol. 2, pp. 213–240). New York: Wiley.

Blazina, C., & Marks, L. I. (2001). College men's affective reactions to individual therapy, psychoeducational workshops, and men's support group brochures: The influence of gender-role conflict and power dynamics upon help-seeking attitudes. *Psychotherapy: Theory, Research, Practice, Training, 38,* 297–305.

Blood, L. & Cornwall, A. (1994). Pretreatment variables that predict completion of an adolescent substance abuse treatment program. *Journal of Nervous and Mental Disease, 182,* 14–19.

Borkovec, T. D., & Castonguay, L. G. (1998). What is the scientific meaning of "Empirically Supported Therapy"? *Journal of Consulting and Clinical Psychology, 66,* 136–142.

Boufous, S., Silove, D., Bauman, A., & Steel, Z. (2005). Disability and health utilization associated with psychological distress: The influence of ethnicity. *Mental Health Services Research, 7,* 171–179.

Brehm, J. W. (1966). *A theory of psychological reactance.* New York: Academic Press.

Callahan, J. L., Swift, J. K. & Hynan, M. T. (2006). Test of the phase model of psychotherapy in a training clinic. *Psychological Services, 3,* 129–136.

Chambless, D. L., Baker, M. J., Baucom, D. H., Beutler, L. E., Calhoun, K. S., Crits-Christoph, P., et al. (1998). Update on empirically validated therapies, ii. *The Clinical Psychologist, 51,* 3–16.

Chambless, D. L., Sanderson, W. C., Shoham, V., Bennett Johnson, S., Pope, K. S., Crits-Christoph, P., et al. (1996). An update on empirically validated therapies. *The Clinical Psychologist, 49,* 5–18.

Chiesa, M., Drahorad, C., & Longo, S. (2000). Early termination of treatment in personality disorder treated in a psychotherapy hospital. *British Journal of Psychiatry, 177,* 107–111.

Ciraulo, D. A., Piechniczek-Buczek, J., & Iscan, E. N. (2003). Outcome predictors in substance use disorders. *The Psychiatric Clinics of North America, 26,* 381–409.

Collins, F. L., Leffingwell, T. R., & Belar, C. D. (2007). Teaching evidence-based practice: Implications for psychology. *Journal of Clinical Psychology, 63*, 657–670.

Cornford, C. S., Morgan, M., Ridsdale, L. (1993). Why do mothers consult when their children cough? *Family Practice, 10*, 193–196.

de Jong, R., Treiber, R., & Henrich, G. (1986). Effectiveness of two psychological treatments for inpatients with severe and chronic depressions. *Cognitive Therapy and Research, 10*, 645–663.

Diener, E., & Lucas, R.E. (2000). Explaining differences in societal levels of happiness: Relative standards, need fulfillment, culture and evaluation theory. *Journal of Happiness Studies, 1*, 41–78.

Duan, C., & Wang, L. (2000). Counseling in the Chinese cultural context: Accommodating both individualistic and collectivistic values. *Asian Journal of Counseling, 7*, 1–21.

Dubrin, J. R., & Zastowny, T. R. (1988). Predicting early attrition from psychotherapy: An analysis of a large private practice cohort. *Psychotherapy, 25*, 393–408.

Emmelkamp, P. M., Brilman, E., & Kuiper, H. (1986). The treatment of agoraphobia: A comparison of self-instructional training, rational emotive therapy, and exposure in vivo. *Behavior Modification, 10*, 37–53.

Fiester, A. R., & Rudestam, K. E. (1975). A multivariate analysis of early dropout process. *Journal of Consulting and Clinical Psychology, 43*, 528–535.

Fiore, M. C., Bailey, W. C., Cohen, S. J., Dorfman, S. F., Goldstein, M. G., Gritz, E. R., et al. (2000). *Treating tobacco use and dependence. Clinical practice guideline*. Rockville, MD: Department of Health and Human Services, Public Health Service.

Floyd, M. R., Lang, F., & McCord, R. S. (2005). Patients with worry: Presentation of concerns and expectations for response. *Patient Education and Counseling, 57*, 211–216.

Furnham, A., & Bochner, S. (1986). *Culture shock: Psychological reactions to unfamiliar environments*. London: Methuen.

Garb, H. N. (1997). Race bias, social class bias, and gender bias in clinical judgment. *Clinical Psychology: Science and Practice, 4*, 99–120.

Garfield, S. L. (1994). Research on client variables in psychotherapy. In S. L. Garfield & A. E. Bergin (Eds.), *Handbook of Psychotherapy and Behavior Change* (4th ed., pp. 72–113). New York: John Wiley.

Gaston, L., Marmar, C. R., Gallagher, D., & Thompson, L. W. (1989). Impact of confirming patient expectations of change processes in behavioral, cognitive, and brief dynamic psychotherapy. *Psychotherapy: Theory, Research, Practice, Training, 26*, 296–302.

Gibbs, J. T. (1985). City girls: Psychosocial adjustment of urban Black adolescent females. *SAGE: A Scholarly Journal on Black Women, 2*, 28–36.

Goodheart, C. D. (2006). Evidence, endeavor, and expertise in psychology practice. In C. D. Goodheart, A. E. Kazdin, & R. J. Sternbert (Eds.), *Evidence-based psychotherapy: Where practice and research meet* (pp. 37–61). Washington, DC: American Psychological Association.

Green, C. A., Polen, M. R., Dickinson, D. M., Lynch, F. L., & Bennett, M. D. (2002). Gender differences in predictors of initiation, retention, and completion in an HMO-based substance abuse treatment program. *Journal of Substance Abuse Treatment, 23*, 285–295.

Griffith, M. S., & Jones, E. E. (1979). Race and psychotherapy: Changing perspectives. In J. H. Masserman (Ed.), *Current Psychiatric Therapies, 18*, New York: Grune & Stratton.

Gunderson, J. G., Frank, A. F., Ronningstam, E. F., Wachter, S., Lynch, V. J., & Wolfe, P. J. (1989). Early discontinuance of borderline clients from psychotherapy. *Journal of Nervous and Mental Disease, 177*, 38–42.

Haaga, D. A., DeRubeis, R. J., Stewart, B. L., & Beck, A. T. (1991). Relationship of intelligence with cognitive therapy outcome. *Behavior Research and Therapy, 29*, 277–281.

Hardisty, D. J., & Haaga, D.A.F. (2008). Diffusion of treatment research: Does open access matter? *Journal of Clinical Psychology, 64*, 821–839.

Horvath, A. O., & Bedi, R. P. (2002). The alliance. In J. C. Norcross (Ed.), *Psychotherapy relationships that work: Therapist contributions and responsiveness to patients* (pp. 37–69). New York: Oxford University Press.

Horvath, A. O., & Greenberg, L. S. (1994). *The working alliance: Theory, research, and practice*. New York: John Wiley.

Howard, K. I., Lueger, R. J., Maling, M. S., & Martinovich, Z. (1993). A phase model of psychotherapy outcome: Causal mediation of change. *Journal of Consulting and Clinical Psychology, 61*, 678–685.

Institute of Medicine (2001). *Crossing the quality chasm: A new health system for the 21st century.* Washington, DC: National Acadmey Press.

Jenkins, A. H. (1997). The empathic context in psychotherapy with people of color. In A. C. Bohart & L. S. Greenberg (Eds.), *Empathy reconsidered: New directions in psychotherapy* (pp. 321–340). Washington, DC: American Psychological Association.

Jensen, J. P., & Bergin, A. E. (1988). Mental health values of professional therapists: A national interdisciplinary survey. *Professional Psychology: Research and Practice, 19,* 290–297.

Joyce, A. S., & Piper, W. E. (1998). Expectancy, the therapeutic alliance, and treatment outcome in short-term individual psychotherapy. *Journal of Psychotherapy Practice and Research, 7,* 236–248.

Kaslow, N. J., Borden, K. A., Collins, F. L., Jr., Forrest, L., Illfelder-Kaye, J., Nelson, P. D., et al. (2004). Competencies conference: Future directions in education and credentialing in professional psychology. *Journal of Clinical Psychology, 60*(7), 699–712.

Keen, A. J. A. & Freeston, M. H. (2008). Assessing competence in cognitive-behavioral therapy. *The British Journal of Psychiatry, 193,* 60–64.

Kypri, K., Saunders, J. B., & Gallagher, S. J. (2003). Acceptability of various brief intervention approaches for hazardous drinking among university students. *Alcohol and Alcoholism, 38,* 626–628.

Lambert, M. J., & Barley, D. E. (2002). Research summary on the therapeutic relationship and psychotherapy outcome. In J. C. Norcross (Ed.), *Psychotherapy relationships that work: Therapist contributions and responsiveness to patients* (pp. 17–32). New York: Oxford University Press.

Lazare A. (1987). Shame and humiliation in the medical encounter. *Archives of Internal Medicine, 147,* 1653–1658.

Lazarus, A. A. (1971). Reflections on behavior therapy and its development: A point of view. *Behavior Therapy, 2,* 369–374.

Leong, F. T. (1986). Counseling and psychotherapy with Asian-Americans: Review of the literature. *Journal of Counseling Psychology, 33,* 196–206.

Lerner, B. (1972). *Therapy in the ghetto.* Baltimore, MD: Johns Hopkins University Press.

Levinson, W., Kao, A., & Kuby, A. (2005). Not all patients want to participate in decision making: A national study of public preferences. *Journal of General Internal Medicine, 20,* 531–535.

Luborsky, L., McLellan, A. T., Diquer, L., Woody, G. & Seligman, D. A. (1997). The psychotherapist matters: Comparison of outcomes across twenty-two therapists and seven patient samples. *Clinical Psychology: Science and Practice, 4,* 53–65.

Maguire, P. (1984). Communication skills in patient care. In M. Steptoe & A. Mathews (Eds.), *Health Care and Human Behavior* (pp. 153–173). London, UK: Academic Press.

Martin, D. J., Garske, J. P., & Davis, M. K. (2000). Relation of the therapeutic alliance with outcome and other variables: A meta-analytic review. *Journal of Consulting and Clinical Psychology, 68,* 438–450.

Mast, M. S., Kindlmann, A., & Langewitz, W. (2005). Recipients' perspective on breaking bad news: How you put it really makes a difference. *Patient Education and Counseling, 3,* 244–251.

McCabe, O. L. (2004). Crossing the quality chasm in behavioral health care: The role of evidence-based practice. *Professional Psychology: Research & Practice, 35,* 571.

McCrady, B. S., Noel, N. E., Abrams, D. B., & Stout, R. L. (1986). Comparative effectiveness of three types of spouse involvement in outpatient behavioral alcoholism treatment. *Journal of Studies on Alcohol, 47,* 459–467.

McDermut, W., & Zimmerman, M. (1998). The effect of personality disorders on outcome in the treatment of depression. In A. J. Rush (Ed.), *Mood & anxiety disorders* (pp. 321–338). Philadelphia: Williams & Wilkins.

McLellan, A. T., Alterman, A. I., Metzger, D. S., Grissom, G. R., Woody, G. E., Luborsky, L., & O'Brien, C. P. (1994). Similarity of outcome predictors across opiate, cocaine, and alcohol treatments: Role of treatment services. *Journal of Consulting and Clinical Psychology, 62,* 1141–1158.

McLellan, A. T., Luborsky, L., Woody, G. E., Druley, K. A., & O'Brien, C. P. (1983). Predicting response to alcohol and drug abuse treatments: Role of psychiatry severity. *Archives of General Psychiatry, 40,* 620–625.

Miller, W. R., Taylor, C. A., & West, J. C. (1980). Focused versus broad-spectrum behavior therapy for problem drinkers. *Journal of Consulting and Clinical Psychology, 48,* 590–601.

Miranda, J. & Borkovec, T. D. (1999). Reaffirming science in psychotherapy research. *Journal of Clinical Psychology, 55,* 191–200.

Murphy, P. M., Cramer, C., Lillie, F. J. (1984). The relationship between curative factors perceived by patients in their psychotherapy and treatment outcome: An exploratory study. *British Journal of Medical Psychology, 57,* 187–192.

National Institute of Drug Abuse. (1999). *Principles of drug addiction treatment* (NIH Publication No. 99–4180). Rockville, MD: Author.

Nezu, C. M., & Nezu, A. M. (1994). Outpatient psychotherapy for adults with mental retardation and concomitant psychopathology: Research and clinical imperatives. *Journal of Consulting and Clinical Psychology, 62,* 34–42.

Oles, P. K. (1991). Value crisis: Measurement and personality correlates. *Polish Psychological Bulletin, 22,* 53–62.

Orlinsky, D. E., Grawe, K., & Parks, B. K. (1994). Process and outcome in psychotherapy: Noch einmal. In A. E. Bergin and S. L. Garfield (Eds.), *Handbook of psychotherapy and behavior change* (4th ed., pp. 270–376). New York: John Wiley.

Orlinsky, D. E., & Howard, K. I. (1978). The relationship of process to outcome in psychotherapy. In S. L. Garfield & A. E. Bergin (Eds.), *Handbook of psychotherapy and behavior change* (2nd ed., pp. 283–329). New York: Wiley.

Ortega, A. N., & Alegría, M. (2002). Self-reliance, mental health need, and the use of mental healthcare among island Puerto Ricans. *Mental Health Services Research, 4,* 131–140.

Passik, S. D., Kirsch, K. L., Donaghy, K., Holtsclaw, E., Theobald, D., Cella, D., et al. (2002). Patient-related barriers to fatigue communication. Initial validation of the fatigue management barriers questionnaire. *Journal of Pain and Symptom Management, 24,* 481–493.

Patkar, A. A., Thornton, C. C., Mannelli, P., Hill, K. P., Gottheil, E., Vergare, M. J. (2004). Comparison of pretreatment characteristics and treatment outcomes for alcohol-, cocaine-, and multisubstance-dependent patients. *Journal of Addictive Diseases, 23,* 93–109.

Pekarik, G. (1983). Improvement in clients who have given different reasons for dropping out of treatment. *Journal of Clinical Psychology, 39,* 909–913.

Petry, N. M., Tennen, H., & Affleck, G. (2000). Stalking the elusive client variable in psychotherapy research. In C. R. Synder & R. E. Ingram (Eds.), *Handbook of psychological change: Psychotherapy processes and practices for the 21st century* (pp. 88–108). New York: John Wiley & Sons.

Piper, M. E., Fox, B. J., Welsch, S. K., Fiore, M. C., & Baker, T. B. (2001). Gender and racial/ethnic differences in tobacco-dependence treatment: A commentary and research recommendations. *Nicotine & Tobacco Research, 3,* 291–297.

Project MATCH Research Group. (1993). Project MATCH: Rationale and methods for a multisite clinical trial matching patients to alcoholism treatment. *Alcoholism: Clinical and Experimental Research, 17,* 1130–1145.

Project MATCH Research Group. (1997). Project MATCH secondary a priori hypotheses. *Addiction, 92,* 1671–1698.

Reid, T. (1999). A cultural perspective on resistance. *Journal of Psychotherapy Integration, 9,* 57–81.

Riedel-Heller, S. G., Matschinger, H., & Angermeyer, M. C. (2005). Mental disorders—Who and what might help? Help-seeking and treatment preferences of the lay public. *Social Psychiatry and Psychiatric Epidemiology, 40,* 167–174.

Rivers, S. M., Greenbaum, R. L., & Goldberg, E. (2001). Hospital-based adolescent substance abuse treatment: Comorbidity, outcomes, and gender. *Journal of Nervous and Mental Disease, 189,* 229–237.

Robertson, J. M., & Fitzgerald, L. F. (1992). Overcoming the masculine mystique: Preferences for alternative forms of assistance among men who avoid counseling. *Journal of Counseling Psychology, 39,* 240–246.

Ross, S. A. (1983). Variables associated with dropping out of therapy. *Dissertation Abstracts International, 44,* 616.

Rossiter, E. M., Agras, W., Telch, C. F., & Schneider, J. A. (1993). Cluster B personality disorder characteristics predict outcome in the treatment of bulimia nervosa. *International Journal of Eating Disorders, 13,* 349–357.

Roth, A., & Fonagy, P. (2004). *What works for whom? A critical review of psychotherapy research* (2nd ed.). New York: Guilford Press.

Sackett, D. L., Rosenberg, W. M., Gray, J. A., Haynes, R. B., & Richardson, W. S. (1996). Evidence based medicine: What it is and what it isn't. *British Medical Journal, 312,* 71–72.

Sackett, D. L., Straus, S. E., Richardson, W. S., Rosenberg, W. M., & Haynes, R. B. (2000). *Evidence based medicine: How to practice and teach EBM* (2nd ed.). London: Churchill Livingstone.

Sagiv, L., & Schwartz, S. H. (2000). Value priorities and subjective well-being: Direct relations and congruity effects. *European Journal of Social Psychology, 30,* 177.

Schwartz, S. H. (1992). Universals in the content and structure of values: Theoretical advances and empirical tests in 20 countries. In M. P. Zanna (Ed.), *Advances in Experimental Social Psychology* (Vol. 25, pp. 1–65). New York: Academic Press.

Schwartz, S. H., & Rubel, T. (2005). Sex differences in value priorities: Cross-cultural and multimethod studies. *Journal of Personality and Social Psychology, 89,* 1010–1028.

Shapiro, D. A., Firth-Cozens, J., & Stiles, W. B. (1989). The question of therapists' differential effectiveness: A Sheffield Psychotherapy Project addendum. *British Journal of Psychiatry, 154,* 383–385.

Shea, M. T., Pilkonis, P. A., Beckham, E., Collins, J. F., Elkin, I., Sotsky, S. M., et al. (1990). Personality disorders and treatment outcome in the NIMH Treatment of Depression Collaborative Research Program. *American Journal of Psychiatry, 147,* 711–718.

Skodol, A. E., Buckley, P., & Charles, E. (1983). Is there a characteristic pattern to the treatment history of clinic outpatients with borderline personality? *Journal of Nervous and Mental Disease, 171,* 405–410.

Sledge, W. H., Moras, K., Hartley, D., & Levine, M. (1990). Effect of time-limited psychotherapy on client dropout rates. *American Journal of Psychiatry, 147,* 1341–1347.

Smith, L. D., Peck, P. L., & McGovern, R. J. (2004). Factors contributing to the utilization of mental health services in a rural setting. *Psychological Reports, 95,* 435–442.

Street, R. L., Krupat, E., Kravitz, R. L., & Haidet, P. (2003). Beliefs about control in the physician–patient relationship. *Journal of General Internal Medicine, 18,* 606–616.

Strupp, H. H. (1980). Humanism and psychotherapy: A personal statement of the therapist's essential values. *Psychotherapy, 17,* 396–400.

Strupp, H. H., Fox, R. E., & Lessler, K. (1969). *Patients view their psychotherapy.* Baltimore, MD: Johns Hopkins Press.

Substance Abuse and Mental Health Services Administration. (2008). *Treatment Improvement Exchange.* Retrieved July 4, 2008 from http://tie.samhsa.gov/Taps/index.html.

Sue, S. & Zane, N. (1987). The role of culture and cultural techniques in psychotherapy: A critique and reformulation, *American Psychologist, 42,* 37–45.

Task Force on Promotion and Dissemination of Psychological Procedures. (1995). Training in and dissemination of psychological treatments. *The Clinical Psychologist, 48,* 3–23.

Tetlock, P. E. (1986). A value pluralism model of ideological reasoning. *Journal of Personality and Social Psychology, 50,* 819–827.

Thase, M. E., Frank, E., Kornstein, S., & Yonkers, K. A. (2000). Gender differences in response to treatments of depression. In E. Frank (Ed.), *Gender and Its Effects on Psychopathology* (pp. 103–129). Washington, DC: American Psychiatric Press.

Thornton, C. C., Patkar, A. A., Murray, H. W., Mannelli, P., Gottheil, E., Vergare, M. J., et al. (2003). High- and low-structure treatments for substance dependence: Role of learned helplessness. *The American Journal of Drug and Alcohol Abuse, 29,* 567–584.

Wampold, B. E. (2001). *The great psychotherapy debate: Models, methods, and findings.* Mahwah, NJ: Lawrence Erlbaum.

Whaley, A.L. (1998). Racism in the provision of mental health services: A social-cognitive analysis. *American Journal of Orthopsychiatry, 68,* 47–57.

Whitehorn, J. C. (1959). Goals of psychotherapy. In E. A. Rubinstein & M. B. Parloff (Eds.), *Research in psychotherapy.* Washington DC: American Psychological Association.

Wong, E. C., Kim, B. S. K., & Zane, N. W. S. (2003). Examining culturally based variables associated with ethnicity: Influences on credibility perceptions of empirically supported interventions. *Cultural Diversity & Ethnic Minority Psychology, 9,* 88–96.

8

From Individual Therapy to Individualized Treatment

Jessica M. Peirce, Van L. King, and Robert Kevin Brooner

Johns Hopkins University School of Medicine

Contents

Mental health providers are the ideal group to inform and guide the treatment of substance use disorder. Mental health treatments are designed to change behaviors that cause problems for patients or others around them. Substance use disorders are characterized by a set of behaviors that are personally devastating and often detrimental to loved ones and the society at large. Unfortunately, there has been a historical divide between mental health and substance use disorder treatment. Indeed, psychologists, psychiatrists, social workers, and professional counselors often believe that they do not have the expertise to treat substance use disorders, so they exclude patients with those problems from their practice. This leaves treatment of substance use disorder to disciplines that possess less knowledge or interest in the use of evidence-based treatments. This chapter describes evidence-based treatment of substance use disorder that can—and should—be directed by mental health professionals.

The purpose of this chapter is primarily to describe a conceptual approach to treatment of substance use disorder (SUD). We distinguish between chronic SUD and milder forms of SUD (e.g., binge drinking) that, while more common, are by definition less problematic and more easily treated in a wide range of settings. Chronic SUD is more difficult to treat and is the focus of the current chapter. We will review some specific individual therapies that are effective for chronis SUD, but do not intend the review to be exhaustive. Several high-quality reviews have already been written on that topic (see Carroll, 2005; Carroll, Ball, & Martino 2004; and Finney, Wilbourne, & Moos, 2007, as well as other chapters included in this volume). The brief review of individual therapies below is designed to provide a framework for discussing the benefits of these therapies and, more importantly, discussing the considerable limitations of relying solely upon traditional individual therapies for treatment of chronic SUD. We will then describe adaptive treatment, which is a relatively new approach to individualized treatment of SUD that is both flexible and responsive to the SUD patient's needs over the course of treatment. A current example of adaptive treatment will be given later in the chapter to demonstrate how an adaptive treatment approach includes the benefits of traditional individual therapies and helps resolves the limitations inherent in them.

Individual Therapies

Individual Therapy is Effective for Substance Use Disorder

Although considerable research supports the conclusion that treatment is helpful for SUD, it is not yet clear which therapies are most effective under which conditions. This section includes brief descriptions of individual therapies that meet established criteria for empirical support in the research literature (Chambless & Ollendick, 2001). It is not our intent to provide an exhaustive review of all proven individual therapies or an in-depth review of any particular approach. Instead, we highlight specific evidence-based individual therapies that can be a useful part of a comprehensive treatment approach. In the strictest sense, individual therapy in the treatment of substance use disorder consists of a prescribed set of sessions (typically 8–12) during which specific content is delivered and explored by a single therapist and a single patient. The next section describes therapies under this strict definition, including cognitive-behavioral therapy, mindfulness-based therapy, and 12-step facilitation therapy, followed by a discussion of the difficulty in choosing one of these specific therapies over another.

Evidence-Based Individual Therapy

Cognitive-behavioral treatments comprise the largest category of evidence-based individual therapies for SUD reported in the literature. Relapse Prevention (Marlatt & Donovan, 2005;

Marlatt & Gordon, 1985) is the oldest and most well-known of this category, but variations on the model have also emerged, such as cognitive-behavioral therapy for cocaine addiction (Carroll, 1998) or coping skills training (Monti, Rohsenow, Michalec, Martin, & Abrams, 1997). This group of therapies focuses on behaviors, affective responses, and maladaptive cognitions that are thought to precipitate and maintain drug use. Common to these interventions are (a) identifying high-risk situations for drug use, (b) recognizing common affective and cognitive responses to a lapse, and (c) training in coping skills to manage a lapse and prevent future lapses. Key concepts include "apparently irrelevant decisions," which are small decisions that place the patient at increased risk for drug use, and the "abstinence violation effect," which describes a set of common cognitions that label the lapse as a failure. Irvin and colleagues (1999) conducted a meta-analysis and found that relapse prevention was consistently effective, across a wide range of substance classes, and in both individual and group therapy formats. One of the advantages of cognitive-behavioral approaches is the potential for a delayed emergence of benefit, thought to be due to solidification of skills through practice (Carroll, Rounsaville, Nich et al., 1994; Rawson et al., 2002, 2006).

The next generation of cognitive-behavioral therapy approaches has also spawned new mindfulness-based individual therapies for SUD, such as Dialectical Behavior Therapy (DBT; Linehan & Dimeff, 1997) and Acceptance and Commitment Therapy (ACT; Hayes, Strosahl, & Wilson, 1999). Such treatments were originally developed for mood or personality disorders and have had significant success (Bauer, 2003). Recently, these treatments have been reformulated to train substance users in mindfulness and radical acceptance strategies. Mindfulness is the state of full awareness of thoughts, feelings, and sensations. The patient is instructed to be aware, but not to avoid or try to change anything he or she notices. In mindfulness-based treatment, accepting all aspects of self and one's experience is considered a necessary foundation for changing behaviors. Mindfulness and acceptance are conceptualized as alternative coping skills for physical and emotional distress, such as drug craving and guilty feelings after using drugs. Mindfulness-based treatments rely heavily on these emotion regulation skills as central to treatment efficacy (Hoppes, 2006).

Although considerably less data are available on the efficacy of mindfulness-based treatments for SUD, early results appear promising. In a nonrandomized study, incarcerated substance users who learned mindfulness-based Vipassana meditation showed a greater decrease in drug use postrelease than inmates who received SUD treatment as usual (Bowen et al., 2006). In addition, Linehan and colleagues conducted two studies of DBT for substance users with comorbid borderline personality disorder. The first study showed that DBT is somewhat more effective at reducing drug use than treatment as usual in the community (Linehan et al., 1999). The second study expanded on the first by using a comparison treatment that was matched in intensity (Linehan et al., 2002). Patients in the comparison treatment increased their drug use whereas DBT patients' substance use remained essentially the same. Enthusiasm for these results is tempered somewhat by the very high rates of continuing drug use present in the intervention groups, although it is noted that the patient population in these studies was severely impaired by both a chronic substance use disorder and a personality disorder. In support of the underlying principle of mindfulness-based treatments, a very large study showed that patients who exhibited more acceptance behaviors, regardless of treatment received, reduced their substance use over time (Gifford, Ritsher, McKellar, & Moos, 2006).

The 12-step facilitation therapies use the 12-step principles in therapy and emphasize attendance to and involvement in Alcoholics Anonymous and other mutual self-help groups outside of therapy (Nowinski & Baker, 1992). This therapy is considered most beneficial when patients thoroughly immerse themselves in the treatment by regularly attending community-based 12-step meetings, obtaining a 12-step sponsor for guidance, working on the steps of the model in the prescribed fashion with the individual therapist, and using the 12-step group fellowship aspect of the program for support. Because of the strong spiritual component of the 12-step philosophy, 12-step therapies and groups do not appeal to some patients, but several studies have found that 12-step facilitation therapy reduces substance use as much as cognitive-behavioral therapies (Brown, Seraganian, Tremblay, & Annis, 2002; Crits-Cristoph et al., 1999; Glasner-Edwards et al., 2007; Ouimette, Finney, & Moos, 1997). Actual participation in self-help groups is important for beneficial outcomes during and after a treatment episode (Fiorentine, 1999; Morgenstern et al., 2003; Weiss et al., 2005).

Three evidence-based treatment approaches have been reviewed here: cognitive-behavioral therapy, mindfulness-based therapy, and 12-step facilitation. In spite of their development as individual therapies (i.e., a single therapist working with a single patient), all of these approaches can be delivered in a group therapy format and this approach has been adopted in many treatment settings as either the primary modality of treatment or as an integral part. Many aspects of a group therapy service delivery platform are advantageous in the treatment of substance use disorder: reducing stigma, modeling of alternative behaviors, and the universality of common experience helping the individual to adhere to treatment goals and commitments. Group therapy is specifically discussed in another chapter, but we note that group therapy compares favorably to individual therapy in efficacy (Graham, Annis, Brett, & Venesoer, 1996; Weiss, Jaffee, de Menil, & Cogley, 2004). There is also considerable overlap in the hypothesized mechanisms of these three categories of therapies, which has prompted several developers to suggest combining effective therapies. Alan Marlatt, for example, has recently proposed adding mindfulness training to traditional Relapse Prevention to capitalize on the benefits of both (Marlatt, 2002; Witkiewitz, Marlatt, & Walker, 2005). Indeed, combining effective treatments may be the most appropriate approach, given that it is so difficult to choose which treatment to offer.

Comparing Individual Therapies

There are several individual therapies for SUD that have documented empirical support, but there are little data to support choosing one of these therapies over another for any given patient. When compared directly, most individual therapy approaches for SUD produce similar efficacy (e.g., Ouimette et al., 1997; Project MATCH Research Group, 1997a). This may be due, in part, to the common elements present in these individual therapies for SUD (Moos, 2007). Efforts to match treatments to patients based on some predefined set of characteristics have unfortunately consistently failed to produce better patient outcomes (Project MATCH Research Group, 1997b; UKATT Research Team, 2008). There are a number of possible reasons why treatment-matching has failed, including problematic study design (Project MATCH Research Group, 1997b), inappropriate statistical analyses (Witkiewitz, van der Maas, Hufford, & Marlatt, 2007), or a limited choice of predictor and outcome variables (Bühringer, 2006). Although all of these explanations make good sense, we offer yet another likely contribution to this finding. Patients in most of these studies consistently received very little of the planned number of therapy sessions. Attrition and nonadherence to scheduled services are common problems in SUD treatment. Poor adherence to scheduled sessions clearly lowers the "dose" of these therapies and likely reduces their effectiveness to some extent, although perhaps not to the same extent across each of them. For example, some of these therapies may be more efficacious than others when all are delivered at the prescribed doses. Unfortunately, poor adherence to therapy schedules is so large a problem that many randomized controlled trials don't even report the proportion of the scheduled amount of treatment that was actually received by patients (e.g., UKATT Research Team, 2005). Poor attendance to these treatment interventions is a major limitation to interpretation of research on evidence-based treatments and patient-treatment matching. These and other limitations to individual therapy are discussed in the next section.

Limitations of Individual Therapy

Advances in clinical research have led to numerous evidence-based treatments, several of which are outlined above. However, significant limitations remain in their application to patients seeking treatment. This is evident in the failure to disseminate evidence-based treatments to front-line treatment. The first limitation is that individual therapy, as designed, is not feasible for most patients. Not only is traditional individual therapy difficult to implement in typical SUD treatment environments, but it will be clearly insufficient for all patients at all times. For patients with moderate to severe chronic substance use disorders, a course of 8–12 weekly sessions of individual therapy can be beneficial, but is unlikely to be all the treatment that patient will need at that time or during his drug-using career. In addition to the amount of therapy offered, the amount of therapy the patient actually receives is often less than that scheduled. This comprises the second limitation: patients' participation in scheduled therapy is typically poor, thereby reducing treatment effectiveness. In combination, these problems result in most patients with difficult-to-treat SUDs coming into contact with very little of the evidence-based therapy. We explore these limitations and their effects in this section.

Standard Individual Therapy is Impractical

Evidence-based individual therapies have not been widely adopted for use in treatment of SUDs. This failure is largely due to two problems with the interventions themselves. Several features of the therapies, as designed, are incompatible with characteristics of the outpatient therapeutic environments in which most patients with SUDs are treated. More important, however, is that individual once-weekly treatment provides an inadequate dose of treatment for many patients with moderate to severe substance use problems. Each of these problems alone weakens the benefit of well-validated individual therapy. Together, they mean that individual therapy alone is often inadequate.

Individual therapies that meet empirical tests for efficacy must, by definition, have clear structure and content. In addition, therapists need to learn the therapy and reliably adhere to the structure and content across patients and over time. Each of these necessary components of therapy poses problems for most environments in which patients with SUD are treated. The structure of most individual therapies for SUD typically includes 8–12 one-hour individual weekly sessions (e.g., Relapse Prevention; Marlatt & Gordon, 1985). The vast majority of SUD treatment in the United States is provided in outpatient treatment facilities wherein individual direct patient care is provided by counselors in sessions lasting 30 minutes. Frequency of scheduled sessions ranges from once weekly to once monthly, and counseling is often offered without a schedule on an "as-needed" basis. Thus, fidelity to the structure of traditional individual therapies is already challenged, because existing therapy sessions would have to increase in length and frequency.

Individual therapy content is usually standardized with the use of a treatment manual, in which detailed instructions are provided about the topics to be covered, how to discuss them, and how to manage typical patient responses (Chambless & Ollendick, 2001). Currently, however, the use of treatment manuals in SUD treatment is very uncommon. This is true even in community-based treatment programs participating in the National Drug Abuse Clinical Trials Network (CTN), the staff of which are considered relatively open to evidence-based practice (McCarty et al., 2008). With little prior experience, counselors will have trouble applying manualized therapies. Counselor education prior to their work experience is also unlikely to have included specific exposure to evidence-based treatments for substance use disorders or training in their application (Ball et al., 2002). Even in the CTN, the highest educational attainment for the majority of counselors is a Bachelor's degree (McCarty et al., 2007), and few college programs provide more than a survey of clinical orientations. For those counselors who are interested in using evidence-based treatments, considerable evidence shows that merely reading the manual is insufficient to fully understand and correctly deliver the therapy (Miller, Yahne, Moyers, Martinez, & Pirritano, 2004; Sholomskas et al., 2005). Current research on training therapists to deliver manual-guided therapy emphasizes extensive didactic training, practice cases with measures of treatment adherence, and ongoing intensive clinical supervision (Carroll et al., 2002). The current structure of most treatment programs likely could not support such intensive training and supervision. Aside from the prohibitive cost of reducing counselors' direct care responsibilities to devote time to training, 42% of supervisors (even in CTN community-based clinics) have no more educational or experiential exposure to evidence-based treatments than counselors (McCarty et al., 2007).

Standard Individual Therapy is Insufficient

Even if treatment could be provided in one-hour weekly sessions given by experienced and well-trained therapists, there remains the problem that individual therapy provided in one session per week is inadequate for many patients. Patients with moderate or severe SUDs will typically have periods of instability in drug use or in drug use-associated problems. Such periods will require at least brief episodes of more intensive treatment, often by both the primary individual therapist and additional providers.

Chronic substance use disorder is similar in many ways to chronic medical illnesses such as adult-onset diabetes and asthma (see McLellan, Lewis, O'Brien, & Kleber, 2000 for more discussion on this point). Chronic SUD and chronic medical illnesses are characterized by periods of relative health interspersed with relapse to disordered functioning. Both types of chronic illnesses require regular ongoing care that needs to fluctuate in intensity in response to the health of the patient. Patients who are extremely unstable in their drug use are likely to need increased amounts and more varied kinds of care than once-weekly individual therapy. For example, patients who are dependent on benzodiazepines or alcohol may require a medically supervised inpatient detoxification to prevent withdrawal-related morbidity or mortality. Outpatient medications such as disulfiram or naltrexone may be helpful for patients trying to stop drug use, but they need to be prescribed by a physician and adherence must be monitored. For any patient who has increased her drug use to one or more daily doses, regardless of the drug used, intensified treatment is recommended to help restabilize drug-free lifestyle patterns that will promote abstinence. More frequent visits to the therapist may be necessary, and the patient's family and friends may be recruited to assist with treatment implementation. With continued drug use, the patient's housing, employment, and financial stability are also likely to be threatened, which may require case management services to help the patient reestablish a safe and drug-free environment.

Unfortunately, intensifying and broadening treatment for unstable SUD patients is often cost- and time-prohibitive. Even mild intensifications, such as increasing from once- to thrice-weekly individual therapy sessions, would greatly increase cost to the patient and health care system as well as increase the time burden on the therapist, who may already have a large caseload. Broadening the scope of therapy to include inpatient care, medication, family therapy, or case management also adds more providers, which in turn increases cost to the patient and time from the therapist's and others' schedules.

Some individual therapists persist in the belief that they can prevent problems related to more severe drug use by refusing to admit unstable substance use disordered patients to their practice. Unfortunately, information provided by the patient at admission is subject to change. Patients seeking treatment will commonly underreport their current drug use, including those who are seeking treatment specifically for chronic SUD (Darke, 1998). Without objective or corroborating measures of drug use severity, the individual therapist will make a decision about accepting a patient into care based on inaccurate information that typically reflects less than actual use. Furthermore, a patient whose drug use is not problematic at treatment entry may not remain stable throughout the course of treatment. Relapse is a central feature of the disorder, and should be expected. In either situation, good therapists will endeavor to provide an appropriate level of care, thus placing them in the same position of needing to intensify treatment for patients.

Significant problems with the application of evidence-based treatments have prevented the SUD treatment community from fully embracing them. SUD treatment developed outside a traditional psychotherapy environment, and many of the structures in place conflict with good individual psychotherapy practice. SUD treatment providers are often ill-equipped to learn and apply individual therapy approaches, and would be hard-pressed to do so in most SUD clinic treatment settings. On the other hand, several aspects of SUD treatment clinic settings are more useful than office-based individual therapy, particularly the ability to intensify treatment for patients in need. However, both types of settings suffer from the other primary limitation to individual therapy for SUD, namely that patients receive so little of the treatment that its efficacy is limited.

Participation in Substance Use Disorder Treatment is Poor

If and when the necessary intensified treatment services can be offered to a patient, it is common for patients to fail to participate fully in treatment. Nonparticipation manifests in two ways: attrition and nonadherence to scheduled services. Attrition occurs when a patient leaves the treatment setting before the treatment plan goals are achieved. It is a problem associated with many psychiatric disorders, but attrition is a central feature of substance use disorders. Nonadherence to scheduled treatment is somewhat different and a much more prevalent problem, in that many patients remain enrolled in treatment but fail to attend the scheduled treatment services. In our experience, nonadherence is rather more frustrating for providers than attrition and a much greater drain on treatment resources, but any form of nonparticipation limits the benefits and success of SUD treatment. Research on the extent of nonparticipation and its effects on treatment response and outcomes is reviewed here.

Attrition is a well-known problem in SUD treatment settings. Attrition rates range widely in treatment, depending upon the treatment modality and patient population, but often occurs at rates as high as 75% over the whole treatment episode, with most attrition occurring within the first three months (Crits-Cristoph et al., 1999; Simpson, Joe, & Rowan-Szal, 1997). Much of the work on attrition has been conducted within clinic settings and less is known about office-based individual therapy attrition, although it is unlikely to be less severe, because clinics have many more resources to re-engage patients in treatment. Attrition occurs at all stages of treatment, but early attrition is potentially the most damaging, because patients leave prior to any experience of treatment benefits, including hope for success if they invest additional time and effort. It is not uncommon for fewer than half of people scheduled for an intake to attend that appointment (Chawdhary et al., 2007), which means that large numbers of drug users who have some interest in treatment do not receive any. The rate of attrition is consistently higher in the first few weeks of treatment even after attending the first appointment, regardless of treatment delivered (Pena et al., 1999). Such high attrition rates have spawned increasing insistence on full disclosure about attrition in research studies and statistical analyses of outcome that include all patients accepted for treatment, otherwise known as the "intention-to-treat" sample (Carroll, Rounsaville, Gordon et al., 1994; Pena et al., 1999).

Nonadherence to scheduled services is less well-studied in SUD treatment settings and rarely reported, but is no less a problem. Without specific intervention, patients regularly attend less than 50% of scheduled counseling sessions (Ball & Ross, 1991; Brooner et al., 2007, 2004) and nonadherence with SUD treatment medications such as disulfiram and naltrexone is very high (Weiss, 2004). Unfortunately, chronic SUD is only one of many chronic illnesses that are characterized by a need for long-term treatment, the success of which is compromised by poor patient adherence. Good long-term management of chronic illnesses such as adult-onset diabetes, hypertension, or schizophrenia require regular health care visits, increased health behaviors such as exercise or scheduled activities, and proper medication administration to maximize and sustain gains in health (McLellan et al., 2000). Nonadherence to any part of the treatment plan increases the risk of symptom recurrence or exacerbation. For example, a patient with schizophrenia who does not adhere to a regular schedule of activities or take psychiatric medication as prescribed will be at risk for increased psychotic symptoms and more frequent hospitalizations (Leucht & Heres, 2006). Similarly, patients with chronic SUD who do not attend all scheduled services or take treatment medication as prescribed are at risk for increased drug use and deterioration in associated medical and psychiatric problems.

As noted earlier, attrition and nonadherence are often related but intrinsically different. Patients who leave treatment early have typically been nonadherent to some or all of the treatment prior to leaving. However, patients can be—and often are—considered to have completed treatment if they remained enrolled for the prescribed length of time, even if they have not adhered to treatment while enrolled. A seminal study by Crits-Cristoph and colleagues (1999) provides a good example of the interaction between attrition and nonadherence to treatment services. Of the 1,777 eligible treatment-seeking cocaine users, 65% ($N=1,148$) failed to attend one or more of the three orientation appointments, which were incorporated into the design to exclude potential participants who likely would not adhere to study requirements. Fewer than one-third (28%) of participants who met enrollment criteria, including the orientation appointments, actually completed the prescribed six months of treatment. These two stages of attrition, in addition to other problems, resulted in the final group of completers comprising less than 8% of the original study sample. Nonadherence was also a problem overall, as participants in the better-attended treatment conditions (cognitive therapy and supportive-expressive therapy) attended less than half of their scheduled sessions (about 16 of 36 individual sessions). The authors did not separate the figures on attrition and nonadherence, so it was impossible for us to determine the rate of nonadherence in those participants considered to be treatment completers. We highlight the Crits-Cristoph et al. study here to demonstrate that both attrition and nonadherence are significant problems in the treatment of patients with SUD, even when high-quality treatments are offered by well-trained providers. Perhaps even more important, nonparticipation can confound the interpretation and our expectations of both the efficacy and effectiveness of SUD treatment. It seems risky to draw conclusions that one treatment is more efficacious than another when both are delivered at much lower rates than prescribed.

The effects of nonparticipation are not well studied, because studying it requires one to compare treatment outcomes of patients who received an adequate dose of treatment with those who receive less exposure. This is more difficult than it sounds. Comparing outcomes of patients who voluntarily attend more treatment to patients who do not participate confounds the results with the possible presence of a third factor related to voluntary participation. That is, patients who voluntarily attend more treatment may be more likely to succeed with any amount of treatment. Although randomization to participation versus nonparticipation would remove the self-selection bias, it is difficult to support ethically when the treatment under study is efficacious. These caveats notwithstanding, studies of nonparticipation have consistently found that treatment retention is associated with better outcomes across treatment modalities (e.g., Hser, Evans, Huang, & Anglin, 2004; Simpson et al., 1997) and that patients who attend more of the scheduled treatment stay in treatment longer (Simpson et al., 1997) and have better outcomes (Schumacher et al., 1995). As discussed earlier, reports of nonadherence are often indistinguishable from attrition, which masks the independent contribution of nonadherence to treatment outcome. The problem of nonadherence is relatively understudied, compared to attrition, and likely has a greater bearing on poor treatment outcomes than has been acknowledged previously. In the next sections, we review causes of nonparticipation as well as the solutions that have been offered for both attrition and nonadherence.

Contributors to Nonparticipation in Substance Use Disorder Treatment

Nonparticipation in SUD treatment can generally be attributed to some combination of patient or organization characteristics. Patient causes of nonparticipation are those that are internal to the patient which inhibit his or her ability to fully engage in treatment. These include low internal motivation for abstinence or treatment, age, race, gender, and comorbid psychiatric disorders. Organizational characteristics that negatively influence participation are often called "barriers to treatment." These are typically features of the organization that make it difficult for a patient to engage in treatment. Examples include long waiting periods for admission, the absence of additional desirable treatment services, high cost, and problems with transportation. Considerable effort has been invested in attempting to determine the most likely causes of nonparticipation so that their influence can be diminished and thereby improve treatment outcomes. We review below the patient-based and organization-based variables that are thought to increase nonparticipation.

The earliest research on sources of nonparticipation focused on patient variables, with a specific emphasis on internal motivation for treatment. It is more accurate to say that nonparticipation was typically interpreted to represent patients' low treatment motivation, because motivation was rarely assessed in any systematic way. Recent work has more rigorously evaluated the influence of several patient variables, including motivation, demography (i.e., age, race, gender), and comorbidity. Although individual studies have found relationships, the preponderance of the literature has failed to find any consistent predictive utility in these variables, with the exception of psychiatric comorbidity, specifically, comorbid Axis II disorders. Personality disorders that are comorbid with SUD, whether or not the patients also carry an additional comorbid Axis I disorder, consistently increase the risk of attrition (Cacciola, Alterman, Rutherford, McKay, & Mulvaney, 2001; Daughters et al., 2008; Martinez-Raga, Marshall, Keaney, Ball, & Strang, 2002) and nonadherence (Neufeld et al., 2008). Preliminary work has also suggested that impulsivity, low distress tolerance, and low cognitive functioning contribute to attrition from SUD treatment (Aharonovich et al., 2006; Daughters et al., 2005, 2008; Moeller et al., 2001; Patkar et al., 2004), although these findings have yet to be consistently replicated.

The finding that motivation has not been related to treatment participation requires further explanation. Standardized measures of motivation such as the URICA (DiClemente & Hughes, 1990) typically do not change much during treatment and have not been predictive of participation in treatment (Blanchard, Morgenstern, Morgan, Labouvie, & Bux, 2003; Carpenter, Miele, & Hasin, 2002; Carroll et al., 2006). It is not our intention to say that motivation does not exist or is not important. Rather, it seems likely that patients have some motivation to participate in treatment, but we are not able to accurately quantify their motivation with the current measures. In addition, efforts to influence changes in motivation that can be measured by questionnaires have been generally unsuccessful, although several interventions can successfully increase participation in treatment (see below).

Apart from motivation, studies that rely solely on patient-related predictors of nonparticipation complicate interpretation of their results. The few studies that have found an influence of patient-related variables such as age or gender have generally failed to include other predictor variables that are known to have greater influence on nonparticipation (Curran, Stecker, Han, & Booth, 2009; Greenfield et al., 2007). Furthermore, the mechanism by which the relevant patient variables increase nonparticipation is not clear. Does a personality disorder itself prevent a patient from attending treatment, or is it that a patient with a personality disorder has difficulty interacting effectively with the organization and leaves frustrated? The latter seems more likely, and increased attention to the interaction of the patient with the treatment should prove more fruitful. Recent studies have found that patients with relatively low risk for attrition have greatly increased risk when they report conflict with treatment staff (Ball, Carroll, Canning-Ball, & Rounsaville, 2006; McKellar, Kelly, Harris, & Moos, 2006). Alternatively, the therapy itself may be difficult for the patient, as with lower-functioning patients enrolled in cognitive-behavioral therapies (Aharonovich et al., 2006).

In contrast, several organizational contributors have been reliably related to nonparticipation, including long waits for admission and the absence of additional treatment services in the treatment setting. An often overlooked but consistent predictor of attrition is the length of time until the first appointment (Claus & Kindleberger, 2002; Festinger, Lamb, Kountz, Kirby & Marlowe, 1995; Stasiewicz & Stalker, 1999). Patients seeking treatment are often asked to wait until the next fixed intake day, which can be days to weeks away. Clinics that require several visits before admission also increase the chances that patients will fail to return during that process. In fact, clinics not infrequently depend on early attrition to drop patients thought to have low motivation. Again, this approach conflicts with the data in that patients required to wait even a few days are at increased risk for attrition, regardless of their measurable motivation for treatment (Chawdhary et al., 2007). Also concerning is the long wait for treatment access because there are insufficient treatment slots available for the need in the area. This problem is particularly acute in rural and suburban settings where a number of societal pressures, including cost and stigmatization, prevent sufficient SUD treatment settings, but it is no less a problem in many large urban settings with substantial numbers of people who need SUD treatment.

Even after a patient is able to access treatment, many providers do not have the range of services many patients need. A particularly acute example is the documented need for psychiatric care. About 50% of patients seeking treatment have at least one comorbid psychiatric disorder (Brooner, King, Kidorf, Schmidt, & Bigelow, 1997; Kessler, 2004), but very few treatment settings provide psychiatric care (McGovern, Xie, Segal, Siembab, & Drake, 2006). Having psychiatric care within the SUD treatment setting increases length of stay and utilization of those services; both of those responses are also associated with better drug use outcomes (Grella & Stein, 2006). The medical literature clearly identifies that poorly treated depressed mood increases medical nonadherence to treatment for coronary heart disease (Gehi, Haas, Pipkin, & Whooley, 2005). Depression or other psychiatric comorbidities that are not treated within the SUD treatment setting seem just as likely to increase nonadherence and ultimately lead to the attrition noted above. Other barriers to treatment often considered clinically important, such as high cost and problems with transportation, have surprisingly not been related to attrition, either in objective comparisons or by patient self-report (Ball et al., 2006).

Relatively few patient- and organization-based characteristics consistently contribute to nonparticipation. In truth, far more is known about what does not cause treatment nonparticipation than what does. The only useful purpose in searching for causes of nonparticipation is to develop responses that will increase participation. With those variables that we know are related to nonparticipation—psychiatric disorders, long admission waiting times, and lack of enhanced treatment services—the solutions are clear: provide assessment and integrated treatment of psychiatric disorders and reduce waiting time. However, there are several interventions that directly address nonparticipation that occurs for any reason. A discussion of these follows.

Current Approaches to Nonparticipation in Substance Use Disorder Treatment

Before methods to reduce nonparticipation are reviewed, a discussion of the current attitudes and approaches to nonparticipation is warranted. As noted in the prior section, there is a strong tendency in clinical settings to interpret attrition and nonadherence as evidence of low motivation. This attitude persists in spite of considerable research that clearly indicates that motivation, per se, is only one contributor to nonparticipation, and a relatively minor one at that. Unfortunately, the problem this fallacy creates is compounded by the dominant provider response to perceived low motivation, which is to dismiss the patient and expect that he or she will return to treatment when "ready." Either the patient or provider then initiates discharge, and often the provider bars the patient from treatment for a set period of time, often six months to a year or longer. This response blames the patient wholly for nonparticipation, does nothing to treat the problem, and draws attention away from those sources of nonparticipation that can be addressed directly. A persistent belief that their efforts are unwanted and unhelpful also likely contributes to the high burnout and turnover rate in SUD treatment professionals (Knudsen, Ducharme, & Roman, 2007).

The transtheoretical "stages of change" model revolutionized attitudes toward patients considered resistant or unmotivated for treatment by introducing the concept of ambivalence as an inherent characteristic of substance use disorders (Prochaska, DiClemente, & Norcross, 1992). A substantial benefit of this approach is that providers are more accepting of patients' nonparticipation and less eager to discharge them. A drawback is that ambivalence is just as difficult to measure as motivation has been, although ambivalence is considered a more viable target for treatment. The "stages of change" provides a framework for addressing ambivalence that is consistent with therapeutic orientations such as Motivational Interviewing (Miller, 1983).

Regardless of the underlying cause of nonparticipation, several interventions have been developed that increase patients' participation in treatment. Three interventions have been reliably effective in reducing attrition and nonadherence: contingency management, Motivational Interviewing, and role induction. Contingency management is the term for providing reinforcers to increase behaviors integral to SUD recovery, such as adhering to counseling sessions, providing drug-negative urine specimens, or adhering to medical or psychiatric care. Contingency management has reliably reduced attrition from treatment and increased adherence to sessions, among a wide range of behavioral targets (see Stitzer and Petry, 2006, for a review). Motivational Interviewing (MI), as described by Miller and Rollnick (2002), is often called an intervention, but is more appropriately considered a therapeutic style (Hettema, Steele, & Miller, 2005). The purpose of MI is to explore ambivalence toward abstinence and treatment, help resolve that ambivalence, and elicit commitments to change. As might be expected based on the description, MI has particular benefit with regard to increasing treatment adherence (see Hettema et al., 2005, for a review). Finally, role induction is a method of orienting patients to what they should expect from treatment and what is expected of them (Zweben & Li, 1981). Role induction interventions were specifically designed to increase retention in psychotherapy, but the approaches had fallen out of favor for many years. Recent work has brought role induction back as a useful method of increasing both retention in and adherence to SUD treatment (Harrison et al., 2007; Katz et al., 2004, 2007). Because they are transtheoretical, these interventions can be added to any treatment. In fact, there is evidence that they are most successful when added to treatment instead of being used as standalone treatments (Miller & Rollnick, 2002).

This section has reviewed the limitations of individual therapy alone for SUD. Not only is high-quality individual therapy difficult to implement in the usual clinic environment, but patients with chronic SUD often need far more care than individual therapists can usually provide. Patients' unwillingness to participate in treatment is one of the signs that establishes their need for more treatment, and places them at high risk of leaving treatment or failing to attend scheduled services at a higher intensity of care. Treatment goals need to be expanded to include attrition and nonadherence and allow increases and decreases in intensity as the patients demonstrate their need. There is an increasing need for adaptive treatment strategies that individualize treatment by addressing the patient's response in real-time. Adaptive treatment is growing in acceptance in the medical and psychiatric care fields, and is the next stage of evidence-based SUD treatment.

The Next Wave in Substance Use Disorder Treatment

Adaptive Treatment Models for Chronic Substance Use Disorder

Although individual therapy alone has limited effectiveness with a large percentage of the patients seeking treatment for SUD, adaptive treatment strategies build on the strengths of individual evidence-based intervention and resolve some of the limitations regarding feasibility and necessary intensity. Adaptive treatment models embody the goals of individualized treatment by establishing structured plans of care that systematically seek to match the intensity and scope of service to well-defined objective indicators of problem severity in a dynamic and flexible fashion over extended periods of time (Murphy, Lynch, Oslin, McKay, & TenHave, 2007). Adaptive treatments have emerged in recent years as the best practice models for many chronic health problems, including obesity (Berkowitz, Wadden, Tershakovec, & Cronquist, 2003), bipolar disorder (Perlis et al., 2006), and depression (Rush et al., 2006). Although the field of SUD treatment has been slower to embrace adaptive treatment models, several groups have expressed support for this type of approach (Carroll & Rounsaville, 2007; Kidorf, King, & Brooner, 2006; McKay 2006; Murphy et al., 2007; Sobell and Sobell, 2000).

Essentially, adaptive treatment for SUD may be particularly well suited to the chronic form of SUD, which constitutes a large proportion of people seeking help for this problem. The long-term nature of chronic SUD necessitates long-term management of the disorder, which increases the risk of poor patient adherence. This problem is compounded by treatments that are inconvenient and often produce unpleasant side effects while improving overall functioning. Adaptive treatment approaches seek to employ the least intrusive and least costly amount of services necessary to achieve and sustain good response to treatment over episodes of care that can last for many months and years. This method is a remarkably efficient way to establish and adjust the intensity and scope of treatment services for people with chronic SUDs, and is flexible enough to readily incorporate a wide range of clinical interventions for a range of clinical problems. With an adaptive approach, new admissions are routinely assigned to lower intensities of care and are only advanced to brief periods of higher intensity and broader scopes of service based upon objective indicators of continued partial or poor treatment response to lower intensities of service (Breslin et al., 1998; Brooner et al., 2004, 2007; McKay, Lynch, Shepard, & Pettinati, 2005). Less treatment is prescribed for patients with good and improving responses to care, and more intensive treatment schedules are employed for brief periods in those with evidence of a partial or poor response.

Aside from the model developed by our group, described below, there are only a few studies of adaptive treatment approaches in the substance abuse treatment literature. Breslin et al. (1998) investigated an adaptive treatment for problem drinkers. In this study, problem drinkers who did not respond to an initial 4-session motivational intervention were randomized either to ongoing evaluation or an additional motivational session. There were no differences in outcome between the two groups at the 6-month follow-up, but this may have been due either to the poor patient adherence or the low intensity of both the patients' problems and the added intervention. A recent telephone-based motivational intervention study conducted in primary care settings compared an adaptive stepped care intervention to reduce problem drinking to a standardized intervention and a no-treatment group (Bischof et al., 2008). The interventions had equivalent outcomes, which were better than the no-treatment outcome, with the adaptive treatment resulting in lower costs because only those patients needing further intervention received it. McKay et al. (2005) used an adaptive continuing care approach for patients who had finished a 4-week episode of intensive outpatient therapy for alcohol or cocaine dependence. A lower-intensity telephone-based continuing care treatment yielded better outcomes for patients who had stabilized adequately during the IOP phase of treatment when compared to patients who were assigned to a standard-care, group therapy intervention. However, patients who demonstrated poor progress in achieving goals in the IOP phase did better in the standard continuing care condition. Kakko et al. (2007) evaluated an adaptive stepped care treatment for heroin dependence in which patients were started on buprenorphine/naloxone and switched to methadone upon evidence of poor response. The adaptive treatment was identical in retention outcomes to the standard methadone maintenance treatment condition (78% over six months), probably because both groups also received high-quality psychosocial interventions with treatment intensification as needed.

In a novel study of a population with comorbid problems, Zatzick et al. (2004) compared an adaptive approach to standard treatment for patients who had experienced acute physical trauma requiring hospitalization. Adaptive treatment patients received ongoing intensive case management, and were assessed for PTSD and alcohol abuse at three months posttrauma. Patients diagnosed with either problem were immediately offered specific treatment by appropriate team members (i.e., care was intensified). Standard treatment patients were given referrals at the end of the initial hospitalization period. The adaptive treatment patients had improved 12-month PTSD and alcohol abuse outcomes compared to the standard treatment patients. Together, these five studies support the benefit of adaptive treatment for SUD, but none presents a comprehensive approach to chronic SUD that fully addresses the limitations of individual therapy.

A comprehensive adaptive treatment for chronic SUD will address the problems with individual therapy described above. It ideally would include methods to increase intensity of treatment with more clinical contact, and would use predefined objective criteria to adjust the intensity of services either upward or downward. These approaches are likely to produce more consistent evidence of increased efficacy when evidence-based treatment interventions are employed. The major problem limiting many of the present examples of adaptive treatment is the well-known problem of poor adherence. Simply scheduling more treatment services of any type has limited therapeutic value unless the service is actually delivered to the patient. A comprehensive adaptive treatment model therefore must incorporate interventions to improve patient attendance to scheduled services, as well as offer several steps of treatment intensity and access to a wide enough scope of services to adequately address the more common problems associated with chronic SUD.

A Real-World Comprehensive Adaptive Treatment Model for Substance Use Disorder

Prior work at our center has focused on the establishment, testing, and refinement of a comprehensive adaptive treatment approach for people with chronic opioid dependence disorder that is routinely complicated by the presence of one or more additional substance use diagnoses (e.g., cocaine, alcohol, cannabis, or sedative use disorders), along with other types of psychiatric and social problems. This treatment approach is commonly referred to as Motivated Stepped Care (MSC; Kidorf et al., 2006), which embodies all of the principles of adaptive care models (Murphy et al., 2007). In a series of studies published over the past decade, we have shown that patients receiving this adaptive MSC have dramatically increased attendance to scheduled counseling sessions at all levels of intensity, reduced substance use, increased social support within the treatment setting and in the community, and demonstrated marked increases in rates of employment (Kidorf, Neufeld, King, Clark, & Brooner, 2007; Kidorf, Neufeld, & Brooner, 2004; King et al., 2006; Brooner et al., 2007, 2004). This treatment model is presented below in greater detail as an example of an adaptive treatment that substantially addresses many of the limitations of treatment plans that rely solely on individual therapy for SUD.

Adaptive Motivated Stepped Care addresses the long-term requirements of chronic SUD patients by matching intensity of service to severity of problem in a dynamic fashion over time using behavioral reinforcement to motivate counseling adherence and treatment plan progress. Figure 8.1 is a schematic diagram of the adaptive MSC model. All new admissions routinely start treatment at Step 2, receiving 0.5 to 1.5 hours of weekly drug counseling with a Bachelor's-trained counselor combined with weekly urine monitoring and individualized clinic-based dispensing of opioid agonist medications (e.g., methadone). Treatment success is defined a priori as the following: (1) random weekly urine toxicology tests negative for all drugs, (2) full adherence to scheduled counseling, and (3) adherence to other parts of the treatment plan (e.g., employment, social functioning). Patients who respond well to this

FIGURE 8.1
Diagram of Adaptive Motivated Stepped Care Treatment.

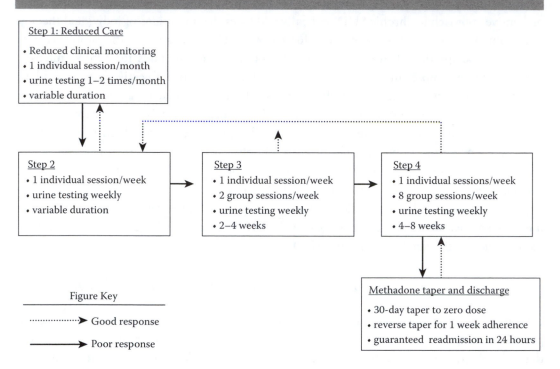

treatment schedule for several months (i.e., meet all objective criteria) are reduced to Step 1, in which patients attend one individual counseling session every 14 to 28 days and provide two urine samples per month for testing. Patients can always request and receive additional services if desired.

Patients with a partial or poor response to Step 2 (i.e., missed counseling sessions or drug-positive urine tests or both for two weeks) are advanced to Step 3 the very next week. Step 3 patients are routinely scheduled for about 3 to 4 hours per week of individual and group counseling. Patients who fail to produce at least two consecutive weeks of attendance to all scheduled counseling sessions or continue to provide drug-positive urine specimens within a period of four weeks are advanced to Step 4, the highest schedule of treatment intensity and scope available in our outpatient setting. In this step, patients are scheduled to attend up to 9 hours of counseling per week including individual counseling, stress management group, relapse control group, coping skills group, cognitive-behavioral therapy group, and a community support group. All of the group treatments are based on evidence-based therapies and are conducted by senior Master's-trained therapists, clinical psychologists, and board-certified psychiatrists.

Behavioral contingencies are active at all steps of care in this treatment model to motivate good progress in the treatment plan, but are adaptively applied such that the more strongly reinforcing contingencies are used at the higher steps of care. For example, patients are expected to attend the clinic on every day scheduled for medication, as well as all scheduled counseling sessions to avoid movement to higher steps of care. Once in Step 4, patients are also asked to identify and bring into the treatment program a drug-free community support person who participates in a community support group. The patient and support person have behavioral homework each week designed to assist the patient to establish or enhance use of positive drug-free social networks. If patients do not adhere to the plan of care, they are subject to a 30-day methadone taper in preparation for discharge. However, the medication taper can be reversed after only one week of attendance to all scheduled sessions along with a single drug-negative urine specimen. Patients who elect to complete the taper are offered rapid readmission as soon as 24 hours if they agree to restart at Step 4 and work toward returning to the lower steps of care. Once four weeks of attendance and drug-negative urine specimens are achieved, patients are returned to Step 2 to continue their care and help solidify the gains accomplished at the higher steps of care. This is a very dynamic treatment process with repeated bidirectional moves across the different steps of care and, as such, a more individualized treatment episode than commonly provided in many SUD treatment settings.

Adaptive Motivated Stepped Care is an adaptive treatment for chronic SUD applied in a real-world community-based treatment setting. Many of the limitations of individual therapy are substantially lessened by an adaptive MSC approach. Most valuable is the ability to intensify treatment as needed by increasing scheduled clinical contact. The use of group therapy in particular maximizes the ability to deliver treatment to a large number of patients with no increase in staff or space necessary. Group therapy is as effective as individual therapy, particularly when the content is empirically based (Graham et al., 1996; Weiss et al., 2004). It is important that Master's-trained and doctoral staff, who have considerably more training and experience in evidence-based treatment provide much of the group therapy. When patients demonstrate clear need for more intensive care, they are systematically exposed both to increased amounts and a broader scope of empirically based therapy with much of the added service provided by the most senior staff in the program. Patients who respond well to the lower intensities of care (e.g., Steps 2 and 1) are never required to participate in more intrusive and costly high-intensity services, which make the overall approach more cost-efficient than if all patients were exposed to the high-intensity steps of care and worked toward lower intensities. Another vital component of the treatment model is the use of predetermined objective criteria to guide changes in treatment intensity. Both drug-positive urine test results and counseling nonadherence are considered evidence of increased need for treatment. Attendance to individual and group counseling sessions is recorded by the provider after the scheduled session, so is just as objective as urine test results. This particular feature of the model reduces the mystery of the treatment planning process for patients, sets clear guidelines for staff, and makes treatment a predictable experience overall.

The considerable problem of patient nonadherence with scheduled treatment services is directly addressed within the MSC model of adaptive treatment. Adherence with scheduled counseling is considered a primary treatment outcome measure and is specifically targeted for improvement by using both positive and negative reinforcement, otherwise described in the context of this treatment approach as behavioral contingencies. The use of behavioral contingencies builds on extensive research showing that contingency management improves treatment outcome for a wide range of targeted behaviors (Stitzer & Petry, 2006). Patients will make substantial gains in reduced drug use and nonparticipation with large cash or voucher payments, but these are less feasible for community-based clinics (Petry, Alessi, Marx, Austin, & Tardif, 2005). Lower-cost positive reinforcement such as chances to win prizes (Peirce et al., 2006; Petry, Peirce et al., 2005) and methadone take-home privileges (Kidorf, Stitzer, Brooner, & Goldberg, 1994) are effective and easier for clinics to implement. The adaptive MSC incorporates incentives already available in the clinic, including methadone take-home doses and clinic time restrictions, avoiding the need for additional funding for monetary-based voucher incentives to deliver behavioral reinforcement. For example, patients who are adherent to scheduled individual and group counseling can earn one methadone take-home, even in Step 4. Nonadherence results in removal of that take-home until the patient attends all sessions for a week.

A unique feature of the adaptive MSC model is the use of higher intensities of care as negative reinforcers. Although we might wish that patients would happily attend as much treatment as they need, the truth is that they do not. Therapy is intrusive, inconvenient, and takes substantial time and effort before results are seen. Once in higher-intensity treatment, patients are motivated to graduate to lower intensities to escape this inconvenience. Negatively reinforcing reduced drug use and increased adherence with higher-intensity care has the additional effect of creating avoidance schedules for patients in lower steps. For example, patients in Step 3 are motivated to attend their individual and group counseling and provide drug-negative urine specimens to avoid going to Step 4, and patients in Step 4 are motivated to succeed to avoid beginning a methadone taper. Although negative reinforcement and avoidance are not often used in SUD treatment, they have been used successfully for years in medicine. Patients can be motivated to diet and exercise and stop smoking if they have had a heart attack or stroke and know they are at risk for another. There can be no question about the effectiveness of both positive and negative behavioral contingencies. Rates of adherence to scheduled counseling are consistently twice as high in the adaptive MSC treatment as in the adaptive stepped care treatment condition without the behavioral reinforcement on attendance (Brooner et al., 2007, 2004). In decreased intensities of care, treatment adherence also includes employment, drug-free social activities, and medical/dental care. We have successfully increased employment rates (Kidorf et al., 2004), decreased cannabis use (Kidorf et al., 2007), and increased social support activities (Kidorf et al., 2005) using modest changes to the basic adaptive MSC model.

Problems associated with SUD treatment attrition are also addressed with the adaptive MSC treatment model. Same-day admission is automatic for new admissions to minimize attrition associated with long waiting times for admission. Furthermore, rapid readmission is encouraged for any patient leaving treatment, especially for Step 4 nonadherence. In the adaptive treatment model, participation in treatment is viewed more broadly to include multiple treatment episodes and readmission is one method to reduce attrition (Dennis, Scott, Funk, & Foss, 2005). Readmitting patients who were unsuccessful in the last treatment episode directly opposes the current standard of care in which nonadherent patients are discharged and often excluded from readmission to the program for several months or longer. Excluding patients from treatment in the hope that they will become more motivated is likely to result in increased time away from treatment. The chronic illness model strongly suggests that a treatment failure simply indicates the need for either more or different treatment, rather than low motivation on the part of the patient. Patients with SUD naturally increase and decrease their drug use and transition into and out of treatment frequently (Scott, Foss, & Dennis, 2005), although there is typically very little continuity between treatment episodes. Multiple readmissions for chronic SUD with a small number of treatment provider groups can help increase the chances of successful outcome (Mertens, Weisner, & Ray, 2005). Accordingly, the adaptive MSC model strongly encourages readmission to the same treatment setting, where a therapeutic relationship already exists and providers know what has and has not worked in prior treatment episodes.

Because the adaptive MSC model provides for several well-trained professionals in our academic medicine setting, we can also enhance care for patients who need it. The clinic employs professionals from a variety of health care fields, including psychiatrists, clinical psychologists, Master's-trained therapists, physician extenders, and registered and licensed practical nurses. Accordingly, we can provide psychiatric care (including medication and psychotherapy), medical monitoring and acute medical care, and administration and monitoring of medication adherence (including medications for SUD, medical illnesses, and psychiatric illnesses). Most individual therapists would be unable to provide all of these services, and those who have the training and experience to provide one or more of the specific interventions would still find it difficult to intensify treatment as needed. The adaptive MSC model has successfully treated patients with severe antisocial personality disorder (Neufeld et al., 2008) and has provided primary psychiatric care to patients with comorbid nonsubstance Axis I and II psychiatric disorders (Brooner et al., 2008). Of course, not all clinics have the resources available to provide these enhanced services, but it may not be necessary. We have recently begun a new program to provide intensified and enhanced care to community-based clinics in our area, called Community Access to Specialized Treatment (CAST; Neufeld, 2008). The CAST program maximizes resource allocation by keeping patients who are successful at lower intensities of care in their home treatment program, but offering brief periods of higher-intensity care based on the adaptive MSC model in our clinic. Patients in CAST can also take advantage of enhanced services, such as psychiatric evaluation and treatment. The CAST program is the evolution of adaptive treatment as applied across multiple unrelated clinics.

Summary

We have endeavored in this chapter to describe the evolution of evidence-based treatment from individual therapy to individualized treatment. Although there are many individual therapies with proven efficacy for SUD, significant problems limit their utility with patients who have chronic and severe forms of the disorder. Individual therapy, as traditionally defined, is both impractical in the majority of treatment settings and insufficient for many patients. In addition, the pervasive problem of SUD patient nonparticipation results in such a low dose of therapy as to render effective therapies nearly inert.

It is no longer a question whether treatment for chronic SUD works, but rather how and when we should apply treatments that work. Chronic SUD is like other chronic illnesses that require more than time-limited single-method isolated treatment episodes. As with any good psychotherapy practice, treatment for chronic SUD should be long-term, readjusted over time to address the patient's needs, and should be delivered in sufficient doses to maximize the benefit to the patient. Adaptive treatment models are flexible and responsive to the needs of the patient as they become clear and, when combined with proven methods to increase patient participation, represent the best practice of SUD treatment. We provided the real-world example of Adaptive Motivated Stepped Care in order to demonstrate the concept of adaptive treatment and a practical application in community-based treatment. Adaptive MSC is by no means the only adaptive treatment model, nor does it address all of the needs SUD patients have. It does, however, vary the intensity of care using objectively defined criteria and address the problems of attrition and nonadherence in new and interesting ways.

This is an exciting time in the field of SUD treatment. There is renewed interest and progress in creating effective individual therapies, which has generated hope for providers and patients alike. The field is ready to reconceptualize treatment as the long-term management of a chronic illness, requiring changes in treatment intensity in response to the demonstrated need. Emerging from individual therapy, adaptive treatment approaches that individualize treatment over time for each patient will be at the forefront of the next generation of substance use disorder treatment.

References

Aharonovich, E., Hasin, D. S., Brooks, A. C., Liu, X., Bisaga, A., & Nunes, E. V. (2006). Cognitive deficits predict low treatment retention in cocaine dependent patients. *Drug and Alcohol Dependence, 81,* 313–322.

Ball, J. C., & Ross, A. (1991). *The effectiveness of methadone maintenance treatment.* New York: Springer-Verlag.

Ball, S., Bachrach, K., DeCarlo, J., Farentinos, C., Keen, M., McSherry, T., et al. (2002). Characteristics, beliefs, and practices of community clinicians trained to provide manual-guided therapy for substance abusers. *Journal of Substance Abuse Treatment, 23,* 309–318.

Ball, S. A., Carroll, K. M., Canning-Ball, M., & Rounsaville, B. J. (2006). Reasons for dropout from drug abuse treatment: Symptoms, personality, and motivation. *Addictive Behaviors, 31,* 320–330.

Bauer, R. A. (2003). Mindfulness training as a clinical intervention: A conceptual and empirical review. *Clinical Psychology: Science and Practice, 10,* 125–143.

Berkowitz, R. I., Wadden, T. A., Tershakovec, A. M., & Cronquist, J. L. (2003). Behavior therapy and sibutramine for the treatment of adolescent obesity: A randomized controlled trial. *The Journal of the American Medical Association, 289,* 1805–1812.

Bischof, G., Grothues, J. M., Reinhardt, S., Meyer, C., John, U., & Rumpf, H.-J. (2008). Evaluation of a telephone-based stepped care intervention for alcohol-related disorders: A randomized controlled trial. *Drug and Alcohol Dependence, 93,* 244–251.

Blanchard, K. A., Morgenstern, J., Morgan, T. J., Labouvie, E., & Bux, D. A. (2003). Motivational subtypes and continuous measures of readiness for change: Concurrent and predictive validity. *Psychology of Addictive Behaviors, 17,* 56–65.

Bowen, S., Witkiewitz, K., Dillworth, T. M., Chawla, N., Simpson, T. L., Ostafin, B. D., et al. (2006). Mindfulness meditation and substance use in an incarcerated population. *Psychology of Addictive Behaviors, 20,* 343–347.

Breslin, F. C., Sobell, M. B., Sobell, L. C., Cunningham, J. A., Sdao-Jarvie, K., & Borsoi, D. (1998). Problem drinkers: Evaluation of a stepped-care approach. *Journal of Substance Abuse, 10,* 217–232.

Brooner, R. K., Kidorf, M. S., King, V. L., Stoller, K. B., Neufeld, K. J., & Kolodner, K. (2007). Comparing adaptive stepped care and monetary-based voucher interventions for opioid dependence. *Drug and Alcohol Dependence, 88,* S14–23.

Brooner, R. K., Kidorf, M. S., King, V. L., Stoller, K. B., Peirce, J. M., Bigelow, G. E., et al. (2004). Behavioral contingencies improve counseling attendance in an adaptive treatment model. *Journal of Substance Abuse Treatment, 27,* 223–232.

Brooner, R. K., King, V., Neufeld, K., Stoller, K., Peirce, J., Kidorf, M., et al. (2008, June). *Integrated psychiatric services are associated with improved service delivery and better treatment response*. Poster session presented at the annual meeting of the College on Problems of Drug Dependence, San Juan, PR.

Brooner, R. K., King, V. L., Kidorf, M., Schmidt, C. W., Jr., & Bigelow, G. E. (1997). Psychiatric and substance use comorbidity among treatment-seeking opioid abusers. *Archives of General Psychiatry, 54,* 71–80.

Brown, T. G., Seraganian, P., Tremblay, J., & Annis, H. (2002). Matching substance abuse aftercare treatments to client characteristics. *Addictive Behaviors, 27,* 585–604.

Bühringer, G. (2006). Allocating treatment options to patient profiles: Clinical art or science? *Addiction, 101,* 646–652.

Cacciola, J. S., Alterman, A. I., Rutherford, M. J., McKay, J. R., & Mulvaney, F. D. (2001). The relationship of psychiatric comorbidity to treatment outcomes in methadone maintained patients. *Drug and Alcohol Dependence, 61,* 271–280.

Carpenter, K. M., Miele, G. M., & Hasin, D. S. (2002). Does motivation to change mediate the effect of *DSM-IV* substance use disorders on treatment utilization and substance use? *Addictive Behaviors, 27,* 207–225.

Carroll, K. M. (1998). *A cognitive-behavioral approach: Treating cocaine addiction*. Rockville, MD: National Institute on Drug Abuse.

Carroll, K. M. (2005). Recent advances in the psychotherapy of addictive disorders. Current Psychiatry Reports, 7, 329–336.

Carroll, K. M., Ball, S. A., & Martino, S. (2004). Cognitive, behavioral, and motivational therapies. In M. Galanter & H. D. Kleber (Eds.), The American Psychiatric Publishing textbook of substance abuse treatment (3rd ed., pp. 365–376). Washington, DC: American Psychiatric.

Carroll, K. M., Ball, S. A., Nich, C., Martino, S., Frankforter, T. L., Farentinos, C., et al. (2006). Motivational interviewing to improve treatment engagement and outcome in individuals seeking treatment for substance abuse: A multisite effectiveness study. *Drug and Alcohol Dependence, 28,* 301–312.

Carroll, K. M., Farentinos, C., Ball, S. A., Crits-Christoph, P., Libby, B., Morgenstern, J., et al. (2002). MET meets the real world: Design issues and clinical strategies in the clinical trials network. *Journal of Substance Abuse Treatment, 23,* 73–80.

Carroll, K. M., & Rounsaville, B. J. (2007). A vision of the next generation of behavioral therapies research in the addictions. *Addiction, 102,* 850–862.

Carroll, K. M., Rounsaville, B. J., Gordon, L. T., Nich, C., Jatlow, P., Bisighini, R. M., et al. (1994). Psychotherapy and pharmacotherapy for ambulatory cocaine abusers. *Archives of General Psychiatry, 51,* 177–187.

Carroll, K. M., Rounsaville, B. J., Nich, C., Gordon, L. T., Wirtz, P. W., & Gawin, F. (1994). One-year follow-up of psychotherapy and pharmacotherapy for cocaine dependence. Delayed emergence of psychotherapy effects. *Archives of General Psychiatry, 51,* 989–997.

Chambless, D. L., & Ollendick, T. H. (2001). Empirically supported psychological interventions: Controversies and evidence. *Annual Review of Psychology, 52,* 685–716.

Chawdhary, A., Sayre, S. L., Green, C., Schmitz, J. M., Grabowski, J., & Mooney, M. E. (2007). Moderators of delay tolerance in treatment-seeking cocaine users. *Addictive Behaviors, 32,* 370–376.

Claus, R. E., & Kindleberger, L. R. (2002). Engaging substance abusers after centralized assessment: Predictors of treatment entry and dropout. *Journal of Psychoactive Drugs, 34,* 25–31.

Crits-Christoph, P., Siqueland, L., Blaine, J., Frank, A., Luborsky, L., Onken, L. S., et al. (1999). Psychosocial treatments for cocaine dependence: National Institute on Drug Abuse collaborative cocaine treatment study. *Archives of General Psychiatry, 56,* 493–502.

Curran, G. M., Stecker, T., Han, X., & Booth, B. M. (2009). Individual and program predictors of attrition from VA substance use treatment. *Journal of Behavioral Health Services Research, 36,* 25–34.

Darke, S. (1998). Self-report among injecting drug users: A review. *Drug and Alcohol Dependence, 51,* 253–263.

Daughters, S. B., Lejuez, C. W., Bornovalova, M. A., Kahler, C. W., Strong, D. R., & Brown, R. A. (2005). Distress tolerance as a predictor of early treatment dropout in a residential substance abuse treatment facility. *Journal of Abnormal Psychology, 114,* 729–734.

Daughters, S. B., Stipelman, B. A., Sargeant, M. N., Schuster, R., Bornovalova, M. A., & Lejuez, C. W. (2008). The interactive effects of antisocial personality disorder and court-mandated status on substance abuse treatment dropout. *Journal of Substance Abuse Treatment, 34,* 157–164.

Dennis, M. L., Scott, C. K., Funk, R., & Foss, M. A. (2005). The duration and correlates of addiction and treatment careers. *Journal of Substance Abuse Treatment, 28,* S51–S62.

DiClemente, C. C., & Hughes, S. O. (1990). Stages of change profiles in outpatient alcoholism treatment. *Journal of Substance Abuse, 2,* 217–235.

Festinger, D. S., Lamb, R. J., Kountz, M. R., Kirby, K. C., & Marlowe, D. (1995). Pretreatment dropout as a function of treatment delay and client variables. *Addictive Behaviors, 20,* 111–115.

Finney, J., Wilbourne, P., & Moos, R. 2007 (in press). Psychosocial treatments for substance use disorders. In P. E. Nathan & J. M. Gorman (Eds.), A guide to treatments that work (3rd ed.). New York: Oxford.

Fiorentine, R. (1999). After drug treatment: Are 12-step programs effective in maintaining abstinence? *American Journal of Drug and Alcohol Abuse, 25,* 93–116.

Gehi, A., Haas, D., Pipkin, S., & Whooley, M. A. (2005). Depression and medication adherence in outpatients with coronary heart disease: Findings from the heart and soul study. *Archives of Internal Medicine, 165,* 2508–2513.

Gifford, E. V., Ritsher, J. B., McKellar, J. D., & Moos, R. H. (2006). Acceptance and relationship context: A model of substance use disorder treatment outcome. *Addiction, 101,* 1167–1177.

Glasner-Edwards, S., Tate, S. R., McQuaid, J. R., Cummins, K., Granholm, E., & Brown, S. A. (2007). Mechanisms of action in integrated cognitive-behavioral treatment versus twelve-step facilitation for substance-dependent adults with comorbid major depression. *Journal of Studies on Alcohol and Drugs, 68,* 663–672.

Graham, K., Annis, H. M., Brett, P. J., & Venesoen, P. (1996). A controlled field trial of group versus individual cognitive-behavioural training for relapse prevention. *Addiction, 91,* 1127–1139.

Greenfield, S. F., Brooks, A. J., Gordon, S. M., Green, C. A., Kropp, F., McHugh, R. K., et al. (2007). Substance abuse treatment entry, retention, and outcome in women: A review of the literature. *Drug and Alcohol Dependence, 86,* 1–21.

Grella, C. E., & Stein, J. A. (2006). Impact of program services on treatment outcomes of patients with comorbid mental and substance use disorders. *Psychiatric Services, 57,* 1007–1015.

Harrison, S. R., Toriello, P., Pavluck, A., Ellis, R., Pedersen, E., Gaiennie, R., et al. (2007). The impact of a brief induction on short-term continuation in a therapeutic community. *American Journal of Drug and Alcohol Abuse, 33,* 147–153.

Hayes, S. C., Strosahl, K. D., & Wilson, K. G. (1999). *Acceptance and commitment therapy: An experiential approach to behavior change.* New York: Guilford.

Hettema, J., Steele, J., & Miller, W. R. (2005). Motivational interviewing. *Annual Review of Clinical Psychology, 1,* 91–111.

Hoppes, K. (2006). The application of mindfulness-based cognitive interventions in the treatment of co-occurring addictive and mood disorders. *CNS Spectrums, 11,* 829–851.

Hser, Y. I., Evans, E., Huang, D., & Anglin, D. M. (2004). Relationship between drug treatment services, retention, and outcomes. *Psychiatric Services, 55,* 767–774.

Irvin, J. E., Bowers, C. A., Dunn, M. E., & Wang, M. C. (1999). Efficacy of relapse prevention: A meta-analytic review. *Journal of Consulting and Clinical Psychology, 67,* 563–570.

Kakko, J., Gronbladh, L., Svanborg, K. D., von Wachenfeldt, J., Ruck, C., Rawlings, B., et al. (2007). A stepped care strategy using buprenorphine and methadone versus conventional methadone maintenance in heroin dependence: A randomized controlled trial. *American Journal of Psychiatry, 164,* 797–803.

Katz, E. C., Brown, B. S., Schwartz, R. P., King, S. D., Weintraub, E., & Barksdale, W. (2007). Impact of role induction on long-term drug treatment outcomes. *Journal of Addictive Diseases, 26,* 81–90.

Katz, E. C., Brown, B. S., Schwartz, R. P., Weintraub, E., Barksdale, W., & Robinson, R. (2004). Role induction: A method for enhancing early retention in outpatient drug-free treatment. *Journal of Consulting and Clinical Psychology, 72,* 227–234.

Kessler, R. C. (2004). The epidemiology of dual diagnosis. *Biological Psychiatry, 15,* 730–737.

Kidorf, M., King, V. L., & Brooner, R. K. (2006). Counseling and psychosocial services. In E. C. Strain & M. L. Stitzer (Eds.) *The treatment of opioid dependence* (2nd ed., pp. 119–150). Baltimore, MD: Johns Hopkins University Press.

Kidorf, M., King, V. L., Neufeld, K., Stoller, K. B., Peirce, J., & Brooner, R. K. (2005). Involving significant others in the care of opioid-dependent patients receiving methadone. *Journal of Substance Abuse Treatment, 29,* 19–27.

Kidorf, M., Neufeld, K., & Brooner, R. K. (2004). Combining stepped-care approaches with behavioral reinforcement to motivate employment in opioid-dependent outpatients. *Substance Use & Misuse, 39,* 2215–2238.

Kidorf, M., Neufeld, K., King, V. L., Clark, M., & Brooner, R. K. (2007). A stepped care approach for reducing cannabis use in opioid-dependent outpatients. *Journal of Substance Abuse Treatment, 32,* 341–347.

Kidorf, M., Stitzer, M. L., Brooner, R. K., & Goldberg, J. (1994). Contingent methadone take-home doses reinforce adjunct therapy attendance of methadone maintenance patients. *Drug and Alcohol Dependence, 36,* 221–226.

King, V. L., Kidorf, M. S., Stoller, K. B., Schwartz, R., Kolodner, K., & Brooner, R. K. (2006). A 12-month controlled trial of methadone medical maintenance integrated into an adaptive treatment model. *Journal of Substance Abuse Treatment, 31,* 385–393.

Knudsen, H. K., Ducharme, L. J., & Roman, P. M. (2007). Research participation and turnover intention: An exploratory analysis of substance abuse counselors. *Journal of Substance Abuse Treatment, 33,* 211–217.

Leucht, S., & Heres, S. (2006). Epidemiology, clinical consequences, and psychosocial treatment of nonadherence in schizophrenia. *Journal of Clinical Psychiatry, 67 Suppl 5,* 3–8.

Linehan, M. M., & Dimeff, L.A., 1997. *Dialectical behavior therapy for substance abuse treatment manual.* Seattle, WA: University of Washington.

Linehan, M. M., Dimeff, L. A., Reynolds, S. K., Comtois, K. A., Welch, S. S., Heagerty, P., et al. (2002). Dialectical behavior therapy versus comprehensive validation therapy plus 12-step for the treatment of opioid dependent women meeting criteria for borderline personality disorder. *Drug and Alcohol Dependence, 67,* 13–26.

Linehan, M. M., Schmidt, H., 3rd, Dimeff, L. A., Craft, J. C., Kanter, J., & Comtois, K. A. (1999). Dialectical behavior therapy for patients with borderline personality disorder and drug-dependence. *American Journal on Addictions, 8,* 279–292.

Marlatt, G. A. (2002). Buddhist psychology and the treatment of addictive behavior. *Cognitive and Behavioral Practice, 9,* 44–49.

Marlatt, G. A., & Donovan, D. (2005). *Relapse prevention: Maintenance strategies in the treatment of addictions* (2nd ed.). New York: Guilford Press.

Marlatt, G. A., & Gordon, J. R. (1985). *Relapse prevention: Maintenance strategies in the treatment of addictive behaviors.* New York: Guilford Press.

Martinez-Raga, J., Marshall, E. J., Keaney, F., Ball, D., & Strang, J. (2002). Unplanned versus planned discharges from in-patient alcohol detoxification: Retrospective analysis of 470 first-episode admissions. *Alcohol and Alcoholism, 37,* 277–281.

McCarty, D., Fuller, B. E., Arfken, C., Miller, M., Nunes, E. V., Edmundson, E., et al. (2007). Direct care workers in the national drug abuse treatment clinical trials network: Characteristics, opinions, and beliefs. *Psychiatric Services, 58,* 181–190.

McCarty, D., Fuller, B., Kaskutas, L. A., Wendt, W. W., Nunes, E. V., Miller, M., et al. (2008). Treatment programs in the national drug abuse treatment clinical trials network. *Drug and Alcohol Dependence, 92,* 200–207.

McGovern, M. P., Xie, H., Segal, S. R., Siembab, L., & Drake, R. E. (2006). Addiction treatment services and co-occurring disorders: Prevalence estimates, treatment practices, and barriers. *Journal of Substance Abuse Treatment, 31,* 267–275.

McKay, J. R. (2006). Continuing care in the treatment of addictive disorders. *Current Psychiatry Reports, 8,* 355–362.

McKay, J. R., Lynch, K. G., Shepard, D. S., & Pettinati, H. M. (2005). The effectiveness of telephone-based continuing care for alcohol and cocaine dependence: 24-month outcomes. *Archives of General Psychiatry, 62,* 199–207.

McKellar, J., Kelly, J., Harris, A., & Moos, R. (2006). Pretreatment and during treatment risk factors for dropout among patients with substance use disorders. *Addictive Behaviors, 31,* 450–460.

McLellan, A. T., Lewis, D. C., O'Brien, C. P., & Kleber, H. D. (2000). Drug dependence, a chronic medical illness: Implications for treatment, insurance, and outcomes evaluation. *Journal of the American Medical Association, 284,* 1689–1695.

Mertens, J. R., Weisner, C. M., & Ray, G. T. (2005). Readmission among chemical dependency patients in private, outpatient treatment: Patterns, correlates and role in long-term outcome. *Journal of Studies on Alcohol, 66,* 842–847.

Miller, W. R. (1983). Motivational interviewing with problem drinkers. *Behavioural Psychotherapy, 11,* 147–172.

Miller, W. R., & Rollnick, S. (2002). *Motivational interviewing: Preparing people for change* (2nd ed.). New York: Guilford Press.

Miller, W. R., Yahne, C. E., Moyers, T. B., Martinez, J., & Pirritano, M. (2004). A randomized trial of methods to help clinicians learn motivational interviewing. *Journal of Consulting and Clinical Psychology, 72,* 1050–1062.

Moeller, F. G., Dougherty, D. M., Barratt, E. S., Schmitz, J. M., Swann, A. C., & Grabowski, J. (2001). The impact of impulsivity on cocaine use and retention in treatment. *Journal of Substance Abuse Treatment, 21,* 193–198.

Monti, P. M., Rohsenow, D. J., Michalec, E., Martin, R. A., & Abrams, D. B. (1997). Brief coping skills treatment for cocaine abuse: Substance use outcomes at three months. *Addiction, 92,* 1717–1728.

Moos, R. H. (2007). Theory-based active ingredients of effective treatments for substance use disorders. *Drug and Alcohol Dependence, 88,* 109–121.

Morgenstern, J., Bux, D. A., Labouvie, E., Morgan, T., Blanchard, K. A., & Muench, F. (2003). Examining mechanisms of action in 12-step community outpatient treatment. *Drug and Alcohol Dependence, 72,* 237–247.

Murphy, S. A., Lynch, K. G., Oslin, D., McKay, J. R., & TenHave, T. (2007). Developing adaptive treatment strategies in substance abuse research. *Drug and Alcohol Dependence, 88,* S24–30.

Neufeld, K. J. (2008, January). Community access to specialized treatment. Paper presented at Johns Hopkins School of Medicine Department of Psychiatry Seminar, Baltimore, MD.

Neufeld, K. J., Kidorf, M. S., Kolodner, K., King, V. L., Clark, M., & Brooner, R. K. (2008). A behavioral treatment for opioid-dependent patients with antisocial personality. *Journal of Substance Abuse Treatment, 34,* 101–111.

Nowinski, J., & Baker, S. (1992). *The twelve-step facilitation handbook.* San Francisco: Jossey-Bass.

Ouimette, P. C., Finney, J. W., & Moos, R. H. (1997). Twelve-step and cognitive-behavioral treatment for substance abuse: A comparison of treatment effectiveness. *Journal of Consulting and Clinical Psychology, 65,* 230–240.

Patkar, A. A., Murray, H. W., Mannelli, P., Gottheil, E., Weinstein, S. P., & Vergare, M. J. (2004). Pre-treatment measures of impulsivity, aggression and sensation seeking are associated with treatment outcome for African-American cocaine-dependent patients. *Journal of Addictive Diseases, 23,* 109–122.

Peirce, J. M., Petry, N. M., Stitzer, M. L., Blaine, J., Kellogg, S., Satterfield, F., et al. (2006). Effects of lower-cost incentives on stimulant abstinence in methadone maintenance treatment: A national drug abuse treatment clinical trials network study. *Archives of General Psychiatry, 63,* 201–208.

Pena, J. M., Franklin, R. R., Rice, J. C., Foulks, E. F., Bland, I. J., Shervington, D., et al. (1999). A two-rate hypothesis for patterns of retention in psychosocial treatments of cocaine dependence: Findings from a study of African-American men and a review of the published data. *American Journal on Addictions, 8,* 319–331.

Perlis, R. H., Ostacher, M. J., Patel, J. K., Marangell, L. B., Zhang, H., Wisniewski, S. R., et al. (2006). Predictors of recurrence in bipolar disorder: Primary outcomes from the systematic treatment enhancement program for bipolar disorder (STEP-BD). *American Journal of Psychiatry, 163,* 217–224.

Petry, N. M., Alessi, S. M., Marx, J., Austin, M., & Tardif, M. (2005). Vouchers versus prizes: contingency management treatment of substance abusers in community settings. *Journal of Consulting and Clinical Psychology, 73,* 1005–1014.

Petry, N. M., Peirce, J. M., Stitzer, M. L., Blaine, J., Roll, J. M., Cohen, A., et al. (2005). Effect of prize-based incentives on outcomes in stimulant abusers in outpatient psychosocial treatment programs: A national drug abuse treatment clinical trials network study. *Archives of General Psychiatry, 62,* 1148–1156.

Prochaska, J. O., DiClemente, C. C., & Norcross, J. C. (1992). In search of how people change: Applications to addictive behaviors, *American Psychologist, 47,* 1102–1114.

Project MATCH Research Group. (1997a). Matching alcoholism treatments to client heterogeneity: Project MATCH posttreatment drinking outcomes. *Journal of Studies on Alcohol, 58,* 7–29.

Project MATCH Research Group. (1997b). Project MATCH secondary a priori hypotheses. *Addiction, 92,* 1671–1698.

Rawson, R. A., Huber, A., McCann, M., Shoptaw, S., Farabee, D., Reiber, C., et al. (2002). A comparison of contingency management and cognitive-behavioral approaches during methadone maintenance treatment for cocaine dependence. *Archives of General Psychiatry, 59,* 817–824.

Rawson, R. A., McCann, M. J., Flammino, F., Shoptaw, S., Miotto, K., Reiber, C., et al. (2006). A comparison of contingency management and cognitive-behavioral approaches for stimulant-dependent individuals. *Addiction, 101,* 267–274.

Rush, A. J., Trivedi, M. H., Wisniewski, S. R., Nierenberg, A. A., Stewart, J. W., Warden, D., et al. (2006). Acute and longer-term outcomes in depressed outpatients requiring one or several treatment steps: A STAR*D report. *American Journal of Psychiatry, 163,* 1905–1917.

Schumacher, J. E., Milby, J. B., Caldwell, E., Raczynski, J., Engle, M., Michael, M., et al. (1995). Treatment outcome as a function of treatment attendance with homeless persons abusing cocaine. *Journal of Addictive Diseases, 14,* 73–85.

Scott, C. K., Foss, M. A., & Dennis, M. L. (2005). Pathways in the relapse—treatment—recovery cycle over 3 years. *Journal of Substance Abuse Treatment, 28,* S63–S72.

Sholomskas, D. E., Syracuse-Siewert, G., Rounsaville, B. J., Ball, S. A., Nuro, K. F., & Carroll, K. M. (2005). We don't train in vain: A dissemination trial of three strategies of training clinicians in cognitive-behavioral therapy. *Journal of Consulting and Clinical Psychology, 73,* 106–115.

Simpson, D. D., Joe, G. W., & Rowan-Szal, G. A. (1997). Drug abuse treatment retention and process effects on follow-up outcomes. *Drug and Alcohol Dependence, 47,* 227–235.

Sobell, M. B., & Sobell, L. C. (2000). Stepped care as a heuristic approach to the treatment of alcohol problems. *Journal of Consulting and Clinical Psychology, 68,* 573–579.

Stasiewicz, P. R. & Stalker, R. (1999). A comparison of three "interventions" on pretreatment dropout rates in an outpatient substance abuse clinic. *Addictive Behaviors, 24,* 579–582.

Stitzer, M., & Petry, N. (2006). Contingency management for treatment of substance abuse. *Annual Review of Clinical Psychology, 2,* 411–434.

UKATT Research Team. (2005). Effectiveness of treatment for alcohol problems: Findings of the randomised UK alcohol treatment trial (UKATT). *British Medical Journal, 331,* 541.

UKATT Research Team. (2008). UK alcohol treatment trial: Client-treatment matching effects. *Addiction, 103,* 228–238.

Weiss, R. D. (2004). Adherence to pharmacotherapy in patients with alcohol and opioid dependence. *Addiction, 99,* 1382–1392.

Weiss, R. D., Griffin, M. L., Gallop, R. J., Najavits, L. M., Frank, A., Crits-Christoph, P., et al. (2005). The effect of 12-step self-help group attendance and participation on drug use outcomes among cocaine-dependent patients. *Drug and Alcohol Dependence, 77,* 177–184.

Weiss, R. D., Jaffe, W. B., de Menil, V. P., & Cogley, C. B. (2004). Group therapy for substance use disorders: What do we know? *Harvard Review of Psychiatry, 12,* 339–350.

Witkiewitz, K., Marlatt, G. A., & Walker, D. (2005). Mindfulness-based relapse prevention for alcohol and substance use disorders. *Journal of Cognitive Psychotherapy: An International Quarterly, 19,* 211–228.

Witkiewitz, K., van der Maas, H. L., Hufford, M. R., & Marlatt, G. A. (2007). Nonnormality and divergence in posttreatment alcohol use: Reexamining the project MATCH data "another way". *Journal of Abnormal Psychology, 116,* 378–394.

Zatzick, D., Roy-Byrne, P., Russo, J., Rivara, F., Droesch, R., Wagner, A., et al. (2004). A randomized effectiveness trial of stepped collaborative care for acutely injured trauma survivors. *Archives of General Psychiatry, 61,* 498–506.

Zweben, A., & Li, S. (1981). The efficacy of role induction in preventing early dropout from outpatient treatment of drug dependency. *American Journal of Drug and Alcohol Abuse, 8,* 171–183.

9

Group Therapy for Substance Abuse

Holly E. R. Morrell and Mark G. Myers

University of California

Contents

What is Group Therapy?

A wide variety of psychotherapeutic treatments for substance abuse and dependence have been adapted for use in a group format (Khantzian, Golden-Schulman, & McAuliffe, 2004). Thus, there are cognitive-behavioral groups, process-oriented groups, relapse prevention groups, psychoeducational groups, and so forth. There are also numerous peer-led self-help groups, such as Alcoholics Anonymous (AA). This diversity can make it difficult to define what group therapy is. For the purposes of the present chapter, we focus on groups that are led by trained professionals and define group therapy as "two or more unrelated clients and a therapist who meet together regularly, with the primary goal of reducing or eliminating substance use, or of addressing behaviors related to substance use" (Weiss, Jaffee, de Menil, & Cogley, 2004). We do not discuss self-help groups such as AA, because the empirical evidence in support of them is equivocal at best despite a widespread belief in their benefits (Mueller, Petitjean, Boening, & Wiesbeck, 2007; Shearer, 2007).

Why Group Therapy?

There are many advantages of group therapy for substance abuse and dependence, which is one of the reasons why it is such a widespread treatment modality (CSAT, 2005). In an age of managed care, group therapy is viewed as more cost-effective than individual therapy because one trained professional can deliver services to multiple clients at once (Washton, 2005). The few studies that have compared group therapy to individual therapy have shown that group therapy is at least as effective as individual therapy (Graham, Annis, Brett, & Venesoen, 1996; Marques & Formigoni, 2001; Schmitz et al., 1997; Weiss et al., 2004), and may actually be more effective than individual therapy in some circumstances (Scheidlinger, 2000; Toseland & Siporin, 1986). It is generally assumed that comparable rates of clinical effectiveness between group and individual therapy translate into better cost-effectiveness for group therapy. However, a recent meta-analysis based on a limited number of studies suggested that at least one type of group therapy for (Substance Use Disorder) SUDs, CBT, might not be more cost-effective than individual therapy, because higher costs were associated with group CBT even though both group and individual therapy were found to be equally efficacious (Tucker & Oei, 2007).

Another advantage of group therapy is that it provides a forum for modeling adaptive behavior. While witnessing the recovery of others, clients can learn which strategies help to maintain abstinence and observe the results of these strategies as they are applied to real-world situations. Clients can also vicariously learn the consequences of maladaptive coping strategies, such as hearing about another group member being expelled from a recovery home after getting caught using substances to alleviate emotional distress. In addition, clients can improve their social skills by observing and participating in healthy social interactions, which may in turn allow them to form better relationships with existing friends, family members, and significant others.

Ideally, groups provide much-needed human contact for individuals who may otherwise be socially isolated. They may help group members to cope with life stressors without turning to substances by providing positive peer support and pressure to abstain from drug use. This support, encouragement, and sense of accountability may carry over into daily life as group members develop relationships with each other that extend beyond the treatment setting. Group leaders and other group members can also provide valuable feedback regarding each client's strengths, weaknesses, values, abilities, and patterns of behavior. Furthermore, the group as a whole may have the capacity to confront an individual about harmful behaviors more effectively than a single therapist, because of the power of receiving feedback from multiple people who have personally experienced and struggled with drug addiction. Confronting others may have the added benefit of helping the individual client recognize his or her own denial.

Watching and participating in others' recovery may instill a sense of hope and purpose in substance users. Newer group members can see that recovery is possible, and they can see what they need to do to succeed. As group members gain seniority, they may begin to act as quasi-therapists in that they help new members acculturate to the treatment environment, give advice based on experience, ask insightful questions, and act as sympathetic guides throughout the recovery process, frequently resulting in the reinforcement of the influence of the group leader. Finally, groups offer a level of structure and discipline that is typically lacking in the lives of substance users, thus replacing chaos with order and stability in at least one area of clients' lives.

There are also several potential disadvantages of group therapy for substance abuse, although most of them can be avoided through awareness, planning, and the use of good therapy skills. One potential disadvantage of group therapy is deviancy training, or the possibility that grouping adolescents with substance and behavior problems together may actually undermine treatment. However, there is little to no empirical evidence in support of deviancy training in adolescents, and it is unknown whether such a process occurs among adults (Kaminer, 2005). Including group members who frequently relapse may also hinder treatment, because other members may become discouraged, frustrated, and noncompliant. To prevent this from happening, groups should have clear, consistently enforced rules and abstinence criteria (assuming the group is abstinence-oriented) that govern eligibility to remain in the group.

The potential for group conflict may be considered another disadvantage in group therapy, but it may be turned into an advantage if handled correctly. Conflict within the group may damage the therapeutic relationship between the group leader and group members, undermine the group leader's authority, harm relationships between group members, create factions within the group, cause clients to drop out of treatment, or precipitate relapse. On the other hand, a well-handled conflict may model effective conflict resolution (and therefore reduce the likelihood of conflict-related relapse), increase group cohesion, and strengthen the positive influence of the group leader.

Frequent and unchecked digression to topics unrelated to the group purpose can impede progress in therapy by taking time away from therapeutic interventions and allowing members to avoid painful subjects, such as underlying reasons for drug use and relapse. Nevertheless, judicious use of digression by the group leader can regulate the intensity of group discussion by allowing members to take a break from emotionally intense topics and enhance group camaraderie by allowing group members to relax and get to know each other better. It should be noted that this problem is not isolated to group therapy, but may be more likely to occur in a group setting as a byproduct of having several closely connected people together in one place.

Another disadvantage of group therapy is that there may be some individuals who feel uncomfortable sharing information about themselves and their habits in a group setting. This problem may be especially prevalent among substance users, who often struggle with being open and with trusting others. These individuals are unlikely to benefit fully from group therapy if they find it difficult to become engaged in treatment. As with most of the disadvantages of group therapy, however, an experienced group leader can use the group process itself to treat the underlying problem, in this case by gradually socializing reticent members to treatment and "drawing them out of their shell." In such cases, the group may become an excellent place to learn about trust, openness, and honesty.

Types of Group Therapy for Substance Abuse

Many treatments that were originally developed in the context of individual therapy for substance use have been formatted for group therapy. Therefore, it would be futile to list every possible permutation of group therapy. Instead, we focus on describing broad categories of group therapy, with the caveat that there is still significant variability within each category. We use a classification scheme developed by the Center for Substance Abuse Treatment (CSAT, 2005) that includes psychoeducational groups, skills development groups, cognitive-behavioral therapy (CBT) groups, support groups, and interpersonal process groups.

The general purpose of the psychoeducational group is to educate clients about the nature and effects of substance abuse. It typically follows a classroom format, with the group leader acting as the instructor and group members acting as students. This type of group is usually quite structured in format and content, but can include facilitated group discussion. The purpose of skills development groups is to help clients develop skills that will aid their recovery, such as social, problem-solving, and coping skills. Techniques may include teaching skills, role-playing the use of these skills in the group, and practicing them as homework assignments.

Cognitive-behavioral groups use cognitive-behavioral theory and techniques to promote recovery from substance abuse or dependence. Clients learn how thoughts, feelings, and behaviors influence one another reciprocally. They learn to challenge and restructure maladaptive thoughts and beliefs that lead to substance use and other harmful behaviors, and they learn to change drug-related behaviors. There can be substantial overlap with skills groups, as many types of skills are presented within a CBT framework (e.g., coping and problem-solving skills). Support groups are designed to provide group members with support and encouragement as they make substantial life changes on their road to recovery, but they do not typically focus on skills building or directly changing thoughts and behaviors. Interpersonal process groups use interpersonal processes within the group to promote and sustain recovery. There is an emphasis on identifying and changing fundamental developmental issues and dysfunctional relationship patterns that have contributed to addiction (CSAT, 2005).

Treatment Matching: Placing Clients in Groups

There is a remarkable amount of individual variability within any mental disorder, including within psychoactive substance use disorders, which implies that different clients may respond more favorably to different types of treatment. Therefore, recent years have seen an increased awareness of the need for treatment matching and a trend toward assessing multiple client factors before recommending or assigning the client to a particular type of group treatment (CSAT, 2005; Emmelkamp & Vedel, 2006). What follows is a description of key factors to consider when placing a client in a group.

It is important to assess where a client is in the recovery process when considering treatment options. Prochaska and DiClemente's stages of change model is frequently used for this purpose (DiClemente et al., 1991). According to this model, substance abusers move through several stages as they progress toward abstinence. Individuals in the first stage (*precontemplation*) are not currently thinking about quitting substances. In the second stage (*contemplation*) individuals begin to think about quitting, and in the third stage (*preparation*) they begin to prepare themselves for an actual quit attempt. In the fourth stage (*action*), individuals make a quit attempt, and in the fifth stage (*maintenance*) they are in the process of maintaining their abstinence. There is a sixth stage, *relapse*, which is not desirable, but is often a natural part of the recovery process. Depending on which stage a client is in, his or her treatment needs may be very different. For example, a client in the contemplation stage may benefit from a psychoeducational group that will expand his or her knowledge of the consequences of addiction, whereas a client in the action phase may benefit more from a CBT group that focuses on skills-building.

A related issue is the client's level of motivation for treatment and recovery. It is not advisable to mix clients who have little motivation for change and clients who are extremely motivated to succeed in their recovery. The focus of therapy needs to be very different for these two types of individuals. For example, clients with little motivation for change are more likely to benefit from motivational enhancement, whereas clients with high levels of motivation can benefit from directly learning and implementing strategies for maintaining abstinence.

In some cases, a client may not be appropriate for group therapy at all, such as if he refuses to participate or makes the therapist uncomfortable (CSAT, 2005). Clients with significant fears of social interaction (e.g., clients with comorbid social anxiety), problems with impulse control and anger management, and difficulties making a commitment to therapy may not be suitable for certain types of groups. For example, a client who struggles with social interaction will probably benefit more from a social skills group than an interpersonal process group; perhaps she could transfer to a process group once her social skills have improved.

Individual client characteristics such as gender, ethnicity, and co-occurring psychopathology, should also be considered when placing someone in a group. Women who have experienced trauma secondary to substance abuse may only feel comfortable with other women. People from a particular ethnic group may feel more comfortable when everyone in the group speaks their language and understands their cultural background. Clients with the same co-occurring psychological disorder may benefit from being grouped together because they are likely to have similar treatment needs. For example, a group designed for individuals with comorbid substance abuse or dependence and major depression could focus on the interaction between depression and addiction. Personality differences, social resources, and level of cognitive functioning may also inform treatment choices. For example, Rosenblum, Cleland, et al. (2005) found that clients with antisocial personality disorder (ASPD), a highly concrete cognitive style, and a social network that is supportive of alcohol and drug use responded better to group CBT than to a group motivational intervention. Nevertheless, both treatments effectively reduced substance use (Rosenblum, Cleland, et al., 2005).

Difficulties in Evaluating the Empirical Evidence for Group Therapy

Despite the apparent advantages and widespread use of group therapy to treat substance use disorders, there are comparatively few studies that directly test its efficacy. Of the studies that do exist, it is difficult to make direct comparisons of treatment outcomes. One reason for this is that group therapy is often included as just one component in a multimodal treatment program: individual psychotherapy, psychopharmacological treatment, and contingency management (CM) programs are often delivered in combination with group therapy (Alessi, Hanson, Wieners, & Petry, 2007; Battjes et al., 2004; Charney, Palacios-Boix, Negrete, Dobkin, & Gill, 2005; el-Guebaly, Cathcart, Currie, Brown, & Gloster, 2002; Latimer, Winters, D'Zurilla, & Nichols, 2003; Smith, Hall, Williams, An, & Gotman, 2006).

Additional group therapies are also frequently included in treatment programs, and they vary widely in type, from motivational interviewing to supportive therapy to psychoeducation. For example, Hillhouse et al. (2007) tested predictors of treatment outcome among 420 methamphetamine users enrolled in a manualized Matrix Model outpatient treatment program. This program comprised CBT groups, family education groups, social support groups, and individual counseling over the course of 16 weeks. Results indicated that this treatment program effectively reduced methamphetamine use, but it was difficult to determine the specific contribution of any given therapy group (Hillhouse, Marinelli-Casey, Gonzales, Ang, & Rawson, 2007).

Other studies evaluate treatments that use a combination of individual and group sessions. For example, Winters, Fals-Stewart, O'Farrell, Birchler, and Kelley (2002) compared a Behavioral Couples Therapy (BCT) package that included individual, group, and couples therapy sessions to individual behavioral therapy (IBT) in female drug abusers. (Participants in the latter condition actually attended individual and group sessions.) The primary difference between treatments was that BCT addressed couples issues and included couples sessions, whereas IBT did not. Participants in the BCT condition reported greater relationship satisfaction during treatment and equal reductions in drug abuse in comparison with participants in the IBT condition. On the other hand, participants in the BCT showed better long-term outcomes: they reported fewer days of substance use, longer periods of continuous abstinence, and lower levels of addiction severity up to 9 months following treatment, but these treatment differences had disappeared within 12 months. Again, it is hard to isolate the effects of group therapy in this study because it was combined with couples and individual therapy.

In addition, there are not enough studies that directly test the effects of treatment intensity (e.g., number or length of therapy sessions) on substance abuse outcomes to allow us to make confident treatment recommendations. In general, less intensive group treatment may be just as effective as more intensive group treatment for cocaine users (Coviello et al., 2001). In some cases, less intensive treatment may even produce better outcomes and therefore be more cost-effective (Dennis et al., 2004; Diamond et al., 2002).

Several studies also mix type and intensity of treatment, further complicating the ability to compare results across studies. For instance, the Cannabis Youth Treatment study was a well-designed randomized clinical trial that evaluated five multimodal treatments for youth with cannabis use disorders. Three of these treatments included a group component: 3 sessions of group CBT combined with 2 sessions of individual MET (MET/CBT5); 12 sessions of group CBT combined with 2 sessions of individual MET (MET/CBT12); and six parent education groups, four therapeutic home visits, case management, and referral to support groups in addition to MET/CBT12 (FSN). Results indicated that all three treatment approaches were similarly effective in promoting abstinence, and there was a trend toward superiority for the MET/CBT5 treatment at follow-up (Burleson, Kaminer, & Dennis, 2006; Dennis et al., 2004; Diamond et al., 2002). Even though the research design allowed the authors to test intensity of CBT (defined by number of sessions) as a predictor of treatment outcome, it restricted their ability to make inferences about the effectiveness of the group therapy component in isolation.

What the Evidence Tells us about Group Therapy

The CSAT system for categorizing group therapy, as outlined previously, provides a useful heuristic for clinicians to classify types of group therapy. Unfortunately, this classification system becomes unwieldy when trying to organize research findings, because of the high degree of content overlap among categories. Therefore, we adapted to our own purposes a classification model from William Miller that is based on type of research design (Weiss et al., 2004): (1) group therapy compared to no group therapy or treatment as usual, (2) group therapy compared to individual therapy, (3) group therapy plus individual/couples therapy compared to individual or group therapy alone, and (4) one type of group therapy compared to another type of group therapy. We excluded studies that did not include a control or comparison group. It should be noted that we are often forced to draw conclusions from a very limited number of studies in any given area; therefore, most conclusions should be viewed as tentative until researchers have collected more data.

Group Therapy Compared to No Group Therapy or Treatment as Usual

Group therapy appears to produce superior outcomes to that of no treatment at all, with one exception. For example, Rosenblum and colleagues found that a combination of group motivational therapy (12 sessions) and CBT (36 sessions) was more successful in reducing alcohol and drug use than information, referral, and peer advocacy services (Rosenblum, Magura, Kayman, & Fong, 2005). In addition, Stephens, Roffman, and Curtin (2000) assigned marijuana users to one of three conditions: 14 group cognitive-behavioral skills training sessions, two brief individual sessions for assessment and MET, or a wait-list control condition. Participants in all three conditions improved over time, but participants in the group CBT condition and the individual sessions condition demonstrated greater reductions in marijuana use and dependence than participants in the wait-list control condition. In contrast, Razavi et al. (1999) assigned smokers who had recently completed a three-month detoxification program to a support group led by a psychologist, a support group led by a former smoker, or a no-group-therapy control condition and found that posttreatment self-reported abstinence rates were the same across all three conditions (i.e., the treatment groups were not superior to the wait-list control group).

Clients who participate in group therapy tend to improve just as much as clients who are engaged in treatment as usual (TAU). Magura, Rosenblum, Fong, Villano, and Richman (2002) compared "enhanced" to standard methadone treatment for cocaine abusers. Enhanced treatment included a combination of individual and group CBT sessions; standard treatment consisted of regular clinic services, which included weekly meetings with a methadone counselor. Both treatment groups showed similar treatment outcomes. Messina, Farabee, and

Rawson (2003) also compared several forms of treatment for cocaine addicts with and without ASPD. Specifically, they compared the effects group CBT, individual CM (CM; a form of behavioral treatment in which clients earn rewards for abstinence), CBT + CM, and standard methadone maintenance (MM). All treatments were associated with reductions in cocaine; however, patients with ASPD showed better in-treatment and long-term outcomes over a one-year follow-up period.

Group Therapy Compared to Individual or Couples Therapy

The limited number of studies that have compared group and individual therapy for substance use disorders suggests that the two treatment modalities are equally effective (Weiss et al., 2004). For instance, Graham et al. (1996) compared a group-based relapse prevention program to an individual-based relapse prevention program for individuals with substance use disorders. Treatment outcomes were the same in both conditions. Schmitz et al. (1997) also investigated treatment outcomes for a CBT-based relapse prevention program delivered in a group or individual format, but in a sample of cocaine users. Both delivery formats reduced cocaine use, but participants in the group-based program reported less cocaine use and fewer cocaine-related problems immediately following treatment. Similarly, Marques and Formigoni (2001) found that individual CBT and group CBT for substance use (in this case alcohol dependence) produced roughly equivalent reductions in drinking. More recently, Li and colleagues found that group BCT was as effective as individual BCT for clients with a variety of substance use disorders (Li, Armstrong, Chaim, Kelly, & Shenfeld, 2007).

Group Therapy Plus Individual/Couples Therapy Compared to Individual or Group Therapy Alone

To our knowledge, no studies have compared group therapy in combination with individual/couples therapy to individual therapy alone, except for one conducted by Linehan et al. (1999), which is discussed later in this chapter. However, there are a few studies that look at a combination of group and individual therapy versus group therapy alone. The evidence that exists suggests that combination therapy and group therapy are at least equally effective, but implies that combination therapy may be more effective in some cases.

Ball et al. (2004) compared group cognitive-behavioral coping skills training, coping skills training plus CM, and coping skills training plus CM and relationship counseling in 115 individuals who were dependent on opiates. The authors were most interested in whether client profiles based on the MCMI-III predicted differential treatment outcomes; however, it is notable that all participants showed a decrease in opiate use over the course of treatment regardless of treatment condition (12 weeks).

McKay et al. (1997) randomly assigned cocaine-dependent men to either standard group therapy, which consisted of a "mix of addictions counseling and 12-step recovery practices," or to standard group therapy plus individual relapse prevention therapy. Participants in standard group therapy alone demonstrated better rates of total abstinence. However, participants in the combined treatment condition who reported using cocaine within the first three months of treatment demonstrated fewer days of cocaine use and a lower relapse rate than participants in the standard group therapy condition who reported using cocaine during the same time frame. In contrast, results from the National Institute on Drug Abuse Collaborative Cocaine Treatment Study (Crits-Christoph et al., 1999) showed that a combination of individual and group drug counseling (GDC) that focused on stages of change, 12-step participation, and general support was more effective than manualized cognitive therapy alone.

Group Therapy Compared to Another Type of Group Therapy

A review of the literature suggests that no particular type of group therapy has consistently demonstrated superior treatment outcomes in adults. Part of the reason may be that treatment implementation varies so widely, even within one specific type of therapy, that it is difficult to make broad inferences about the effectiveness of any single group therapy model. For example, cognitive-behavioral group therapies may primarily address coping skills, relapse prevention, or cognitive restructuring while still being identified as CBT groups. This flexibility in group content is often advantageous in clinical settings because it allows practitioners to cope with individual variability in client and group needs that to some extent may be ignored in strictly manualized treatments. Such flexibility may even be necessary due to client population or clinic resources. One of the disadvantages of such variability is that we lack multiple treatment studies evaluating the same group therapy package against other similarly well-defined group therapies, across treatment settings and substance use disorders. However, Carroll and Onken (2005) reviewed behavioral therapies for substance use disorders and concluded that, despite the lack of well-controlled trials, treatments such as motivational interviewing, CBT, and CM appear to treat this population effectively.

Research indicates that several types of group therapy are effective when the group is open to individuals with a variety of substance use disorders, rather than focusing on a single substance. Multimodal milieu treatment for male inmates has been shown to improve AA attendance and reduces alcohol and drug use (Annis, 1979). Drug psychoeducation groups and recovery groups based on the stages of change model appear to improve substance abuse outcomes, although drug psychoeducation may be linked to greater treatment retention and satisfaction (Martin, Giannandrea, Rogers, & Johnson, 1996). In a more recent study, Greenfield, Trucco, McHugh, Lincoln, and Gallup (2007) conducted a randomized clinical trial to compare a newly developed women's recovery group (WRG) to mixed-gender GDC in women diagnosed with a variety of substance use disorders. The WRG was a 12-session relapse prevention group based on cognitive-behavioral theory, whereas the GDC was a 12-session psychoeducational and supportive group (Crits-Christoph et al., 1999; Daley, Mercer, & Carpenter, 2002). Women in both groups significantly reduced amount and frequency of substance use, as well as substance-related problems. However, only women in the WRG maintained these gains and actually continued to improve at nine-month follow-up.

Much of the research on adults with substance use disorders has focused on the treatment of alcohol use disorders (AUDs). Behavioral group treatment and psychodynamic group therapy appear to perform equally well, depending on their specific treatment goals. Pomerleau, Pertschuk, Adkins, and Brady (1978) assigned predominantly male alcoholics to either behavioral group treatment, which included stimulus control and CM strategies, or a "traditional" group therapy that was psychodynamic and insight-oriented. Treatment goals were controlled drinking in the behavioral group and abstinence in the psychodynamic group. Participants in the behavioral group had a lower dropout rate and better reductions in drinking, but participants who completed treatment in the psychodynamic group had better overall abstinence rates. Each group outperformed the other with respect to its own treatment goals. However, transactional analytic group therapy, another type of treatment stemming from the psychoanalytic tradition, may be less effective than 12-step and behavioral approaches unless it is combined with behavioral therapy (Olson, Ganley, Devine, & Dorsey, 1981). Finally, supportive group therapy may be associated with a greater decrease in daily drinking than group covert sensitization (a behavioral intervention) or nonspecific group therapy, even though all three therapies have been linked to similar blood alcohol levels two weeks after treatment (Telch, Hannon, & Telch, 1984).

Group social skills training may be superior to a discussion group for alcohol-dependent males, with respect to reduced alcohol consumption, increased number of days abstinent, and increased number of working days for at least one year after treatment (Eriksen, Bjornstad, & Gotestam, 1986). However, evidence for the effectiveness of group coping skills training in comparison to interactional groups (i.e., interpersonal process groups) is somewhat unclear. Both types of group therapy are associated with an increase in proportion of days abstinent from alcohol and a decrease in number of heavy drinking days through 18 months posttreatment, but coping skills training appears more effective for alcoholics with higher levels of psychopathology, sociopathy, and cognitive impairment (Cooney, Kadden, Litt, & Getter, 1991; Kadden, Cooney, Getter, & Litt, 1989; Kadden, Litt, Cooney, Kabela, & Getter, 2001; Litt, Kadden, Cooney, & Kabela, 2003).

Group CBT- based interventions appear to be as effective as other types of treatment for AUDs. Six months into treatment, male alcoholics in cognitive-behavioral relapse prevention therapy demonstrated similar levels of alcohol use to male alcoholics in interpersonal process groups (Ito, Donovan, & Hall, 1988). Similarly, Swedish alcoholics derived equal benefit from CBT and psychodynamic therapy groups, although participants in psychodynamic group therapy reported more days abstinent at nine-month follow-up (Sandahl, Gerge, & Herlitz, 2004). Group CBT was also found to be as effective as group coping skills training among German alcoholics over a two-year follow-up period, and both treatments produced better outcomes than nondirective, supportive group therapy (Burtscheidt, Wolwer, Schwarz, Strauss, & Gaebel, 2002; Burtscheidt et al., 2001). In some cases, CBT-based interventions for AUDs may be superior to other types of treatment. Easton et al. (2007) evaluated a new group cognitive-behavioral treatment program (Substance Abuse–Domestic Violence treatment approach, or SADV) for alcohol-dependent males who also engaged in interpersonal violence with their significant others. The authors compared this treatment to a 12-step facilitation group, and found that number of days abstinent increased and number of violent episodes decreased among individuals in the SADV group.

Limited evidence also supports the efficacy of group therapy for heroin and cocaine use disorders, with theoretically based treatments being more advantageous than treatment as usual or drug education. A study of heroin-addicted mothers showed that support group therapy was associated with better substance use and mother–child relationship outcomes than standard drug counseling typically used in methadone clinics (Luthar & Suchman, 2000). In addition, MET and coping skills training has been shown to be more effective than drug education in female, but not male, cocaine abusers (Rohsenow et al., 2004).

Vaughn and Howard (2004) reviewed the adolescent substance abuse treatment literature from 1988 to 2003, and critically analyzed treatment studies according to both outcome and strength of research design. With regard to group therapy, their results indicated that group CBT produced the best outcomes with the strongest research designs, as compared to undifferentiated adolescent group treatment, supportive group counseling, interactional group treatment, parent group treatment, and general group counseling. The authors were careful to note, however, that their results must be considered cautiously, as they were only able to find 15 studies to evaluate.

As with adults, some group treatment is likely to be better than no treatment at all for adolescents. Smith (1983) compared a school-based group treatment for adolescent marijuana users to a no-treatment control condition. The group treatment consisted of psychoeducation about marijuana, problem-solving training, and interpersonal skills training. Substance use, as well as peer and academic functioning, were all significantly improved among adolescents in the group treatment condition.

When adolescents with different types of SUDs are included in the same group, most forms of therapy are equally effective, with a couple of exceptions (Waldron & Kaminer, 2004). Research by Liddle and colleagues (2001) indicated that group CBT was as effective as multidimensional family therapy and group family education, with a couple of caveats: multi-family therapy produced more immediate benefits than CBT in one study, and was associated with continued improvements relative to CBT over 6- and 12-month follow-up in another study. Other studies have shown that group CBT is as effective as group psychoeducation in this population (Burleson & Kaminer, 2005; Kaminer, Burleson, & Goldberger, 2002). Two studies by Azrin and colleagues have shown that behavioral treatment may be superior to group supportive counseling for adolescent substance users in reducing drug use and drug-related problems (Azrin, Donohue, et al., 1994; Azrin, McMahon, et al., 1994). Furthermore, Joanning, Thomas, Quinn, and Mullen (1992) have found that family systems therapy may produce better treatment outcomes than process-oriented group therapy or family drug education for adolescents with a variety of SUDs.

Clients with Co-Occurring Disorders

Rates of comorbidity among substance use disorders and other psychiatric disorders are high. Clients who have co-occurring disorders are likely to experience additional problems related to the interaction between their substance use and other mental disorder, and they may suffer from poorer treatment outcomes than clients without comorbid disorders (McGovern, Wrisley, & Drake, 2005). Recent empirical evidence supports the use of integrated treatments that address substance use and psychiatric symptomatology simultaneously (Goldsmith & Garlapati, 2004; Tiet & Mausbach, 2007), and several integrated group treatments have already been developed for clients who struggle with co-occurring PTSD, Borderline Personality Disorder, psychosis, Bipolar Disorder, and other mood disorders.

One of the most frequently studied integrated therapies for clients with comorbid SUDs and PTSD is Seeking Safety, which has been successfully adapted to a group format (Cook, Walser, Kane, Ruzek, & Woody, 2006; Hien, Cohen, Miele, Litt, & Capstick, 2004; Najavits, 2002; Najavits, Weiss, Shaw, & Muenz, 1998; Zlotnick, Najavits, Rohsenow, & Johnson, 2003). The primary goals of this treatment program are to reduce substance use and symptoms of PTSD, with an emphasis on safety as the main priority. It comprises 25 topics within four content areas: cognitive, behavioral, interpersonal, and case management. There is also an emphasis on the impact of therapist processes on treatment. Even though Seeking Safety has been studied more than most other integrated treatments for individuals with co-occurring disorders, it should be noted that the majority of studies on group-based Seeking Safety are uncontrolled pilot trials. One exception is a study conducted by Gatz and colleagues (2007), in which the authors compared group Seeking Safety to treatment as usual for women with SUDs and a history of trauma. At 12 months, participants in the Seeking Safety group showed better treatment retention, greater improvement in PTSD symptoms, and better coping skills. Both groups demonstrated improvements on substance-related problems.

Dialectical Behavior Therapy (DBT) for female clients with Borderline Personality Disorder and any SUD may be more effective than TAU, as defined by alternate substance abuse or mental health treatment in the community (Linehan et al., 1999). Linehan and colleagues found that the DBT intervention was associated with better treatment retention, drug use outcomes, and global/social adjustment outcomes.

The treatment of individuals with co-occurring psychosis and substance use disorders has not been comprehensively investigated (Barrowclough, Haddock, Fitzsimmons, & Johnson, 2006; Barrowclough, Haddock, Lobban, et al., 2006). However, many researchers and clinicians state the need for integrated treatment for individuals with both conditions, whether the format is individual- or group-based. It is not clear at this point whether integrated treatments will produce better treatment outcomes than nonintegrated treatments (e.g., Hellerstein, Rosenthal, & Miner, 1995).

Integrated group therapy for clients with co-occurring SUDs and Bipolar Disorder may be superior to no treatment at all or treatment as usual. For example, adult substance users with Bipolar I Disorder demonstrated fewer days of drug use following integrated group treatment for substance use and bipolar disorder in comparison to a no-treatment control group (Weiss et al., 2002). Interestingly, the integrated treatment did not reduce number of drinking days relative to the control condition. In an earlier study, Weiss et al. (2000) compared up to 20 weeks of integrated group CBT for Bipolar Disorder and substance abuse to treatment as usual. They found that integrated CBT was associated with lower addiction severity ratings and longer periods of abstinence.

Carroll (2004) reviewed behavioral treatments for individuals with co-occurring substance use and mood disorders. She concluded that, despite the lack of well-controlled trials, treatments such as motivational interviewing, CBT, and CM appear to treat this population effectively. In addition, Brown et al. (2001) compared a standard group cognitive-behavioral smoking cessation program to a combined cognitive-behavioral treatment for smoking cessation and depression in a sample of adult smokers with a history of major depressive disorder. In general, both treatments produced similar increases in abstinence, but neither treatment influenced levels of depression. The combined treatment was more effective for heavier smokers with a history of recurrent depression.

Summary and Conclusions

Group therapy, defined as two or more unrelated clients and a therapist who meet together regularly with the primary goal of reducing or eliminating substance use, or of addressing behaviors related to substance use, may be the most widely used treatment modality for substance use disorders (Weiss et al., 2004). This treatment modality is associated with both advantages and disadvantages. With regard to advantages, it is cost-effective, provides a forum for modeling adaptive behavior, provides much-needed human contact for individuals who may otherwise be socially isolated, fosters positive peer support and pressure to abstain from drug use, allows group members to give and receive valuable feedback from group leaders and other group members, allows the group as a whole to confront an individual about harmful behaviors more effectively than a single therapist, and may instill a sense of hope and purpose in substance users by giving members the opportunity to watch and participate in others' recovery. With regard to disadvantages, there is typically the potential for group conflict or for digression to topics unrelated to the group purpose. In addition, some individuals may not benefit as much from group therapy because they feel uncomfortable sharing information about themselves and their habits in a group setting. These disadvantages can present serious problems to the extent that they hinder the achievement of group goals, trigger relapse, and engender social withdrawal among group members. However, these problems can be remedied or even used for the good of the group by an experienced therapist.

According to the CSAT, group therapies for SUDs can be placed into one of five categories: psychoeducational groups, skills development groups, CBT groups, support groups, and interpersonal process groups. The prevailing opinion, which is based on some empirical evidence, is that clients should be matched with a type of group therapy that would best serve their treatment needs. Clients can be matched to the most appropriate group according to numerous factors, which may include but are not limited to level of motivation for treatment, stage of recovery, presence or absence of a co-occurring disorder, and personality characteristics.

Despite the widespread use of group therapy to treat SUDs, there is a surprising lack of empirical evidence that consistently supports any one type of group therapy. In addition, it is hard to make specific treatment recommendations based on the existing research because of variations in population, control/comparison groups, treatment modality, and treatment protocol. Nevertheless, it appears that group therapy is effective for a variety of substance use disorders in adult and adolescent populations. It tends to produce better treatment outcomes than no treatment at all, and similar outcomes to TAU.

Group and individual therapy appear equally effective. A combination of group and individual therapy is at least as effective as group therapy alone, and may be more effective in some cases. Integrated treatments for patients with co-occurring substance abuse and other psychiatric disorders also produce good treatment outcomes. In fact, integrated treatments such as Seeking Safety for individuals with co-occurring PTSD, DBT for individuals with co-occurring BPD, and Weiss's treatment for co-occurring SUDs and Bipolar Disorder are associated with better treatment outcomes than nonintegrated treatments. Behavioral treatments for individuals with co-occurring substance use and mood disorders, such as motivational interviewing, CBT, and CM, also reduce substance use and its negative consequences, whether integrated or not. In general, the empirical evidence does not indicate that one type of group therapy is superior to any other. However, group CBT appears to consistently demonstrate positive outcomes, perhaps because it is one of the most frequently studied types of treatment.

References

Alessi, S. M., Hanson, T., Wieners, M., & Petry, N. M. (2007). Low-cost contingency management in community clinics: Delivering incentives partially in group therapy. *Experimental and Clinical Psychopharmacology, 15,* 293–300.

Annis, H. M. (1979). Group treatment of incarcerated offenders with alcohol and drug problems: A controlled evaluation. *Canadian Journal of Criminology, 21,* 3–15.

Azrin, N. H., Donohue, B., Besalel, V. A., Kogan, E. S., & Acierno, R. (1994). Youth drug abuse treatment: A controlled outcome study. *Journal of Child & Adolescent Substance Abuse, 3,* 1–16.

Azrin, N. H., McMahon, P. T., Donohue, B., Besalel, V. A., Lapinski, K. J., Kogan, E. S., et al. (1994). Behavior therapy for drug abuse: A controlled treatment outcome study. *Behaviour Research and Therapy, 32,* 857–866.

Ball, S. A., Nich, C., Rounsaville, B. J., Eagan, D., & Carroll, K. M. (2004). Millon Clinical Multiaxial Inventory-III subtypes of opioid dependence: Validity and matching to behavioral therapies. *Journal of Consulting and Clinical Psychology, 72,* 698–711.

Barrowclough, C., Haddock, G., Fitzsimmons, M., & Johnson, R. (2006). Treatment development for psychosis and co-occurring substance misuse: A descriptive review. *Journal of Mental Health: New advancements in the study of co-occurring substance use and psychiatric disorders* [Special Issue] *15*(6), 619–632.

Barrowclough, C., Haddock, G., Lobban, F., Jones, S., Siddle, R., Roberts, C., et al. (2006). Group cognitive-behavioural therapy for schizophrenia. *British Journal of Psychiatry, 189,* 527–532.

Battjes, R. J., Gordon, M. S., O'Grady, K. E., Kinlock, T. W., Katz, E. C., & Sears, E. A. (2004). Evaluation of a group-based substance abuse treatment program for adolescents. *Journal of Substance Abuse Treatment, 27,* 123–134.

Brown, R. A., Kahler, C. W., Niaura, R., Abrams, D. B., Sales, S. D., Ramsey, S. E., et al. (2001). Cognitive-behavioral treatment for depression in smoking cessation. *Journal of Consulting and Clinical Psychology, 69,* 471–480.

Burleson, J. A., & Kaminer, Y. (2005). Self-efficacy as a predictor of treatment outcome in adolescent substance use disorders. *Addictive Behaviors: Trends in the treatment of adolescent substance abuse* [Special Issue], *30,* 1751–1764.

Burleson, J. A., Kaminer, Y., & Dennis, M. L. (2006). Absence of iatrogenic or contagion effects in adolescent group therapy: Findings from the Cannabis Youth Treatment (CYT) Study. *The American Journal on Addictions. Advances in the assessment and treatment of adolescent substance use disorders* [Special Issue] *15*(Suppl. 1), 4–15.

Burtscheidt, W., Wolwer, W., Schwarz, R., Strauss, W., & Gaebel, W. (2002). Out-patient behaviour therapy in alcoholism: Treatment outcome after 2 years. *Acta Psychiatrica Scandinavica, 106,* 227–232.

Burtscheidt, W., Wolwer, W., Schwarz, R., Strauss, W., Loll, A., Luthcke, H., et al. (2001). Out-patient behaviour therapy in alcoholism: Relapse rates after 6 months. *Acta Psychiatrica Scandinavica, 103,* 24–29.

Carroll, K. M. (2004). Behavioral therapies for co-occurring substance use and mood disorders. *Biological Psychiatry, 56*, 778–784.

Carroll, K. M., & Onken, L. S. (2005). Behavioral therapies for drug abuse. *American Journal of Psychiatry, 162*, 1452–1460.

Charney, D. A., Palacios-Boix, J., Negrete, J. C., Dobkin, P. L., & Gill, K. J. (2005). Association between concurrent depression and anxiety and six-month outcome of addiction treatment. *Psychiatric Services, 56*, 927–933.

Cook, J. M., Walser, R. D., Kane, V., Ruzek, J. I., & Woody, G. (2006). Dissemination and feasibility of a cognitive-behavioral treatment for substance use disorders and posttraumatic stress disorder in the Veterans Administration. *Journal of Psychoactive Drugs, 38*, 89–92.

Cooney, N. L., Kadden, R. M., Litt, M. D., & Getter, H. (1991). Matching alcoholics to coping skills or interactional therapies: Two-year follow-up results. *Journal of Consulting and Clinical Psychology, 59*, 598–601.

Coviello, D. M., Alterman, A. I., Rutherford, M. J., Cacciola, J. S., McKay, J. R., & Zanis, D. A. (2001). The effectiveness of two intensities of psychosocial treatment for cocaine dependence. *Drug and Alcohol Dependence, 61*, 145–154.

Crits-Christoph, P., Siqueland, L., Blaine, J., Frank, A., Luborsky, L., Onken, L. S., et al. (1999). Psychosocial treatments for cocaine dependence: National Institute on Drug Abuse Collaborative Cocaine Treatment Study. *Archives of General Psychiatry, 56*, 493–502.

CSAT. (2005). *Substance abuse treatment: Group therapy* (No. DHHS Publication No. (SMA) 05-3991). Rockland, MD: Substance Abuse and Mental Health Services Administration.

Daley, D. C., Mercer, D., & Carpenter, G. (2002). *Drug counseling for cocaine addiction: The Collaborative Cocaine Treatment Study Model.* Bethesda, MD: U.S. Department of Health and Human Services.

Dennis, M., Godley, S. H., Diamond, G., Tims, F. M., Babor, T., Donaldson, J., et al. (2004). The Cannabis Youth Treatment (CYT) Study: Main findings from two randomized trials. *Journal of Substance Abuse Treatment, 27*, 197–213.

Diamond, G., Godley, S. H., Liddle, H. A., Sampl, S., Webb, C., Tims, F. M., et al. (2002). Five outpatient treatment models for adolescent marijuana use: A description of the Cannabis Youth Treatment Interventions. *Addiction, 97*(Suppl. 1), 70–83.

DiClemente, C. C., Prochaska, J. O., Fairhurst, S. K., Velicer, W. F., et al. (1991). The process of smoking cessation: An analysis of precontemplation, contemplation, and preparation stages of change. *Journal of Consulting and Clinical Psychology, 59*, 295–304.

Easton, C. J., Mandel, D. L., Hunkele, K. A., Nich, C., Rounsaville, B. J., & Carroll, K. M. (2007). A cognitive behavioral therapy for alcohol-dependent domestic violence offenders: An integrated substance abuse-domestic violence treatment approach (SADV). *The American Journal on Addictions, 16*, 24–31.

el-Guebaly, N., Cathcart, J., Currie, S., Brown, D., & Gloster, S. (2002). Smoking cessation approaches for persons with mental illness or addictive disorders. *Psychiatric Services, 53*, 1166–1170.

Emmelkamp, P. M. G., & Vedel, E. (2006). *Evidence-based treatment for alcohol and drug abuse.* New York: Routledge.

Eriksen, L., Bjornstad, S., & Gotestam, K. G. (1986). Social skills training in groups for alcoholics: One-year treatment outcome for groups and individuals. *Addictive Behaviors, 11*, 309–329.

Gatz, M., Brown, V., Hennigan, K., Rechberger, E., O'Keefe, M., Rose, T., et al. (2007). Effectiveness of an integrated, trauma-informed approach to treating women with co-occurring disorders and histories of trauma: The Los Angeles site experience. *Journal of Community Psychology, 35*, 863–878.

Goldsmith, R. J., & Garlapati, V. (2004). Behavioral interventions for dual-diagnosis patients. *Psychiatric Clinics of North America, Addictive Disorders* [Special Issue], *27*, 709–725.

Graham, K., Annis, H. M., Brett, P. J., & Venesoen, P. (1996). A controlled field trial of group versus individual cognitive-behavioural training for relapse prevention. *Addiction, 91*, 1127–1140.

Greenfield, S. F., Trucco, E. M., McHugh, R. K., Lincoln, M., & Gallop, R. J. (2007). The women's recovery group study: A stage I trial of women-focused group therapy for substance use disorders versus mixed-gender group drug counseling. *Drug and Alcohol Dependence, 90*, 39–47.

Hellerstein, D. J., Rosenthal, R. N., & Miner, C. R. (1995). A prospective study of integrated outpatient treatment for substance-abusing schizophrenic patients. *The American Journal on Addictions, 4*, 33–42.

Hien, D. A., Cohen, L. R., Miele, G. M., Litt, L. C., & Capstick, C. (2004). Promising treatments for women with comorbid PTSD and substance use disorders. *American Journal of Psychiatry, 161*, 1426–1432.

Hillhouse, M. P., Marinelli-Casey, P., Gonzales, R., Ang, A., & Rawson, R. A. (2007). Predicting in-treatment performance and post-treatment outcomes in methamphetamine users. *Addiction, 102*(Suppl. 1), 84–95.

Ito, J. R., Donovan, D. M., & Hall, J. J. (1988). Relapse prevention in alcohol aftercare: Effects on drinking outcome, change process, and aftercare attendance. *British Journal of Addiction, 83*, 171–181.

Joanning, H., Quinn, W., Thomas, F., & Mullen, R. (1992). Treating adolescent drug abuse: A comparison of family systems therapy, group therapy, and family drug education. *Journal of Marital & Family Therapy, 18*, 345–356.

Kadden, R. M., Cooney, N. L., Getter, H., & Litt, M. D. (1989). Matching alcoholics to coping skills or interactional therapies: Posttreatment results. *Journal of Consulting and Clinical Psychology, 57*, 698–704.

Kadden, R. M., Litt, M. D., Cooney, N. L., Kabela, E., & Getter, H. (2001). Prospective matching of alcoholic clients to cognitive-behavioral or interactional group therapy. *Journal of Studies on Alcohol, 62*, 359–369.

Kaminer, Y. (2005). Challenges and opportunities of group therapy for adolescent substance abuse: A critical review. *Addictive Behaviors: Trends in the treatment of adolescent substance abuse* [Special Issue], *30*, 1765–1774.

Kaminer, Y., Burleson, J. A., & Goldberger, R. (2002). Cognitive-behavioral coping skills and psycho-education therapies for adolescent substance abuse. *Journal of Nervous and Mental Disease, 190*, 737–745.

Khantzian, E. J., Golden-Schulman, S. J., & McAuliffe, W. E. (2004). *Group therapy*. Washington, DC: American Psychiatric.

Latimer, W. W., Winters, K. C., D'Zurilla, T., & Nichols, M. (2003). Integrated family and cognitive-behavioral therapy for adolescent substance abusers: A Stage I efficacy study. *Drug and Alcohol Dependence, 71*, 303–317.

Li, S., Armstrong, M. S., Chaim, G., Kelly, C., & Shenfeld, J. (2007). Group and individual couple treatment for substance abuse clients: A pilot study. *American Journal of Family Therapy, 35*, 221–233.

Liddle, H. A., Dakof, G. A., Parker, K., Diamond, G. S., Barrett, K., & Tejeda, M. (2001). Multidimiensional family therapy for adolescent drug abuse: Results of a randomized clinical trial. *American Journal of Drug and Alcohol Abuse, 27*, 651–688.

Linehan, M. M., Schmidt, H., III, Dimeff, L. A., Craft, J. C., Kanter, J., & Comtois, K. A. (1999). Dialectical behavior therapy for patients with borderline personality disorder and drug-dependence. *The American Journal on Addictions, 8*, 279–292.

Litt, M. D., Kadden, R. M., Cooney, N. L., & Kabela, E. (2003). Coping skills and treatment outcomes in cognitive-behavioral and interactional group therapy for alcoholism. *Journal of Consulting and Clinical Psychology, 71*, 118–128.

Luthar, S. S., & Suchman, N. E. (2000). Relational psychotherapy mothers' group: A developmentally informed intervention for at-risk mothers. *Development and Psychopathology, 12*, 235–253.

Magura, S., Rosenblum, A., Fong, C., Villano, C., & Richman, B. (2002). Treating cocaine-using methadone patients: Predictors of outcomes in a psychosocial clinical trial. *Substance Use & Misuse, 37*, 1927–1953.

Marques, A. C. P. R., & Formigoni, M. L. C. O. S. (2001). Comparison of individual and group cognitive-behavioral therapy for alcohol and/or drug-dependent patients. *Addiction, 96*, 835–846.

Martin, K., Giannandrea, P., Rogers, B., & Johnson, J. (1996). Group intervention with pre-recovery patients. *Journal of Substance Abuse Treatment, 13*, 33–41.

McGovern, M. P., Wrisley, B. R., & Drake, R. E. (2005). Special section on relapse prevention: Relapse of substance use disorder and its prevention among persons with co-occurring disorders. *Psychiatric Services, 56*, 1270–1273.

McKay, J. R., Alterman, A. I., Cacciola, J. S., Rutherford, M. J., O'Brien, C. P., & Koppenhaver, J. (1997). Group counseling versus individualized relapse prevention aftercare following intensive outpatient treatment for cocaine dependence: Initial results. *Journal of Consulting and Clinical Psychology, 65,* 778–788.

Messina, N., Farabee, D., & Rawson, R. (2003). Treatment responsivity of cocaine-dependent patients with antisocial personality disorder to cognitive-behavioral and contingency management interventions. *Journal of Consulting and Clinical Psychology, 71,* 320–329.

Mueller, S. E., Petitjean, S., Boening, J., & Wiesbeck, G. A. (2007). The impact of self-help group attendance on relapse rates after alcohol detoxification in a controlled study. *Alcohol and Alcoholism, 42,* 108–112.

Najavits, L. M. (2002). *Seeking safety: A treatment manual for PTSD and substance abuse.* New York, NY: Guilford Press.

Najavits, L. M., Weiss, R. D., Shaw, S. R., & Muenz, L. R. (1998). "Seeking safety": Outcome of a new cognitive-behavioral psychotherapy for women with posttraumatic stress disorder and substance dependence. *Journal of Traumatic Stress, 11,* 437–456.

Olson, R. P., Ganley, R., Devine, V. T., & Dorsey, G. C. (1981). Long-term effects of behavioral versus insight-oriented therapy with inpatient alcoholics. *Journal of Consulting and Clinical Psychology, 49,* 866–877.

Pomerleau, O., Pertschuk, M., Adkins, D., & Brady, J. P. (1978). A comparison of behavioral and traditional treatment for middle-income problem drinkers. *Journal of Behavioral Medicine, 1,* 1573–3521.

Razavi, D., Vandecasteele, H., Primo, C., Bodo, M., Debrier, F., Verbist, H., et al. (1999). Maintaining abstinence from cigarette smoking: Effectiveness of group counselling and factors predicting outcome. *European Journal of Cancer, 35,* 1238–1247.

Rohsenow, D. J., Monti, P. M., Martin, R. A., Colby, S. M., Myers, M. G., Gulliver, S. B., et al. (2004). Motivational enhancement and coping skills training for cocaine abusers: Effects on substance use outcomes. *Addiction, 99,* 862–874.

Rosenblum, A., Cleland, C., Magura, S., Mahmood, D., Kosanke, N., & Foote, J. (2005). Moderators of effects of motivational enhancements to cognitive behavioral therapy. *American Journal of Drug and Alcohol Abuse, 31,* 35–58.

Rosenblum, A., Magura, S., Kayman, D. J., & Fong, C. (2005). Motivationally enhanced group counseling for substance users in a soup kitchen: A randomized clinical trial. *Drug and Alcohol Dependence, 80,* 91–103.

Sandahl, C., Gerge, A., & Herlitz, K. (2004). Does treatment focus on self-efficacy result in better coping? Paradoxical findings from psychodynamic and cognitive-behavioral group treatment of moderately alcohol-dependent patients. *Psychotherapy Research, 14,* 388–397.

Scheidlinger, S. (2000). The group psychotherapy movement at the millennium: Some historical perspectives. *International Journal of Group Psychotherapy, 50,* 315–339.

Schmitz, J. M., Oswald, L. M., Jacks, S. D., Rustin, T., Rhoades, H. M., & Grabowski, J. (1997). Relapse prevention treatment for cocaine dependence: Group vs. individual format. *Addictive Behaviors, 22,* 405–418.

Shearer, J. (2007). Psychosocial approaches to psychostimulant dependence: A systematic review. *Journal of Substance Abuse Treatment, 32,* 41–52.

Smith, D. C., Hall, J. A., Williams, J. K., An, H., & Gotman, N. (2006). Comparative efficacy of family and group treatment for adolescent substance abuse. *The American Journal on Addictions: Advances in the assessment and treatment of adolescent substance use disorders* [Special Issue], *15*(Suppl. 1), 131–136.

Smith, T. E. (1983). Reducing adolescents' marijuana abuse. *Social Work in Health Care, 9,* 33–44.

Stephens, R. S., Roffman, R. A., & Curtin, L. (2000). Comparison of extended versus brief treatments for marijuana use. *Journal of Consulting and Clinical Psychology, 68,* 898–908.

Telch, M. J., Hannon, R., & Telch, C. F. (1984). A comparison of cessation strategies for the outpatient alcoholic. *Addictive Behaviors, 9,* 103–109.

Tiet, Q. Q., & Mausbach, B. (2007). Treatments for patients with dual diagnosis: A review. *Alcoholism: Clinical and Experimental Research, 31,* 513–536.

Toseland, R. W., & Siporin, M. (1986). When to recommend group treatment: A review of the clinical and the research literature. *International Journal of Group Psychotherapy, 36*, 171–201.

Tucker, M., & Oei, T. P. S. (2007). Is group more cost effective than individual cognitive behaviour therapy? The evidence is not solid yet. *Behavioural and Cognitive Psychotherapy, 35*, 77–91.

Vaughn, M. G., & Howard, M. O. (2004). Adolescent substance abuse treatment: A synthesis of controlled evaluations. *Research on Social Work Practice, 14*, 325–335.

Waldron, H. B., & Kaminer, Y. (2004). On the learning curve: The emerging evidence supporting cognitive-behavioral therapies for adolescent substance abuse. *Addiction, 99*(Suppl. 2), 93–105.

Washton, A. M. (2005). Group therapy. In J. H. Lowinson, P. Ruiz, R. B. Millman, & J. G. Langrod (Eds.), *Substance abuse: A comprehensive textbook* (4th ed., pp. 671–680). Philadelphia: Lippincott, Williams, & Wilkins.

Weiss, R. D., Griffin, M. L., Greenfield, S. F., Najavits, L. M., Wyner, D., Soto, J. A., et al. (2000). Group therapy for patients with bipolar disorder and substance dependence: Results of a pilot study. *Journal of Clinical Psychiatry, 61*, 361–367.

Weiss, R. D., Jaffee, W. B., de Menil, V. P., & Cogley, C. B. (2004). Group therapy for substance use disorders: What do we know? *Harvard Review of Psychiatry: The neurobiology and treatment of substance use disorders* [Special Issue], *12*, 339–350.

Weiss, R. D., Kolodziej, M., Griffin, M. L., Najavits, L. M., Jacobson, L. M., & Greenfield, S. F. (2002). Substance use and perceived symptom improvement among patients with bipolar disorder and substance dependence. *Journal of Affective Disorders, 79*, 279–283.

Winters, J., Fals-Stewart, W., O'Farrell, T. J., Birchler, G. R., & Kelley, M. L. (2002). Behavioral couples therapy for female substance-abusing patients: Effects on substance use and relationship adjustment. *Journal of Consulting and Clinical Psychology, 70*, 344–355.

Zlotnick, C., Najavits, L. M., Rohsenow, D. J., & Johnson, D. M. (2003). A cognitive-behavioral treatment for incarcerated women with substance abuse disorder and posttraumatic stress disorder: Findings from a pilot study. *Journal of Substance Abuse Treatment, 25*, 99–105.

10

Community Reinforcement Approach: CRA and CRAFT Programs

Loren Gianini, S. Laura Lundy, and Jane Ellen Smith

University of New Mexico

Contents

The Community Reinforcement Approach (CRA: Hunt & Azrin, 1973) is a comprehensive behavioral intervention for treating individuals with substance abuse problems (Meyers & Smith, 1995). The reinforcing aspects of the substance user's family, social, vocational, and recreational interests are strengthened throughout CRA with the goal of facilitating a lifestyle that is more rewarding and enjoyable than one in which the client is using drugs or alcohol. The Community Reinforcement and Family Training (CRAFT) program is based on these same principles, but it is a treatment that is conducted instead with the loved ones of treatment-refusing substance abusers (Smith & Meyers, 2004).

CRA: Treatment for the Substance User

CRA Overview

CRA is rooted in the idea that the substance user's community (e.g., family, friends, job, church) plays an essential role in the recovery process. CRA relies heavily on positive reinforcement and operant techniques while specifically avoiding confrontation (Azrin, 1976; Hunt & Azrin, 1973). CRA is a menu-driven program that typically begins with a functional analysis of the triggers for substance use, as well as the positive and negative consequences. The functional analysis allows the therapist and client to determine what the client is gaining from the substance use, so they can identify healthy, enjoyable alternative activities that can compete with the drinking or drug use. Following the functional analysis, the client and therapist negotiate a commitment to a manageable period of sobriety that is not experienced as overwhelming by the client. This procedure is referred to as "sobriety sampling." A fundamental strategy of the CRA program involves identifying and setting goals of the client's choosing, including a number of different life areas. In the process of setting goals it often becomes apparent that the client is lacking the skills necessary to achieve these goals. The therapist can then employ various techniques (e.g., problem-solving, communication skills, drink/drug refusal, etc.) to increase the chance that the client will be successful. Job counseling, relapse prevention, and relationship therapy are examples of useful treatment approaches that may be employed. The use of specific techniques listed above is optional depending upon the client's needs, and thus, treatment is quite individualized (see Meyers & Smith, 1995; Smith & Meyers, 2001, 2004; Smith, Meyers, & Miller, 2001).

CRA Functional Analyses

The functional analysis, a fundamental procedure in CRA, is a way of identifying the function of certain behaviors. CRA uses two types of functional analyses: one for substance use, and one for pro-social behaviors. A semi-structured interview designed to identify both the antecedents and consequences of problem behaviors is typically used (Meyers & Smith, 1995, pp. 20–29). It is a method for placing the substance user's drinking or drug-using behavior into a larger, more comprehensive context, and for then developing the CRA treatment plan. The functional analysis is typically done in one of the first sessions, but is often referred to throughout treatment, and may even be repeated if a client experiences a relapse.

The CRA *Functional Analysis for Substance Use* interview (Table 10.1) forms the framework for treatment. However, rather than simply going through each question sequentially, the therapist begins by asking the client to describe a typical or recent using episode for his substance of choice. This allows one to gather critical information without appearing somewhat mechanical and distant to the client. Specific questions can then be asked to fill in any gaps. It is important to keep in mind that the desired outcome of the functional analysis is not to have every question on the chart answered, but to garner a solid understanding of the client's typical using behavior.

The first two columns address the antecedents, or triggers, associated with substance use. External triggers (column 1) are aspects of the client's environment, and include people, places, and times that typically accompany a substance-using episode. Internal triggers (column 2) are the thoughts and feelings that the client experiences before engaging in substance use. The specific using behavior itself (type, quantity, frequency, duration) is identified in the third column. The last two columns are devoted to exploring the consequences of the using behavior. The short-term positive consequences (column 4) provide reasons for client continued use. It is important to remember that the reasons the client initially began using may differ from those that maintain the use. Positive consequences of substance use can include pleasant physical and emotional feelings, such as relaxation or increased self-confidence, as well as the ability to avoid negative thoughts and feelings, such as anxiety. It is rather unusual for therapists to acknowledge and inquire about the positive aspects of a client's drinking or drug use, and thus many clients respond with appreciation and respect. Long-term negative consequences (column 5) are probed in such areas as physical health, legal issues, and interpersonal relationships.

Because the functional analysis contains a wealth of information, therapists need to summarize what they have learned before incorporating this information into a CRA treatment plan. Remember, the functional analysis can remain helpful throughout treatment, as the triggers represent high-risk occasions that should be anticipated, and the negative consequences serve as motivators for the client. Furthermore, the positive consequences must be kept at the forefront, because essentially CRA therapists will need to help their clients find ways to obtain the positive consequences in a healthier manner.

The second functional analysis, for pro-social behavior, is designed to identify healthy pleasant activities that are occurring occasionally now, and which the client would like to increase in frequency. Ideally the activity will compete directly with times during which the

TABLE 10.1
Functional Analysis for Substance Use

External Triggers	Internal Triggers	Using Behavior	Short Term Consequences	Long Term Consequences
1. Who are you usually with when you use?	1. What are you thinking about right before you use?	1. What do you usually use?	1. What do you like about using with (whom)?	1. What are the negative results of your using in each of these areas?
			2. What do you like about using (where)?	(a) Family members: (b) Friends:
			3. What do you like about using (when)?	(c) Emotional feelings:
2. Where do you usually use?	2. What are you usually feeling physically right before you use?	2. How much do you usually use?	4. What are the pleasant thoughts you have while using?	(d) Physical feelings: (e) Job/school situation:
			5. What are the pleasant physical feelings you have while using?	(f) Legal situation:
3. When do you usually use?	3. What are you feeling emotionally right before you use?	3. Over how long a period of time do you usually use?	6. What are some of the pleasant emotion feelings you have while using?	(g) Financial situations: (h) Other situations:

Source. Clinical Guide to Alcohol Treatment: The Community Reinforcement Approach (pp. 34–35) by R. J. Meyers & J. E. Smith, 1995, New York: Guilford Press. Adapted by permission.

client is likely to engage in substance use, and will offer some of the positive consequences previously associated with that use. The CRA *Functional Analysis for Pro-Social Behavior* (see Meyers & Smith, 1995, pp. 34–35) is very similar in structure to the one for using behaviors. However, rather than identifying short-term positive and long-term negative consequences of the behavior, the pro-social functional analysis focuses on short-term negative and long-term positive outcomes. Short-term negative consequences are akin to roadblocks that currently are preventing the client from engaging in the activity more often. For example, if a client wishes to start working out three times a week, he may list transportation problems or lack of money as reasons that he has not begun. It often becomes evident at this point that the client lacks the skills to find solutions to these obstacles, and the treatment plan should incorporate skill-building steps to address these issues. The last category, long-term positive consequences, examines the outcomes the client hopes to achieve by engaging in the pro-social activity. Referring back to these reasons throughout treatment will reinforce the client's desire to make healthy changes in his or her life.

Sobriety Sampling

The idea that total abstinence is the only measure of success forms the basis for most traditional alcohol and drug treatment programs (see McCrady, Horvath, & Delaney, 2003; Miller & Hester, 2003). In contrast, the philosophy of CRA is that therapists are more likely to successfully engage clients in treatment by convincing them initially to "sample" sobriety for a limited period of time, rather than by imposing unyielding and overwhelming expectations of abstinence. The concept of sobriety sampling is often more attractive to clients, especially those who simply want to moderate their alcohol or drug use, and they are thus more willing to participate in treatment.

When introducing the idea of sobriety sampling, it is helpful to inform clients of the many advantages of a period of sobriety. Examples include: (a) it allows clients to see what it feels like to be sober for a more extended period of time than is common for them, during which time they may begin to notice positive changes in physical and emotional feelings; (b) it demonstrates to the client's family members that a commitment has been made, which in turn elicits their indispensable support; and (c) it promotes self-esteem and paves the way for future success.

Sobriety sampling is comprised of two stages: first, the therapist must get the client to agree to a period of abstinence. It is useful to begin by suggesting an overly ambitious period of time, such as 90 days. Most clients will balk at a time period this long, feeling unsure or unwilling to make such a commitment. At this point, the process of negotiation begins. Through discussion and acceptance, the therapist and the client can agree upon a period of time for which the client feels abstinence is attainable. Depending on the client, this period can range from one day to many weeks. Nonetheless, it is necessary to schedule another session prior to the end-date of the period.

The second step of sobriety sampling involves devising specific strategies for accomplishing the sobriety goal. A number of CRA procedures are designed for just this purpose, but because sobriety sampling will occur early in treatment, it is likely that the client will not yet have been taught these skills. Consequently, the therapist should refer back to the triggers on the functional analysis so that alternative responses to them can be developed. It is worthwhile to devise back-up plans as well, inasmuch as many high-risk situations may be unavoidable (e.g., a businessman may be expected to entertain clients with dinner and drinks). It is also helpful to schedule multiple sessions in quick succession so that there is time to teach the client basic skills such as problem-solving and drink/drug refusal.

Treatment Plan: Happiness Scale and Goals of Counseling

One of the basic objectives of CRA is to help the client develop a rewarding life without the use of substances. This notion suggests that clients should be encouraged to set goals that address and improve many areas of their lives, and not just the substance-abusing behavior itself. *The Happiness Scale* and *Goals of Counseling* forms (see Meyers & Smith, 1995, pp. 98–99) comprise the foundation of the CRA treatment plan, and they can be used for just these purposes.

The Happiness Scale (Table 10.2) asks about current levels of happiness in 10 life areas. Clients rate each area on a scale of 1 (*completely unhappy*) to 10 (*completely happy*). In explaining the Happiness Scale it is important to emphasize to clients that it will give them an opportunity to identify areas of their lives in which they would like to set and work toward achieving personal goals. Once the scale is completed, therapists should briefly review the ratings, thereby getting an idea of the client's "big picture."

Although therapists generally should allow clients to choose which categories they would like to work on first, it is important for clients to meet with early success so that they are motivated to continue with treatment. Therefore, it is prudent to have clients select areas that they have rated in the medium-to-high range. In order to engage clients in the process of devising goals, therapists might begin by asking clients to operationalize the changes they would like to see. For example, the therapist could say, "You rated the 'communication' category a 5. What would need to be different in your life in order for you to rate it a 7 or 8?" Discussions such as this lend themselves nicely to beginning to develop a treatment plan using the *Goals of Counseling* form (Meyers & Smith, 1995, pp. 98–99).

Goals typically should be targeted for a one-month time frame. Strategies that take steps toward achieving these goals are made on a week-to-week basis in the form of "homework" assignments. Goals tend to be more manageable when they are stated in brief, positive, and specific terms. Goals should also be reasonable and measurable (observable by others). Strategies for achieving these goals should possess these same characteristics. The following are examples of problematic and improved goals and strategies.

> *Problematic goal:* "My goal is to stop hanging out with my drinking friends on Saturday nights." (Not stated positively; what will the person do instead?)
> *Problematic goal:* "My goal is to feel better." (Not specific)
> *Problematic goal:* "My goal is to think about ways to earn more money." (Not measurable)
> *Improved goal:* "My goal is to lose 2 lbs. this month.

A good strategy for accomplishing this goal would be "I'll walk the dog for 30 minutes 4 days this week, and I'll keep track of how many sodas I drink each day." (Brief, specific, positive, and measurable).

TABLE 10.2
Happiness Scale

This scale is intended to estimate your _current_ happiness with your life in each of the ten areas listed below. Ask yourself the
following question as you rate each area:
How happy am I with this area of my life?
You are to circle one of the numbers (1–10) beside each area.
Numbers toward the left indicate various degrees of unhappiness, while numbers toward the right reflect various levels of
happiness. In other words, state according to the numerical scale (1–10) exactly how you feel **today**. Also try not to allow one
category to influence the results of the other categories.

	Completely Unhappy						_Completely Happy_			
Substance Use	1	2	3	4	5	6	7	8	9	10
Job or Education	1	2	3	4	5	6	7	8	9	10
Money Management	1	2	3	4	5	6	7	8	9	10
Social Life	1	2	3	4	5	6	7	8	9	10
Personal Habits	1	2	3	4	5	6	7	8	9	10
Romantic Relationships	1	2	3	4	5	6	7	8	9	10
Family Relationships	1	2	3	4	5	6	7	8	9	10
Emotional Life	1	2	3	4	5	6	7	8	9	10
Communication	1	2	3	4	5	6	7	8	9	10
Spirituality	1	2	3	4	5	6	7	8	9	10
General Happiness	1	2	3	4	5	6	7	8	9	10

Source.   Clinical Guide to Alcohol Treatment: The Community Reinforcement Approach (p. 95) by R. J. Meyers & J. E.
Smith, 1995, New York: Guilford Press. Adapted by permission.

Another important but often neglected component of setting goals and devising strategies
is to explore and address obstacles that might interfere with achieving these goals. Throughout
the development of the treatment plan it is important to remind clients that achieving these
goals will allow them to build the foundation for a life that is satisfying and reinforcing without the use of drugs or alcohol, even if they are not specifically setting goals regarding their
drug or alcohol use.

Monitored Disulfiram

When a client is having great difficulty achieving even short periods of abstinence, adding
a disulfiram (Antabuse) component to treatment can help. Disulfiram, a medication that
causes acute physical illness when it interacts with alcohol, can serve as an effective deterrent to drinking. Disulfiram can be especially useful if a client tends to drink impulsively or
has difficulty identifying triggers, or if the negative consequences of drinking are extremely
serious (e.g., loss of job or incarceration.). Because the effects of disulfiram can range from
mild to serious sickness, it is essential to have a physician involved in its prescription and
management.

Clients may express some doubts or anxiety about beginning a course of disulfiram, so it is
helpful to explain some of its advantages; for example, (a) clients' families may see their willingness to try disulfiram as a commitment to treatment, (b) clients will be forced to develop
coping skills other than drinking, (c) it may help clients experience a period of sobriety that

they previously were unable to achieve, thereby proving that sobriety is possible. Describing the time-limited nature of disulfiram use will further alleviate the client's qualms.

Once a client has agreed to sample disulfiram, it is essential to identify a family member, friend, or significant other who is willing to act as the "monitor." This monitor will attend a therapy session with the client in order to be properly trained to administer the disulfiram daily. The client and monitor will develop a routine for taking the disulfiram, and the monitor will be instructed about ways to help make the ritual both supportive and reinforcing for the client.

Communication Skills Training

If it becomes apparent that a client lacks the skills to communicate positively and effectively, an exercise in positive communication skills is warranted. The purpose of the exercise is to enhance their communication so that it increases the likelihood that clients will get what they want. Communication skills are taught by reviewing the components of effective communication while supplying examples, and then by conducting a series of role-plays wherein these new skills are honed. The components of positive communication are: (a) be brief; (b) refer to specific behaviors; (c) use positive wording; (d) state your feelings; (e) give an understanding statement; (f) take partial responsibility; and (g) offer to help. Clients may not be familiar with some of these concepts, and thus it is important to explain them thoroughly.

Once the seven components have been presented, it is imperative that they be practiced in role-plays of conversations that clients are likely to have. While conducting these role-plays it is important to reinforce clients for their efforts, and to offer constructive criticism. Role-plays should be repeated several times in a session so that clients can incorporate the feedback into their conversation comfortably. This exercise lends itself to homework assignments in which clients would make an effort to use these new skills with their loved ones.

Problem-Solving Skills

Problem solving is another skills area in which substance-abusing clients are likely to have deficits. Alcohol and illicit drugs are often relied upon as the coping strategy when problematic situations arise, and so an emphasis on teaching new problem-solving skills is indicated. CRA's problem-solving work is based upon D'Zurilla and Goldfried's (1971) approach.

1. *Define the problem* as specifically as possible so that it can be experienced as manageable and addressed directly.
2. *Brainstorm* potential solutions to this problem. The goal is to generate as many solutions as possible without initial regard to how likely they are to work or how doable they are. If this activity is done in a group setting it is important to emphasize that solutions offered by others should not be criticized.
3. *Select a potential solution* by having clients eliminate all of the suggested solutions that they cannot see themselves doing. The clients should not be required to give an explanation for why they are eliminating particular solutions. Clients should pick one solution they would like to try in the upcoming week, and should explicitly describe how they will enact this solution.

4. *Identify potential obstacles* that could get in the way of following through with the chosen solution. Clients need assistance first in identifying obstacles, and then in troubleshooting solutions. Back-up plans must be established as well. Clients should then agree to try out this solution as an assignment for the upcoming week.

5. *Evaluate the outcome* of this solution during the next session. Clients should be asked how the assignment went, and praise should be offered for their efforts. Any unforeseen obstacles that stood in the way of task completion should be addressed in the event that the plan is to repeat the assignment for the next week.

Drink/Drug Refusal Skills

Regardless of the stage in treatment or follow-up, many clients face situations in which they are offered alcohol or drugs. Thus it is essential to teach specific skills for successful refusal. Oftentimes when clients are asked how they will avoid taking drugs offered by others, they give responses such as, "I just won't do it," or, "I'll just say no." Although clients should be encouraged to use whatever reasonable means are necessary in order to avoid relapsing, CRA provides several specific drink/drug refusal strategies. Prior to practicing assertive refusal, it is useful to help clients identify friends or family members who will be supportive of their decision to quit drinking/using drugs. A role-play should be conducted in which the client asks for their support. The practiced conversation typically would be assigned as part of the homework. In preparation for the refusal training it also is helpful to review high-risk situations. This might entail referring back to the client's *Functional Analysis of Substance Using Behavior* interview as a starting point for identifying triggers, but there may be other risky situations as well. Although ideally the client would plan to avoid these situations, one cannot count on this strategy 100%.

In terms of actually teaching the client assertive refusal skills, CRA offers five basic options as a starting point: (a) saying, "No, thanks"… and accompanying this with strong, "no-nonsense" assertive body language; (b) suggesting alternatives (e.g., "No thanks. I'd love a strong cup of coffee though"); (c) changing the topic (e.g., "No, I don't want anything. Hey, I can't believe that the Bulls traded. …"); (d) "confronting" the aggressor (e.g., "I've told you three times that I don't want a beer. I'm curious; why is it so important for you to get me to drink?"); and (e) walking away. Repeated role-playing will help clients feel comfortable using these or other assertive responses.

Job Club

A client's job community is an important factor in his or her overall satisfaction, as it has valuable potential to provide reinforcement (e.g., earning an income, advancing in a career, offering opportunities for social interactions). Furthermore, a satisfying job can compete with substance use in a number of ways, such as providing a structured daily routine that obviously would be disrupted by alcohol or drug use. The main components of CRA's successful job acquisition are: (a) developing a resume; (b) generating job leads; (c) obtaining and completing job applications; (d) learning to make appropriate telephone inquiries and follow-up calls; and (e) rehearsing for job interviews. A full description of the job club procedures can be found in Azrin and Besalel (1980) and in Meyers and Smith (1995, pp. 121–126).

Relapse Prevention

Relapse prevention is really the focus of CRA from the start of treatment, as all CRA procedures are designed to promote relapse prevention. For example, functional analyses in the early stages of treatment identify triggers and high-risk situations, and skills training (communication, problem-solving, and social/recreational counseling) provides clients with the necessary resources to navigate potentially risky situations. In addition, CRA employs the *early warning system* as an adjunct to other relapse prevention methods. Those clients with families or close friends may find that these significant others can recognize the danger signs of substance use, such as frustration, boredom, or anger, long before the clients can themselves. CRA takes advantage of this dynamic by setting up the early warning system. The therapist helps the client and significant other to devise a specific plan for discussing and dealing with high-risk behavior when either party notices it. The plan will vary with each client and may involve problem-solving techniques that both parties have practiced, or in some cases, contacting the therapist to set up an emergency session. If a relapse does occur, a modified version of the *Functional Analysis for Substance Using Behavior* interview can be used to identify the specific events associated with this relapse, and that information can be incorporated into the treatment plan.

Social/Recreational Counseling

Social reinforcement can be one of the most rewarding aspects of a client's life. However, by the time most clients seek treatment, it is likely that the vast majority of their social or recreational activities and friendships center on or around drugs or alcohol. Because these relationships and activities are going to be strong triggers for relapse, it is essential to enhance the client's social life with healthy alternatives. Many clients have been immersed in a culture of drinking or drug use for a significant period of time, therefore they will feel stymied by the apparent lack of social opportunities that do not involve substance use. At this point, it is useful to employ such methods as a pro-social functional analysis to examine barriers to healthy social activities in which the client occasionally participates, or problem solving to help the client come up with alternatives to social substance use. The goal is to help the client find activities that are enjoyable and accessible enough to initially compete with using times, and eventually to replace using altogether.

Despite understanding the necessity of forming new social outlets, many clients will find it difficult to try something new, especially when sober. In these cases, systematic encouragement procedures may be warranted. Systematic encouragement is based on the idea that many clients will not possess either the knowledge or skills required to initiate new activities, and thus will need specific assistance. There are three major components of systematic encouragement. First, if clients are having trouble making the first contact on their own, they should make the call during the session after repeated rehearsals or role-plays. This should afford clients basic information about the activity in which they want to engage. The second component of systematic encouragement is to locate a contact person for the activity. Clients should make specific arrangements to meet this contact person at the event, preferably at the door before entering the room. The final step in systematic encouragement is to discuss the experience in the next session, including what the client did and did not like about the activity and any problems that came up. Problem solving can be used to address any obstacles or to find another activity to sample.

For group settings or when a substantial number of individual clients are involved, a social club is often a worthwhile endeavor (see Hunt & Azrin, 1973; Mallams et al., 1982; Smith et al., 1998). This can be especially valuable for clients who have become isolated because of their drinking/drug use and are nervous about participating in social events, or for clients who simply have not been sober at a social event in a long time. The CRA social club provides an opportunity for clients to practice social skills in a substance-free, nonthreatening environment before engaging in more stressful "real-life" situations. Ideally, the club would hold activities that compete with typical high-risk times, such as weekend nights. Other advantages of a social club are: (a) clients are more likely to attend a social club rather than church groups or AA because there are no specific religious tenets or treatment beliefs involved; (b) functions are typically low-cost or free, and are organized around the members' schedules; (c) therapists' presence at the functions provide clients with support and feedback in vivo, to complement the practice work done in treatment sessions; and (d) the club is designed to be a safe environment in which clients can become more comfortable with abstinence in social settings before moving on to more risky venues.

Relationship Therapy

If a substance user's partner is willing to come to sessions, it is often a good idea to include her or him in some portions of the treatment. Partners can learn effective ways to support the client, and the couple can also work toward improving their relationship. CRA's relationship therapy focuses on enhancing communication and problem-solving skills, setting mutually agreed-upon goals, and increasing pleasant interactions between the couple.

CRA's relationship therapy begins with the administration of the *Relationship Happiness Scale* (see Smith & Meyers, 2004, p. 39). A variation of the Happiness Scale mentioned earlier, the Relationship Happiness Scale measures individuals' happiness with their partner in 10 areas related to relationship functioning: household responsibilities, raising the children, social activities, money management, communication, sex and affection, job or school, emotional support, partner's independence, and general happiness. This instrument can be useful in highlighting areas on which the couple would like to work. The *Perfect Relationship Form* (see Meyers & Smith, 1995, pp. 174–176) is introduced next, as it is well suited for setting specific goals in the areas that the couple would like to address. Because experiencing early success in making positive changes in the relationship is useful for continued motivation, it is wise to choose areas that will lend themselves to relatively quick improvement. For instance, it is best to avoid "sex and affection" as an initial area within which to set goals, as it can be a particularly sensitive topic. Clients are asked to list behaviors they would like to see changed or modified in their partner in the area chosen. Like the Goals of Counseling, requests of partners should be brief, positive, specific, and measurable. Examples include the following.

Problematic goal: "I want my husband to stop complaining about everything in the world from the minute he walks through the door each night." (Neither positive nor specific)

Improved goal: "I would like my husband to give me a hug when he walks through the door each night and then tell me one positive thing that happened to him that day." (Positive, specific, measurable)

Communication skills training is a major part of couples' sessions. The format is virtually identical to those taught in the individual sessions (see Communication Skills Training section), except that the therapist obviously does not need to play the role of the partner as they practice the skills. Couples are encouraged to use these skills when formulating goals using the Perfect Relationship Form. For example, the therapist would teach the wife (mentioned above) how to ask her husband for the desired change in his after-work behavior in a very upbeat manner. The wife would practice incorporating elements of CRA's positive communication skills into her request. For example, the "improved goal" above could easily be turned into a request that uses several of CRA's positive communication elements by coaching the wife to say, "I know you're really tired when you get home from work (understanding statement), but I would absolutely love it (feeling statement) if you'd give me a quick hug and tell me something positive about your day. Is there anything I could do to make it easier for you to do that?"(offer to help). The therapist should ask the clients for feedback regarding how this new style of communication feels, while also offering the couple constructive criticism for how they might improve communication further. This exercise lends itself nicely to homework assignments wherein the couple practices these communication skills before the next session.

Couples in therapy often find that they do not have as many pleasant interactions with their partners as they had in the past. The *Daily Reminder to Be Nice* form (see Meyers & Smith, 1995, p. 179) can be introduced to increase the frequency of agreeable behaviors, such that the number of enjoyable interactions outweighs the number of negative interactions. This form has seven categories, which include: expressing appreciation for something the partner does, offering compliments, giving a pleasant surprise, visibly expressing affection, devoting complete attention to a pleasant conversation, initiating pleasant conversations, and offering to help. First, the couple should talk about examples of these various behaviors and should then make a commitment to do at least one of these behaviors every day. The therapist should check in on the couples' progress in increasing these behaviors and help troubleshoot any problems that arise. As the home atmosphere begins to change with the continued and even increased use of these "pleasantries," the couple is often more inclined to be ready to tackle some of the larger issues in their relationship.

Scientific Support for CRA

Reviews

A number of meta-analytic reviews specifically of the alcohol treatment outcome literature have been conducted over the past decade. In each review of over 30 intervention approaches, CRA was ranked in the top five (Finney & Monahan, 1996; Holder, Longabaugh, Miller, & Rubonis, 1991; Miller, Wilbourne, & Hettema, 2003; Miller et al., 1995). Although each of these reviews relied on somewhat different methodologies, the findings consistently suggested that CRA was one of the most effective treatments for alcohol use disorders available.

Inpatient Alcohol Trials

The first CRA studies, which were conducted with alcohol-dependent inpatients, revealed that CRA was superior to standard 12-step-based treatment protocols. In the first matched-pairs study (Hunt & Azrin, 1973), participants in the CRA condition were taught to identify and access nondrinking reinforcers, and were given job and social counseling. Patients in the CRA condition fared much better than those who participated in the hospital's standard Alcoholics Anonymous treatment. They spent significantly less time drinking and hospitalized, and spent more time employed and with their families. Improvements were still noted at 6-month follow-up. The second inpatient study again compared CRA to standard 12-step treatment, but also included a disulfiram component, an early warning system, and a buddy system in the CRA condition (Azrin, 1976). The results were similar to the original study: the CRA group showed significantly more improvement. At the 6-month follow up, CRA participants were drinking only 2% of the time, compared to 55% of the time for the AA group. It is important to note that these outcomes were maintained over two years.

Outpatient Alcohol Trials

Studies with outpatient alcohol-dependent participants echoed the results of inpatient studies. The first outpatient study (Azrin et al., 1982) randomly assigned participants to one of three conditions: the traditional group, which received 12-step counseling and a disulfiram prescription; the Antabuse Assurance group, which received 12-step counseling, a disulfiram prescription, and disulfiram compliance training; or the CRA + Antabuse Assurance group, which received CRA procedures, including disulfiram compliance training and sobriety sampling. The two Antabuse Assurance groups initially had the highest abstinence rates. After six months, the CRA + Antabuse Assurance group still had 97% abstinence, followed by the Antabuse Assurance group with 74%. The traditional group only had 45% abstinence. Miller et al. (2001) conducted an extension of this study with a much larger sample, taking into account eligibility for disulfiram. Although the results were not as robust as some of the earlier CRA studies, participants in CRA conditions still had an advantage over the participants in the traditional conditions on several variables.

In a relatively recent study by Smith, Meyers, and Delaney (1998), homeless individuals were assigned either to a CRA condition or to the homeless shelter's standard 12-step-based treatment. CRA procedures were modified to fit a group format. As expected, participants in the CRA condition significantly outperformed those in the standard treatment in terms of drinking outcomes for a period that included a 12-month follow-up.

Illicit Drug Studies

CRA is typically combined with contingency management programs (e.g., voucher programs) when used in treating cocaine and opiate dependence. Several studies have demonstrated the efficacy of CRA + voucher protocols (e.g., Bickel et al., 1997; Higgins et al., 1993, 1995). Another study (Abbott et al., 1998) found that CRA without a complementary voucher program still improved abstinence in methadone-maintained participants, compared to standard drug counseling procedures. An adolescent version of CRA (A-CRA) has been used recently with teens with problematic marijuana use. Both of the research projects found A-CRA to be highly promising both in terms of marijuana outcomes and cost-effectiveness ratings (Dennis et al., 2004; Godley, Godley, Dennis, Funk, & Passetti, 2002).

CRAFT: Treatment for the Family Members of Treatment-Refusing Substance Users

CRAFT Overview

CRAFT evolved out of the need for a method to work with family members of a treatment-refusing substance abuser. Substance-abuse treatment centers regularly receive calls from these desperate family members, and traditionally there were few options to offer these concerned significant others (CSOs). Most would have been referred to Al-Anon, the companion group to Alcoholics Anonymous, which stresses loving detachment from the drinker/drug user (Al-Anon Family Groups, 1984). Others would have been encouraged to confront the substance user (the identified patient; IP) in a Johnson Institute intervention "surprise party," wherein a group of loved ones gathers to explain how the substance user's behavior negatively affects each of them (Johnson, 1986). Not surprisingly, many CSOs were reluctant to engage in these options, either because they were unwilling to step aside, as directed by Al-Anon, or because they were uncomfortable with the harsh confrontational style of the Johnson Institute intervention.

The researchers who were involved in the development of CRA recognized this dilemma, and began testing a unique type of "family" therapy that was originally called *Community Reinforcement Training* (*CRT*) (Sisson & Azrin, 1986). They realized that CSOs could play an important role in getting resistant substance users into treatment. CSOs had already proven highly useful within the CRA program (e.g., as disulfiram monitors, partners in relationship therapy), and they tended to have extensive contact with the IP and were highly motivated to support positive changes in the IP's behavior. More support for working with CSOs came from the numerous testimonies of substance-abusing individuals that pressure from family and friends was a main reason they eventually sought treatment. Finally, the CRA researchers were concerned for the CSO's psychological health. Living with a substance-abusing individual is considered a chronic stressor. CSOs often experience depression, anxiety, and low self-esteem in response to the violence, constant arguing, financial problems, and disrupted family relationships commonly found in these situations. Consequently it was believed that the CSOs might benefit from behavior therapy themselves.

Now referred to as CRAFT, the program these researchers developed is an outgrowth of CRA. CRAFT is a comprehensive behavioral program that recognizes an individual's community as being instrumental in encouraging or discouraging substance use. Like CRA, CRAFT uses positive reinforcement and skills training as its basis. The difference is that in CRAFT, the CSO is the primary client. Because their IPs are not yet in treatment themselves, CRAFT teaches the CSOs how to rearrange contingencies in the IP's environment to reinforce sober behavior and discourage substance use. In doing so, most CSOs are able to reach their goals of getting their IP into treatment, and improving their own psychological well-being and their relationship with the IP.

Building Rapport and Increasing Motivation

As with most treatment approaches, establishing rapport and building trust with CSOs is a necessary foundation for effective treatment. It is important for therapists to allow the CSOs an adequate amount of time to express their frustration with the IP's substance use, and to assure them that their feelings are normal in light of a very difficult situation. And although CSOs need time to vent, it is essential to begin moving clients in a positive direction and increasing motivation for the CRAFT program.

Motivation for the CRAFT program can be increased in several ways. First, therapists should explain the success the CRAFT program has had in getting treatment-refusing substance-users to enter therapy (i.e., 64% to 86% successful; see the Scientific Support for CRAFT section). Second, the fact that most CRAFT-trained CSOs feel happier with their own lives regardless of the outcome with their IP should be stressed. Finally, the CSO's reasons for pursuing therapy in the first place should be reviewed, and a discussion should take place concerning how life for the CSO and the IP will change in a desirable way if the CSO's goals are achieved.

Functional Analyses

The functional analyses used in CRAFT are essentially the same as those used in CRA, but are modified so that the CSO rather than the IP provides the information (see Smith & Meyers, 2004, pp. 74–75). Antecedents (triggers) and consequences of the behavior, both positive and negative, are outlined in a series of columns, just as in CRA. But whereas in CRA the IPs can use the information laid out in the functional analysis to modify their own behavior to effect changes, in CRAFT the CSOs use this information to alter their reactions to the IPs' behavior to effect similar changes. By using the Functional Analysis for Substance Using Behavior to identify common triggers and patterns, CSOs can learn ways to tailor their actions on many different occasions (e.g., when they notice the immediate antecedents of substance use) to selectively reinforce positive healthy behavior and help eliminate negative behaviors.

For example, suppose a woman completes a functional analysis regarding her husband's drinking. Assume she notices both that arguments with the children about doing their chores (external trigger) often precedes a heavy drinking episode, and that her husband tends to drink when he is feeling frustrated with his job performance (internal trigger). She notes that on those days he comes home and immediately heads to the kitchen to grab a six-pack of beer, and then goes downstairs into the den, where he drinks alone for two or three hours. Figuring out the short-term positive consequences requires a bit of educated guesswork, but she thinks that being able to escape from the stress of work and relax by himself are key motivators for his drinking. She reports that she has heard him say, "I work really hard at a job where I'm not appreciated, so I deserve to relax and not worry about anything once I come home" (positive consequence).

As far as emotions, he has even told her that he feels progressively calmer as the evening passes (positive consequence). She identifies a number of negative consequences, including frequent arguments with his boss and with her, mid-week hangovers which make it harder for him to do his job, guilty feelings about yelling at the children, and fewer social outings.

At the conclusion of the functional analysis, it is important to show CSOs how they can use the information to help the IPs begin changing their behavior. In this example, the wife could problem-solve around the issue of the children arguing about doing their chores. She could also address the positive consequences of drinking by brainstorming other ways her husband might be able to relax, such as taking a walk together or reading a book. It is important to teach the CSOs communication skills as well, because they will need to be able to effectively reinforce positive behavior in their IPs. In this example, the wife might agree to take a walk with her husband every night after work to relax, but only if he is sober.

These early efforts to reduce the IP's substance use are important for several reasons. First, research has shown a correlation between a decrease in use and the IP's acceptance of treatment (Miller et al., 1999; Sisson & Azrin, 1986). Second, some IPs will never agree to enter treatment. In these cases, the CSOs have at the very least learned some effective procedures for reducing the IP's substance use. In presenting these options to CSOs, it is important to remind them that although even minor changes in their actions can help reshape their IP's behavior, it is the IP who is responsible for his or her own substance use. So although ideally the IP would be involved in treatment and would provide the information for the functional analysis, the next best thing is the involvement of a person who is in close contact and has much knowledge about the IP.

The *Functional Analysis for Enjoyable, Healthy Behavior* (See Smith & Meyers, 2004, p. 161) follows the same guidelines as those for substance-using behavior. It should be introduced in later sessions if CSOs are having difficulty coming up with a pleasurable social/recreational activity to sample, either with their IPs or by themselves.

Domestic Violence Precautions

Evidence suggests that there is a significant relationship between alcohol use and violent behavior (Collins, 1981; Greenfeld, 1998). Specifically, more than half of female partners of men seeking alcohol treatment report being physically victimized in the past year (Gondolf & Foster, 1991; Stith, Crossman, & Bischof, 1991). Although research has shown that it is important to take steps to remedy domestic violence situations, it also is essential that precautions be taken so as to secure the abused partner's safety. This is a particular concern for the CRAFT program, as much of it entails assisting CSOs to change their behavior toward the IP in a manner which the IP will perceive as unpleasant. Thus, all attempts must be made to minimize the chance that violent behavior will be directed toward the CSO. It is important to note that the empirical studies that support the efficacy of CRAFT excluded CSOs if ongoing severe domestic violence was reported. This decision to exclude some CSOs was due to concern that the CRAFT program might possibly exacerbate violent situations.

In an effort to reduce the chance that the CSO's new way of interacting with the IP will result in violence, the therapist must first assess any past or current violent behavior on the part of the IP. This can be done with the help of the *Conflict Tactics Scale* (Straus, 1979).

Additionally, a functional analysis of the violent behavior can help the CSO identify triggers that often result in violence. Once these triggers are identified, it may be possible for the CSO to devise new ways of interacting with the IP when these triggers are present, so as to diffuse the situation. Depending upon the severity of the violent behavior, a safety plan may be warranted wherein CSOs have a bag packed with essential items in case they need to leave home quickly. It is also important to encourage the CSO to solicit social supports, so that there are several people who can be involved in this safety plan if need be.

Positive Communication Training

Communication skills training may be especially helpful to couples in which one of the members has a substance-abuse problem. Nagging, defensiveness, and accusations may have become a routine part of conversation, to the detriment of the relationship. Communication skills training in CRAFT is similar to those taught in CRA; however, in this case only the CSO is present for the training. The same seven components of positive effective communication are introduced (see Communication Skills Training in CRA section), and rehearsed in role-plays.

Learning positive communication skills is a necessary precursor to implementing many of the other CRAFT procedures. For example, it will be important for the CSO to explain changes in behavior toward the IP in a manner that will mitigate defensiveness on the part of the IP. Some of these changes may seem aversive to the IP (e.g., not making up excuses for the boss when the IP is too hungover to go to work), and so it is very important that the CSO feel comfortable explaining these behaviors using positive communication skills. Certainly, practicing the best possible way to eventually invite the IP to attend treatment requires excellent communications skills as well. Beyond knowing how to talk about difficult topics with the IP, CRAFT's positive communication training also helps CSOs identify when to have these difficult conversations. For example, IPs may be less receptive to having a conversation when they are upset or stressed, and they should never be approached to discuss an important topic if they are high or hungover.

Use of Positive Reinforcement

CSOs can influence the IPs' behavior by modifying how they interact with them. CSOs may be skeptical of this assertion at first, because they feel that they have put an enormous amount of effort into getting the IP to stop drinking/using substances with little success. However, in all probability the CSOs have employed many "negative" techniques in this pursuit (e.g., nagging and pleading) and the attempts have been delivered both sporadically and without consistent follow-through. It may also be the case that the CSOs tried to have these difficult conversations when the IP was intoxicated or hung over. The therapist's job is to help CSOs carefully plan how they will reward sober behavior. Many CSOs initially balk at this idea because they feel as if they would be "enabling" their IP. Therefore, it needs to be made explicit that only the IP's sober behavior will be rewarded.

A positive reinforcer is something that increases the behavior it follows. The therapist should review this definition with the CSO and explain how the IP's substance use is positively reinforced in some way, which is part of the reason why the IP continues to drink or use drugs. The "Short Term Positive Consequences" section of the CRAFT Functional Analysis should be referenced at this time so that the CSO can review the pleasant thoughts and feelings the IP has as a result of using substances. The therapist and CSO should begin working on ways to help the IP access some of these same positive consequences when the IP is not using. As mentioned above, one of the goals of CRAFT is to attempt to modify the IP's environment, such that the IP can have a satisfying and rewarding life without the use of drugs or alcohol.

Once CSOs are on board with this rationale, they can begin devising a list of rewards to be given to the IP when sober. For the most part, rewards should be small and easy to deliver. For example, offering a compliment, making a special meal, or spending quality time together can all be helpful rewards. When a reward is given (e.g., watching a movie together), it may be useful for CSOs to verbally acknowledge why the reward is being given, as well as how much they enjoy spending time with the sober IP. For instance, a CSO might say, "I'm really having fun watching TV with you tonight. I love spending time with you when you're 'yourself'; when you're not high." As such, it is important to work with CSOs to be able to recognize when their IP has been drinking or using drugs. It is also important to discuss what kinds of nonusing behaviors should be rewarded.

Additionally, CSOs should begin sampling previously enjoyable or new, pleasant, sober social activities with the IP. These activities can compete with substance-using activities and will allow CSOs more chances to reward sober time spent together. It is possible that the IP may suspect that the CSO is "up to something" in introducing these new activities and behaviors. If this is the case, it may be warranted for the CSO to invite the IP to attend a session.

Allowing the Negative Consequences of the Substance Use to Occur

The CRAFT program encourages CSOs not only to provide positive reinforcement for clean/sober behavior, but also to allow the naturally occurring negative consequences of substance abuse to occur. It is not uncommon for good-intentioned CSOs to respond to the using behavior of the IP in ways that prevent the natural negative consequences of drinking/drug using from occurring, and as a result, to unintentionally support the IP's substance use. For example, a CSO might wake an intoxicated IP who has fallen asleep at the foot of the stairs and walk him to his bed.

In training CSOs how not to reward undesirable behaviors, the therapist must be careful to discuss the IP's potential reactions to the CSO's new behaviors. IPs sometimes respond with anger and criticism, and there is even a chance the IP may become violent. If violence is likely, it may be best to target changing the IP's behavior in a less risky situation. In any case, domestic violence precautions should be reviewed. In addition, although some new behaviors on the part of CSOs may not result in the IP experiencing severe negative consequences for abusing drugs, others may (e.g., refusing to pick up an inebriated IP, with the result that the IP drives home drunk). In weighing the pros and cons of allowing a particular negative consequence to occur, CSOs should decide if it is really safe and comfortable enough to do so in the specific situation. In some cases it may be appropriate for the CSOs to tell their IPs what they now intend to do in various situations in which the IP has been drinking or using drugs.

For those CSOs who decide to inform their IP of these changes in their behavior in advance, it is important to help the CSOs choose an appropriate time to do so, and to practice this conversation in a role-play.

Teaching CSOs How to Reward Themselves

As stated earlier, one objective of CRAFT involves improving the quality of CSOs' lives regardless of what happens to their IP. The frequent occurrence of depression and anxiety in CSOs may be due to the fact that living with a substance user makes CSOs vulnerable to assorted problems. These include legal issues, parenting problems, emotional and sexual relationship issues, financial problems, and domestic violence (Collins, Leonard, & Searles, 1990; Jacob, Krahn, & Leonard, 1991; O'Farrell & Birchler, 1987; Paolino & McCrady, 1977; Zweben, 1986).

The Happiness Scale and Goals of Counseling forms described in the CRA section of this chapter are used to help CSOs target different life areas in which they would like to make improvements. As many CSOs become isolated from social support systems as a result of dealing with their IP's drug or alcohol use, focusing on the "social life" category of the Happiness Scale may be particularly warranted. At the same time, it is important for CSOs to have the skills required to reach their goals, and therefore some skills training may be necessary. Furthermore, it is important to process the guilt that some CSOs experience at the prospect of working on their own happiness instead of focusing exclusively on the IPs' problems, and to help CSOs anticipate and plan for the reaction of the IP to these planned changes.

Getting the Substance User into Treatment

In terms of CRAFT's goal of getting a treatment-refusing IP to engage in treatment, it is worthwhile to review past unsuccessful CSO attempts. It is likely that these attempts were confrontational or threatening, and they may have occurred while the IP was under the influence. The therapist should emphasize that in contrast to these earlier ineffective methods, the CSO will now be using positive communication skills and critical timing. Furthermore, the groundwork will have been laid in other ways as well, because CSOs will already have altered their interactions with their IP in ways that support sobriety. This notable change in the CSOs' behavior is reflected in the fact that oftentimes IPs have already significantly reduced their alcohol or drug use by the time they agree to enter treatment.

It is likely that CSOs will be advocating for IP engagement into a cognitive-behavioral or behavioral treatment program, such as CRA. As IPs may be wary of beginning treatment, CSOs should encourage IPs to "sample" one or two treatment sessions before making a long-term commitment. IPs may be encouraged to hear from CSOs that programs such as CRA allow IPs to choose various life areas to work on and improve, rather than focusing solely on reducing substance-using behavior. CSOs might also ask IPs to enter treatment as a means by which to demonstrate their support for the CSOs' decision to address their own problems in therapy.

Determining when a CSO should ask an IP to sample treatment is also critical. Sometimes IPs will inquire as to why CSOs are acting differently toward them (e.g., using positive communication and reinforcement), and this may be an opportune time to describe the CRAFT program and invite IPs to attend a few sessions. In other cases, IPs may already know that their CSOs are in treatment and may express curiosity about what CSOs are doing during their sessions. When this happens, it is an ideal time for CSOs to ask IPs to find out for themselves by attending a session. Other CSOs wait until IPs are in the midst of dealing with very negative consequences of their drinking or drug use to extend the invitation. Regardless, CSOs should ask IPs to sample treatment only when they are sober and generally in good spirits. Despite perfect timing, IPs may refuse to enter treatment. It is important to prepare CSOs for this outcome, discuss its normality, and highlight the fact that it often takes several requests on the parts of CSOs before IPs agree to enter treatment.

Once IPs agree to enter treatment it is essential that the intake process begin quickly. In order to make sure treatment options are sufficiently lined up, therapists should help CSOs select one or two programs that will be available for immediate intakes. Because IPs probably will be ambivalent about entering treatment to begin with, it is important to increase the chance that they will follow through by making sure they can begin in a timely manner. CRAFT therapists should let CSOs know that even when IPs have entered therapy they will still need the help and support of CSOs. Couples therapy may be an appropriate option during this time. Finally, CSOs should be informed that IPs may terminate treatment early, but nevertheless they often return. If IPs do drop out of treatment, CSOs should continue to use the techniques they have learned throughout the CRAFT program in order to increase the likelihood that IPs will make further attempts to get professional help.

Scientific Support for CRAFT

Alcohol Treatment Studies

CRT, the earliest form of CRAFT, was originally tested by Sisson and Azrin (1986). In teaching the CSOs of treatment-refusing drinkers modified CRA procedures, it was believed the CSOs could, in turn, influence their IPs to enter treatment. CSOs in this study were assigned to one of two groups. Those in the traditional group (N = 5) were encouraged to attend Al-Anon meetings and were educated about the disease model of alcoholism. The CRT (CRAFT) group participants (N = 7) were trained in the basic CRAFT procedures. Although none of the CSOs in the 12-step-based traditional program were able to engage their IPs in treatment, six of the seven CSOs (86%) in the CRT group were able to do so. Treatment engagement among IPs in the CRT group occurred after approximately 7.2 CSO sessions. In addition, IPs of CSOs in the CRT group cut their average number of drinking days by more than half during the period when only the CSO was in treatment. Once the IPs actually entered treatment, their number of drinking days dropped even further. In contrast, IPs associated with the traditional group were drinking about the same amount three months into treatment as they had at baseline.

The second CRAFT alcohol study took place at the University of New Mexico's Center on Alcoholism, Substance Abuse, and Addictions (CASAA). This trial was funded by the National Institute on Alcohol Abuse and Alcoholism (NIAA), and involved 130 CSOs (Miller et al., 1999). This sample was primarily female (91%) and was composed of spouses (59%), parents

(30%), and romantic partners, children, or grandparents (11%) of the IPs. The sample mainly consisted of Anglo, non-Hispanic (53%), and Hispanic (39%) participants. Individuals generally were recruited via newspaper advertisements offering free treatment to the loved ones of treatment-refusing individuals with alcohol problems. Eligible CSOs were randomly assigned to one of three conditions: Al-Anon Facilitation Therapy (Al-Anon FT), the Johnson Institute intervention, or CRAFT. Al-Anon FT was an individual therapy version of Al-Anon that was modeled after the 12-step facilitation modality used in Project MATCH (Nowinski, Baker, & Carroll, 1992). The Johnson Institute intervention trained CSOs to hold confrontational surprise meetings with the IP. All conditions offered participants 12 therapy hours.

IPs were said to have engaged in treatment if they completed the assessment battery and scheduled a therapy session within six months of the CSO's own intake. Rates of engagement for CSOs in CRAFT (64%) were significantly higher than those of CSOs in the Johnson Institute intervention (30%) and the Al-Anon FT (13%) conditions. Furthermore, CRAFT CSOs were able to engage their IPs after an average of less than five CSO sessions. As described in earlier research (Liepman, Nirenberg, & Begin, 1989), CSOs who actually delivered the Johnson Institute intervention were quite successful (75%) at engaging their IPs. However, 70% of the CSOs in this condition dropped out prior to the surprise party session, reporting that it was uncomfortably confrontational. Parents engaged their IPs at significantly higher rates (51%) than spouses (32%) across all three conditions. For all treatments, CSOs' own psychological functioning improved, as anger and depression decreased. In addition, the CSO/IP relationship improved and family conflict decreased as family cohesion and overall relationship happiness increased. These changes were not dependent upon whether the CSO's IP entered treatment.

Drug Treatment Studies

Research has demonstrated that CRAFT also successfully engages treatment-refusing illicit drug users (Kirby et al., 1999; Meyers et al., 1999, 2002). An uncontrolled pilot study achieved a 74% engagement rate among 62 culturally diverse CSOs (Meyers et al., 1999). In a controlled study by Kirby and colleagues, CRT (CRAFT) had significantly higher engagement rates (64%) than a 12-step intervention (17%) among its 32 CSOs. A randomized trial conducted by Meyers and colleagues assigned 90 CSOs of treatment-refusing illicit drug users to CRAFT, CRAFT plus an aftercare group, or Al-Anon/Nar-Anon Facilitation Therapy (Al-Anon FT; Meyers et al., 2002). The CRAFT aftercare sessions did not significantly improve outcomes that were achieved by CRAFT alone. Engagement rates for the combined CRAFT conditions (67%) were significantly higher than that for Al-Anon FT (29%). As with the research done among alcohol users, CSO's psychosocial functioning improved independent of their treatment condition and whether their IPs entered treatment. Once IPs did enter treatment they tended to average about eight sessions.

References

Abbott, P., Weller, S., & Delaney, H. D. (1998). Community reinforcement approach in the treatment of opiate addicts. *American Journal of Drug and Alcohol Abuse, 24,* 17–30.

Al-Anon Family Groups (1984). *Al-anon faces alcoholism.* New York: Author.

Azrin, N.H. (1976). Improvements in the community reinforcement approach to alcoholism. *Behavioral Research and Therapy, 14,* 339–348.

Azrin, N. H. & Besalel, V. A. (1980). *Job club counselor's manual.* Baltimore: University Press.

Azrin, N. H., Sisson, R. W., Meyers, R., & Godley, M. (1982). Alcoholism treatment by disulfiram and community reinforcement therapy. *Journal of Behavior Therapy and Experimental Psychiatry, 13,* 105–112.

Bickel, W. K., Amass, L., Higgins, S. T., Badger, G. J., & Esch, R. A. (1997). Effects of adding behavioral treatment to opioid detoxification with buprenorphine. *Journal of Consulting and Clinical Psychology, 65,* 803–810.

Collins, J. J., Jr. (1981). Alcohol use and criminal behavior: An empirical, theoretical, and methodological overview. In J. J. Collins, Jr. (Ed.), *Drinking and crime: Perspectives on the relationships between alcohol consumption and criminal behavior.* New York: Guilford Press.

Collins, R. L., Leonard, K., & Searles, J. (Eds.). (1990). *Alcohol and the family.* New York: Guilford Press.

Dennis, M. L., Godley, S. H., Diamond, G. S., Tims, F. M., Babor, T., Donaldson, J., et al. (2004). Cannabis Youth Treatment (CYT) Study: Main findings from two randomized trials. *Journal of Substance Abuse Treatment, 27,* 197–213.

D'Zurilla, T., & Goldfried, M. (1971). Problem solving and behavior modification. *Journal of Abnormal Psychology, 78,* 107–126.

Finney, J. W., & Monahan, S. C. (1996). The cost-effectiveness of treatment for alcoholism: A second approximation. *Journal of Studies on Alcohol, 57,* 229–243.

Godley, M. D., Godley, S. H., Dennis, M. L., Funk, R. R., & Passetti, L. L. (2002). Preliminary outcomes from the assertive continuing care experiment for adolescents discharged from residential treatment. *Journal of Substance Abuse Treatment, 23,* 21–32.

Gondolf, E. W., & Foster, R. A. (1991). Wife assault among VA alcohol rehabilitation patients. *Hospital and Community Psychiatry, 42,* 74–79.

Greenfeld, L.A. (1998). *Alcohol and crime: An analysis of national data on the prevalence of alcohol involvement in crime.* Report prepared for Assistant Attorney General's National Symposium on Alcohol Abuse and Crime. Washington, DC: U.S. Department of Justice.

Higgins, S. T., Budney, A. J., Bickel, W. K., Hughes, J. R., Foerg, F., & Badger, G. (1993). Achieving cocaine abstinence with a behavioral approach. *American Journal of Psychiatry, 150,* 763–769.

Higgins, S. T., Budney, A. J., Bickel, W. K., Badger, G., Foerg, F., & Ogelen, D. (1995). Outpatient behavioral treatment for cocaine dependence: One-year outcome. *Experimental and Clinical Psychopharmacology, 3,* 205–212.

Holder, H., Longabaugh, R., Miller, W. R., & Rubonis, A. V. (1991). The cost-effectiveness of treatment for alcoholism: A first approximation. *Journal of Studies on Alcohol, 52,* 517–540.

Hunt, G. M., & Azrin, N. H. (1973). A community-reinforcement approach to alcoholism. *Behavioral Research and Therapy, 11,* 91–104.

Jacob, T., Krahn, G. L., & Leonard, K. (1991). Parent–child interactions in families with alcoholic fathers. *Journal of Consulting and Clinical Psychology, 59,* 176–181.

Johnson, V. E. (1986). *Intervention: How to help those that don't want help.* Minneapolis, MN: Johnson Institute.

Kirby, K. C., Marlowe, D. B., Festinger, D. S., Garvey, K. A., & LaMonaca, V. (1999). Community reinforcement training for family and significant others of drug abusers: A unilateral intervention to increase treatment entry of drug users. *Drug and Alcohol Dependence, 56,* 85–96.

Liepman, M. R., Nirenberg, T. D., & Begin, A. M. (1989). Evaluation of a program designed to help family and significant others to motivate resistant alcoholics into recovery. *American Journal of Drug and Alcohol Abuse, 15,* 209–221.

Mallams, J. H., Godley, M. D., Hall, G. M., & Meyers, R. J. (1982). Social-systems approach to resocializing alcoholics in the community. *Journal of Studies on Alcohol, 43,* 1115–1123.

McCrady, B. S., Horvath, A. T., & Delaney, S. I. (2003). Self-help groups. In R. K. Hester & W. R. Miller (Eds.), *Handbook of alcoholism treatment approaches: Effective alternatives* (3rd ed., pp. 165–187). Boston: Allyn & Bacon.

Meyers, R. J., Miller, W. R., Hill, D. E., & Tonigan, J. S. (1999). Community Reinforcement and Family Training (CRAFT): Engaging unmotivated drug users into treatment. *Journal of Substance Abuse, 10,* 1–18.

Meyers, R. J., Miller, W. R., Smith, J. E., & Tonigan, J. S. (2002). A randomized trial of two methods for engaging treatment-refusing drug users through concerned significant others. *Journal of Consulting and Clinical Psychology, 70,* 1182–1185.

Meyers, R. J., & Smith, J. E. (1995). *Clinical guide to alcohol treatment: The community reinforcement approach.* New York: Guilford Press.

Meyers, R. J., & Wolfe, B. L. (2004). *Get your loved one sober: Alternatives to nagging, pleading, and threatening.* Center City, Minnesota: Hazelden Press.

Miller, W. R., Brown, J. M., Simpson, T. L., Handmaker, N. S., Bien, T. H., Luckie, L. F., et al., (1995). What works? A methodological analysis of the alcohol treatment outcome literature. In R. K. Hester & W. R. Miller (Eds.), *Handbook of alcoholism treatment approaches: Effective alternatives* (2nd ed., pp. 12–44). Boston: Allyn & Bacon.

Miller, W. R., & Hester, R. K. (2003). Treating alcohol problems: Toward an informed eclecticism. In R. K. Hester & W. R. Miller (Eds.), *Handbook of alcoholism treatment approaches: Effective alternatives* (3rd ed., pp. 1–12). Boston: Allyn & Bacon.

Miller, W. R., Meyers, R. J., & Tonigan, J. S. (1999). Engaging the unmotivated in treatment for alcohol problems: A comparison of three strategies for intervention through family members. *Journal of Consulting and Clinical Psychology, 67,* 688–697.

Miller, W. R., Meyers, R. J., Tonigan, J. S., & Grant, K. A. (2001). Community reinforcement and traditional approaches: Findings of a controlled trial. In R. J. Meyers & W. R. Miller (Eds.), *A community reinforcement approach to addiction treatment* (pp. 79–103). London: Cambridge University Press.

Miller, W. R., Wilbourne, P. L., & Hettema, J. E. (2003). What works? A summary of alcohol treatment outcome research. In R. K. Hester & W. R. Miller (Eds.), *Handbook of alcoholism treatment approaches: Effective alternatives* (3rd ed., pp. 13–63). Boston: Allyn & Bacon.

Nowinski, J., Baker, S., & Carroll, K. (1992). *12-step facilitations therapist manual: A clinical research guide for therapists treating individuals with alcohol abuse and dependence* (Vol. 1, Project MATCH Monograph Series). Rockville, MD: National Institute on Alcohol Abuse and Alcoholism.

O'Farrell, T. J., & Birchler, G. R. (1987). Marital relationships of alcoholic, conflicted, and nonconflicted couples. *Journal of Marital and Family Therapy, 13,* 259–274.

Paolino, T. J., & McCrady, B. S. (1977). *The alcoholic marriage: Alternative perspectives.* New York: Grune and Stratton.

Sisson, R.W., & Azrin, N. (1986). Family-member involvement to initiate and promote treatment of problem drinkers. *Journal of Behavioral Therapy and Experimental Psychiatry, 17,* 15–21.

Smith, J. E., & Meyers, R. J. (2001). The treatment. In R. J. Meyers & W. R. Miller (Eds.), *A community reinforcement approach to addiction treatment* (pp. 28–61). London: Cambridge University Press.

Smith, J. E., & Meyers, R. J. (2004). *Motivating substance abusers to enter treatment: Working with family members.* New York: Guilford Press.

Smith, J. E., Meyers, R. J., & Delaney, H. D. (1998). The Community Reinforcement Approach with homeless alcohol-dependent individuals. *Journal of Consulting and Clinical Psychology, 66,* 541–548.

Smith, J. E., Meyers, R. J., & Miller, W. R. (2001). The Community Reinforcement Approach to the treatment of substance use disorders. *The American Journal of Addictions, 10* (Suppl.), 51–59.

Stith, S. M., Crossman, R. K., & Bischof, G. P. (1991). Alcoholism and marital violence: A comparative study of men in alcohol treatment programs. *Alcoholism Treatment Quarterly, 8,* 3–20.

Straus, M. A. (1979). Measuring intrafamily conflict and violence: The Conflict Tactics (CT) Scales. *Journal of Marriage and the Family, 41,* 75–88.

Zweben, A. (1986). Problem drinking and marital adjustment. *Journal of Studies on Alcohol, 47,* 167–172.

11

Prevention Science

Lori K. Holleran Steiker, Jeremy T. Goldbach, Dean Sagun, and Laura M. Hopson

The University of Texas at Austin School of Social Work

Justin M. Laird

Columbia University

Contents

Prevention is an important element in the continuum of care for substance abuse. Therefore, significant time has been spent developing and implementing various prevention programs, as well as monitoring their effectiveness. Most programs are targeted at children and adolescents, as this is the time when most people initiate use of alcohol and other drugs (AODS).

Readily understood is the fact that there is no need to treat something that has never occurred. However, examining the prevalence of use can help frame the urgency for these strategies. Prevalence data represent the extent of a condition in a population and this helps to assess the need for intervention (Friis & Sellers, 1999). This is not to be confused with incidence, which is the number of new cases in a population over time.

Each year, numerous studies are conducted in order to determine the prevalence of substance use across the United States. Each of these works to determine trends in drug use, and helps identify specific prevention targets, particularly in adolescents. *Monitoring the Future* (MTF) is a study conducted by the University of Michigan (Johnston, O'Malley, Bachman, & Schulenberg, 2007), and is funded by the National Institute on Drug Abuse (NIDA). Because it has been conducted annually since 1975, it reveals trends in use over time. Table 11.1 outlines trends regarding respondents' use in the last 30 days, and can be generalized to a national average.

The MTF data (Johnston, O'Malley, Bachman, & Schulenberg, 2006) are useful for understanding the effectiveness of generalized and specific prevention programs. The high rates at which students report using substances, especially alcohol, point to a need for prevention strategies. Prevention programs can be helpful for youth by preventing use altogether, delaying the onset of use, and, among those who are already using substances, reducing the frequency and quantity of use and preventing the use of progressively more harmful and addictive substances.

It has long been recognized that research on age of initiation (i.e., at first use) has shown that later onset can help lessen substance-related consequences (Gonzales, 1983). Gonzales found that students who had their first use of alcohol in high school or college had substantially lower alcohol-related problems than those who began using earlier, such as in middle or elementary school. This finding is not limited solely to alcohol use. Hawkins, Catalano, and Miller (1992) also found that age of first use is a predictor of further drug-related problems encountered by adolescents, regardless of the substance that was used. Many in the substance

TABLE 11.1
Prevalence of 30-Day Use, Percentages

	Year	8th Graders	10th Graders	12th Graders
Marijuana	2004	6.4	15.9	19.9
	2005	6.6	15.2	19.8
	2006	6.5	14.2	18.3
Alcohol	2004	18.6	35.2	48.0
	2005	17.1	33.2	47.0
	2006	17.2	33.8	45.3
Other Illicit	2004	4.1	6.9	10.8
	2005	4.1	6.4	10.3
Drugs	2006	3.8	6.3	9.8

Source. Adapted from Johnston, L. D., O'Malley, P. M., Bachman, J. G., & Schulenberg, J. E. Teen Drug Use Continues Down in 2006, Particularly Among Older Teens; But Use of Prescription-Type Drugs Remains High. Ann Arbor: University of Michigan News and Information Services, December 21, 2006.

abuse treatment field maintain that this is due to the fact that once an adolescent experiences substance use as a coping mechanism, other important social and problem-solving skills are either not learned or fall by the wayside. Although there is agreement about the importance of delaying onset of first use, there is no consensus on the best strategy for prevention.

History of Substance Prevention

Law of Prevention in the United States

In the early twentieth century, alcohol use was common because it was regarded primarily as a benign, joy-invoking substance with health benefits and even preventative powers (Miller, Beckles, Maude, & Carson, 1990). Despite two temperance movements in the 1800s, alcohol-related problems received little significant attention. In 1920, Congress added the Eighteenth Amendment and the Volstead Act in an attempt to outlaw alcohol use definitively. However, this Prohibition led to social unrest and Congress repealed the Eighteenth Amendment in 1933.

In the 1960s, the increase in alcohol consumption coupled with the use of illegal drugs garnered the attention of the public and government officials. New information was available on the nature, magnitude, and incidence of alcohol and other problems, raising public awareness. A decade later, the 1970 Controlled Substances Act noted that drugs are classified according to their medical use, their potential for abuse, and their likelihood of producing dependence. The increase in awareness culminated with the creation of the National Institute on Alcohol Abuse and Alcoholism (NIAAA) in 1970 and the NIDA in 1974. Both of these government agencies introduced prevention components to national programs that, up until that point, primarily concentrated on treatment.

Slowly, prevention came to be recognized as a multifaceted and viable option in the battle against substance abuse. The Anti-Drug Abuse Act of 1986 led to the creation of the United States Office for Substance Abuse Prevention (OSAP), which consolidated AOD activities under the Alcohol, Drug Abuse, and Mental Health Administration (ADAMHA). The ADAMHA block grant mandated that 20% of alcohol and drug funds be utilized for prevention, and the remaining 80% be appropriated for treatment services. Six years later in 1992, OSAP transformed into the Center for Substance Abuse Prevention (CSAP), part of the newly founded Substance Abuse and Mental Health Services Administration (SAMHSA).

History of Prevention as a Science

Historically, prevention strategies have focused strictly on education and early intervention. The 1920s through the 1950s was a time of scare tactics and the first media campaigns. *Reefer Madness*, a movie about a group of teenagers who use marijuana and go insane, typifies this trend. Nationally the belief was that drugs were a problem of low-income areas, used to escape pain and avoid reality. In the 1960s, there was a shift in national perspective. Although still used to escape pain, there was a new emphasis on the psychedelic experience. In the late 1960s, prevention scientists introduced a new educational model which consisted of drug information, affective education, and alternatives to drug use (Hogan, Gabrielsen, Luna, & Grothaus, 2003).

These approaches assumed that once adults make adolescents aware of the health hazards of substances and reinforce attitudes, they will develop anti-drug attitudes and subsequently make choices not to use. Scared Straight became a popular intervention where youth were exposed to the potential legal consequences of continued and escalated drug use (Petrosino, Turpin-Petrosino, & Buehler, 2005).

In many of these programs, education alone was intended to inform society about the ills of drugs and alcohol and they attempted to teach people about the early warning signs so that they might initiate treatment as soon as possible (Hogan et. al, 2003). Such information-only prevention programs have failed to produce a reduction in adolescent drug use and in some cases increased use after implementation (Clayton, Leukefeld, Harrington, & Cattarello, 1996; Harmon, 1993). One such program, the Drug Abuse Resistance Education (DARE), is the most popular and prevalent program with over three million participants in the United States. Not only has DARE failed to reduce drug use, but in a number of cases, researchers have noted a subsequent increase in participant substance abuse (Clayton et al., 1996; Harmon, 1993; Lynam, 1999).

With time, information provision models such as DARE (Becker, Agopian, & Yeh, 1992; Clayton et al., 1996; Harmon, 1993; Lynum, 1999; Ringwalt, Ennett, & Holt, 1991) and Health Belief Models (Albert & Simpson, 1985) evolved into more complex Social Influence models including Life Skills Training (Botvin, Baker, Dusenbury, Tortu, & Botvin, 1990; Botvin, Baker, & Dusenbury, 1995) and the Social Competence Program (Caplan et al., 1992) as well as Drug Resistance Strategies Training such as Project SMART (Hansen et al., 1988), Project ALERT (Ellickson & Bell, 1990; Ellikson, Bell, & McGuigan, 1993), and DRS (Hecht et al., 2003).

The 1980s prevention curricula were focused on communication, decision making, and self-esteem building. The focus on effective education and alternatives to drug use became popular. In these years, Project Adolescent Experiences in Resistance Training (ALERT) began. Also in the 1980s, parent groups such as Mothers Against Drunk Drivers (MADD) began to form in order to combat drug abuse. Family interventions also became popular, such as Brief Strategic Family Therapy (BSFT). It is important to note that during the late 1980s a shift in perception became apparent. Society began to view substance abuse and drug use as highly complex, and a new understanding of the disorder became evident. As the 1990s and new millennium approached, the research-based curriculum became more common and peer-based programs also grew. One strong research-supported program that grew out of these interventions is Karol Kumpfer's Strengthening Families program. This program has a strong evidence base and has been culturally adapted for unique groups as well (Kumpfer, Molgaard, & Spoth, 1996).

Although the educational, information-based programs have generally been found to be ineffective, social influence models have been identified as best practice prevention programs by NIDA and CSAP. Meta-analyses of resistance skills training programs also support their effectiveness (Tobler & Stratton, 1997). Today, replication and application of evidence-based models are prevalent in the field of substance abuse prevention and treatment. These attempts tend to be cross-disciplinary, with aspects being explored by social workers, psychologists, nurses, sociologists, and mental health agencies.

Current trends show the gap between research and application is being bridged. Technology transfer is becoming more important and evidence-based interventions are becoming standard. Drug Resistance Strategies training, such as Keepin' it REAL, are also examining the importance of culturally grounded interventions on effectiveness (Holleran & Hopson, 2007).

Classifications of Prevention

Institute of Medicine (IOM) Classification System

In 1994, the IOM created a new framework for classifying strategies in prevention. This was based on a pre-existing classification of disease prevention already in use by the NIDA. In this proposal, prevention was divided into three types: universal, selective, and indicated. All prevention strategies can be categorized based on the population they serve.

Universal Prevention Strategies   These programs address an entire population (country, state, community, school, or neighborhood). The goal is to deter use of substances by providing each member of the community with information and skills to prevent the problem. There is no prescreening for risk in a universal strategy. The entire population is determined to be at risk, and therefore able to benefit from the program. Although this is the primary mode of intervention in school-based prevention, there is some concern that universal interventions miss the youth that may need it most due to their tendency to be marginal, absent, or already engaged in substance use or abuse.

Selective Prevention Strategies   These programs are designed to target specific at-risk subsets of the general population. Risk groups may be identified on the basis of biological, psychological, social, or environmental risk factors known to be associated with substance abuse. These are groups that are determined to be at higher risk for substance abuse due to determinants such as students who are doing poorly academically, incarcerated youth, children who are abused, and children of alcoholics and addicts (Hawkins et al., 1992).

The selective prevention program is administered to members of the subgroup who are deemed to be at higher risk for substance use than others. A selective prevention program would be appropriate for a neighborhood that has a high incidence of admissions for drug treatment, for example, because youth living in this neighborhood may have a higher risk of drug involvement than those in the general population.

Indicated Prevention Strategies   These programs are the most specific in their target. They are administered directly to individuals who have shown themselves to be at high risk for substance abuse based on behaviors. An example would be a juvenile who drops out of school or is caught by the police with marijuana. It is important to recognize that non-drug-related behaviors also create heightened risk for the individual. The mission of the indicated prevention program is to target individuals who are at a subclinical level, but are exhibiting substance abuselike behavior or are initiating problematic use patterns. Specific family counseling or drug education to a habitually truant teenager are examples of indicated strategies.

Classification by Strategy

The CSAP and the SAMHSA created another method of classifying prevention strategies. Because any of the following six methods can be utilized in conjunction with universal, selective, or indicated populations, this model is not in conflict with the IOM system.

Information Dissemination   This strategy provides an awareness and understanding of the nature of substance use, abuse, and addiction. It gives information on the effects of misuse on the individual, the family, and the community. It also informs the target of available community resources for prevention and treatment. In this strategy, there is limited communication between the source and the audience. When used alone, information dissemination has not been shown to be effective prevention.

Education   In this strategy, there is communication between the source and the audience. It is characterized by this communication, and the involvement of the participants is the basis of the intervention. The activities involved are skill building in areas such as decision making, assertiveness, and critical thinking. Recently, in early prevention interventions, educating youth about their brain chemistry and the potential dangers of drugs to their brains have shown promise (Padget, Bell, Shamblen, & Ringwalt, 2006).

Alternatives   This strategy engages the participant in alternative activities to drugs and alcohol. The belief is that by providing a healthy outlet for activities that are not compatible with the use of substances, a reduction in use will occur. Although this method has not been proven effective alone, it is an important component for the relief of boredom (a common assumption as to the cause of youth substance use).

Problem Identification and Referral   In this strategy, individuals are identified who have already engaged in the use of tobacco, alcohol, or other substances. The goal is to utilize education in order to change the participants' previously held beliefs about substances, therefore changing behavior. This is an important component of any prevention program, especially those designed for and implemented in community settings with high-risk youth.

Community-based Process   In this strategy, communities are organized in order to more effectively provide prevention services, as well as substance abuse treatment services for their members. This strategy may encourage community mobilization through coalition building, networking, and interagency agreements among other community-based practices. Participatory Action Research (PAR) is a promising approach for actively collaborating with community members in implementing prevention strategies. This approach is helpful for ensuring that a prevention program incorporates the culture and learning styles of participants (Gosin, Dustman, Drapeau, & Harthun, 2003; Hopson, 2006).

Although PAR has been used as a label for many studies with varying levels of researcher–community member collaboration, the goal of PAR is to achieve active collaboration at every phase of the research including defining goals and methods, gathering and analyzing data, and implementing a change process (Kidd & Kral, 2005). The researcher takes on the role of consultant and lends expertise on methods and theoretical foundations rather than directing the entire research process (Gosin et al., 2003). PAR methods have the advantage of building the capacity among participants to implement and evaluate prevention strategies to meet their own needs (Hughes, 2003).

PAR methods that may be useful in implementing prevention strategies include:

- Interviewing youth about their life experiences, substance use, and strategies for resisting drug use
- Conducting focus groups with youth and staff in schools or community agencies to explore substances that are problematic in their community, patterns of substance use, and previous attempts to address the problem
- Engaging youth in creating or adapting a prevention program
- Collaborating with staff and youth in determining methods for an evaluation of a prevention program
- Maintaining ongoing communication and consultation among researchers, program implementers, and youth
- Obtaining feedback from staff and youth about a prevention program (Hopson, 2006; & Hopson & Holleran Steiker, 2008)

Environmental This strategy involves the establishment or changing of policy, written laws, codes, and standards. It also involves the unwritten codes of conduct and attitudes that the community promotes regarding substance use. The goal is to influence incidence of substance abuse through a change in community attitude. An example may be banning billboards that advertize (and glamorize) the use of cigarettes by young people.

Model of Risk and Resiliency

Data and statistics can provide us with trends in substance use and misuse, however, they do not provide a clear explanation for the factors that influence its occurrence. They also do not provide us with implementation techniques for the previously defined strategies. Social science researchers have worked to provide a better understanding of what factors increase risk (risk factors), and those that encourage resistance (protective factors) to substance abuse. In this prevention model, the risk factors of each community are assessed, and a prevention intervention is designed to reduce these risks while utilizing and fostering protective factors that are present (Hawkins et al., 1992).

Risk and protective factors can be organized by the following domains: individual, peer relational, family, school, or by community influence. Factors can be either a risk or protective. For example, intelligence (specifically, the ability to problem solve) is a protective factor to substance abuse. Conversely, low intelligence (or a low problem-solving ability) may result in social disconnectedness, which is a risk factor. Familial influences include abuse, conflict, and substance abuse history. Alternatively, parental substance resistance role-modeling and positive family communications are protective. The ability to achieve academically and engage with peers in school positively are examples of school protective factors, whereas poor grades and negative school behaviors such as fighting or learning disabilities may result in risk. Finally, each community holds different beliefs about the use of substances and alcohol, and community bylaws and norms can affect individual decision making.

Research on risk and protective factors, however, has been hindered by small sample sizes and inadequate validation studies (Ellickson, 1999). When studies do have a large enough national sample, background characteristics (e.g., education, family structure, region, etc.) do not account for most of the racial/ethnic or SES differences found in drug use (Wallace & Bachman, 1991).

Harm-Reduction Debate

Many substance abuse counselors, social workers, psychologists, politicians, and other professionals believe the goal of prevention should be solely to promote abstinence. Abstinence refers to general prohibition against use of any drug by an individual. Other professionals believe that the goal should be the reduction of suffering, and long-term consequences. This alternative approach has been labeled a *harm-reduction* approach (Marlatt, 1996). Potentially, there are settings such as schools, for which non-abstinence-based prevention messages are not accepted. Parents, teachers, and school administrators often fear that exposure to harm-reduction methods would come across as drug and alcohol promotion (Dodge, Dishion, & Lansford, 2006).

Harm-reduction programs emphasize the identification and reduction of harmful consequences related to the use of alcohol, tobacco, and other drug use rather than only focusing on abstinence. Harm-reduction models are not mutually exclusive of abstinence-based models. From a harm-reduction perspective, abstinence is viewed as the ideal way to minimize harm from personal use of substances, but pragmatically this ideal goal may be unrealistic for many individuals. Harm-reduction models typically encourage abstinence but acknowledge that some patterns of substance use and associated behaviors are more harmful than others (Beyers, Toumbourou, Catalano, Arthur, & Hawkins, 2004).

Despite common resistance to non-abstinence-based interventions, for many youth, a harm-reduction approach to prevention may be more developmentally and culturally appropriate than an abstinence-based curriculum. Youth who have begun to experiment with substances know from experience that drug use does not always result in the dire consequences presented in many abstinence-based prevention programs. These curricula have little credibility for youth who are already using drugs because their experiences are more likely to tell them that drug use improves concentration or relieves anxiety (MacMaster, Holleran, & Chaffin, 2005; Newcomb, Chou, Bentler, & Huba, 1988). Literature suggests that some experimentation with drugs is considered normal for the developmental stage of adolescence (MacMaster & Holleran, 2005; Shedler & Block, 1990). For youth who are experimenting with drugs, harm-reduction models are likely to more accurately reflect their goals and life experiences than abstinence-based models (Neighbors, Dillard, Lewis, Bergstrom, & Neil, 2006).

Any discussion of harm reduction must acknowledge the difficulty of implementing such programs. In the United States, harm-reduction models are politically unpopular and are unlikely to be implemented in schools and community-based organizations (Beyers, Toumbourou, Catalano, Arthur, & Hawkins, 2004). Because substance use is illegal, any program that normalizes substance use is likely to be received with strong opposition (Hopson, 2006). It may be necessary to explore new creative ways of integrating harm-reduction and abstinence messages so that a curriculum can emphasize abstinence while acknowledging the extent to which youth experiment with substances (Hopson, 2006; MacMaster et al., 2005).

Ethnicity, Culture, and Prevention

Conceptualizing Culture

The word *culture* implies the established patterns of human behavior that include thoughts, communications, actions, customs, beliefs, values, and institutions of racial, ethnic, religious, or social groups (National Association of Clinicians, 2001). In the United States, culture has mainly been associated with race and ethnicity, but diversity is taking on a more expansive meaning to include the sociocultural experiences of people. This can include differences in gender, social class, religion and spiritual beliefs, sexual orientation, age, and physical and mental ability. This can also include noting the uniqueness of cultural settings such as 12-step programs (see MacMaster & Holleran, 2005, alternative schools (Hopson, 2006; Hopson & Holleran Steiker, 2008), juvenile justice settings (Garland, 2001), low-income housing (MacLoed, 2004), and centers for LGBTQ youth (Welle, 2003).

Most drug prevention programs are created by and for European-Americans and tested primarily on this Anglo ethnic group. In addition, most community-based drug prevention programs have focused on primarily white communities or ones that represent primarily one ethnic group (Pentz, Rothspan, Skara, & Voskanian, 1999). It has been suggested that the failure of some prevention programs can be traced to their lack of cultural sensitivity (Hansen, Miller, & Leukefeld, 1995; Palinkas, Atkins, Jerreira, & Miller, 1996). Current findings indicate that tailoring an intervention to a target population can increase its effectiveness (Marsiglia, Holleran, & Jackson, 2000). Recently, there has been a shift to ethnically sensitive programs (Botvin et al., 1995; Galan, 1988; Griswold-Ezekoye, Kumpfer, & Bukoski, 1986; Schinke et al., 1985, 1988), based on the argument that cultural sensitivity enhances prevention efforts and that ethnic matching maximizes program impact (Botvin et al., 1995). However, "culture" and "ethnicity" have been defined in various ways, and at times the constructs are problematic. For example, many studies approach ethnicity in a "glossed" fashion, which denies the heterogeneity within groups and other contextual factors (Collins, 1995; Trimble, 1995). Definitions have often ignored the issue of acculturation (Koss-Chioino & Vargas, 1999).

In addition, although ethnic variables are important considerations, it is also important to not make the assumption that ethnicity equates with risk (Pentz et al., 1999). In most cases, research shows that minority/ethnicity as a risk factor is most likely a proxy for socioeconomic status; the Native American population's above-average drug use has been linked directly to this variable (Johnson et al., 1990; Wallace & Bachman, 1991). According to Ellikson, McGuigan, Adams, Bell, and Hays (1996) African-Americans and some Asian groups had significantly lower rates of risky drinking and related problems when family income, education, and family structure were held constant, thus supporting SES as a proxy.

It is true, however, that ethnic groups vary widely as to their susceptibility to drugs, their attitudes regarding drugs, and their resistance strategies (Moon, Hecht, Jackson, & Spellers, 1999). Mexican-American youth in some parts of the country, for example, have reported receiving drug offers at a significantly higher rate than European-Americans or African-Americans (Hecht, Trost, Bator, & McKinnon, 1997). Some Latino subgroups and African-Americans have lower overall rates of alcohol use than Anglos (Vega, Gil, & Wagner, 1998).

In addition, recent research has found that "more acculturated" Latinos have demonstrated higher rates of drug use than their "less acculturated peers (Gilbert & Cervantes, 1986; Zapata & Kaims, 1994). Although Gil, Wagner, & Vega (2000) note that acculturation is a critical factor in examining Latino substance use and "may be an important variable in the planning and implementation of prevention and/or treatment programs" (p. 445), this area has not yet been studied. Acculturative stress is a critical factor in prevention as well (see Marsiglia & Hecht, 2005). It is clear that personal, cultural, and community influences play an important role in an individual's ability to maintain resilience to substance abuse.

Most prevention research is conducted in school settings with students (Hansen, 1992). However, community settings other than schools often give the opportunity for intervening with the youth that need the prevention messages the most. For example, lifetime rates of AOD use are higher among homeless and street youth than among sheltered or household youth (Greene, Ennett, & Ringwalt, 1997). Seventy to eighty percent of street youth report daily use of alcohol and 35 to 55% report weekly or greater use of cocaine, crack, heroin, and/or amphetamines (Greene et al., 1997; Kipke, Montgomery, Simon, & Iverson, 1997; Koopman, Rosario, & Rotheran-Borus, 1994). Koopman and colleagues (1994) report Hispanic homeless youth are more likely than other ethnic groups (White and Black) to continue use of AOD after leaving home. However, a recent study conducted in an urban Texas community did not support this finding (Rew, Taylor-Seehafer, & Fitzgerald, 2001). The prevalence of AOD use was similar to that reported in other studies of homeless youth, however, no significant differences were found between White and Hispanic street youth in AOD use at age of onset or use in the past 30 days (Rew et al., 2001).

Culturally Grounded Substance Prevention

The NIDA funded Drug Resistance Strategies Project (DRS; 1997–2001) in Phoenix, Arizona, was implemented with 4,224 youths, starting in 1997. Caucasian, Latino/Latina, and African-American high school youths from a large city high school were included in the creation of culturally grounded substance abuse prevention videos. Previous studies suggest that videos as prevention tools are not only important for engaging African-American and Latino youth (Schinke et al., 1992) but are also an effective mode of intervention with these groups (Hecht, Corman, & Miller-Rassulo, 1993; Polansky, Buki, Horan, Ceperich, & Burows, 1999). The DRS curriculum is based on established social mediators (e.g., cultural norms supporting substances and economic deprivation) and protective factors (e.g., strong role models, educational successes, school bonding, adaptation to stresses, and positive attitudes; Clayton, Leukefeld, Donohew, Barto, & Harrington, 1995; Hawkins et al., 1992; Moon, Jackson, & Hecht, 2000).

The DRS project made the important contribution of combining the core aspects of social influence models with the added integral component of cultural-groundedness. The DRS study findings confirm the theoretical rationale for involvement of minority adolescents in the development of substance abuse prevention projects (Holleran, Reeves, Marsiglia, & Dustman, 2002). The study utilized an experimental design utilizing videos as tools for depicting resistance strategies (Alberts, Miller-Rassulo, & Hecht, 1991; Hecht, Alberts, & Miller-Rassulo, 1992). The videos, with protagonists of Anglo, Latino, and African-American culture, emphasized values and morals of these cultures. For example, whereas the video depicting Anglo culture portrays individuality, independence from family, and identification with Anglo peers, the Latino video emphasizes familism, ethnic identification with Latino peers and family, traditional Latino rituals, and language.

Analyses of the DRS project (14 months postintervention) indicated that students in the experimental schools had gained greater confidence in the ability to resist drugs, increased use of the strategies taught by the curriculum to resist substance offers (control schools reported a decrease in the use of these resistance strategies), more conservative norms adopted in both school and at home, reduction in the use of alcohol (a decrease of nearly 16% in the experimental group and an increase of slightly more than 20% in the control group), and less positive attitudes toward drug use. The most pointed implication for this study, however, was that the curricula/videos that integrated elements of minority sociocultural norms were more successful than the Anglo curricula/videos with significant effects on drug norms, attitudes, and use, particularly alcohol use. These findings support the importance of culturally grounded information in substance abuse prevention programs. Prevention messages that incorporate cultural elements and are presented within the social context of the participant are more likely to have a positive impact.

Fidelity Versus Adaptation Debate

Although many studies maintain that outcomes of effective prevention interventions do not have a differential impact based on ethnicity, it is important to note that research design limitations keep us from definitively establishing whether prevention interventions are equally effective with different ethnic groups. The core interventions seem to be effective with multi-ethnic youth, however, some research shows that culturally grounded versions of interventions have increased effects, especially in recruitment and retention (Kumpfer, Alvarado, Smith, & Bellamy, 2002; Holleran et al., 2005; Hopson & Holleran Steiker, 2008). Other adaptations, especially those that compromise "dosage" tend to reduce positive outcomes. Although there has been a dearth of research on fidelity of implementation in the social sciences, research in drug abuse prevention provides evidence that poor implementation results in a loss of program effectiveness (Dusenbury, Brannigan, Falco, & Hansen, 2003).

In preliminary research, researchers have found that agencies on the Texas border found some information in the original, universal curriculum irrelevant, outdated, and even, on some occasions, offensive (Holleran Steiker, 2006; Hopson & Holleran Steiker, 2008). In addition, youth felt that curricula needed to reflect their actual language, life events, music, style, and surroundings in order to capture their attention and to resonate with their experiences (Holleran Steiker, 2006).

Much more research is needed in the area of cultural adaptation of drug prevention programming (Hopson & Holleran Steiker, 2008). Clinicians in the field often find themselves adapting the language and activities of a curriculum due to knowledge of the culture of the youth with whom they work. In fact, findings suggest that a significant number of teachers of substance use prevention curricula did not use a curriculum guide at all, whereas only 15% reported they followed one very closely (Ringwalt et al., 2003). In preliminary focus groups,

Hopson & Holleran Steiker (2008) found that prevention interventions on the U.S.–Mexico border were tailored by agency staff to fit the culture of the youth in that setting. Controlling for a variety of school and teacher characteristics, teachers in high-minority schools were instructed to adapt curricula particularly in the areas of youth violence, limited English proficiency, and nuances of various racial/ethnic or cultural groups (Ringwalt, Vincus, Ennett, Johnson, & Rohrbach, 2004). Ultimately, it is crucial that preventionists work in close collaboration with agency staff to assure the fit of the program culturally (Botvin, 2004).

Prevention over the Life Course

Interventions exist for a variety of developmental stages. Early intervention strategies utilize life skills training techniques aiming primarily at delaying onset of use of substances. For example, a team at John's Hopkins utilized classroom-centered and family–school partnerships to assess impact on first-graders (Ialongo et al., 1999). Middle-schools are usually targeted universally for prevention and resistance strategies, as utilized by the original Keepin' It REAL program in Phoenix, Arizona (Hecht et al., 2003). High school interventions are needed to interrupt transitions from experimentation and mild use to more serious use and substances (NIDA, 2006). Relapse prevention is another mode of prevention utilized with recovering alcoholics/addicts to help prevent return to substance use (Marlatt & Donovan, 2005).

Prevention of substance abuse in the college population is analogous to other populations in complexity. Arnett (2000) uses the term emerging adulthood to characterize those between the ages of 18 and 25, and suggests that significant identity exploration takes place and other unique developmental experiences occur. Contextually, the college campus may lend itself to more permissive attitudes and perceptions toward testing boundaries and experimentation. Substance use often peaks during this period, with marked risk associated with binge drinking and related consequences on campuses across the country. Recent data from the American College Health Association's National College Health Assessment (ACHA-NCHA) indicates that 21% of female and 24% of male respondents engaged in binge drinking one to two times per week (ACHA, 2006). Key associations with binge drinking and abuse of other substances in the college population include: negative academic consequences, nonvolitional or unsafe sex, drunk driving, police involvement, fighting, injury, and death. On a broad level, efforts to reduce these consequences have met with little success. According to the NIAAA, "one reason for the lack of success of prevention efforts is that, for the most part, schools have not based their prevention efforts on strategies identified and tested for effectiveness by research" (NIAAA, 2002).

Prevention efforts targeting college students must be theoretically grounded and evidence-based. Some of the most consistently used prevention strategies fail to meet one or both of these requirements. In particular, educational components that solely focus on facts and harm have not been deemed effective (NIAAA, 2002). One of the most consistent theoretical approaches used with this population is based on social norms. Programs and interventions grounded in this framework are based on the assumption that students frequently overestimate peer use and when given the actual norm will align their own behaviors with more moderate use. However, an examination of research on social norm campaigns offers mixed results ranging from equivocal to negative outcomes (Thombs, Dotterer, Olds, Sharp, & Giovanne, 2004). Although evidence suggests that the social norms approach may not effectively target users with varying levels of perceived risk and use, some programs such as one SAMHSA Model Program, Challenging College Alcohol Abuse program at the University of Arizona, have accomplished measurable positive results. This program is classified as both a universal and indicated program and is framed as an environmental intervention type.

Secondary prevention also occurs at the college level with growing evidence of success for programs that focus on teaching useful skills such as blood alcohol level estimation and setting drinking limits (Kivlahan, Marlatt, Fromme, Coppel, & Williams, 1990). Contemporary preventive intervention programs such as Brief Alcohol Screening and Intervention of College Students (BASICS) show promising results for measurable changes in high-risk drinking behaviors from baseline to 4-year follow-up (Marlatt, 2003). BASICS is a harm-reduction-based SAMHSA model program.

In addition to SAMHSA, The U.S. Department of Education's Higher Education for Alcohol and Drug Prevention makes several recommendations for prevention efforts with this population (DeJong et al., 1998):

1. Changing people's knowledge, attitudes, and behavioral intentions regarding alcohol consumption
2. Eliminating or modifying environmental factors that contribute to the problem
3. Protecting students from the short-term consequences of alcohol consumption (health protection or harm reduction strategies)
4. Intervening with and treating students who are addicted

The ecological perspective must be applied to prevention of substance use and abuse among college students. Best practice programs must be supported by assessment which should occur at a local and national level. Individual campuses may examine personal and environmental determinants that may be unique to their population, and must also look to data sources such as the NCHA and CORE Institutes AOD Survey. Additionally, prevention efforts should be inclusive of subpopulations of the campus community, including the special needs of minority groups, women, athletes, "Greeks," nontraditional-aged students, and LGBTQ students (NIAAA, 2002). Successful prevention campaigns must take into account the student, peers, the institution, surrounding community, and public policy factors.

Adult prevention interventions exist in workplaces, provided usually by Employee Assistance Programs (or EAPs; Cook, Back, & Trudeau, 1996). A few programs have recognized the risk to the elderly with regard to alcohol (Atkinson, 1984) and substance abuse, particularly in the area of medication abuse (Abrams & Alexopoulos, 1988). Problems with regard to overuse of medications and over-the-counter remedies were common, and risk factors included retirement, loss of loved ones, and health problems.

Summary

In summary, prevention of drug and alcohol abuse is an important piece of the treatment continuum. Most programs are targeted at children and adolescents, as this is the most common onset age. Due to a high incidence of use, especially with alcohol, prevention stratagems are necessary. Research has shown that the prevention of onset, or later onset, can help lessen substance-related consequences (Gonzales, 1983).

Historically substance use has been viewed in many contexts. Despite two temperance movements, alcohol use and abuse received little attention until the 1920s, when scare tactics became the primary mode of prevention and campaigning. This continued until the 1960s when the national perspective shifted to educational models which were not very effective. Interventions have evolved into more complex, social influence models that concentrate on skills training and resistance strategies. Evidence-based (i.e., empirically supported) interventions have most recently become the gold standard.

Harm reduction is an alternative approach to substance abuse prevention that emphasizes the reduction of harmful consequences related to use of substances, rather than only focusing on abstinence. In this model abstinence is still viewed as ideal, but recognizes that this may be an unrealistic goal for all individuals. However, because substance use is illegal, any program normalizing the behavior is often received with strong opposition (Hopson, 2006).

In addition to considering abstinence- versus non-abstinence-based models, one must choose the target population for an intervention. There is a variety of interventions that fit varied target groups. Universal prevention programs address an entire population. Selective strategies are designed to target a specific at-risk subset of the general population. Indicated strategies are administered directly to individuals who have shown themselves to be at higher risk for substance use and abuse. One must carefully weigh out goals, target population expectations, and agency objectives when deciding on the best model of intervention. It is recommended that decisions about prevention be made, not only by agency administrators, but also by line staff, constituents, and clients receiving services.

Several methods have been identified as appropriate interventions for substance abuse prevention. Six techniques that are identified by NIDA, and recommended to be used in combination with one another, include information dissemination, teaching alternatives, problem identification and referral, community-based processes, and environmental strategies.

Much of the success of prevention interventions relates to recruitment, engagement, and retention. It has been established that culturally grounded interventions not only accomplish these goals, but also may improve the outcomes, such as reducing alcohol use (Holleran Steiker & Hopson, 2007).

It is important to note that ethnicity does not equate with risk (Pentz et al., 1999) and that protective factors can be found in all cultures. In addition, although culture is generally defined as interchangeable with ethnicity, culture can also include the uniqueness of community, such as the 12-step program, alternative schools, juvenile justice settings, and centers for alternative youth.

This chapter has emphasized prevention with youth. However, prevention interventions with youth, college students, and adults have much in common. They are all based in risk and protective factors; all should be based in empirically supported, theory-driven research; and all benefit from collaborative input among researchers, clinicians, recipients, and stakeholders alike. It is recommended that all prevention interventions be based in needs assessment and that they be evaluated proximally (as they unfold) and distally (once they are complete and over time). It has been maintained that "an ounce of prevention is worth a pound of cure," however, prevention scientists might add that if an ounce of prevention works, cure is unnecessary.

References

Abrams, R. C., & Alexopoulos, G. S. (1988). Substance abuse in the elderly: Over-the-counter and illegal drugs. *Hospital Community Psychiatry, 39*, 822–829.

Albert, W. G., & Simpson, R. I. (1985). Evaluating an educational program for the prevention of impaired driving among grade 11 students. *Journal of Drug Education, 15*, 57–71.

Alberts, J. K., Miller-Rassulo, & Hecht, M. L. (1991). A typology of drug resistance strategies. *Journal of Applied Communication Research, 19*, 129–151.

American College Health Association (2006). American College Health Association – National College Health Assessment (ACHA-NCHA) Web Summary. Retrieved from http://www.acha-ncha.org/data_highlights.html.

Arnett, J. J. (2000). Emerging adulthood. A theory of development from the late teens through the twenties. *American Psychologist, 55*(5), 469–480.

Atkinson, R. M., (1984). Substance use and abuse in late life. In: R. Atkinson, (Ed.) *Alcohol and drug abuse in old age*. Washington, DC: American Psychiatric Press, pp. 1–21.

Becker, H. K., Agopian, M. W., & Yeh, S. (1992). Impact evaluation of drug abuse resistance education (DARE). *Journal of Drug Education, 22*, 283–292.

Beyers, J., Toumbourou, J., Catalano, R. M, Arthur, M., & Hawkins, J. (2004). A cross-national comparison of risk and protective factors for adolescent substance use: The United States and Australia. *Journal of Adolescent Health, 35*, 3–16.

Botvin, G. J. (2004). Advancing prevention science and practice: Challenges, critical issues, and future directions. *Journal Prevention Science, 5*, 69–72.

Botvin, G. J., Baker, E., & Dusenbury, L. (1995). Long-term follow-up results of a randomized drug abuse prevention trial in a white middle class population. *Journal of the American Medical Association 27*, 1106–1112.

Botvin, G. J., Baker, E., Dusenbury, L., Tortu, S., & Botvin, E. M. (1990). Preventing adolescent drug abuse through a multimodal cognitive-behavioral approach: Results of a 3-year study. *Journal of Consulting and Clinical Psychology 58*, 437–446.

Botvin, G. J., Baker, E., Filazzola, A., & Botvin, E. M. (1990). A cognitive-behavioral approach to substance abuse prevention: A 1-year followup. *Addictive Behavior 15*, 47–63.

Caplan, M., Weissberg, R. P., Grober, J. S., Sivo, P. J., Grady, K., & Jacoby, C. (1992). Social competence promotion with inner-city and suburban young adolescents: Effects on social adjustment and alcohol use. *Journal of Consulting and Clinical Psychology, 60*, 56–63.

Clayton, R. R., Leukefeld, C. G., Donohew, L., Barto, M., & Harrington, N. G. (1995). Risk and protective factors: A brief review. *Drugs & Society, 8*, 7–14.

Clayton, R. R., Leukefeld, C. G., Harrington, N. G., & Cattarello, A. (1996). DARE Drug Abuse Resistance Education: Very popular but not very effective (pp. 101–109). In C. B. McCoy, L. R. Metsch, & J. A. Inciardi (Eds.), *Intervening with Drug-Involved Youth*. Thousand Oaks, CA: Sage.

Collins, R. L. (1995). Issues of ethnicity in research on prevention of substance abuse. In G. J. Botvin, S. Schinke, & M. A. Orlandi. (1995). *Drug abuse prevention with multiethnic youth*. Thousand Oaks, CA: Sage.

Cook, R. F., Back, A., & Trudeau, J. (1996). Substance abuse prevention in the workplace: Recent findings and an expanded conceptual model. *Journal of Primary Prevention, 16*, 319–339.

DeJong, W., Vince-Whitman, C., Colthurst, T., Cretella, M., Gilbreath, M., Rosati, M., et al. (1998) *Environmental management: A comprehensive strategy for reducing alcohol and other drug use on college campuses*. Newton, MA: Higher Education Center for Alcohol and Other Drug Prevention.

Dodge, K. A., Dishion, T. J., & Lansford, J. E. (2006). Deviant peer influences in intervention and public policy for youth. *Social Policy Report*, vol. XX, pp. 1–19.

Dusenbury, L., Brannigan, R., Falco, M., & Hansen, W. B. (2003). A review of research on fidelity of implementation: Implications for drug abuse prevention in school settings. *Health Education Research, 18*, 237–256.

Ellickson, P. (1999). School-based substance abuse prevention: What works, for whom, and how? In S. B. Kar (Ed.), *Substance abuse prevention: A multicultural perspective*. Amityville, NY: Baywood.

Ellickson, P. L., & Bell, R. M. (1990). Drug prevention in junior high: A multi-site longitudinal test. *Science, 247,* 1299–1305.

Ellickson, P. L., Bell, R. M., & McGuigan, K. (1993). Preventing adolescent drug use: Long-term results of a junior high program. *American Journal of Public Health, 83,* 856–861.

Ellickson, P. L., McGuigan, K. A., Adams, V., Bell, R. M., & Hays, R. D. (1996). Teenagers and alcohol misuse: By any definition, it's a big problem. *Addiction, 91,* 1489–1503.

Friis, R. H. & Sellers, T. A. (1999). *Epidemiology for public health practice* (2nd ed.), Aspen.

Galan, F. J. (1988). Alcoholism prevention and Hispanic youth. *Journal of Drug Issues, 18,* 49–68.

Garland, D. (2001). *The culture of control: Crime and social order in contemporary society.* Chicago: University of Chicago Press.

Gil, A. G., Wagner, E. F., & Vega, W. A. (2000). Acculturation, familism, and alcohol use among Latino adolescent males: Longitudinal relations. *Journal of Community Psychology, 28,* 443–458.

Gilbert, M. J., & Cervantes, R. C. (1986). Patterns and practices of alcohol use among Mexican Americans: A comprehensive review. *Hispanic Journal of Behavioral Sciences, 8*(1), 1–60.

Gonzales, G. M. (1983). Time and place of first drinking experience and parental knowledge as predictors of alcohol use and misuse in college. *Journal of Alcohol and Drug Education, 27,* 1–13.

Gosin, M. N., Dustman, A. E., Drapeau, A. E., & Harthun, M. L. (2003). Participatory action research: Creating an effective prevention curriculum for adolescents in the Southwestern US. *Health Education Research, 18,* 363–379.

Greene, J. M., Ennett, S. T., & Ringwalt, C. L. (1997). Substance use among runaway and homeless youth in three sample. *American Journal of Public Health, 87,* 229–235.

Griswold-Ezekoye, S., Kumpfer, K. L., & Bukoski, W. J. (1986). *Childhood and chemical abuse: Prevention and intervention.* New York: Haworth Press.

Hansen, W. B. (1992). School-based substance abuse prevention: A review of the state of the art in curriculum, 1980–1990. *Health Education Research, 7,* 403–430.

Hansen, W. B., Graham, J. W., Wolkenstein, B. H., Lundy, B. Z., Pearson, J., Flay, B. R., et al. (1988). Differential impact of three alcohol prevention curricula on hypothesized mediating variables. *Journal of Drug Education, 18,* 143–153.

Hansen, W. B., Miller, T. W., & Leukefeld, C. G. (1995). Prevention research recommendations: Scientific integration for the 90's. *Drugs & Society, 8,* 161–167.

Harmon, M. A. (1993). Reducing the risk of drug involvement among early adolescents: An evaluation of drug abuse resistance education (DARE). *Evaluation Review, 17,* 221–239.

Hawkins, J. D., Catalano, R. E., & Miller, J. Y. (1992). Risk and protective factors for alcohol and other drug problems in adolescence and early adulthood: Implications for substance abuse prevention. *Psychological Bulletin, 112,* 64–105.

Hecht, M. L., Alberts, J. K., & Miller-Rassulo, M. (1992). Resistance to drug offers among college students. *International Journal of the Addictions, 27,* 995–1017.

Hecht, M. L., Corman, S., & Miller-Rassulo, M. (1993). An evaluation of the drug resistance project: A comparison of film versus live performance. *Health Communication, 5,* 75–88.

Hecht, M. L., Marsiglia, F. F., Elek, E., Wagstaff, D. A., Kulis, S., & Dustman, P. (2003). Culturally-grounded substance use prevention: An evaluation of the keepin' it REAL 75–97 curriculum. *Prevention Science, 4,* 233–248.

Hecht, M. L., Trost, M., Bator, R., & McKinnon, D. (1997). Ethnicity and gender similarities and difference in drug resistance. *Journal of Applied Communication Research, 25,* 1–23.

Hogan, J., Gabrielsen, K., Luna, N., & Grothaus, D. (2003) *Substance abuse prevention: The intersection of science and practice,* Boston, MA: Pearson Education.

Holleran, L. K., Castro, F., Coard, S., Kumpfer, K., Nyborg, V., & Stephenson, H. (2005, May). *Moving towards state of the art, culturally relevant prevention interventions for minority youth.* Presented at the Society for Prevention Research annual meeting, May 27.

Holleran, L. K., Reeves, L., Marsiglia, F. F., & Dustman, P. (2002). Creating culturally grounded videos for substance abuse prevention: A dual perspective on process. *Journal of Social Work Practice in the Addictions, 2,* 55–78.

Holleran Steiker, L. K. (2006). Consulting with the experts: Utilizing adolescent input in substance use prevention efforts. *Social Perspectives/Perspectivas Sociales, 8,* 53–66.

Holleran Steiker, L. K., & Hopson, L. M. (2007, February). *Evaluation of culturally adapted, evidence-based substance abuse prevention programs for older adolescents in diverse community settings.* Advancing Adolescent Health Conference. The University of Texas at Austin, Center for Health Promotion Research. February 28.

Hopson, L. M. (November, 2006). Effectiveness of culturally grounded adaptations of an evidence-based substance abuse prevention program with alternative school students. Unpublished dissertation. University of Texas at Austin School of Social Work.

Hopson, L. M., & Holleran Steiker, L. K. (2008). Methodology for evaluating an adaptation of evidence-based drug abuse prevention in alternative schools. *Children in Schools, 30,* 116–127.

Hughes, J. (2003). Commentary: Participatory action research leads to sustainable school and community improvement. *School Psychology Review, 32,* 38–43.

Ialongo, N. S., Werthamer, L., Kellam, S. G., Hendricks Brown, C., Wang, S., & Lin, Y. (1999). Proximal impact of two first-grade preventive interventions on the early risk behaviors for later substance abuse, depression, and antisocial behavior. *American Journal of Community Psychology, 27,* 599–641.

Johnson, C. A., Pentz, M. A., Weber, M. D., Dwyer, J. H., MacKinnon, D. P., Flay, B. R., et al. (1990). The relative effectiveness of comprehensive community programming for drug abuse prevention with risk and low risk adolescents. *Journal of Consulting and Clinical Psychology, 58,* 4047–4056.

Johnston, L. D., O'Malley, P. M., Bachman, J. G., & Schulenberg, J. E. (December 21, 2006). *Teen drug use continues down in 2006, particularly among older teens; but use of prescription-type drugs remains high.* Ann Arbor: University of Michigan News and Information Services.

Johnston, L. D., O'Malley, P. M., Bachman, J. G., & Schulenberg, J. E. (2007). *Monitoring the future national results on adolescent drug use: Overview of key findings, 2006* (NIH Publication No. 07-6202). Bethesda, MD: National Institute on Drug Abuse, 71.

Kidd, S. A., & Kral, M. J. (2005). Practicing participatory research. *Journal of Counseling Psychology, 52,* 187–195.

Kipke, M. D., Montgomery, S. B., Simon, R. R., & Iverson, E. F. (1997). Substance abuse disorders among runaway and homeless youth. *Substance Use and Misuse, 32,* 965–982.

Kivlahan, D., Marlatt, G., Fromme, K., Coppel., D., & Williams, E. (1990). Secondary prevention with college drinkers: Evaluation of an alcohol skills training program. *Journal of Consulting and Clinical Psychology, 58,* 805–810.

Koopman, C., Rosario, M., & Rotheram-Borus, M. J. (1994). Alcohol and drug use and sexual behaviors placing runaways at risk for HIV infection. *Addictive Behaviors, 19,* 95–103.

Koss-Chioino, J. D., & Vargas, L. A. (1999). *Working with Latino youth: Culture, development, and context.* San Francisco: Jossey-Bass.

Kumpfer, K. L., Alvarado, R., Smith, P., & Bellamy, N. (2002). Cultural sensitivity and adaptation in family-based prevention interventions. *Journal Prevention Science, 3,* 241–246.

Kumpfer, K. L., Molgaard, V., & Spoth, R. (1996). The Strengthening Families Program for prevention of delinquency and drug use in special populations. In R. Peters & R. J. McMahon (Eds.), *Childhood disorders, substance abuse, and delinquency: Prevention and early intervention approaches.* Newbury Park, CA: Sage.

Lynam, D. R. (1999). Project DARE: No effects at 10-year follow-up. *Journal of Consulting and Clinical Psychology, 67,* 590.

MacLeod, J. (2004). *Ain't no makin' it: Aspirations and attainment in a low-income neighborhood.* Oxford: Westview Press.

MacMaster, S. A., & Holleran, L. K. (2005). Incorporating 12-step group attendance in addictions courses: A cross-cultural experience. *Journal of Teaching in the Addictions, 4,* 79–91.

MacMaster, S. A., Holleran, L., & Chaffin, K. (2005). Empirical and theoretical support for non-abstinence-based prevention services for substance using adolescents. *Journal of Evidence-Based Social Work, 2,* 91–111.

Marlatt, G. A. (1996). Harm reduction: Come as you are. *Journal of Addictive Behavior, 21*(6), 779–788.

Marlatt, G. A. (May, 2003). BASICS – Brief alcohol screening and intervention for college students. In SAMHSA Model Programs, Retrieved June 20, 2007 from http://modelprograms.samhsa.gov.

Marlatt, G. A., & Donovan, D. M. (2005). *Relapse prevention: Maintenance strategies in the treatment of addictive behaviors.* New York: Guilford Press.

Marsiglia, F., & Hecht, M. (2005). *Keepin it REAL: Drug resistance strategies: Teacher guide.* Santa Cruz, CA: ETR Associates.

Marsiglia, F. F., Holleran, L. & Jackson, K. M. (2000). The impact of internal and external resources on school-based substance abuse prevention. *Social Work in Education, 22,* 145–161.

Miller, G. J., Beckles, G. L. A., Maude, G. H., & Carson, D. C. (1990). Alcohol consumption: Protection against coronary heart disease and risks to health. *International Journal of Epidemiology, 19,* 923–930.

Moon, D. G., Hecht, M. L., Jackson, K. M., & Spellers, R. E. (1999). Ethnic and gender differences and similarities in adolescent drug use and refusals of drug offers. *Substance Use & Misuse, 34,* 1059–1083.

Moon, D. G., Jackson, K. M., & Hecht, M. L. (2000). Family risk and resiliency factors, substance use, and the drug resistance process in adolescence. *Journal of Drug Education, 30,* 373–398.

National Association of Clinicians (2001). NASW Standards for Cultural Competence in Social Work Practice. Retrieved February 6, 2007 from http://www.socialworkers.org/sections/credentials/cultural_comp.asp.

National Institute on Alcohol Abuse and Alcoholism (2002). A Call to Action: Changing the Culture of Drinking on College Campuses. Task Force of the National Advisory Council on Alcohol Abuse and Alcoholism. Retrieved from http://www.collegedrinkingprevention.gov/media/TaskForceReport.pdf.

National Institute on Drug Abuse (NIDA; 2006). Drug Abuse Prevention Intervention Research: Program Announcement Number: PA-05-118. Retrieved from Website, June, 2007. http://grants.nih.gov/grants/guide/pa-files/PA-05-118.html.

Neighbors, C., Dillard, A. J., Lewis, M. A., Bergstrom, R. L., & Neil, T. A. (2006). Normative misperceptions and temporal precedence of perceived norms and drinking. *Journal of Studies on Alcohol, 67,* 290–299.

Newcomb, M. D., Chou, C., Bentler, P. M., & Huba, G. J. (1988). Cognitive motivations for drug use among adolescents: Longitudinal tests of gender differences and predictors of change in drug use. *Journal of Counseling Psychology, 35,* 426-438.

Padget, A., Bell, M. L., Shamblen, S. R., & Ringwalt, C. L. (2006). Does learning about the effects of alcohol on the developing brain affect children's alcohol use? *Journal Prevention Science, 7,* 293–302.

Palinkas, L. A., Atkins, C. J., Jerreira, D., & Miller, C. (1996). Effectiveness of social skills training form primary and secondary prevention of drug use in high-risk female adolescents. *Preventive Medicine, 25,* 692–701.

Pentz, M. A., Rothspan, G. T., Skara, S., & Voskanian, S. (1999). Multi-ethnic considerations in community-based drug abuse prevention research. In S. B. Kar (Ed.), *Substance abuse prevention: A multicultural perspective.* Amityville, NY: Baywood.

Petrosino A., Turpin-Petrosino C., & Buehler J. (2005) "Scared Straight" and other juvenile awareness programs for preventing juvenile delinquency (Cochrane Review). In: *The Cochrane Library,* Issue 4, 2003. Chichester, UK: John Wiley & Sons.

Polansky, J. M., Buki, L. P., Horan, J. J., Ceperich, S. D., & Burows, D. D. (1999). The effectiveness of substance abuse prevention videotapes with Mexican-American adolescents. *Hispanic Journal of Behavioral Sciences, 21,* 186–198.

Rew, L., Taylor-Seehafer, M., & Fitzgerald, M. L. (2001). Sexual abuse, alcohol and other drug use, and suicidal behaviors in homeless adolescents. *Issues in Comprehensive Pediatric Nursing, 24,* 225–240.

Ringwalt, C., Ennett, S. T., & Holt, K. D. (1991). An outcome evaluation of project DARE (drug abuse resistance education). *Health Education Research, 6,* 327–337.

Ringwalt, C. L., Ennett, S., Johnson, R., Rohrbach, L. A., Simons-Rudolph, A., Vincus, A., et al. (2003). Factors associated with fidelity to substance use prevention curriculum guides in the nation's middle schools. *Health Education & Behavior, 3,* 75–391.

Ringwalt, C. L., Vincus, A., Ennett, S., Johnson, R., & Rohrbach, L. A. (2004). Reasons for teachers' adaptation of substance use prevention curricula in schools with non-white student populations. *Journal Prevention Science, 5,* 61–67.

Schinke, S., Orlandi, M., Botvin, G., Gilchrist, L. D., Trimble, J. E., & Locklear, V. S. (1988). Preventing substance abuse among American-Indian adolescents: A bicultural competence skills approach, *Journal of Counseling Psychology, 35*, 87–90.

Schinke, S., Orlandi. M., Vaccaro, D., Espinoza, R., McAlister, A., & Botvin, G. (1992). Substance use among Hispanic and non-Hispanic adolescents. *Addictive Behaviors, 17,* 117–124.

Schinke, S. P., Gilchrist, L. D., Schilling, R. F., Walker, R. D., Kirkham, M. A. Bobo, J. K., et al. (1985). Strategies for preventing substance abuse with American Indian youth. *White Cloud Journal, 3,* 12–18.

Shedler, J., & Block, J. (1990). Adolescent drug use and psychological health: A longitudinal inquiry, *American Psychologist, 45,* 612–630.

Thombs, D., Dotterer, S., Olds, S., Sharp., K., & Giovanne, R. (2004). A close look at why one social norms campaign did not reduce student drinking. *Journal of American College Health,* 53, 61–68.

Tobler, N. S., & Stratton, H. H. (1997) Effectiveness of school-based drug prevention programs: A meta-analysis of the research. *Journal of Primary Prevention. 18,* 71–128.

Trimble, J. (1995). Toward an understanding of ethnicity and ethnic identity, and their relationship with drug use research. In G. J. Botvin, S. Schinke, & M. A. Orlandi (Eds.), *Drug abuse prevention with multiethnic youth* (pp. 28–45). Thousand Oaks, CA: Sage.

Vega, W. A., Gil, A. G., & Wagner, E. (1998). Cultural adjustment and Hispanic\adolescent drug use. In W. A. Vega & A. G. Gil (Eds.), *Drug use and ethnicity in early adolescence* (pp. 125–148). New York: Plenum Press.

Wallace, J. M., & Bachman, J. G. (1991). Explaining racial/ethnic differences in adolescent drug use: The impact of background and lifestyle. *Social Problems, 38,* 333–357.

Welle, D. L. (2003). LGBTQ youth: Research on developmental complexity. *Society for Research on Adolescence Newsletter, Fall, 1,* 7–8.

Zapata, J. T., & Kaims, D. S. (1994). Antecedents of substance use among Mexican-American school-age children. *Journal of Drug Education, 24,* 233–251.

Part III

Assessment and Treatment of Substance Abuse

Katrina L. Cook
Texas Tech University

Lee M. Cohen
Texas Tech University

Introduction

The aim of Part III is to provide an overview of the assessment and treatment of commonly abused substances. Chapters focus on different substances of abuse providing both the historical background and the contemporary conceptualization of the use of, abuse of, and/or dependence upon each substance. Prevalence of use and contemporary assessment and treatment strategies are highlighted. In addition, colorful case presentations and helpful resources are included.

Blume, Resor, Villanueva, and Braddy emphasize the use of evidence-based practice to treat problems with alcohol in Chapter 12. This chapter promotes the use of validated measures in assessing alcohol use, as well as some of the interventions discussed in the previous section within the context of the treatment of alcohol abuse. Additionally, relapse prevention and harm reduction strategies are discussed. The authors provide suggestions on individualizing therapy for diverse clientele including treatment matching, culturally relevant treatment, and clients with comorbid disorders.

Chapter 13 depicts the variety of assessment and treatment options available in tackling nicotine use. Brandon, Drobes, Ditre, and Elibero identify and describe measures including demographic information, the client's motivation to quit, nicotine dependence and withdrawal, and social learning variables. Interventions of interest include those derived from social and/or behavioral orientations, as well as specific, FDA-approved nicotine-based pharmacotherapies. The authors also highlight a mismatch between assessment and treatment in that measures of nicotine use are often superficial and do not adequately inform decisions regarding treatment.

The assessment and treatment of marijuana use disorders is the focus of Chapter 14. Looby and Earleywine point out that most options used to assess and treat marijuana use have been adapted from those utilized within the context of other substance use disorders. It is not surprising that measures of marijuana use include those related to severity of dependence, patterns of use, problems associated with substance use, and the client's readiness to change. Empirical evidence is provided in support of treatment efficacy in adult and adolescent marijuana users and programs are presented that may be useful in working with nontreatment-seeking adults and adolescents. Finally, additional treatment variables are considered.

In Chapter 15, Barry, Petry, and Alessi tackle the assessment and treatment of cocaine abuse and dependence. Interviews have proved useful in measuring tolerance and withdrawal symptoms, as well as patterns and consequences of cocaine use. Evidence-based treatments included in this chapter are cognitive-behavioral, 12-step/self help, and/or motivational in nature. Contingency management interventions are presented as efficacious in promoting abstinence from cocaine use and a viable option when working in community settings.

Behavioral and pharmacological approaches to the assessment and treatment of amphetamine dependence are discussed by Rush, Vansickel, Lile, and Stoops in Chapter 16. Contemporary assessment guidelines are outlined. Although the authors state that few studies have been conducted in an effort to identify effective treatments, contingency management and agonist replacement therapies are highlighted as potentially effective strategies in treating methamphetamine dependence, although the latter have elicited some controversy among clinicians. Future directions are provided.

Marsch and Bickel address the assessment and treatment of heroin and other opioid use in Chapter 17. Opioid abuse and dependence is described in terms of physiological, interpersonal, and behavioral presentation. The authors recognize the effective combination of psychosocial and pharmacotherapies as those dependent upon heroin and other opioids often demonstrate a variety of maladaptive behaviors and psychiatric problems.

The focus of Chapter 18 is the assessment and treatment of inhalant abuse. Crano, Ting, and Hemovich emphasize the importance of classifying inhalant users and abusers based on demographics, use, and intention once they have been identified as this classification proves useful in treatment. It is of particular importance in the case of inhalants to assess for both psychological and physical issues. The authors elaborate upon the specifics of neurocognitive rehabilitation to address impairments that can result from inhalant abuse. Other considerations and components of treatment include detoxification, peer advocates, and family and community involvement. Methods to prevent initiation of inhalant use are also described.

Hallucinogen use, assessment, and treatment constitute the topic of Chapter 19. Suzuki, Halpern, Passie, and Huertas describe the unique psychological and physiological effects of hallucinogens and differentiate between the various hallucinogen use and hallucinogen-induced disorders. In turn, the authors address details pertaining to the criteria, assessment, differential diagnoses, and treatments of each.

Finally, in Chapter 20, Echeverry and Nettles define the term "Club Drug," list those that are most commonly used in the United States, and describe populations that are most at risk for club drug use. Drugs of interest include Ecstasy, Rohypnol, ketamine, GHB, crystal methamphetamine, and poppers. The authors address each club drug in turn regarding its nature, prevalence, effects, typical user, most effective treatment approach, and research trends related to behaviors resulting from its use. Other considerations that are mentioned include the influence of music on club drug use, legislation and law enforcement, and future research directions.

12

Evidence-Based Practices to Treat Alcohol Problems

Arthur W. Blume, Michelle R. Resor, Michael R. Villanueva, and Leslie D. Braddy

University of North Carolina at Charlotte

Contents

Historical Overview and Prevalence

The term "alcoholic" is generally used colloquially to refer to someone whose drinking behavior is thought to exceed "normal" alcohol consumption levels (Skog, 2006). Although many scientists used this terminology through the 1960s, in current times practitioners and researchers use specific criteria to assess for alcohol use disorders. The *Diagnostic and Statistical Manual of Mental Disorders–IV* (*DSM–IV*; American Psychiatric Association, 1994) defines alcohol use disorders as either alcohol abuse or alcohol dependence. To meet criteria for the diagnosis of alcohol abuse, an individual must experience clinically significant impairment or distress resulting from recurrent alcohol use such as difficulties at home, school, or work; exposure to dangerous situations; legal problems; and continued drinking even when drinking is negatively affecting social relationships. These consequences can indicate alcohol dependence as well, but this diagnosis is additionally characterized by the presence of tolerance and withdrawal, drinking more than intended, trying unsuccessfully to cut back or quit, spending a significant amount of time drinking and accessing alcohol, and continued drinking despite physical or psychological disorders that are worsened by alcohol consumption.

Using diagnostic criteria from the *DSM–IV*, prevalence of lifetime alcohol abuse in U.S. adults has been estimated at 17.8%, with 4.7% reporting alcohol abuse within the past year (Hasin, Stinson, Ogburn, & Grant, 2007). Approximately 12.5% adults have met criteria for alcohol dependence in their lifetimes and 3.8% have met criteria within the past year. Factors associated with risk for alcohol use disorders include being white or Native American, male, young, and unmarried. Treatment rates for those with alcohol use disorders have declined slightly over the past several years.

Historically, drinking alcoholic beverages has been convenient for a variety of reasons and was often safer than drinking water (Hyman, 2004). Alcohol use was typically viewed as a personal choice. Before the 1800s, if an individual drank to the point of drunkenness it may have been interpreted as an indication of poor morality or character but would likely not be viewed as a significant health concern (e.g., Levine, 1978). In the late 1700s some groups began to see drinking as a disease, and by the early 1800s temperance movements began in the United States. In 1870, a group of American physicians created an association to promote empirical investigation of the disease concept of alcohol use disorders (Babor, 1996; Lender, 1979). The Eighteenth amendment prohibiting alcohol use and trade was passed in 1919; however, following significant problems resulting from this prohibition, the amendment was repealed in 1933. By that time focus had begun to shift toward a psychodynamic view of addictions, with scholars commonly describing problem drinking as a manifestation of underlying neuroses (Knight, 1938; Wingfield, 1919). Bowman and Jellinek (1941) published a synthesis of numerous typologies classifying different types of alcohol use. Jellinek built on this work and published a book in 1960 that described different categories of problematic alcohol use from the disease model perspective that assumes alcohol use disorders are progressive and outside one's control, and abstinence is necessary for recovery (Babor, 1996; Jellinek, 1960; Levine, 1978).

The disease model of alcohol use disorders was generally accepted as the only scientific conceptualization of alcohol abuse and dependence until the 1970s, when researchers began to examine other possible explanations for the addictive process. Controversial studies investigated controlled drinking as a goal for individuals receiving treatment for alcohol use disorders (Marlatt, 1983; Sobell & Sobell, 1973). Results not only showed that controlled drinking was possible in this population, but they also demonstrated that working toward this goal may be a better fit for some people with alcohol use disorders than focusing on abstinence as the only acceptable outcome. These results stood in stark contrast with the disease model that had dominated the field for several decades and the belief that following treatment for an alcohol use disorder, an individual who has a drink has fallen back into the disease of addiction that will only become progressively worse until he or she can attain complete sobriety again. Studies continued to support the Sobells' findings that moderate drinking is possible and at times a more desirable alternative for people who have been diagnosed with alcohol use disorders, and in 1990 the Institute of Medicine (1990) released a report stating that the diverse nature of alcohol use disorders necessitates a variety of treatment options rather than a "one size fits all" approach. This report described alcohol use disorders as cyclical and episodic rather than progressive.

Contemporary Assessment and Treatment

Researchers have identified variables that appear to affect therapy outcomes, and assessment of these variables aids in the development of treatment plans and interventions. For example, neuropsychological problems or other psychological disorders seem to place clients at risk for poorer treatment outcomes (e.g., Bates, Pawlak, Tonigan, & Buckman, 2006; Bradizza, Stasiewicz, & Paas, 2006). Therapists working with clients who have alcohol problems should conduct comprehensive diagnostic and neuropsychological assessments. Behavioral analyses of drinking events are important to determine the function and context of drinking behavior. Consumption patterns including frequency, quantity, and peak events should be assessed using empirically validated semi-structured interviews such as the Steady Pattern Chart from the Form 90 (Miller, 1996) and the Timeline Follow-back Interview (Sobell & Sobell, 1995).

Alcohol outcome expectancies and self-efficacy in drinking situations have been found to be significant predictors of changes in drinking behavior over time (Ilgen, Tiet, Finney, & Moos, 2006; Jones, Corbin, & Fromme, 2001) and can be assessed using one of several instruments. Assessments developed within the Transtheoretical Stages of Change Model (Prochaska, DiClemente, & Norcross, 1992) can help determine if a client is aware of his or her problematic drinking behavior, motivated to change it, and in the process of taking steps to do so. Examples include the Brief Readiness to Change Questionnaire (Heather, Rollnick, & Bell, 1993; Rollnick, Heather, Gold, & Hall, 1992) to more comprehensive measures such as the University of Rhode Island Change Assessment (or URICA; McConnaughy, DiClemente, Prochaska, & Velicer, 1989; McConnaughy, Prochaska, & Velicer, 1983) are available. Emotional states and moods also predict drinking behavior (e.g., Cooper, Frone, Russell, & Mudar, 1995) and may be assessed by self-monitoring of thoughts and emotions prior to and during drinking events.

Brief Interventions

Interventions of short duration can be effective means to change drinking behavior. Because many people with alcohol problems will not seek psychotherapeutic help for alcohol problems voluntarily (Cohen, Feinn, & Arias, 2007), alcohol interventions have been used successfully in emergent and primary care medical facilities (Babor, Higgins-Biddle, Dauser, Higgins, & Burleson, 2005; Heather, 1998; Minugh et al., 1997; Saitz, Svikis, D'Onofrio, Kraemer, & Perl, 2006). Physical problems may provide a moment of pause in which clients are open to examining alcohol use. One highly effective brief intervention is the Brief Drinker Check-up (Miller, Sovereign, & Krege, 1988), which uses assessment and personalized feedback with motivational interviewing (Miller & Rollnick, 2002; see Chapter 29) to motivate change.

Motivational Enhancement Therapy (Miller, Zweben, DiClemente, & Rychtarik, 1999), an evidence-based four-session therapy, was developed as a result of this research.

Face-to-face and Web-based brief interventions using assessment and personalized feedback have been used to intervene upon high-risk drinking by adolescents or young adults (Borsari & Carey, 2001; Carey, Carey, Maisto, & Henson, 2006; Kypri et al., 2004; Walters & Bennett, 2000). Recent studies conducted by Carey, Borsari, and colleagues (2006) and Epstein and colleagues (2005) found that assessment without personalized feedback was associated with drinking reductions among college students and adults.

Social Norms Interventions

The use of normative data to modify drinking, referred to as social norm campaigns or interventions, has been employed as a standalone intervention targeting drinking behavior on college campuses by confronting students with evidence that their drinking is abnormally high when compared to peers (Perkins & Berkowitz, 1986). Social norms interventions may vary from social marketing campaigns that present data to campuses through a variety of media in public forums about what normative alcohol use is on campus (e.g., Gomberg, Schneider, & DeJong, 2001) to more individualized interventions comparing individual alcohol use to drinking patterns of college peers (e.g., Agostinelli, Brown, & Miller, 1995), and can be completed with a therapist, on a computer, or on the Internet.

Research on the efficacy of social norms as a standalone intervention has produced mixed results (Clapp, Lange, Russel, Shillington, & Voas, 2003; Perkins & Craig, 2006; Stamper, Smith, Gant, & Bogle, 2004; Wechsler et al., 2003). Two different classes of norms seem to influence drinking behavior: descriptive norms, in which students compare their drinking with the perceived consumption patterns of peers, and injunctive norms, in which students compare personal drinking with what they perceive to be peer group dictates for normative drinking behavior (Carey, Borsari, Carey, & Maisto, 2006). Intervening upon descriptive norms may be effective but inconsistent methodologies in these studies make the interpretation of results difficult (Borsari & Carey, 2001; Lewis & Neighbors, 2006).

Alcohol Skills Training Program (ASTP), Lifestyle Management Classes, and Brief Alcohol Screening and Intervention for College Students (BASICS)

Several evidence-based interventions targeting college student drinking behavior incorporate cognitive-behavioral change strategies in addition to assessment and personalized feedback. The Alcohol Skills Training Program (ASTP), originally conducted as an eight-session program (Fromme, Marlatt, Baer, & Kivlahan, 1994; Kivlahan, Marlatt, Fromme, Coppel, & Williams, 1990), has been found to be effective in a two-session format (e.g., Miller, 1999). ASTP also has been used successfully among Spanish-speaking college students (Hernandez et al., 2006). Lifestyle Management Classes (Fromme & Corbin, 2004; Fromme & Orrick, 2004) emphasize broader objectives of personal growth and empowerment by teaching skills to manage desires to participate in a variety of risky behaviors and learning from risky drinking experiences.

Common elements in these interventions include normative feedback, evidence-based cognitive modification strategies (e.g., expectancy and drinking myth challenges), the use of motivational interviewing techniques, and education about the research on consequences (i.e., physical, psychological, and social) of moderate versus heavy alcohol use. In addition, these programs teach harm reduction techniques as well as drink refusal and assertiveness skills to decrease the risks of overdrinking and subsequent consequences, how to calculate blood alcohol levels by means of weight- and gender-adjusted charts that are often provided in the manual and on a wallet-sized card, as well as self-monitoring of drinking events between sessions.

Brief Alcohol Screening and Intervention for College Students (BASICS; Dimeff, Baer, Kivlahan, & Marlatt, 1999) is an evidence-based two-session program that intervenes upon college student drinking behavior (Baer, Kivlahan, Blume, McKnight, & Marlatt, 2001). The format is similar to the one used in the Drinkers Check-up (Miller et al., 1988); motivational interviewing is used to enhance the therapeutic alliance and promote change, and assessment and feedback are used to develop discrepancy and enhance the change process. If warranted, BASICS may use the cognitive-behavioral strategies mentioned above that are part of ASTP.

Evidence-Based Therapy

In addition to brief interventions, many evidence-based therapies have been developed in the cognitive-behavioral therapy model and are described subsequently. Following review of cognitive-behavioral therapies, Twelve-Step Facilitation Therapy is discussed, followed by interventions targeting relationships and environmental factors that influence drinking behavior.

Stimulus Control, Cue Exposure, and Response Management Therapists use stimulus control methods with clients, such as emptying the home of alcohol and avoiding old drinking friends and favorite bars or taverns, to limit or avoid exposure to cues that may trigger cravings or urges to drink alcohol (e.g., Marlatt, 1985). However, many drinking-related cues in the environment cannot be avoided or even anticipated. Under these conditions, exposure to those cues under controlled conditions may be a useful strategy in learning to cope effectively in their presence. Cue exposure draws upon the rich tradition of exposure therapy that has been found to be extremely effective in extinguishing anxiety, worry, and fear responses (e.g., Barlow, Raffa, & Cohen, 2002). Cue exposure targets a variety of stimuli paired with alcohol consumption including situations or items that generate cravings for alcohol as well as tastes and smells associated with alcohol consumption. Therapists also teach clients effective ways to cope with exposure to cues and cravings without drinking. Homework assignments can be used to generalize the skills to real-world exposure to drinking cues.

Cue exposure that involves tasting alcohol has been controversial among those who have postulated client loss of control when consuming alcohol, but several cue exposure trials that included tasting have been associated with reduced consumption of alcohol (Drummond & Glautier, 1994; Monti et al., 1993; Rohsenow et al., 2001). Conklin and Tiffany (2002) have challenged the efficacy of cue exposure for substance abuse, but their meta-analysis included cue exposure studies for a variety of substances. The four longitudinal studies cited by the authors that tested cue exposure for alcohol problems all showed positive outcomes. Current evidence suggests that cue exposure can be an effective means to intervene upon alcohol problems regardless of their severity (Dawe, Rees, Mattick, Sitharthan, & Heather, 2002).

Coping Skills Project MATCH, a large-scale study funded by the National Institute on Alcohol Abuse and Alcoholism (NIAAA; Project MATCH, 1998), found that three highly regarded therapies to intervene upon alcohol problems showed evidence of being effective. One of the three modalities tested in this study was Cognitive-Behavioral Coping Skills Therapy, a manualized therapy conducted over 12 sessions (Kadden et al., 1999). Coping skills therapy, designed to strengthen client competence and confidence to respond skillfully to achieve their treatment goals and avoid temptations of alcohol use, includes instruction on craving management, drink refusal, assertiveness training, emotion management, and life skills training, as well as techniques for problem solving and cognitive modification. Craving management skills teach clients how to use distraction techniques such as ceasing current behavior and switching to a new activity, thought-stopping techniques, counting activities (such as number of breaths), or engaging in a highly structured intellectual or physically taxing task that keeps the mind occupied. Engaging in pleasurable activities without opportunities to drink, such as relaxation training, meditation, or physical exercise, also can be helpful.

Drink refusal skills teach clients how to avoid drinking in situations where alcohol may be present or where there may be peer pressure to drink. Assertiveness training, related to drink refusal, teaches clients to effectively ask for what they need from others. Emotion management skills (e.g., anger management) help clients negotiate emotional extremes without drinking. Teaching life skills helps clients to handle everyday problems and satisfy basic needs such as maintaining employment and managing budgets.

Clients also learn to modify interpretation of life situations, unrealistic expectations (including alcohol expectancies), thoughts about cravings, and decision-making processes. Problem-solving skills are taught to aid clients in negotiating difficult situations without drinking, prioritize life goals, and formulate plans to reach those goals. The therapy also includes relapse prevention (described later in the chapter). Homework encourages skillset generalization to real-world situations (Kadden et al., 1999).

Contingency Management Contingency management uses behavioral contracts that specify expectations and rewards for meeting expectations to modify behavior. Behaviors targeted include adhering to and completing therapy, engaging in appropriate social interactions, adhering to medication regimens, reducing alcohol consumption, and maintaining longer abstinence after completion of therapy (Higgins & Petry, 1999; Petry, 2000; Petry, Martin, Cooney, & Kranzler, 2000). Potential reinforcers include cash, vouchers for goods or services during treatment, and drawings for cash or vouchers.

Behavioral Economics Behavioral economics (see Chapter 27) conceptualizes alcohol use as a function of access (availability), use of limited commodities such as time and money, and operant conditioning principles. If drinking activities are accessible, a beneficial use of time and money, and reinforcing, then an individual will likely choose to engage in these activities (Bickel, Madden, & Petry, 1998; Vuchinich & Tucker, 1988). Conversely, time-consuming nondrinking activities that are reinforcing (Murphy, Correia, Colby, & Vuchinich, 2005), facilitating changes in spending habits (Tucker, Vuchinich, Black, & Rippens, 2006), or manipulating beverage prices (Murphy & MacKillop, 2006) appear to influence alcohol consumption.

Expectancy Challenges   Challenging alcohol expectancies has been shown to lead to reduced alcohol use (Darkes & Goldman, 1998). Positive alcohol expectancies are challenged by placing clients in socially and sexually stimulating situations while drinking alcohol or a placebo beverage using a balanced placebo design (Marlatt, Demming, & Reid, 1973) in which clients are blinded to whether the drink contains alcohol. The client reports expectancies of the drinking event before consuming the beverages. Later, those expectancies are contrasted by drinking condition in order to provide data on whether the expected effects of drinking were in fact experienced while drinking and whether the placebo condition provided positive experiences errantly attributed to alcohol (Darkes & Goldman, 1993). Cognitive modification methods such as data collection and hypothesis testing can be used to challenge expected drinking results in real-world conditions. However, it is unclear whether it is more helpful to reduce positive expectancies or increase those that are negative (Jones et al., 2001).

Relapse Prevention   Relapse prevention is an evidence-based practice (Carroll, 1996; Irvin, Bowers, Dunn, & Wang, 1999; McCrady, 2000) intended to promote maintenance of behavior change. The initial relapse model proposed by Marlatt (1985) posited that relapses occur in a predictable linear chain of events, but recent research suggests that events preceding relapse are dynamic rather than linear and involve risk factors such as family history, symptom severity, and withdrawal symptoms that influence subsequent cognitions and behavior (Marlatt & Witkiewitz, 2005). Relapse prevention incorporates many cognitive-behavioral change strategies including self-monitoring, assessment of relapse patterns including context and emotions associated with events, assessment of relapse fantasies and alcohol expectancies, cognitive restructuring to modify beliefs related to drinking, and meditation to foster acceptance. Relapse prevention can reduce the likelihood of use of alcohol or moderate relapses.

Relapse chains often begin in the context of lifestyle imbalances or apparently irrelevant decisions that may cause vulnerability to risky circumstances. Lifestyle imbalances occur when a client engages in certain activities excessively that diminish the ability to engage in other healthy and perhaps necessary activities. Apparently irrelevant decisions place a client in a risky situation where he or she may be tempted to return to alcohol use. Risky situations may include the experience of extreme emotional states, interpersonal or environmental stressors, or personal conflict (Marlatt, 1996). Often, clients are unaware of or tend to underestimate the level of risk. Other times, the decisions may reflect a desire by the client to self-indulge (e.g., "I have been doing really well and one drink will not be a problem for me"). Lifestyle imbalances are addressed by use of pleasurable and healthy nondrinking activities and the use of time management strategies to structure balance into daily schedules.

When a client encounters a high-risk situation, the goal of relapse prevention is to empower the client with skills that will enable her to successfully negotiate the situation without returning to alcohol use. Stimulus control may be utilized to aid the client in learning to avoid prolonged exposure to high-risk situations that may lead to temptation. Cue exposure and response prevention are used to teach clients to successfully cope with unavoidable high-risk situations without drinking.

Relapse prevention trains clients to use effective skills, such as drink refusal or assertiveness, to cope successfully without drinking, and to enhance self-efficacy in maintaining treatment gains. Relaxation training and meditation skills, such as focusing on breath and

using urge surfing imagery to ride out cravings, are taught to reduce stress and increase tolerance to environmental stressors. Therapists use role play to assess adequacy of skills and self-
efficacy to succeed in particular high-risk situations and homework to develop confidence
and competence.

If a client does not cope effectively, then the positive expected effects of drinking increase
concurrently with a decrease in self-efficacy to cope without alcohol use. Relapse prevention
teaches clients how to respond effectively when they encounter a crisis. All means are used to
challenge alcohol expectancies in a client and to promote self-efficacy to negotiate high-risk
situations. A relapse plan is developed that in effect provides a roadmap for how to respond
in case of emergency or crisis that threatens therapeutic gains and goals. The plan, written on
a wallet-sized card, serves as a reminder to the client about what to do in the event of a crisis.
The therapist and client jointly identify warning signs of an impending crisis so that the client
learns cues (i.e., past relapse triggers and apparently irrelevant decisions) to prompt implementation of the emergency plan. The client and therapist practice identifying the warning
signs and utilizing the plan in session to make client responses habitual prior to the experience
of a crisis. A relapse contract may be included as an agreement that client and therapist are
committed to act in specific ways should a lapse or relapse occur. The therapist may conduct
rehearsal drills in session to see if the client utilizes the relapse plan effectively.

If the client does experience a lapse, a common response is to feel angry, guilty, or ashamed,
referred to as an abstinence or goal violation effect. Relapse prevention attempts to circumvent
this negative emotional response by teaching that relapses are normative and informative,
providing clues on how to improve the relapse prevention plans (Marlatt, 1985). The goal is to
avoid a toxic response that contributes to client resignation and discourages return to maintenance of previous behavior change, and to promote a return to therapeutic goals as quickly as
possible by moderating the duration and severity of alcohol use.

Harm Reduction Strategies   Harm reduction strategies do not require abstinence as a precondition for receiving therapy and are used to reduce the risk of aversive consequences among
clients (Marlatt, 1998). Therapy is focused on aiding clients in meeting self-determined
drinking goals. In support of this effort, clients self-monitor drinking behavior in order to
provide a clear picture of the baseline presentation (Larimer et al., 1998). Self-monitoring
provides data on changes that can be made to reduce the harmful consequences associated
with alcohol use and to allow clients to make an informed choice about goals for alcohol use.
The therapist provides advice when requested and works with the client to plan how to reach
the client's goals.

Harm reduction utilizes a variety of behavior modification strategies aimed at lowering
the risks of alcohol abuse that can be built into the change plan. For example, harm reduction plans often involve structuring time in such a way that it precludes the use of substances
(Blume & Marlatt, 2003). Time management skills may be taught in order to facilitate this
effort. Alternative activities that preclude the possibility of drinking are encouraged and structured into the client's daily schedule (Blume, Anderson, Fader, & Marlatt, 2001). Clients may
be encouraged to switch from hard liquor to wine or beer or from high alcohol content malt
liquors or specialty beers to lower alcohol content beer to reduce the ethanol per drink being
consumed.

A related strategy is to encourage alternating alcoholic beverages with nonalcoholic beverages, for example, drinking a full glass of water after drinking a beer and finishing the water prior to drinking another beer. Eating food between sips is also an effective method for slowing and reducing the consumption of alcohol. Tapering the amounts of alcohol consumed also may be suggested if the client goal is reduction (Blume & Marlatt, 2003). The tapering process allows a stepwise and gradual reduction in drinking that may prevent extreme discomfort when compared to complete immediate cessation. Controlling the size of drinks through measured reductions and sipping of drinks rather than gulping can aid efforts to taper amounts consumed. Another strategy is to limit access to alcoholic beverages. One idea is to reduce ease of access by keeping only small amounts of alcohol in the home, perhaps linked to daily drinking goals, rather than stockpiling beverages. This encourages daily shopping trips to buy the daily allotments that in effect make drinking inconvenient (Blume et al., 2001). Harm reduction therapists will often recommend a period of cessation commonly referred to as trial abstinence (Blume & Marlatt, 2003). The rationale for such a recommendation is to allow the body time to heal itself while lowering tolerance levels to alcohol. Many clients will commit to a time-limited period of trial abstinence and find benefits they had not imagined. Some clients may return to drinking after abstinence but often at more modest levels.

Many cognitive-behavioral strategies used in relapse prevention (Larimer & Marlatt, 1990) can be used effectively in harm reduction to help clients meet their goals. Distress management skills that include urge surfing and other tolerance strategies (Marlatt & Witkiewitz, 2005) and meditation (Marlatt & Kristeller, 1999) may be used to aid clients in meeting treatment goals. In addition, pharmacotherapy (see Chapter 28) is often used in harm reduction in conjunction with behavior modification. Medications are used to control cravings and withdrawal symptoms during tapers from alcohol use. In addition, psychotropic and mood-stabilizing medications can aid clients with co-occurring disorders in reducing drinking once psychiatric symptoms are managed.

Twelve-Step Facilitation Therapy   Although 12-step-based counseling has been the standard of care in the United States for many years, the development and testing of Twelve-Step Facilitation Therapy in Project MATCH represented the first sincere effort to codify a 12-step therapy and test it scientifically (Nowinski, Baker, & Carroll, 1995). The study found that the therapy compared favorably to both Cognitive-Behavioral Coping Skills Therapy and Motivational Enhancement Therapy in intervening on alcohol abuse (Project MATCH Research Group, 1998). The 12-session Twelve-Step Facilitation Therapy incorporates many principles from Alcoholics Anonymous (AA) including completion of Steps 1–3 and accompanying sessions on acceptance of powerlessness over alcohol and surrender to a higher power that can restore balance and sanity, work on becoming involved in AA and other community-based sobriety activities, and optional units focused upon alcohol dependence as a family disease.

Many treatment centers still do not specifically use the Twelve-Step Facilitation Therapy. Because Twelve-Step Facilitation Therapy has been developed with a manual to guide therapist activities, it can be conducted much more consistently than 12-step counseling conducted without a manual. Facilities operating under the 12-step model certainly would enhance their level of care by using the scientifically validated Project MATCH-tested therapy manual.

Relationship and Environmental Interventions Behavioral couples therapy (BCT) and behavioral marital therapy (BMT) have been associated with reduced drinking (Maisto, McKay, & O'Farrell, 1998; Walitzer & Dermen, 2004) and improvement in partner interactions, fewer negative consequences (Fals-Stewart, Birchler, & Kelley, 2006), improved psychosocial adjustment of children (Kelley & Fals-Stewart, 2002), and reduced intimate partner violence (O'Farrell, Murphy, Stephan, Fals-Stewart, & Murphy, 2004; O'Farrell, Van Hutton, & Murphy, 1999) as well as increased positive relationship functioning (Maisto et al., 1998).

Targeting environmental factors (see also Chapter 11) that influence the drinking behavior of clients also can be quite effective, even if the client is not fully engaged in therapy. For example, the Community Reinforcement Approach (CRA) is an evidence-based practice that intervenes upon reinforcement systems in order to make abstinence or moderate drinking more rewarding than disordered drinking (Hunt & Azrin, 1973; Meyers & Smith, 1995; Meyers, Villanueva, & Smith, 2005). Treatment components include functional analysis to identify antecedents to and consequences of alcohol use, trial abstinence, behavioral and occupational skills training, social and recreational counseling, relapse prevention, and relationship counseling. Community Reinforcement and Family Training enlists family members and concerned friends and peers to shape the client's drinking behavior (Meyers & Smith, 1997).

Multisystemic therapy (MST; Swenson, Henggeler, Taylor, & Addison, 2005) stems from social-ecological theory emphasizing the transactional nature of an adolescent's relationship with his or her environment (Bronfenbrenner, 1979). MST has been used to reduce alcohol consumption among youth involved in the criminal justice system (Henggeler et al., 2006; Henggeler, Pickrel, & Brondino, 1999). MST intervenes on a youth's home life, school, neighborhoods, and workplace in order to modify systems of interactions. MST typically consists of 20–30 sessions lasting 4–6 months.

Individualizing Alcohol Therapy to Serve Diverse Clientele

Treatment Matching Clinical evidence suggests that individualized treatment contributes to successful outcomes, and treatment matching arguably is a systematic method for individualizing care. Interestingly, research studies that have tested treatment matching have found little support for their matching hypotheses (Ouimette, Finney, Gima, & Moos, 1999; Project MATCH Research Group, 1998). However, these studies randomly assigned clients to a therapy and subsequently examined how clients with certain characteristics did within those therapies, rather than an intentional (nonrandom) assignment to a therapy based on client characteristics. Because of the methodological controls employed by the studies, actual matching of individual clients to therapies was not done. In fairness to investigators of matching studies, true treatment matching would be extraordinarily difficult to test in large controlled trials.

Research findings have suggested that matching change strategies to a client's level of motivation to change may enhance the change process (e.g., Perz, DiClemente, & Carbonari, 1996). Project MATCH tested whether readiness to change measures would predict better outcomes in one of the three therapies but no significant long-term relationships between these measures and specific therapy outcomes were found (Project MATCH Research Group, 1998). However, Project MATCH did not specifically assign clients according to their stage of change to specific intervention strategies, but rather randomly assigned clients to therapy and then tested whether motivation to change was associated with positive outcomes in those therapies. One interesting study that linked clients' stages of change with their preference for treatment strategies found evidence that clients prefer the stage-matched interventions proposed by Transtheoretical Model theorists (Giovazolias & Davis, 2005). Individualizing therapy according to client motivation to change seems to be a prudent course.

Culturally Relevant Treatment   Mortality due to behaviors related to alcohol abuse, such as acts of violence toward others or self, physical trauma, or liver diseases is quite high among some minority populations when compared to Whites in the United States (National Center for Injury Prevention and Control, 2007). However, great disparities between treatment need and rates of access and utilization among these high-risk ethnic groups has been documented (NIAAA, 2001). An implicit assumption has been made by researchers that evidence-based therapy developed for use among majority populations will be transportable and effective among ethnic minority communities but little research has been conducted in those communities to test these assumptions (e.g., Blume & Escobedo, 2005). However, evidence exists that minority groups have different responses to well-established treatment practices and utilize different methods for drinking reduction than Whites (e.g., Arroyo, Miller, & Tonigan, 2003; Arroyo, Westerberg, & Tonigan, 1998; Flores, 1986; Tonigan, 2003). Furthermore, controlled intervention trials for alcohol problems may be excluding members of minority groups at disproportionately high rates, raising concerns about generalizability to those populations (Humphreys, 2000).

Basic assumptions behind the beliefs of transportability and effectiveness are flawed. Socialization of minority clients may occur in cultures where majority culture assumptions do not operate. Psychological constructs described and assessed in majority culture (e.g., self-efficacy or autonomy) may not be the same or even exist in minority cultures (see Blume, Morera, & García de la Cruz, 2005, for a comprehensive review in this area). In addition, the life experiences of minority clients may be fundamentally different from those of the majority. Many minority clients face prejudice, discrimination, and racism, which in turn have been linked to greater psychological problems including alcohol abuse (Carter, 1994; Wingo, 2001). These concerns extend to sexual minority clients who often face widespread prejudice including in therapy (Cochran, 2004).

To address these concerns, successful alcohol treatment for minority clients often includes traditional cultural, spiritual, and healing practices commonly practiced within the community being served to make it more culturally relevant. As an example, therapy for alcohol problems among American Indians and Alaska Native communities may use sweat ceremonies and other traditional activities linked to community identity (Abbott, 1998; Marlatt et al., 2003). Development of culturally enhanced evidence-based therapy requires great sensitivity to history, traditions, and language in addition to appropriate use of evidence-based strategies (e.g., Andrés, Wagner, & Tubman, 2004). Including community stakeholders in the development, implementation, and dissemination of culturally relevant therapy is necessary to ensure that client and community values are protected (e.g., Hernandez et al., 2006; Marlatt et al., 2003).

Clients with Co-occurring Disorders   Recent national data have estimated that 5.2 million adults in the United States have co-occurring substance abuse and another psychological disorder but less than 9% of these adults have received treatment targeting both or multiple disorders

(Substance Abuse and Mental Health Services Administration, 2006). Clients with alcohol problems and co-occurring psychological disorders often have poorer treatment outcomes and higher relapse rates (McCarthy et al., 2005; Tomlinson, Brown, & Abrantes, 2004). Evidence-based practices for treating co-occurring disorders have included cognitive-behavioral therapy (e.g., Moak et al., 2003) or motivational interviewing (e.g., Martino, Carroll, Nich, & Rounsaville, 2006) combined with psychiatric medications. Clients with co-occurring disorders may benefit from extended stepped-up care that provides intensive services to address their multiple needs.

Theoretically speaking, using a combination of therapies that show evidence of improving outcomes for each of the presenting disorders may be helpful. For example, with clients who have co-occurring anxiety and alcohol problems, use of evidence-based practices for anxiety in conjunction with evidence-based practices for alcohol should in theory be helpful for a client who presents with both problems (Kushner et al., 2006). However, the research evidence supporting the use of such combinations is limited and has produced mixed results (e.g., Bowen, D'Arcy, Keegan, & Senthilselvan, 2000; Schadé et al., 2005). In spite of the mixed findings, clinical expertise suggests that effectively treating clients with co-occurring disorders should incorporate evidence-based practices with concurrent use of medications that have been found to be effective in the treatment of the disorders in question.

Case Presentation

Jason is an 18-year-old American Indian male who presented for therapy after concerns were expressed by his mother for his well-being and safety. In addition to his mother, he lives with his two brothers and his maternal grandmother. At intake, he reported binge drinking alcohol three to four times a week for the last six months with a small group of peers. He also occasionally smokes marijuana and uses peyote.

At intake, Jason was experiencing academic problems related to his drinking and was in danger of dropping out of high school. This is a radical change because he had been on the honor roll for every semester prior to the current one. He attends a high school that includes both American Indian and Caucasian students, and sometimes there is tension between the different groups. He also reports having been detained by tribal police for drunken behavior along with his friends, but released after being escorted home. He argues with his mother when drinking but the pattern of belligerence does not persist when he is sober. Recently he drove his mother's car off the road into an arroyo and smashed the headlights and front end of the car so it would not drive. He experienced a few cuts on his face and forehead that looked worse than they were and was able to walk the four miles home, leaving the disabled car behind. His mother was very distraught to see Jason with blood all over his face and hair, which caused Jason to feel very badly. Because the car was disabled, Jason's mother had to walk to work (three miles) for the past several weeks. Jason's grandmother has recently expressed her displeasure over his behavior, telling Jason he is letting his family down with his drinking and setting bad examples for his brothers, and suggesting he talk to a community spiritual leader.

Jason also reports feeling very depressed and hopeless, with suicidal ideations daily but with no concrete or proximal plan in place. His father committed suicide when Jason was in middle school, and one of Jason's cousins attempted suicide without success in the last year. He thinks about both of those events when he is drinking and tries to kill the thoughts by drinking more. Although Jason thinks about suicide, he also expresses hope that he could some day go to a local tribal college and help his mother financially after graduation. Because he is quite bright and has a history of good academic performance previous to this year, it seems likely that Jason would achieve the goal of enrolling in college if he reduced drinking and improved his grades.

As Jason's therapist, you would want to take into consideration several important factors as you developed a treatment plan. Jason's age makes it likely that traditional treatment efforts that work for some older adults will not be successful with him. For example, 12-step therapies are not typically appealing or effective with young adults and adolescents who do not feel powerless over drinking. He also may not be receptive to the idea of the need for changing his drinking behavior, so the initial stages of therapy at the least should utilize strategies that will address ambivalence about behavior change. Many adolescents and young adults have not experienced the depth of consequences that adults have and as a result usually are not necessarily aware of the need for change or highly motivated to change. A comprehensive behavioral analysis will yield important information about the context, function, and reinforcement history of the drinking episodes. His therapist will also want to assess whether Jason has experienced racism and prejudice in school and if these experiences have played a part in his drinking, as well as the relationship of depression and alcohol abuse.

In addition, addressing Jason's drinking behavior will require use of culturally relevant practices. Respecting his culture and the importance of his family in the treatment process will be critical to overall success. Jason's depression also will be important to treat, and this will require a creative approach that merges evidence-based practices to treat alcohol problems with evidence-based practices to treat depression.

The initial stages of therapy would use motivational interviewing to help Jason explore his ambivalence about his current pattern of alcohol use and its relationship to a number of recent critical events. Use of the BASICS intervention model of assessment and personalized feedback would be potentially effective to reduce drinking behavior if used in conjunction with traditional tribal spiritual healing practices. Jason's therapist will want to collaborate with the tribal healer as much as possible in order to ensure sensitivity to the cultural practices of the tribal community. As an example, a therapist would want to consider whether the use of peyote is part of the spiritual practices of the community and tribal healers could provide this information. The therapist would want to include the extended family in therapy as much as possible if the client and family were willing, because family support will be critical to his success.

When it is clear that Jason is committed to behavior change, therapy will shift to use of cognitive-behavioral therapy change strategies, using motivational interviewing to enhance commitment to change when needed. He will likely need to learn drink refusal skills including assertiveness, and emotion regulation skills to deal with anger and depression. Structuring his time with alternative nondrinking activities would be useful as would cue exposure techniques related to encounters with friends and the availability of alcohol. He will benefit from role play in session and practice of these new skills between sessions as part of homework assignments. If it is clear that Jason will not abstain from alcohol and the other substances, then it will be helpful to include harm reduction goals and strategies.

Concurrently, the therapist will also want to use empirically based therapy for depression, which may include adjunct pharmacotherapy if deemed necessary after consultation with a physician. The use of pharmacotherapy will depend greatly upon his response to the cognitive-behavioral therapy for depression to moderate his suicidal ideations and increase behavioral activity and mood. Another method to consider is to intervene on the environmental systems that may be contributing to stress and depression in Jason's life, and potentially intervening on those systems by use of CRA or MST to shape Jason's drinking behavior and reduce environmental stressors, including from interactions at school and in the family.

Depending upon the goals for drinking reduction, relapse prevention methods will be used with Jason to encourage maintenance of gains in therapy, and to promote further improvements in quality of life after termination. Relapse prevention methods will work well to maintain changes in drinking behavior as well as encourage reduction in depressive symptoms and suicidal ideations. If abstinence is not a realistic outcome for Jason, then relapse prevention strategies can be used to promote management of moderate substance use over the long-term. Therapy would likely include booster sessions after termination in order to check up on progress and modify the relapse prevention plan if necessary. The net result is that Jason has been provided with quality care that respected his culture, his treatment goals, and his own personal values. Because of the use of culturally relevant evidence-based practices, he overcame his depression and moderated his drinking, eventually enrolling in the local tribal college.

Conclusions

Providing evidence-based therapy for alcohol problems begins with comprehensive assessment using validated measures. A variety of evidence-based interventions exists to treat alcohol problems after needs have been assessed (please see Table 12.1 for more information about evidence-based resources). The use of evidence-based therapy ensures that clients receive the highest quality care. Clinical expertise allows therapists to individualize care in order to meet

| TABLE 12.1 |
| Resources for the Assessment and Treatment of Alcohol Use Disorders |

Resources

1. Alcohol—Problems and Solutions: http://www2.potsdam.edu/hansondj/index.html.
2. Alcoholics Anonymous: http://www.alcoholics-anonymous.org.
3. Daley, D. C., & Marlatt, G. A. (2006). *Overcoming your alcohol or drug problem: Effective recovery strategies.* New York: Oxford University Press.
4. Marlatt, G. A. (2002). *Harm reduction: Pragmatic strategies for managing high-risk behaviors.* New York: Guilford Press.
5. Marlatt, G. A., & Donovan, D. M. (2007). *Relapse prevention: Maintenance strategies in the treatment of addictive behaviors* (2nd ed.). New York: Guilford Press.
6. Monti, P. M., Kadden, R. M., Rohsenow, D. J., & Cooney, N. L. (2002). *Treating alcohol dependence: A coping skills training guide.* New York: Guilford Press.
7. National Institute on Alcohol Abuse and Alcoholism: http://www.niaaa.nih.gov/.
8. Project MATCH Materials: http://pubs.niaaa.nih.gov/publications/match.htm.
9. Rotgers, F., & Davis, B. A. (2006). *Treating alcohol problems.* New York: John Wiley.
10. Research Society on Alcoholism: http://www.rsoa.org/.
11. Sobell, M. B. (1987). *Moderation as a goal or outcome of treatment for alcohol problems.* New York: Haworth Press.

specific needs of clients and act effectively even when evidence-based practices for presenting problems are absent or inconclusive. Respecting client values in general will likely enhance the therapeutic alliance which in turn may improve outcomes. A client may be more likely to be motivated when working with a therapist who shows visible evidence of acceptance and compassion. In addition, respecting the cultural values and special needs of minority clients and clients with co-occurring disorders is essential to successful outcomes.

An important next step for addiction science is to study relationships among evidence-based change strategies, clinical expertise, and client values. Understanding these relationships may provide guidance on how to effectively match care with client needs, increasing the likelihood of positive outcomes in therapy for clients that present with increasingly diverse and complex problems associated with alcohol misuse.

References

Abbott, P. J. (1998). Traditional and Western healing practices for alcoholism in American Indians and Alaska Natives. *Substance Use & Misuse, 33,* 2605–2646.

Agostinelli, G., Brown, J. M., & Miller, W. R. (1995). Effects of normative feedback on consumption among heavy drinking college students. *Journal of Drug Education, 25,* 31–40.

American Psychiatric Association. (1994). *Diagnostic and statistical manual of mental disorders* (4th ed.). Washington, DC: Author.

Andrés, G. G., Wagner, E. F., & Tubman, J. G. (2004). Culturally sensitive substance abuse intervention for Hispanic and African American adolescents: Empirical examples from the Alcohol Treatment Targeting Adolescents in Need (ATTAIN) Project. *Addiction, 99 (S2),* 140–150.

Arroyo, J. A., Miller, W. R., & Tonigan, J. S. (2003). The influence of Hispanic ethnicity on long-term outcome in three alcohol-treatment modalities. *Journal of Studies on Alcohol, 64,* 98–104.

Arroyo, J. A., Westerberg, V. S., & Tonigan, J. S. (1998). Comparison of treatment utilization and outcome for Hispanics and non-Hispanic Whites. *Journal of Studies on Alcohol, 59,* 286–291.

Babor, T. F. (1996). The classification of alcoholics: Typology theories from the 19th century to the present. *Alcohol Health & Research World, 20,* 6–17.

Babor, T. F., Higgins-Biddle, J., Dauser, D., Higgins, P., & Burleson, J. A. (2005). Alcohol screening and brief intervention in primary care settings: Implementation models and predictors. *Journal of Studies on Alcohol, 66,* 361–368.

Baer, J. S., Kivlahan, D. R., Blume, A. W., McKnight, P., & Marlatt, G. A. (2001). Brief intervention for heavy drinking college students: Four-year follow-up and natural history. *American Journal of Public Health, 91,* 1310–1316.

Barlow, D. H., Raffa, S. D., & Cohen, E. M. (2002). Psychosocial treatments for panic disorders, phobias, and generalized anxiety disorder. In P. E. Nathan & J. M. Gorman (Eds.), *A guide to treatments that work* (2nd ed., pp. 301–335). New York: Oxford Press.

Bates, M. E., Pawlak, A. P., Tonigan, J. S., & Buckman, J. F. (2006). Cognitive impairment influences drinking outcome by altering therapeutic mechanisms of change. *Psychology of Addictive Behaviors, 20,* 241–253.

Bickel, W. K., Madden, G. J., & Petry, N. M. (1998). The price of change: The behavioral economics of drug consumption. *Behavior Therapy, 29,* 545–565.

Blume, A. W., Anderson, B. K., Fader, J. S., & Marlatt, G. A. (2001). Harm reduction programs: Progress rather than perfection. In R. H. Coombs (Ed.), *Addiction recovery tools: A practical handbook.* Thousand Oaks, CA: Sage.

Blume, A. W., & Escobedo, C. (2005). Best practices for substance abuse treatment among American Indians and Alaska Natives: Review and critique. In E. H. Hawkins & R. D. Walker (Eds.), *Best practices in behavioral health services for American Indians and Alaska Natives,* (pp. 77–93). Portland, OR: One Sky National Resource Center for American Indian and Alaska Native Substance Abuse Prevention and Treatment Services.

Blume, A. W., & Marlatt, G. A. (2003). Harm reduction. In W. O'Donohue, J. E. Fisher, & S. C. Hayes (Eds.), *Cognitive behavior therapy: Applying empirically supported techniques in your practice* (pp. 196–201). New York: John Wiley & Sons.

Blume, A. W., Morera, O. F., & García de la Cruz, B. (2005). Assessment of addictive behaviors in ethnic-minority populations. In D. M. Donovan & G. A. Marlatt (Eds.), *Assessment of addictive behaviors* (2nd ed., pp. 49–70). New York: Guilford Press.

Borsari, B., & Carey, K. B. (2001). Peer influences on college drinking: A review of the literature. *Journal of Substance Abuse, 13,* 391–424.

Bowen, R. C., D'Arcy, C., Keegan, D. & Senthilselvan, A. (2000). A controlled trial of cognitive behavioral treatment of panic in alcoholic inpatients with comorbid panic disorder. *Addictive Behaviors, 25,* 593–597.

Bowman, K. M., & Jellinek, E. M. (1941). Alcohol addiction and its treatment. *Quarterly Journal of Studies on Alcohol, 2,* 98–176.

Bradizza, C. M., Stasiewicz, P. R., & Paas, N. D. (2006). Relapse to alcohol and drug use among individuals diagnosed with co-occurring disorders: A review. *Clinical Psychology Review, 26,* 162–178.

Bronfenbrenner, U. (1979). *The ecology of human development: Experiments by nature and design.* Cambridge, MA: Harvard University Press.

Carey, K. B., Borsari, B., Carey, M. P., & Maisto, S. A. (2006). Patterns and importance of self-other differences in college drinking norms. *Psychology of Addictive Behaviors, 20,* 385–393.

Carey, K. B., Carey, M. P., Maisto, S. A., & Henson, J. M. (2006). Brief motivational interventions for heavy college drinkers: A randomized controlled trial. *Journal of Consulting and Clinical Psychology, 74,* 943–954.

Carroll, K. M. (1996). Relapse prevention as a psychosocial treatment: A review of controlled trials. *Experimental and Clinical Psychopharmacology, 4,* 46–54.

Carter, J. H. (1994). Racism's impact on mental health. *Journal of the American Medical Association, 86,* 543–547.

Clapp, J. D., Lange, J. E., Russel, C., Shillington, A., & Voas, R. B. (2003). A failed social norms marketing campaign. *Journal of Studies on Alcohol, 64,* 409–414.

Cochran, B. N. (2004). Sexual minorities in substance abuse treatment: The impact of provider biases and treatment outcomes. Unpublished dissertation, University of Washington.

Cohen, E., Feinn, R., & Arias, A. (2007). Alcohol treatment utilization: Findings from the National Epidemiologic Survey on Alcohol and Related Conditions. *Drug and Alcohol Dependence, 86,* 214–221.

Conklin, C. A., & Tiffany, S. T. (2002). Applying extinction research and theory to cue-exposure addiction treatments. *Addiction, 97,* 155–167.

Cooper, M. L., Frone, M. R., Russell, M., & Mudar, P. (1995). Drinking to regulate positive and negative emotions: A motivational model of alcohol use. *Journal of Personality and Social Psychology, 69,* 990–1005.

Darkes, J., & Goldman, M. S. (1993). Expectancy challenge and drinking reduction: Experimental evidence for a mediational process. *Journal of Consulting and Clinical Psychology, 61,* 344–353.

Darkes, J., & Goldman, M. S. (1998). Expectancy challenge and drinking reduction: Process and structure in the alcohol expectancy network. *Experimental and Clinical Psychopharmacology, 6,* 64–76.

Dawe, S., Rees, V. W., Mattick, R., Sitharthan, T., & Heather, N. (2002). Efficacy of moderation-oriented cue exposure for problem drinkers: A randomized controlled trial. *Journal of Consulting and Clinical Psychology, 70,* 1045–1050.

Dimeff, L. A., Baer, J. S., Kivlahan, D. R., & Marlatt, G. A. (1999). *Brief alcohol screening and intervention for college students (BASICS): A harm reduction approach.* New York: Guilford Press.

Drummond, D. C., & Glautier, S. (1994). A controlled trial of cue exposure treatment in alcohol dependence. *Journal of Consulting and Clinical Psychology, 62,* 809–817.

Epstein, E. E., Drapkin, M. L., Yusko, D. A., Cook, S. M., McCrady, B. S., & Jensen, N. K. (2005). Is alcohol assessment therapeutic? Pretreatment change in drinking among alcohol-dependent women. *Journal of Studies on Alcohol, 66,* 369–378.

Fals-Stewart, W., Birchler, G. R., & Kelley, M. L. (2006). Learning sobriety together: A randomized clinical trial examining behavioral couples therapy with alcoholic female patients. *Journal of Consulting and Clinical Psychology, 74,* 579–591.

Flores, P. J. (1986). Alcoholism treatment and the relationship of Native American cultural values to recovery. *International Journal of the Addictions, 11–12,* 1707–1726.

Fromme, K., & Corbin, W. (2004). Prevention of heavy drinking and associated negative consequences among mandated and voluntary college students. *Journal of Consulting and Clinical Psychology, 72,* 1038–1049.

Fromme, K., Marlatt, G. A., Baer, J. S., & Kivlahan, D. R. (1994). The alcohol skills training program: A group intervention for young adult drinkers. *Journal of Substance Abuse Treatment, 11,* 143–154.

Fromme, K., & Orrick, D. (2004). The lifestyle management class: A harm reduction approach to college drinking. *Addiction Research and Theory, 12,* 335–351.

Giovazolias, T., & Davis, P. (2005). Matching therapeutic interventions to drug and alcohol abusers' stage of motivation: The clients' perspective. *Counseling Psychology Quarterly, 18,* 171–182.

Gomberg, L., Schneider, S. K., & DeJong, W. (2001). Evaluation of social norms marketing campaign to reduce high-risk drinking at the University of Mississippi. *American Journal of Drug and Alcohol Abuse, 27,* 375–389.

Hasin, D. S., Stinson, F. S., Ogburn, E., & Grant, B. F. (2007). Prevalence, correlates, disability, and comorbidity of *DSM–IV* alcohol abuse and dependence in the United States. *Archives of General Psychiatry, 64,* 830–842.

Heather, N. (1998). Using brief opportunities for change in medical settings. In W. R. Miller & N. Heather (Eds.), *Treating Addictive Behaviors* (2nd ed., pp. 133–147). New York: Plenum Press.

Heather, N., Rollnick, S., & Bell, A. (1993). Predictive validity of the Readiness to Change Questionnaire. *Addiction, 88,* 1667–1677.

Henggeler, S. W., Halliday-Boykins, C. A., Cunningham, P. B., Randall, J., Shapiro, S. B., & Chapman, J. E. (2006). Juvenile drug court: Enhancing outcomes by integrating evidence-based treatments. *Journal of Consulting and Clinical Psychology, 74,* 42–54.

Henggeler, S. W., Pickrel, S. G., & Brondino, M. J. (1999). Multisystemic treatment of substance abusing and dependent delinquents: Outcomes, treatment fidelity, and transportability. *Mental Health Services Research, 1,* 171–184.

Hernandez, D. V., Skewes, M. C., Resor, M. R., Villanueva, M. R., Hanson, B. S., & Blume, A. W. (2006). A pilot test of an alcohol skills training programme for Mexican-American college students. *International Journal of Drug Policy, 17,* 320–328.

Higgins, S. T., & Petry, N. M. (1999). Contingency management: Incentives for sobriety. *Alcohol Research and Health, 23,* 122–127.

Humphreys, K. (2000). Use of exclusion criteria in selecting research subjects and its effect on the generalizability of alcohol treatment outcome studies. *American Journal of Psychiatry, 157,* 588–594.

Hunt, G. M., & Azrin, N. H. (1973). A community-reinforcement approach to alcoholism. *Behaviour Research and Therapy, 11,* 91–104.

Hyman, Z. (2004). Historical interpretations of alcohol use & misuse: Implications for nursing curricula. *Journal of Psychosocial Nursing & Mental Health Services, 42,* 46–57.

Ilgen, M. A., Tiet, Q., Finney, J. W., & Moos, R. H. (2006). Self-efficacy, therapeutic alliance, and alcohol-use disorder treatment outcomes. *Journal of Studies on Alcohol, 67,* 465–472.

Institute of Medicine (1990). *Broadening the base of treatment for alcohol problems.* Washington, DC: National Academy Press.

Irvin, J. E., Bowers, C. A., Dunn, M. E., & Wang, M. C. (1999). Efficacy of relapse prevention: A meta-analytic review. *Journal of Consulting and Clinical Psychology, 67,* 563–570.

Jellinek, E. M. (1960). *The disease concept of alcoholism.* New Haven, CT: College and University Press.

Jones, B. T., Corbin, W., & Fromme, K. (2001). A review of expectancy theory and alcohol consumption. *Addiction, 96,* 57–72.

Kadden, R., Carroll, K., Donovan, D., Cooney, N., Monti, P, Abrams, D., Litt, M., & Hester, R. (1999). *Cognitive-behavioral coping skills therapy manual.* Project MATCH Monograph Series, Vol. 3, M. E. Mattson, (Ed.), Rockville, MD: National Institute on Alcohol Abuse and Alcoholism.

Kelley, M. L., & Fals-Stewart, W. (2002). Couples- versus individual-based therapy for alcohol and drug abuse: Effects on children's psychosocial functioning. *Journal of Consulting and Clinical Psychology, 70,* 417–427.

Kivlahan, D. R., Marlatt, G. A., Fromme, K., Coppel, D. B., & Williams, E. (1990). Secondary prevention with college drinkers: Evaluation of an alcohol skills training program. *Journal of Consulting and Clinical Psychology, 58,* 805–810.

Knight, P. R. (1938). Psychoanalytic treatment in a sanatorium of chronic addiction to alcohol. *Journal of the American Medical Association, 111,* 1443–1448.

Kushner, M. G., Donahue, C., Sletten, S., Thuras, P., Abrams, K., Peterson, J., & Frye, B. (2006). Cognitive behavioral treatment of comorbid anxiety disorder in alcoholism treatment patients: Presentation of a prototype program and future directions. *Journal of Mental Health, 15,* 697–707.

Kypri, K. Saunders, J. B., Williams, S. M., McGee, R. O., Langley, J. D., Cashell-Smith, M. L., & Gallagher, S. J. (2004). Web-based screening and brief intervention for hazardous drinking: A double-blind randomized controlled trial. *Addiction, 99,* 1410–1417.

Larimer, M. E., & Marlatt, G. A. (1990). Applications of relapse prevention with moderation goals. *Journal of Psychoactive Drugs, 22,* 189–195.

Larimer, M. E., Marlatt, G. A., Baer, J. S., Quigley, L. A., Blume, A. W., & Hawkins, E. H. (1998). Harm reduction for alcohol problems: Expanding access to and acceptability of prevention and treatment services. In G. A. Marlatt (Ed.), *Harm reduction: Pragmatic strategies for managing high risk behaviors* (pp. 69–121). New York: Guilford Press.

Lender, M. E. (1979). Jellinek's typology of alcoholism: Some historical antecedents. *Journal of Studies on Alcohol, 40,* 361–375.

Levine, H. G. (1978). The discovery of addiction: Changing conceptions of habitual drunkenness in America. *Journal of Studies on Alcohol, 39,* 143–174.

Lewis, M. A., & Neighbors, C. (2006). Social norms approaches using descriptive norms education: A review of the research on personalized normative feedback. *Journal of American College Health, 54,* 213–218.

Maisto, S. A., McKay, J. R., & O'Farrell, T. J. (1998). Twelve-month abstinence from alcohol and long-term drinking and marital outcomes in men with severe alcohol problems. *Journal of Studies on Alcohol, 59,* 591–598.

Marlatt, G. A. (1983). The controlled drinking controversy: A commentary. *American Psychologist, 38,* 1097–1110.

Marlatt, G. A. (1985). Relapse prevention: Theoretical rationale and overview of the model. In G. A. Marlatt & J. R. Gordon (Eds.), *Relapse prevention: Maintenance strategies in the treatment of addictive behaviors* (1st ed., pp. 3–70). New York: Guilford Press.

Marlatt, G. A. (1996). Taxonomy of high-risk situations for alcohol relapse: Evolution and development of a cognitive-behavioral model. *Addictions, 91(S),* S37–S49.

Marlatt, G. A. (1998). Basic principles and strategies of harm reduction. In G. A. Marlatt (Ed.), *Harm reduction: Pragmatic strategies for managing high risk behaviors* (pp. 49–66). New York: Guilford Press.

Marlatt, G. A., Demming, B., & Reid, J. B. (1973). Loss of control drinking in alcoholics: An experimental analogue. *Journal of Abnormal Psychology, 81,* 223–241.

Marlatt, G. A., & Kristeller, J. (1999). Mindfulness and meditation. In W. R. Miller (Ed.), *Integrating spirituality into treatment.* Washington, DC: American Psychological Association. Marlatt, G. A., Larimer, M. E., Mail, P. D., Hawkins, E. H., Cummins, L. H., Blume, A. W., Lonczak, H. S., Burns, K. M., Chan, K. K., Cronce, J. M., LaMarr, J. Radin, S., Forquera, R., Gonzales, R., Tetrick, C., & Gallion, S. (2003). Journeys of the circle: A culturally congruent life skills intervention for adolescent Indian drinking. *Alcoholism: Clinical and Experimental Research, 27,* 1327–1329.

Marlatt, G. A., & Witkiewitz, K. (2005). Relapse prevention for alcohol and drug problems. In G. A. Marlatt & D. M. Donovan (Eds.), *Relapse prevention: Maintenance strategies in the treatment of addictive behaviors* (2nd ed., pp. 1–44). New York: Guilford Press.

Martino, S., Carroll, K. M., Nich, C., & Rounsaville, B. J. (2006). A randomized controlled pilot study of motivational interviewing for patients with psychotic and drug use disorders. *Addiction, 101,* 1479–1492.

McCarthy, D. M., Tomlinson, K. L., Anderson, K. G., Marlatt, G. A., & Brown, S. A. (2005). Relapse in alcohol- and drug-disordered adolescents with comorbid psychopathology: Changes in psychiatric symptoms. *Psychology of Addictive Behaviors, 19,* 28–34.

McConnaughy, E. A., DiClemente, C. C., Prochaska, J. O., & Velicer, W. F. (1989). Stages of change in psychotherapy: A follow-up report. *Psychotherapy, 26,* 494–503.

McConnaughy, E. A., Prochaska, J. O., & Velicer, W. F. (1983). Stages of change in psychotherapy: Measurement and sample profiles. *Psychotherapy: Theory, Research and Practice, 20*, 368–375.

McCrady, B. S. (2000). Alcohol use disorders and the Division 12 task force of the American Psychological Association. *Psychology of Addictive Behaviors, 14*, 267–276.

Meyers, R. J., & Smith, J. E. (1995). *Clinical guide to alcohol treatment: The community reinforcement approach.* New York: Guilford Press.

Meyers, R. J., & Smith, J. E. (1997). Getting off the fence: Procedures to engage treatment resistant drinkers. *Journal of Substance Abuse Treatment, 14*, 467–472.

Meyers, R. J., Villanueva, M., & Smith, J. E. (2005). The Community Reinforcement Approach: History and new directions. *Journal of Cognitive Psychotherapy, 19*, 247–260.

Miller, E. T. (1999). Preventing alcohol abuse and alcohol-related negative consequences among freshmen college students: Using emerging computer technology to deliver and evaluate the effectiveness of brief intervention efforts. Unpublished doctoral dissertation, University of Washington, Seattle.

Miller, W. R. (1996). *Form 90: A structured interview for drinking and related behaviors.* Project MATCH Monograph Series, Vol. 5, M. E. Mattson, (Ed.), Bethesda, MD: National Institute on Alcohol Abuse and Alcoholism.

Miller, W. R., & Rollnick, S. (2002). *Motivational interviewing* (2nd ed.). New York: Guilford Press.

Miller, W. R., Sovereign, R. G., & Krege, B. (1988). Motivational interviewing with problem drinkers: II. The Drinker's Check-up as a preventive intervention. *Behavioural Psychotherapy, 16*, 251–268.

Miller, W. R., Zweben, A., DiClemente, C. C., & Rychtarik, R. G. (1999). *Motivational enhancement therapy manual: A clinical research guide for therapists treating individual with alcohol abuse and dependence.* Project MATCH Monograph Series, Vol. 2, M. E. Mattson, (Ed.), Rockville, MD: National Institute on Alcohol Abuse and Alcoholism.

Minugh, P. A., Nirenberg, T. D., Clifford, P. R., Longabaugh, R., Becker, B. M., & Woolard, R. (1997). Analysis of alcohol use clusters among subcritically injured emergency department patients. *Academy of Emergency Medicine, 11*, 1059–1067.

Moak, D. H., Anton, R. F., Latham, P. K., Voronin, K. E., Waid, R. L., & Durazo-Arvizu, R. (2003). Sertraline and cognitive behavioral therapy for depressed alcoholics: Results of a placebo-controlled trial. *Journal of Clinical Psychopharmacology, 23*, 553–562.

Monti, P. M., Rohsenow, D. J., Rubonis, A. V., Niaura, R. S., Sirota, A. D., Colby, S. M., Goddard, P., & Abrams, D. B. (1993). Cue exposure coping skills treatment for male alcoholics: A preliminary investigation. *Journal of Consulting and Clinical Psychology, 61*, 1011–1019.

Murphy, J. G., Correia, C. J., Colby, S. M., & Vuchinich, R. E. (2005). Using behavioral theories of choice to predict drinking outcomes following a brief intervention. *Experimental and Clinical Psychopharmacology, 13*, 93–101.

Murphy, J. G., & MacKillop, J. (2006). Relative reinforcing efficacy of alcohol among college student drinkers. *Experimental and Clinical Psychopharmacology, 14*, 219–227.

National Center for Injury Prevention and Control. (2007). 10 leading causes of death, United States. http://webappa.cdc.gov/sasweb/ncipc/leadcaus10.html.

National Institute on Alcohol Abuse and Alcoholism. (2001). *Forecast for the future: Strategic plan to address health disparities.* Bethesda, MD: Author.

Nowinski, J., Baker, S., & Carroll, K. (1995). *Twelve Step Facilitation Therapy Manual.* Project MATCH Monograph Series, Vol. 2, M. E. Mattson (Ed.). Rockville, MD: National Institute on Alcohol Abuse and Alcoholism.

O'Farrell, T. J., Murphy, C. M., Stephan, S. H., Fals-Stewart, W., & Murphy, M. (2004). Partner violence before and after couples-based alcoholism treatment for male alcoholic patients: The role of treatment involvement and abstinence. *Journal of Consulting and Clinical Psychology, 72*, 202–217.

O'Farrell, T. J., Van Hutton, V., & Murphy, C. M. (1999). Domestic violence before and after alcoholism treatment: A two-year longitudinal study. *Journal of Studies on Alcohol, 60*, 317–321.

Ouimette, P. C., Finney, J. W., Gima, K., & Moos, R. H. (1999). A comparative evaluation of substance abuse treatment: III. Examining mechanisms underlying patient-treatment matching hypotheses for 12-step and cognitive-behavioral treatments for substance abuse. *Alcoholism: Clinical and Experimental Research, 23*, 545–551.

Perkins, H. W., & Berkowitz, A. D. (1986). Perceiving the community norms of alcohol use among students: Some research implications for campus alcohol education programming. *International Journal of the Addictions, 21,* 961–976.

Perkins, H. W., & Craig, D. W. (2006). A successful social norms campaign to reduce alcohol misuse among college student-athletes. *Journal of Studies on Alcohol, 67,* 880–889.

Perz, C. A., DiClemente, C. C., & Carbonari, J. P. (1996). Doing the right thing at the right time? The interaction of stages and processes in successful smoking cessation. *Health Psychology, 15,* 462–468.

Petry, N. M. (2000). A comprehensive guide to the application of contingency management procedures in clinical settings. *Drug and Alcohol Dependence, 58,* 9–25.

Petry, N. M., Martin, B., Cooney, J. L., & Kranzler, H. R. (2000). Give them prizes, and they will come: Contingency management for treatment of alcohol dependence. *Journal of Consulting and Clinical Psychology, 68,* 250–257.

Prochaska, J. O., DiClemente, C. C., & Norcross, J. C. (1992). In search of how people change. *American Psychologist, 47,* 1102–1114.

Project MATCH Research Group. (1998). Matching alcoholism treatments to client heterogeneity: Project MATCH three-year drinking outcomes. *Alcoholism: Clinical and Experimental Research, 22,* 1300–1311.

Rohsenow, D. J., Monti, P. M., Rubonis, A. V., Gulliver, S. B., Colby, S. M., Binkoff, J. A., & Abrams, D. B. (2001). Cue exposure coping skills training and communication skills training for alcohol dependence: 6- and 12-month outcomes. *Addiction, 96,* 1161–1174.

Rollnick, S., Heather, N., Gold, R., & Hall, W. (1992). Development of a short 'readiness to change' questionnaire for use in brief, opportunistic interventions among excessive drinkers, *British Journal of Addiction, 87,* 743–754.

Saitz, R., Svilkis, D., D'Onofrio, G., Kraemer, K. L., & Perl, H. (2006). Challenges applying alcohol brief intervention in diverse practice settings: Populations, outcomes, and costs. *Alcoholism: Clinical and Experimental Research, 30,* 332–338.

Schadé, A., Marquenie, L. A., van Balkom, A. J. L. M., Koeter, M. W. J., de Beurs, E., van den Brink, W., & van Dyck, R. (2005). The effectiveness of anxiety treatment on alcohol-dependent patients with a comorbid phobic disorder: A randomized controlled trial. *Alcoholism: Clinical and Experimental Research, 29,* 794–800.

Skog, O. J. (2006). The historical roots of Ledermann's theory of the distribution of alcohol consumption. *Contemporary Drug Problems, 33,* 143–174.

Sobell, L., & Sobell, M. (1995). Alcohol consumption measures. In J. Allen & M. Columbus (Eds.), *Assessing alcohol problems: A guide for clinicians and researchers* (pp. 55–73). Rockville, MD: National Institute on Alcohol Abuse and Alcoholism.

Sobell, M. B., & Sobell, L. C. (1973). Individualized behavior therapy for alcoholics. *Behavior Therapy 4,* 49–72.

Stamper, G. A., Smith, B. H., Gant, R., & Bogle, K. E. (2004). Replicated findings of an evaluation of a brief intervention designed to prevent high-risk drinking among first-year college students; Implications for social norming theory. *Journal of Alcohol and Drug Education, 48,* 53–72.

Stinchfield, R., & Owen, P. (1998). Hazelden's model of treatment and its outcome. *Addictive Behaviors, 23,* 669–683.

Substance Abuse and Mental Health Services Administration. (2006). *Results from the 2005 National Survey on Drug Use and Health: National Findings* (Office of Applied Studies, NSDUH Series H-30, DHHS Publication No. SMA 06-4194). Rockville, MD: Author.

Swenson, C. C., Henggeler, S. W., Taylor, I. S., & Addison, O. W. (2005). *Multisystemic therapy and neighborhood partnerships: Reducing adolescent violence and substance abuse.* New York: Guilford Press.

Tomlinson, K. L., Brown, S. A., & Abrantes, A. (2004). Psychiatric comorbidity and substance use treatment outcomes of adolescents. *Psychology of Addictive Behaviors, 18,* 160–169.

Tonigan, J. S. (2003). Project MATCH treatment participation and outcome by self-reported ethnicity. *Alcoholism: Clinical and Experimental Research, 27,* 1340–1344.

Tucker, J. A., Vuchinich, R. E., Black, B. C., & Rippens, P. D. (2006). Significance of a behavioral economic index of reward value in predicting drinking problem resolution. *Journal of Consulting and Clinical Psychology, 74,* 317–326.

Vuchinich, R. E., & Tucker, J. A. (1988). Contributions from behavioral theories of choice to an analysis of alcohol abuse. *Journal of Abnormal Psychology, 92,* 408–416.

Walitzer, K. S., & Dermen, K. H. (2004). Alcohol-focused spouse involvement and behavioral couples therapy: Evaluation of enhancements to drinking reduction treatment for male problem drinkers. *Journal of Consulting and Clinical Psychology, 72,* 944–955.

Walters, S. T., & Bennett, M. E. (2000). Reducing alcohol use in college students: A controlled trial of two brief interventions. *Journal of Drug Education, 30,* 361–372.

Wechsler, H., Nelson, T. F., Lee, J. E., Seibring, M., Lewis, C., & Keeling, R. P. (2003). Perception and reality: A national evaluation of social norms marketing interventions to reduce college students' heavy alcohol use. *Quarterly Journal of Studies on Alcohol, 64,* 484–494.

Wingfield, H. (1919). *The forms of alcoholism and their treatment.* London: Oxford University Press.

Wingo, L. K. (2001). Substance abuse in African American women. *Journal of Cultural Diversity, 20,* 23–37.

13

Nicotine

Thomas H. Brandon, David J. Drobes, Joseph W. Ditre, and Andrea Elibero

University of South Florida

Contents

Germany, 1946: "In disregard of considerations of personal dignity, conventional decorum, and esthetic-hygienic feelings, cigarette butts were picked up out of the street dirt by people who, on their own statements, would in any other circumstances have felt disgust at such contact."

(Arntzen, 1948)

Wisconsin, 1987: The first author led a smoking cessation group of mostly educated, upper-middle class professionals in which one member mentioned that when he ran out of cigarettes during snowstorms, he would go to a sheltered bus stop and collect unfinished cigarette butts previously dropped by boarding passengers. Several other group members volunteered that they had also used that tactic during "cigarette emergencies."

The above vignettes illustrate the powerfully addictive nature of nicotine delivered via cigarettes, an addiction that is most clearly revealed when supplies are limited, whether due to production shortages after WWII or severe blizzards in the Upper Midwest. Because in contemporary times there has been easy access to cigarettes, the nature of nicotine dependence has often been underappreciated. Yet a range of animal and human laboratory and survey research has demonstrated that nicotine is highly addictive (Baker et al., 2004; USPHS, 1988). Although approximately 70% of smokers indicate a desire to quit smoking (CDC, 2002), only about 2.5% successfully quit each year (CDC, 1999), despite now widely-circulated statistics that smoking kills an estimated 440,000 Americans annually (CDC, 2005), and 5 million worldwide (Ezzati & Lopez, 2003).

Historical Overview & Prevalence

In the United States, smoking prevalence accelerated greatly beginning in the 1920s with the development of milder tobacco and industrial cigarette rolling machines, peaking in the 1950s, when the majority of adult men smoked. Prevalence has been declining over the past 30 years, often attributed to the nonsmokers' rights movement; however the rate of decline has slowed considerably in the new century, with current prevalence estimates of 24 and 18% for men and women, respectively (CDC, 2007). It has been postulated that those smokers who have yet to quit despite the health warnings and social sanctions might be more tobacco dependent than earlier populations of smokers (Hughes, 2001), although this selectivity hypothesis is controversial (Warner & Burns, 2003). Nevertheless, analyses of published clinical trials have revealed a steady drop in reported cessation rates over the past two decades, consistent with the notion that the smoking population is becoming increasingly challenging to treat (Irvin & Brandon, 2000; Irvin et al., 2003).

Approximately 90% of self-quitters eventually return to smoking, and the relapse rate of even the best cessation programs remains about 70% (Fiore et al., 2008). Thus, tobacco dependence can best be conceptualized as a chronic relapsing disorder that may require intensive and repeated care. It is noteworthy that the daily rate of smoking (cigarettes per day) has apparently been dropping in recent years, most likely due to increasing environmental constraints (e.g., nonsmoking workplaces). At the extreme is a class of low-frequency smokers, often referred to as "chippers," who do not appear to develop dependence on nicotine (Shiffman & Paty, 2006).

This chapter provides an introduction to and overview of the assessment and treatment of tobacco dependence, followed by a case example. We emphasize techniques for which there is an evidence base, but the nature and strength of the evidence will differ considerably across techniques. Although nicotine can be delivered through a variety of products and routes of administration, by far the most common is cigarette smoking, so it is the primary focus of this chapter.

Contemporary Assessment of Nicotine Use and the Nicotine-Related Disorders

In this section, we describe various methods for assessment of cigarette smokers. Rather than provide comprehensive coverage of the available assessment techniques, we focus on contemporary methods with demonstrated validity, and those that are most likely to aid evidence-based treatment planning. Assessment is an important step in the context of providing evidence-based treatment, both in terms of treatment planning and tracking treatment progress, although it has not been clearly established that individualized assessment of smokers is associated with improved treatment efficacy, this is an active area of current research. We recommend that providers collect assessment data to the extent possible, within practical constraints such as time and financial considerations.

This section is organized around several assessment domains that we consider central for providing evidence-based smoking cessation treatment. Aside from collecting basic demographic and smoking-related information, the domains we consider most important include motivation to quit, nicotine dependence, nicotine withdrawal, urges/cravings to smoke, and social learning variables. Within each domain, we provide descriptions of widely used and readily available assessment methods, including brief versions, where available. A summary of measures is provided in Table 13.1. Of course, the choice of assessment method will vary according to individual circumstances, as well as the perceived importance of a particular domain for a given smoker.

Basic Demographic and Smoking Information

No one approach to smoking cessation is likely to be effective for all smokers. Thus, awareness of basic demographic variables could be useful during treatment planning. For instance, cessation counseling or self-help materials should take into account the distinguishing cultural characteristics of targeted groups. Indeed, several demographic variables have shown a relationship with smoking cessation outcomes, including age, gender, ethnicity, education, and socio-economic status. These are straightforward variables to assess via self-report or interview, and should be obtained prior to initiation of treatment.

Smoking and quitting history is the next crucial area that should be assessed. Basic information to obtain is the age at which smoking began, the length of time as a smoker, and changes in smoking rate since smoking initiation. Information about prior quit attempts should be collected,

TABLE 13.1
Summary of Smoking Assessment Measures

Measures	# of Items	Scores	Citation
Motivation to Quit			
Stages of Change	3	Overall stage	Prochaska, DiClemente, & Norcross, 1992
Contemplation Ladder	1	Overall score	Beiner & Abrams, 1991
Reasons for Quitting	12	2 subscales	Curry et al., 1990
Nicotine Dependence			
Diagnostic and Statistical Manual, IV	7	Overall score	APA, 1994
Heaviness of Smoking Index	2	Overall score	Heatherton et al., 1989
Fagerström Tolerance Questionnaire	8	Overall score	Fagerström, 1978
Fagerström Test of Nicotine Dependence	6	Overall score	Heatherton, Kozlowski, Frecker, & Fagerström, 1991
Hooked on Nicotine Checklist	10	Overall score	Wellman et al., 2005
Cigarette Dependence Scale-12	12	Overall score	Etter et al., 2003
Cigarette Dependence Scale-5	5	Overall score	Etter et al., 2003
Nicotine Dependence Syndrome Scale	19	5 subscales	Shiffman, Waters, & Hickox, 2004
Wisonsin Smoking Dependence Motives Scale	68	13 subscales	Piper et al., 2004
Nicotine Withdrawal			
Shiffman–Jarvik Withdrawal Scale	23	5 subscales	Shiffman & Jarvik, 1976
Minnesota Withdrawal Scale	13	Overall score	Hughes & Hatsukami, 1986
Wisconsin Smoking Withdrawal Scale	28	Overall score & 7 subscales	Welsch et al., 1999
Urge/Craving			
Shiffman Craving Scale	4	Overall score	Shiffman et al., 2003
Questionnaire of Smoking Urges	32	Overall score & 2 subscales	Tiffany & Drobes, 1991
Questionnaire of Smoking Urges – Brief	10	Overall score & 2 subscales	Cox, Tiffany, & Christen, 2001
Tobacco Craving Questionnaire	47	Overall score & 4 subscales	Heishman, Singleton, & Moolchan, 2003
Social Learning Constructs			
Self-Efficacy/Temptations Scale	20	Overall score & 2 subscales	Velicer et al., 1990
Relapse Situation Efficacy Questionnaire	74	7 subscales	Gwaltney et al., 2001
Smoking Consequences Questionnaire	50	4 subscales	Brandon & Baker, 1991
Smoking Consequences Questionnaire-Adult	55	10 subscales	Copeland et al., 1995
Smoking Consequences Questionnaire-Short Form	21	4 subscales	Myers et al., 2003
Coping with Temptations Inventory	48	Overall score	Shiffman, 1988

including the number and relative success of past attempts, especially recent attempts. It is particularly useful to determine the techniques employed (if any) during past quit attempts, the perceived benefits of each approach used, and the conditions that led to relapse.

Current cigarette consumption can be assessed with simple questions such as "How much do you smoke per day?" This question may specify a particular timeframe (e.g., over the past week, month, year). For a more detailed analysis of smoking rate and pattern, a Timeline Follow-Back (TLFB) interview can be employed (Sobell & Sobell, 1992). Although originally developed for assessment of alcohol consumption, the TLFB method is now widely used for smoking assessment (Brown et al., 1998). The TLFB is a retrospective recall of cigarettes consumed over a specified length of time (e.g., 30 days). The interviewer provides a calendar, probes for special events (e.g., birthdays, holidays, etc.), and the number of cigarettes per day is recorded. The TLFB may take 10 or more minutes to administer; yet this may be a worthwhile investment for getting a more detailed and accurate retrospective recall of smoking amount and patterns.

If prospective data collection regarding smoking is feasible, then self-monitoring using paper-and-pencil diaries can be used. These diary forms can be quite brief, limited to recording the number of cigarettes smoked during particular time periods, or they can obtain more detailed information regarding the situational or affective precursors to smoking. One potential pitfall associated with paper-and-pencil diary recording is the "waiting room effect," in which the smoker completes diaries some time after the behavior occurred (e.g., just prior to meeting with a smoking cessation counselor). In addition, this method does not take base rates into account when attempting to establish the situational or affective precursors to smoking. That is, somebody who reports smoking when depressed may, in fact, be depressed most of the time, even when not smoking.

Some of the problems with diary keeping are avoided with Ecological Momentary Assessment (EMA; Stone & Shiffman, 1994), a more complex method of obtaining real-time smoking data in real-world environments. Smokers carry palm-top computers and enter electronic diary (ED) assessments, which are time-stamped. The ED can initiate assessments at random times and/or when certain events occur, and can record a range of information. For example, EMA can be used to record details about the natural history of coping during smoking cessation. EMA techniques are still relatively expensive and technologically sophisticated, and not used widely outside of research settings.

Biochemical indices can be used to objectively characterize smoking status prior to and over the course of treatment. Expired air (breath) sampling of carbon monoxide (CO) is frequently used to validate abstinence in smoking cessation. CO is a product of combustion during the smoking process and is, therefore, insensitive to nicotine that may be in the system during use of nicotine replacement therapy (NRT). It is relatively simple to obtain after an initial investment in a monitoring devise (approximately $1000). However, given its short half-life, CO is only accurate for detecting smoking that occurred over the prior 12 hours. A more stable estimate of nicotine intake is cotinine, which is the major metabolite of nicotine and can be detected in the blood, urine, or saliva. Cotinine has a relatively long half-life (up to 24 hours), and can be detected up to 96 hours after smoking occurs. Cotinine is not a good measure of smoking among persons who are using NRT.

Motivation to Quit

Motivation to quit is a key element of the smoking cessation process, and one of the best predictors of cessation outcome. However, because most treatment-seeking smokers exhibit a relatively high level of motivation to quit, it may be difficult to discriminate among these smokers using available measures. Nonetheless, smokers seek treatment for various reasons, and it is important to establish and reinforce their motivation to quit in order to sustain the effort required for successful cessation. It may also be useful to conceptualize motivation to quit smoking as a dynamic construct, and interventions may benefit if designed to maintain high levels of motivation throughout the quitting process.

The most prominent measure of motivation to quit smoking is based on the Transtheoretical Model of behavior change, and the stages of changes that are embedded within this model (Prochaska, DiClemente, & Norcross, 1992). According to this model, ongoing smokers can be placed into one of three stages. In the precontemplation stage, the smoker is not seriously considering quitting within the next six months. In the contemplation stage, the smoker is seriously considering quitting in the next six months, but not within the next 30 days. In the preparation stage, the smoker intends to quit smoking in the next 30 days and has made an attempt to quit within the past year. A 3-item questionnaire is used to place a smoker into one of the stages. According to the model, smokers in the preparation stage will benefit most from immediate action oriented smoking cessation treatment, whereas smokers in the precontemplation stage would benefit more from low intensity interventions designed to increase motivation to change. This model has received mixed support to date and is rather controversial.

Another measure of motivation to quit smoking is the Contemplation Ladder (CL; Biener & Abrams, 1991), which consists of a single 11-point scale that measures readiness to quit smoking along a continuum. The CL is depicted as a ladder with higher rungs representing greater motivation to quit. CL scores are significantly associated with reported intention to quit, number of previous quit attempts, perceived co-worker encouragement to quit, and socioeconomic status. CL scores have also been found to predict subsequent participation in programs designed to educate workers about their smoking habit and its contingent risks (Biener & Abrams, 1991).

It may also be fruitful to assess factors that motivate a given quit attempt. The Reasons for Quitting scale (Curry, Wagner, & Grothaus, 1990) is a 12-item measure that includes scales that address both intrinsic and extrinsic sources of motivation. Intrinsically motivated behaviors are driven by the desire to achieve rewards that are internal to the person, and this scale includes dimensions of health concern and self-control. Extrinsically motivated behaviors are driven by external rewards or punishment, and this scale includes dimensions of immediate reinforcement and social influence. Intrinsically motivated behavior is more likely to persist over time, and smokers with higher baseline levels of intrinsic relative to extrinsic motivation are more likely to achieve and maintain smoking abstinence (Curry, Grothaus, & McBride, 1997).

Nicotine Dependence

Information pertaining to the presence, extent, and nature of nicotine dependence may be particularly useful for guiding the selection and intensity of smoking cessation treatment. According to the *DSM-IV* (American Psychiatric Association, 1994), dependence is present if a smoker has at least three of the following symptoms: tolerance (i.e., smoking more over time to obtain the same effects), withdrawal, smoking more or longer than intended, persistent desire or unsuccessful attempts to quit or control tobacco use, spending a great deal of time obtaining or using cigarettes, giving up important activities due to smoking, and continued smoking despite knowledge of harmful consequences. This diagnosis can be established through checklists or standardized clinical interviews, such as the Composite International Diagnostic

Interview (Kessler & Üstün, 2004) or the Diagnostic Interview Schedule (Robins, 1986). Use of such checklists or structured interviews rarely occurs in clinical practice, as it is typically assumed that the majority of treatment-seeking smokers meet *DSM-IV* criteria for dependence. Nonetheless, an increasing proportion of smokers exhibit features of non-dependent use, so it is reasonable to assess for the presence of nicotine dependence.

Beyond the presence of nicotine-related diagnosis, a number of self-report scales are available to assess the severity and nature of nicotine dependence. A brief measure of nicotine dependence is the Heaviness of Smoking Index (HSI; Heatherton, Kozlowski, Frecker, Rickert, & Robinson, 1989), which contains two items: smoking amount and time to first cigarette in the morning. The HSI is derived from the Fagerström Tolerance Questionnaire (FTQ; Fagerström, 1978), an 8-item self-report measure of nicotine dependence. Smokers with higher FTQ scores are less likely to maintain long-term abstinence, and generally show higher biochemical indices of smoking. The Fagerström Test of Nicotine Dependence (FTND; Heatherton, Kozlowski, Frecker, & Fagerström, 1991) is a refined version of the FTQ, with six items and somewhat improved psychometric characteristics. The FTND emphasizes time to first cigarette of the day, morning smoking, difficulty in refraining from smoking, and number of cigarettes smoked. The FTQ and FTND are the most widely used measures of dependence, despite recent criticisms over their psychometric characteristics and a limited assessment of only the physical aspect of nicotine dependence.

The Hooked on Nicotine Checklist (Wellman et al., 2005) is a 10-item measure of the loss of autonomy over tobacco use. The number of positive responses is proposed to reflect the degree of dependence. The Cigarette Dependence Scale (CDS; Etter, Le Houezec, & Perneger, 2003) is a brief, self-administered, continuous measure covering *DSM-IV* criteria of dependence that has been shown to predict smoking abstinence (Etter et al., 2003). It emphasizes compulsion to smoke, withdrawal, loss of control, time allocation, neglect of other activities, and persistence despite harm, but does not address tolerance. In addition to the original 12-item instrument, there is also a 5-item version that has similar properties, but is less comprehensive (Etter et al., 2003). These instruments can be useful for tracking progress in cessation treatment.

Several multidimensional scales of nicotine dependence have recently been developed. The 19-item Nicotine Dependence Syndrome Scale (NDSS; Shiffman, Waters, & Hickox, 2004) is a theory-based scale designed to measure five factors: Drive (craving and withdrawal in abstinence), Priority (behavioral preference of smoking), Tolerance (reduced sensitivity to the effects of smoking), Continuity (regularity of smoking), and Stereotypy ("sameness" of smoking factors). The Wisconsin Smoking Dependence Motives Scale (WISM-68; Piper et al., 2004) is a 68-item theory-based scale that addresses 13 separate motives for smoking that are thought to reflect mechanisms underlying dependence. The NDSS and WISDM complement and extend the FTND and other brief scales, providing a more complex and broad assessment of nicotine dependence.

Nicotine Withdrawal

Nicotine withdrawal is an especially salient feature of nicotine dependence. According to many models of smoking behavior, avoidance of withdrawal is thought to be a primary motivator of ongoing smoking behavior, and one of the main reasons that smokers often relapse shortly after a cessation attempt. Indeed, withdrawal severity appears to be among the best predictors of cessation success, with lower severity predictive of greater success. The primary symptoms of nicotine withdrawal include dysphoric or depressed mood; insomnia; irritability, frustration, or anger; anxiety; difficulty concentrating; restlessness; decreased heart rate; and increased appetite or weight gain (*DSM-IV*; APA, 1994). The time course for these symptoms is highly variable across individuals, but some symptoms may begin within the first hour after the last cigarette (Hendricks, Ditre, Drobes, & Brandon, 2006). Symptoms typically peak within 48 hours, and are largely resolved within 7-10 days after smoking, although in some cases withdrawal may last substantially longer. Relief of withdrawal is a primary target of several of the pharmacotherapies discussed later in this chapter. In addition to tracking withdrawal over the course of a current quit attempt, assessment of prior withdrawal experiences may help in preparing for an upcoming quit attempt; for instance, by informing decisions regarding the utilization of pharmacotherapy.

Several scales are available for assessing nicotine withdrawal. The Shiffman-Jarvik Withdrawal Scale (Shiffman & Jarvik, 1976) is a 23-item measure that asks respondents to indicate the degree to which several aspects of withdrawal are currently being experienced. Although this scale is widely used, several of its dimensions are no longer considered central to nicotine withdrawal. The Minnesota Withdrawal Scale (Hughes & Hatsukami, 1986) is a 13-item checklist of common withdrawal symptoms that were derived from *DSM-III* (APA, 1980) nicotine withdrawal criteria. More recently, the Wisconsin Smoking Withdrawal Scale was developed to address DSM-IV withdrawal criteria (Welsch et al., 1999). This measure contains 28 items, and can be scored for seven factor-derived scales (i.e., craving, anxiety, sadness, anger, concentration, sleep, and hunger) or a single overall withdrawal scale.

Urges/Cravings to Smoke

Smoking urges (or "cravings") are key aspects of nicotine dependence. Major theoretical models of addiction assign a central role to urges, which are typically defined as a subjective motivational state of desire that drives drug-use behavior. Many smokers claim that unmanageable urges are what ultimately end their quit attempts. Various cognitive-behavioral and pharmacological treatment methods, as discussed below, are specifically geared to address urges in the cessation process. Thus, it is appropriate that treating clinicians assess urges to smoke before, during, and after a quit attempt. It is especially important to assess urges on an ongoing basis as they can change frequently over the course of a quit attempt, and in response to particular situational or affective cues. Research has shown that strong urges immediately following cessation are associated with an increased likelihood of eventual smoking relapse (e.g., Killen & Fortman, 1997).

It is only in recent years that adequate attention has been paid to the measurement of urge. Previously, urge assessment almost always consisted of a single-item visual analog scale, with limited content and unknown psychometric properties. There are now a number of validated multi-item measures that address diverse aspects of tobacco-related urge. Shiffman and colleagues (2003) have used a 4-item scale, including items that assess desire, urge, and craving.

This and similar brief scales consider urge to be a unidimensional construct. In contrast, the 32-item Questionnaire of Smoking Urges (QSU; Tiffany & Drobes, 1991) has a factor structure consisting of two subscales. The first factor measures positive reinforcement from smoking, and the second factor measures negative reinforcement from smoking, as well as urges that are urgent and overwhelming. A shorter 10-item version of this scale has also been developed, with the same two factors (QSU-Brief; Cox, Tiffany, & Christen, 2001). The Tobacco Craving Questionnaire (TCQ; Heishman, Singleton, & Moolchan, 2003) is a 47-item questionnaire that is quite similar to the QSU, with the addition of items that address a lack of control over tobacco use. It should be noted that only 17 of the 47 TCQ items load onto its four-factor solution, whereas 26 of the 32 QSU items load onto its two factors.

Social Learning Variables: Self-Efficacy, Coping, and Expectancies

Several constructs derived from social learning theory have proven to be useful in terms of defining smoker characteristics, and for predicting cessation outcomes. We will briefly describe three of these constructs and the primary measures to obtain them: self-efficacy, outcome expectancies, and coping.

Self-efficacy (Bandura, 1977) in the present context refers to confidence in being able to abstain from smoking. This is often assessed via a single item that asks how confident one is in being able to avoid smoking over a particular period of time (e.g., month, year). A more detailed and clinically useful assessment of self-efficacy involves an assessment of confidence in being able to avoid smoking in a number of specific situations. An example of such a measure is the 20-item Self-Efficacy/Temptations Scale, which includes subscales that measure confidence to avoid smoking in positive affect/social, negative affect, and habit/craving situations (Velicer, DiClemente, Rossi, & Prochaska, 1990). Similarly, the Relapse Situation Efficacy Questionnaire (Gwaltney et al., 2001) is a longer form (74 items) that addresses confidence in being able to resist smoking in a number of specific situations, which can be scored for seven domains: negative affect, positive affect, restrictive situations, idle time, social-food situations, low arousal, and craving. Subscale scores on this measure have been predictive of the types of situations in which smokers lapse, which suggests a high degree of clinical utility.

Outcome expectancies refer to the expected effects or consequences from smoking, which are in turn thought to be key motivators of smoking behavior. The Smoking Consequences Questionnaire (Brandon & Baker, 1991) is a 50-item measure that captures the multidimensional nature of smoker's expectancies, including four subscales: positive reinforcement/sensory satisfaction, negative reinforcement/negative affect reduction, negative consequences, and appetite/weight control. The original SCQ was developed with a college student sample. A subsequent SCQ-Adult was developed with older, more experienced smokers, and has ten subscales: negative affect reduction, stimulation/state enhancement, health risk, taste/sensorimotor manipulation, social facilitation, weight control, craving/addiction, negative physical feelings, boredom reduction, and negative social impression (Copeland, Brandon, & Quinn, 1995). Several of these subscales have been shown to predict withdrawal symptoms upon quitting, as well as smoking cessation success. Administration of this scale could improve the relevance of counseling strategies aimed at modifying expectancies regarding positive and/or negative effects of smoking. There is also a brief version (SCQ-Short Form; Myers, MacPherson, McCarthy, & Brown, 2003), developed with adolescents and young adults, which contains 21 items and can be scored for the four subscales of the original SCQ.

Coping with tempting situations is a major feature within the highly influential relapse prevention model of Marlatt & Gordon (1985). According to this model, successful coping leads to increased self-efficacy and abstinence, whereas lack of coping leads to decreased self-efficacy, positive outcome expectancies for smoking, negative emotional states, lapse, and (potentially) relapse. Stemming from this model, development of adequate coping skills is the primary emphasis in cognitive-behavioral forms of smoking cessation counseling. The assessment of coping resources among smokers can be important prior to quitting and throughout the quitting process. Informally, the smoker can be asked open-ended questions about how they manage not to smoke in particular situations. More formally, the Coping with Temptation Inventory (Shiffman, 1988) addresses the presence or absence of specific behavioral and cognitive coping strategies using a 48-item questionnaire. EMA techniques have also been used to assess coping among smokers in the naturalistic environment (O'Connell et al., 1998).

Other Assessment Issues

The brevity of this chapter requires that we cover only the most crucial areas of tobacco assessment. There are several other areas that could be important to assess in clinical settings. For instance, social support for non-smoking should be considered, as other smokers present in the household are generally associated with poorer outcomes. Also, mood and stress levels prior to and during the course of a smoking cessation attempt. Importantly, the presence of psychiatric and other substance use disorders may complicate or interfere with treatment if not addressed, and should be assessed if suspected. Indeed, comorbidity between smoking and a number of other disorders is an active area of research in the smoking field. The next few years should offer improved validated methods for assessing and treating comorbid conditions along with smoking cessation. Finally, there is a growing appreciation of the genetic basis for nicotine dependence, and several candidate genes have been examined in relation to various smoking-related indices (see Munafò, Clark, Johnstone, Murphy, & Walton, 2004). In addition, ongoing research is attempting to determine whether the efficacy of existing and novel pharmacotherapies is moderated by genetic factors (e.g., Berrettini & Lerman, 2005; Uhl et al., 2008). In the future, it may be possible to direct smokers to treatment modalities that have the greatest likelihood for success based on individual genetic profiles.

Contemporary Treatment of Nicotine Use and the Nicotine-Related Disorders

This section on treatments for nicotine dependence is divided into two subsections: broadly defined social/behavioral interventions and FDA-approved pharmacotherapies. Within the social/behavioral section, interventions are organized from the least intensive (i.e., self-help) to the most intensive (i.e., face-to-face counseling). We rely primarily on qualitative and meta-analytic reviews as the evidence base for our overview.

Social/Behavioral Treatments

Self-Help   Self-help refers to very minimal types of interventions, such as print materials, videotapes, or audiotapes that are provided to smokers. The best-known examples are the American Lung Association's "Freedom from Smoking" booklets. Because few smokers seek more intensive interventions, self-help materials have the potential for high public health impact if they can reach large numbers of smokers and aid them in achieving cessation. Unfortunately, recent meta-analyses indicate little efficacy for self-help interventions. Both the US Public Health Service's Clinical Practice Guideline for Treating Tobacco Use and Dependence (Fiore et al., 2008) and a Cochrane Review (Lancaster & Stead, 2005) concluded that self-help materials have marginal efficacy, improving cessation rates by about 1% compared to no-treatment controls. However, because self-help information is so widely available, control participants may have also benefited from self-help information outside of the studies, minimizing observed group differences in these studies.

A relatively recent advance in self-help involves "tailoring" the materials to the characteristics of individual smokers, often based upon measures and algorithms associated with the Transtheoretical Model (Prochaska et al., 1992). The Cochrane meta-analysis found that tailored materials produced slightly superior outcomes over standard, non-tailored materials. However, many of these studies were not adequately controlled, and there is also some evidence that the benefits of tailoring may be due to expectancy (i.e., "placebo") effects associated with tailored materials rather than to the theory-based tailored content (Webb, Hendricks, & Brandon, 2007; Webb, Simmons, & Brandon, 2005).

Although it appears that self-help smoking cessation materials produce very small effects, two controlled studies indicate that print materials have more substantial effects on preventing smoking relapse (Brandon et al., 2000, 2004). Based upon relapse-prevention theory (Marlatt, 1985), these materials were designed to be delivered to individuals shortly after they quit smoking, with the purpose of improving the maintenance of abstinence. They have produced significant reduction in relapse through two years of follow-up, and appear to be highly cost-effective. It may be that written self-help materials are not sufficiently potent to overcome the barriers associated with smoking cessation itself, but they are sufficient for maintaining abstinence that has already been achieved.

Telephone Quit Lines   All Americans now have access to state-supported telephone "quit lines." One number (1-800-QUITNOW) serves as a central access point that automatically routes calls to the appropriate state or federal quit line service. Telephone counseling services differ in the amount and frequency of counseling offered, the provision of ancillary materials, referrals to local smoking cessation agencies, the provision of free or subsidized pharmacotherapies, and whether calls are proactive (call-out), reactive (call-in), or both. Quit lines have the advantage of providing more personal and intensive help than self-help materials, while also having greater potential reach than face-to-face counseling. Two recent meta-analyses concluded that quit lines were effective (Fiore et al., 2008; Stead, Perera, & Lancaster, 2006), with odds ratios of 1.2 – 1.4 compared to control conditions, which translates into differential abstinence rates of 3-5%. Stead et al. found evidence of a dose-response effect, with the most effective quit lines providing 3 or more telephone counseling sessions.

Moreover, there was greater evidence for proactive compared to reactive quit lines, partially due to few controlled studies of the latter. Finally, despite the variability of provided services, there is evidence for the applied effectiveness of the telephone counseling component per se (Zhu et al., 2002).

Brief Interventions Continuing the progression of increasing treatment intensity, the next step comprises relatively brief face-to-face interventions, often delivered by a health-care provider. Given the dire health consequences of smoking, it would appear obvious that health professionals should provide their patients with advice about quitting, yet research consistently shows that this is done no more than 50% of the time by physicians (e.g., Ellerbeck et al., 2001). The data are similarly disappointing for other professions, including psychologists (Phillips & Brandon, 2004).

Meta-analyses indicate that physician advice to quit smoking produces small, but significant, effects on smoking cessation. Both the Clinical Practice Guideline (Fiore et al., 2008) and a Cochrane Review (Lancaster & Stead, 2004) concluded that physician advice increased abstinence rates by approximately 2.3–2.5%. Thus, physician advice will result in about one new quitter for every 40 smokers advised to quit. Although this per-patient effect appears small (and the low rate of reinforcement no doubt adversely affects the maintenance of physician behavior), because 70% of smokers visit their physician each year, the potential cumulative effect is sizable. Consistent quitting advice by physicians could yield an additional 1 million quitters annually. When other health professionals are considered—including psychologists, dentists, physical therapists, pharmacists, and nurses—the public health potential is magnified. Moreover, the Clinical Practice Guideline analyses found a dose-response relationship between contact time and abstinence outcomes, with minimal counseling (< 3 minutes) yielding 13.4% abstinence, low-intensity counseling (3–10 minutes) yielding 16.0%, and higher intensity counseling (> 10 minutes) yielding 22.1% abstinence. Similarly higher abstinence rates were found with greater number of meetings and greater number of clinician types delivering the cessation messages.

With respect to the content of brief interventions, the Clinical Practice Guideline recommends the "5 A's": Asking every patient if he or she is currently a smoker; Advising smokers, in a clear, strong, and personalized way, to quit smoking; Assessing their willingness to make a quit attempt within the next 30 days; Assisting those patients willing to quit in developing a quit plan, providing practical counseling, providing social support, recommending pharmacotherapy, and providing supplementary materials; and Arranging an additional follow-up contact, preferably within the first week after the target quit date. For the patient who is unwilling to attempt to quit smoking, the guideline recommends a motivational intervention built around the "5 R's": emphasizing the personal Relevance of quitting; identifying the acute and long-term Risks of continued smoking to the patient and family; identifying the potential Rewards associated with cessation (e.g., improved health, improved sense of taste and smell); addressing barriers or Roadblocks that could impede quitting (e.g., withdrawal symptoms, weight gain, depression); and Repeating this motivational intervention at every opportunity with the patient.

Intensive Interventions The Clinical Practice Guideline concluded that treatment intensity and duration were highly related to treatment efficacy. At the upper end of this continuum are multisession treatments typically offered through smoking cessation clinics associated with health foundations (e.g., American Lung Association), hospitals, public health departments, and occasionally private therapists and commercial clinics. In this section, we review several of the most prominent and efficacious types of smoking cessation counseling.

Cognitive Behavioral Counseling   The key components of this approach include patient education regarding the nature of tobacco dependence and withdrawal, advice for surviving the withdrawal syndrome without smoking, identifying high-risk situations ("triggers") that produce urges to smoke, teaching and practicing cognitive and behavioral responses for coping with urges, discussion of long-term risk factors such as depression and weight gain; and discussion of how to respond in the event of an initial "slip" or "lapse." This general approach has multiple names, including Coping Skills Training, Practical Counseling, General Problemsolving, Multicomponent Behavior Therapy, and Relapse Prevention Training. Counseling usually occurs over the course of 6-12 sessions offered over 2-12 weeks. There may or may not be counseling sessions prior to the target quit day. Therapy may be provided in group or individual formats. The most comprehensive description of this general approach is provided by Perkins, Conklin, and Levine (2007). The Clinical Practice Guideline analysis found Practical Counseling to be effective, with an odds ratio of 1.5 compared to no counseling and an average abstinence rate of 16.2% compared to 11.2%. A Cochrane Review found that cognitive-behavioral components of group smoking cessation counseling produced marginal, but significant improvements in outcome (Stead & Lancaster, 2005). Also, a meta-analysis of relapse-prevention therapies for a range of addictions found that relapse-prevention was efficacious for treating smoking, but less so than for other addictions (Irvin, Bowers, Dunn, & Wang, 1999). Finally, a review of interventions within health psychology identified multicomponent behavior therapy as the only smoking cessation intervention that met criteria to be labeled "empirically supported" (Compas et al., 1998).

Aversion Therapy   Aversion therapy is a Pavlovian counterconditioning approach designed to produce conditioned aversive responses to smoking-related stimuli. Most common is rapid smoking, which involves inhaling on cigarettes at 6-sec signaled intervals for up to 3 min until 3 cigarettes are consumed or the patient is too ill to continue, with the procedure repeated up to 2 additional times per session, for multiple sessions (Lichtenstein et al., 1973). Other, less aversive variations have also been developed, included rapid puffing (without inhaling), and focused smoking (smoking at one's own pace while focusing on negative sensations). Rapid smoking reached maximum popularity during the 1980's, including use by some commercial cessation programs, but Zelman et al. (1992) reported equivalent outcomes with nicotine gum. Now that multiple pharmacotherapies are available, rapid smoking is rarely used. Nevertheless, the Clinical Practice Guideline reported rapid smoking as the most efficacious of the counseling and behavior therapies, with an odds ratio of 2.0. Hajek and Stead (2001) reported a similar odds ratio. However, rapid smoking is not recommended at this time due to the methodological limitations of the these older studies and side effects of the procedure. There is a need to reevaluate rapid smoking using contemporary standards of research methodology.

Scheduled Reduced Smoking   Methods of gradually reducing nicotine exposure by reducing the number of cigarettes smoked per day, or switching to progressively lower nicotine-containing brands of cigarettes have generally not been found to be efficacious (Fiore et al., 2008). However, a variation on this strategy has garnered some empirical support. Scheduled reduced smoking differs from other gradual reduction techniques in that the determination of when to have a cigarette is made by the therapist (using a computer algorithm) rather than by the smoker. In this way, smoking is thought to become disassociated with personally relevant cues and periods of potentially high reinforcement from tobacco use. Compas et al. (1998) included scheduled reduced smoking as a "possibly efficacious" treatment, with the endorsement limited because of only two published studies, both by the same research team. The second of these studies (Cinciripini et al., 1995) found that the technique produced 44% abstinence at one year, which was superior to multiple control conditions, including nonscheduled reduced smoking (18%), and scheduled nonreduced smoking (32%), supporting the contribution of both scheduled smoking and smoking reduction. Importantly, these scheduled reduced smoking interventions also included cognitive behavioral counseling.

Cue Exposure Therapy   Because smokers report strong urges to smoke in response to cues previously paired with smoking, and because relapse often occurs in response to such exteroceptive (e.g., the presence of other smokers) and interoceptive cues (e.g., negative affect states), classical conditioning models have been invoked to explain smoking motivation and relapse (Niaura et al., 1988). It follows that extinction-based therapies (cue exposure with response prevention) should be effective at reducing the risk of cue-provoked relapse. These therapies involve exposing smokers to in vivo, imaginal, video-based, or virtual reality generated cues associated with smoking, without allowing the patient to smoke. However, results from the few clinical trials to date have been discouraging (Conkin & Tiffany, 2002). Contemporary learning models suggest that extinction is highly context dependent and that treatments may need to include additional steps to extend extinction beyond the clinic or lab (Bouton, 2002; Collins & Brandon, 2002; Conklin & Tiffany, 2002). Research on such steps is ongoing, so despite its potential, cue exposure cannot yet be recommended.

Pharmacotherapy

According to the Clinical Practice Guideline for Treating Tobacco Use and Dependence, all smokers who are attempting to quit should be encouraged to use one or more FDA-approved pharmacologic aids (Fiore et al., 2008). Current first-line agents include five forms of NRT, the antidepressant bupropion (*Zyban*), and the partial nicotine agonist/antagonist varenicline tartrate (*Chantix*). Each of these medications has been documented to significantly increase rates of long-term smoking abstinence, essentially doubling (or tripling, in the case of varenicline) the rates of successful quitting relative to placebo (Fiore et al., 2008). However, special consideration is required for some populations, including those with medical contraindications, those smoking fewer than 10 cigarettes per day, pregnant or breastfeeding women, and adolescent smokers.

FDA-Approved Nicotine-Based Pharmacotherapies

Overview   Nicotine-based medications are the most widely investigated and utilized pharmacotherapy for the treatment of tobacco dependence and withdrawal. NRT supports smoking cessation by partially replacing nicotine in circulation, thereby reducing symptoms of withdrawal. NRT is typically administered over the initial period of abstinence (i.e., the first 8–12 weeks) when tobacco withdrawal symptoms are most pronounced. NRT is available in a range of forms including chewing gum, transdermal patches, intranasal spray, inhaler devices, and lozenges. These products vary in administration method, daily dosages, and delivery duration. The overall duration of treatment also varies, and treatment strategies may integrate concurrent therapies. Table 13.2 summarizes some important characteristics of each FDA-approved NRT. In general, NRT delivers 1/3–1/2 of the plasma nicotine levels achieved by smoking (Balfour & Fagerstrom, 1996). Of the five NRT dosage forms, the nicotine nasal spray reaches its peak concentration most rapidly, followed by the gum, lozenge, and oral inhaler, which have similar concentration curves. The nicotine transdermal patch has the slowest onset, but provides more consistent blood levels of nicotine over a longer period of time.

Empirical Support   A meta-analysis of 103 randomized, controlled trials of nicotine replacement for smoking cessation revealed that each commercially available form of NRT significantly improved abstinence rates and increased the odds of quitting approximately 1.5 to 2 fold over placebo or no NRT (Silagy et al., 2004). These odds were largely independent of the duration of therapy, the intensity of additional support provided, or the setting in which the NRT was offered. Moreover, these nicotine replacement agents do not appear to differ in their effects on withdrawal discomfort, urges to smoke, perceived helpfulness, or rates of abstinence (Hajek et al., 1999). It should be noted, however, that most reviews and meta-analyses only examine treatment outcomes for approximately 6–12 months post-cessation. A systematic review of the long-term effect of NRT revealed that although the relative efficacy of a single course of NRT remains constant over many years, the extant literature tends to overestimate the lifetime benefit and cost-efficacy by about 30% (Etter & Stapleton, 2006).

Mechanisms of Action   Nicotine replacement medications deliver nicotine to the bloodstream in a relatively safer form by eliminating exposure to the harmful carcinogens and toxic gases found in cigarette smoke. There are at least three mechanisms of action by which NRT medications enhance smoking cessation (Henningfield et al., 2005; Lerman et al., 2005). First, NRTs reduce the severity of nicotine withdrawal symptoms by providing a lower dose of nicotine, making it easier for people to feel better when attempting to quit. Second, the nicotine provided by NRT may reduce the rewarding effects of nicotine derived from tobacco. Finally, NRTs may facilitate the development of more adaptive coping strategies for dealing with the psychological and behavioral aspects of nicotine addiction (e.g., coping with stress or boredom, managing hunger and weight gain).

Precautions and Considerations   Although each form of nicotine replacement is associated with specific precautions, the clinical guideline recommends that special consideration

TABLE 13.2
FDA-Approved Pharmacotherapies for the Treatment of Nicotine Dependence

Pharmacotherapy/Availability	Advantages (A)/Disadvantages (D)	Dosing	Duration	Adverse Effects	Precautions/Contraindications
FDA-Approved Nicotine-Based Pharmacotherapies					
Nicotine Patch[OTC/G] 24-hour patch (7, 14, 21 mg) 16-hour patch (5, 10, 15 mg)	A: easy to use (apply once per day), few side effects; D: slow onset, no acute dosing	> 10 cpd: 21 mg/day for 4–6 wk; 14 mg/day for 2 wk; 7 mg/day for 2 wk	8–10 wk (varies by patch product and strength)	Local skin reaction (50% mild, 10% causing discontinuation); vivid dreams or insomnia (can occur if worn overnight)	Caution in unstable cardiac disease (e.g., recent heart attack)
Nicotine Gum[OTC/G] regular, mint, orange (2, 4 mg)	A: flexible dosing, faster onset than patches; D: often used incorrectly	> 20 cpd: 4 mg gum < 20 cpd: 2 mg gum (every 1–2 hrs)	Up to 12 wk	Mouth soreness; jaw ache; nausea; hiccups; extra salivation	Acidic food/drink 15 min before/during use decreases absorption
Nicotine Nasal Spray[Rx] metered spray (0.5 mg)	A: flexible dosing, rapid onset; D: side effects, poor compliance	1–2 sprays/hr (up to 5 times/hr or 40 times/day)	3–6 mos (gradually decrease)	Nasal irritation (80–90%); possible dependence (10–20%)	Caution with asthma, rhinitis, sinusitis, and nasal polyps
Nicotine Oral Inhaler[Rx] 10 mg cartridge (4 mg inhaled vapor)	A: mimics hand–mouth behavior; D: costly, frequent use required	6–16 cartridges/d	Up to 6 mos	Cough; local irritation of mouth and throat (40%), usually mild	Avoid acidic food/drink 15 min before/during use
Nicotine Lozenge[OTC] mint, cherry (2, 4 mg)	A: flexible dosing, ease of use; D: poor compliance	2v4 mg based on time to first AM cig; Up to 24 pieces/d	Up to 12 wk (6 wks then taper)	Nausea (12–15%), hiccups, cough, heartburn, insomnia, headache, mouth soreness	Avoid acidic food/drink 15 min before/during use
FDA-Approved Non-Nicotine Pharmacotherapies					
Bupropion SR[Rx/G] Zyban (150 mg)	A: ease of use (pill form), can be combined with NRT; D: medical contraindications	Start 1–2 wk before TQD (150 mg/d for 3 days, then 150 mg twice/d)	Up to 12 wk (maintenance up to 6 mos)	Insomnia, dry mouth, nervousness, difficulty concentrating, seizure risk (0.1%)	Caution with history of seizures, eating disorders, significant head trauma
Varenicline[Rx] Chantix (0.5, 1 mg)	A: ease of use (pill form); no known drug interactions; D: nausea	Start 1–2 wk before TQD (0.5 mg/d for 3 days, then 0.5 mg twice/d for 4 days, then 1 mg twice/d)	Up to 12 wk (maintenance up to 6 mos)	Nausea (30%), sleep disturbance, constipation, flatulence, vomiting	Monitor for neuropsychiatric symptoms. Adjust dose if kidney function is impaired, safety of use with NRT is unknown

Note. The information in this table is not comprehensive. Please see package inserts for additional information. Adapted from Fiore et al., *Treating tobacco use and dependence. Clinical Practice Guideline.* Rockville, MD: US Department of Health and Human Services, Public Health Service. May 2008; Fould, et al., Developments in pharmacotherapy for tobacco dependence: Past, present and future. *Drug and Alcohol Review, 25,* 2006; and Frishman et al., Nicotine and non-nicotine smoking cessation pharmacotherapies. *Cardiology in Review, 14,* 2006.
OTC = available over-the-counter; Rx = available by prescription only; G = generic form available; cpd = cigarettes per day; TQD = target quit date; d = day; wk = week; mos = mo.

be given before using NRT with patients who present with acute cardiovascular disease or who may be pregnant. However, there is currently no empirical evidence of increased cardiovascular risk with NRT use, even among high-risk outpatients with cardiac disease (Fiore et al., 2008; Joseph et al., 1996). Also, because none of these medications has been tested in pregnant women for efficacy in treating tobacco dependence, the relative ratio of risks to benefits remains unknown (Dempsey & Benowitz, 2001; Fiore et al., 2008). In general, most experts would agree that the risks associated with continued smoking outweigh those associated with NRT use, but no product is FDA-approved for pregnant women.

FDA-Approved Non-Nicotine Pharmacotherapies

Bupropion sustained-release (SR) (Zyban)

Overview   Bupropion relieves the symptoms of craving and nicotine withdrawal, and attenuates the weight gain that often occurs after smoking cessation. Currently available in two sustained-release (SR) forms, bupropion was initially marketed as an antidepressant (Wellbutrin). In 1997, bupropion became the first non-nicotine medication to gain FDA approval for the long-term maintenance of smoking cessation (Zyban). See Table 13.2 for additional important characteristics of bupropion.

Empirical Support   Bupropion, like NRT, has been shown to double quit rates when compared with placebo (Hughes et al., 1999). A recent meta-analysis of 31 randomized trials of bupropion for smoking cessation revealed that the odds ratio of abstinence at six or more months was 1.94 for bupropion SR relative to placebo (Hughes et al., 2007). There is also evidence that bupropion can be effective when offered in a primary care-oriented healthcare system setting, where a combination of bupropion and minimal or moderate counseling was associated with 12-month quit rates of 23.6% to 33.2% (Swan et al., 2003). Finally, the results of a double-blind, placebo-controlled comparison of bupropion to nicotine transdermal patch indicated that treatment with bupropion alone resulted in significantly greater long-term rates of smoking cessation (30.3% vs. 16.4%) than did use of the nicotine patch alone (Jorenby et al., 1999).

Mechanisms of Action   Bupropion's exact mechanism of action in tobacco cessation is currently unknown. However, there is evidence that bupropion has a specific effect on neural pathways believed to underlie nicotine addiction (Dwoskin et al., 2006). For example, bupropion inhibits the neuronal reuptake of dopamine and norepinephrine (neurotransmitters believed to be important in maintaining nicotine dependence) in the central nervous system. There is also evidence that bupropion antagonizes nicotinic receptors in the brain and blocks nicotine's reinforcing effects. The fact that only some antidepressants aid long-term smoking cessation (e.g., bupropion and nortriptyline), whereas others do not (e.g., selective serotonin reuptake inhibitors), suggests that their mechanisms of action may be independent of antidepressant effects (Hughes et al., 2007). Indeed, studies have shown bupropion to be equally efficacious in smokers with or without a history of depression (Hayford et al., 1999).

Precautions and Considerations   Treatment with bupropion SR should be initiated while the patient is still smoking, because approximately one week of treatment is necessary to achieve steady-state blood levels. Bupropion is contraindicated, or to be used with caution, among smokers with a history of seizure disorders or a history of factors known to increase the risk of seizures (e.g., bulimia or anorexia nervosa, serious head trauma, alcoholism). There is a risk of about 1 in 1,000 of seizures associated with bupropion use (Hughes et al., 2007). Bupropion SR may be preferable for smokers who favor oral medications or have a history of depressive symptomotology. The safety of bupropion for use in human pregnancy has not been established.

Varenicline (Chantix)

Overview   Varenicline is an orally administered partial agonist of α4β2 nicotinic acetyl-choline receptors (nAChRs). Varenicline was developed from the naturally occurring alkaloid compound cytisine, a drug derived from the plant Cytisus Laburnum L. (Golden Rain). Evidence to date suggests that varenicline can increase the odds of successful long-term smoking cessation approximately threefold when compared to placebo. The main adverse effect of varenicline is mild to moderate nausea. See Table 13.2 for additional important characteristics of varenicline.

Empirical Support   A recent meta-analysis of six randomized controlled trials of varenicline for smoking cessation ($N = 4924$) revealed that the odds ratio for continuous abstinence at 12 months was 3.22 for varenicline relative to placebo (Cahill et al., 2007). In three of these trials, varenicline was also shown to increase the probability of quitting relative to bupropion by an odds ratio of 1.66. When compared to placebo, varenicline appears to attenuate cravings to smoke, negative affect withdrawal symptoms, and some reinforcing effects of smoking (Keating & Siddiqui, 2006).

Mechanisms of Action   Varenicline is a specific α4β2 nicotinic receptor partial agonist that stimulates dopamine and simultaneously blocks nicotinic receptors (Foulds, 2006). As a partial agonist, varenicline is hypothesized to alleviate craving and withdrawal symptoms by stimulating and maintaining moderate levels of dopamine in the mesolimbic region of the brain. The antagonist properties of varenicline are hypothesized to reduce nicotine-mediated activation of the dopaminergic system by blocking nicotine binding, thus reducing smoking satisfaction and psychological reward in those who continue to smoke while taking the drug (Coe et al., 2005).

Precautions and Considerations   The most frequently reported adverse effect of varenicline in clinical trials was dose-dependent nausea, which was generally mild to moderate, diminished over time, and was associated with low discontinuation rates. However, postmarketing reports by patients have led the FDA in early 2008 to warn of serious neuropsychiatric symptoms including "changes in behavior, agitation, depressed mood, suicidal ideation, and attempted and completed suicide." Patients are advised to discontinue the drug if these symptoms appear. Unlike bupropion and some nicotine-based medications, varenicline does not appear to reduce postcessation weight gain (Jorenby et al., 2006). Whether varenicline is more effective than nicotine-based pharmacotherapies remains unclear (Cahill et al., 2007). Varenicline is not approved for use with pregnant women.

Additional Pharmacotherapy Considerations

Efficacy Versus "Real World" Effectiveness

Despite the demonstrated efficacy of pharmacotherapies for the treatment of nicotine dependence, some apprehension remains about their "real world" effectiveness (Shiffman et al., 2002). For example, early efficacy trials took place in controlled environments, usually excluding participants with low quitting motivation and comorbid diagnoses. Also, compliance with pharmacotherapy may be superior in research settings because they generally offer free or paid treatment, and often incorporate careful instruction, psychosocial support, and multiple contacts. Indeed, population-based pharmacotherapy effectiveness trials conducted in more typical treatment settings (e.g., primary care, over-the-counter) have obtained lower rates of smoking abstinence (Hughes et al., 2003; Pierce & Gilpin, 2002; Velicer et al., 2006). However, most "real-world" studies with adequate sample sizes to detect small effect sizes have demonstrated a significant improvement over placebo at long-term follow-up (Foulds et al., 2006).

Combination Pharmacotherapies

Combination NRT involves the use of a long-acting product that delivers relatively constant levels of nicotine (e.g., nicotine patch) in combination with a short-acting product that permits acute nicotine delivery (e.g., nasal spray). Although research indicates that NRT combinations may provide greater efficacy in relieving withdrawal and enabling cessation than monotherapy, these findings are not robust and additional studies are needed (Sweeney et al., 2001). There is also some evidence that NRT can be combined with bupropion to achieve greater rates of smoking abstinence than with either treatment alone (Jorenby et al., 1999; Prochazka, 2000). However, the authors of a recent review concluded there was insufficient evidence that adding bupropion to NRT provides any additional long-term benefit (Hughes et al., 2007). Nevertheless, some researchers suggest that bupropion in combination with the nicotine patch may be appropriate for patients who have high levels of nicotine dependence, have a history of psychiatric problems, or who have previously failed to quit (Frishman et al., 2006). No research to date has examined the utility of adding varenicline to NRT.

Second-Line Agents

Pharmacologic agents that have not received FDA approval for smoking cessation but are recommended as second-line agents if first-line pharmacotherapies are not effective include clonidine and nortriptyline (Fiore et al., 2008). Clonidine is a centrally acting α_2-adrenergic agonist that reduces sympathetic outflow from the central nervous system and is approved for use as an anti-hypertensive agent. A recent meta-analysis concluded that clonidine was an effective agent for tobacco cessation with a pooled odds ratio of 1.89 relative to placebo (Gourlay et al., 2004). Nortriptyline, a tricyclic antidepressant, has also demonstrated efficacy for smoking cessation in five long-term studies with a 2.34 odds ratio compared with placebo (Hughes et al., 2007). The high incidence of side effects (e.g., sedation and dizziness for clonidine, and risk of arrhythmias and postural hypotension for nortriptyline) relegates each to second-line status.

Pharmacotherapies Under Investigation

Novel nicotine delivery systems currently under investigation include rapid-release nicotine gum, buccal adhesive nicotine tablets, a pulmonary nicotine inhaler, and nicotine-based straws, lollipops, wafers, and drops (see reviews by Foulds et al., 2006; Frishman et al., 2006). Also of interest to researchers are (a) medications capable of blocking the CYP2A6 enzyme (an enzyme that accounts for individual differences in the rate of nicotine metabolism), (b) agents such as lobeline that produce pharmacologic effects similar to but weaker than those of nicotine, and (c) nicotine vaccines, which are designed to reduce the distribution of nicotine to the brain.

Treatment Conclusions

Our separate reviews of the behavioral and pharmacological treatments might imply that these are alternatives, or mutually exclusive options. Unfortunately, many smokers and their physicians tend to view them in this way as well, with pharmacotherapy as the more attractive choice due to the relative ease of taking medication versus attending multiple counseling sessions. It should be noted, however, that the effect sizes for pharmacotherapy and the better behavioral therapies are approximately equal, with both yielding odds ratios around 2.0 according to the Clinical Practice Guideline (Fiore et al., 2008). More important, however, is that they have complementary, and additive, effects. The combination of behavioral counseling and pharmacotherapy produces outcomes that are approximately double those of either approach alone (Hughes, 1995).

It is also noteworthy that, with respect to the behavioral approaches, there is a strong dose-response effect, with the more intensive treatments producing better cessation outcomes. Given the high mortality rates associated with smoking, a high-intensity counseling program (combined with pharmacotherapy) would appear to be justified, despite the short-term inconvenience. This is a public health message that has not yet been communicated effectively to either smokers or health providers.

A final point is that smoking cessation treatments are highly cost-effective health interventions. In the health economic metric of each quality-adjusted life-year saved, smoking cessation typically costs under $10,000 (Cromwell, Bartosch, Fiore, Baker, & Hasselblad, 1997), with self-help relapse-prevention costing under $100 (Brandon et al., 2004). This compares to other well-accepted interventions (e.g., annual mammography, neonatal intensive care, universal precautions for HIV) with costs in the hundreds of thousands of dollars per year of life saved (Tengs et al., 1995).

Case Presentation

Ben is a 28-year-old graduate student at a major university. He began smoking at age 17, during his final year of high school. His wife is pregnant with their first child, and together they decided that Ben should quit smoking prior to the birth of the baby. Ben had seen postings for the campus smoking cessation clinic, so he called to arrange an appointment. Upon arrival at the clinic, he provided demographic information, and completed a smoking history form, a measure of motivation to quit (CL), a nicotine dependence scale (FTND), as well as a more detailed assessment of his individualized motives for smoking (WISDM).

The assessment revealed that Ben never attempted to quit smoking previously, but that he is highly motivated to quit at present (CL = 9). He smokes 30 cigarettes per day, his level of nicotine dependence is in the high range (FTND = 8), and his afternoon CO reading is 35 parts per million (ppm). He reported that he smokes primarily to reduce negative affect and withdrawal, and in response to situations that include cues or reminders of smoking (elevations on negative reinforcement and cue exposure/associative processes subscales of the WISDM). Based on his high level of nicotine dependence, and his patterns of smoking motives, the intake counselor recommended pharmacotherapy combined with behavioral counseling. Two days later, Ben has an initial meeting with a smoking cessation counselor, during which a quit date is planned for one week later. During the meeting, the counselor reviews medication options with Ben, and they decide that nicotine patch therapy would be affordable and likely to increase his chance for a successful quit attempt. They review his reasons for quitting, and begin to discuss ways for Ben to reduce his urges to smoke during the early stages of quitting. This includes getting rid of his cigarettes and reminders of smoking (lighters, ashtrays), avoiding alcohol and social situations with smokers for the time being, and trying to reduce his stress. Ben purchased an 8-week supply of nicotine patches.

On the morning of the quit day, he placed a 24-hour nicotine patch (21 mg) on his upper back. The next day, he met with the smoking cessation counselor for approximately 30 minutes. They discussed his use of the nicotine patch, withdrawal symptoms, and high risk (or, trigger) situations they he has encountered or may encounter over the next week. The focus was on generating ways to minimize urges during this first week, and on developing plans to anticipate, avoid, and/or cope with situations that tend to trigger his smoking. Several behavioral and cognitive coping techniques are discussed and practiced, including finding distractions from and substitutes for smoking, as well as increasing awareness of and counteracting thought processes that may lead to smoking. Another meeting was scheduled for the following week to reinforce Ben's development of active coping skills for avoiding smoking, and to troubleshoot any issues that may develop with the patch. At each appointment, Ben was asked to complete brief ratings of his withdrawal (WSWS) and cravings (QSU-Brief), and to report his confidence in quitting. He reports that he is utilizing methods discussed during counseling, and that he has generated a number of other useful strategies. His motivation to

TABLE 13.3 **Internet Resources**	

Web Address	Content
www.surgeongeneral.gov/tobacco	Health and Human Services site dedicated to tobacco use. Includes all surgeon general's reports, the Clinical Practice Guideline, and consumer materials
www.smokefree.gov	Online guide to quitting smoking, sponsored by the National Cancer Institute (NCI) and the Centers for Disease Control and Prevention (CDC). Includes several self-help manuals that can be downloaded
Cancercontrolplanet.cancer.gov	NCI site providing links to evidence-based cancer control interventions, including tobacco prevention and cessation programs
www.cancer.gov/cancerinfo/tobacco	NCI site with multiple tobacco-related links
www.cdc.gov/tobacco	CDC tobacco site with multiple resources
www.srnt.org	Society for Research on Nicotine and Tobacco (SRNT)
www.treatobacco.net	Database and educational resource for treating tobacco dependence, sponsored by SRNT and other organizations
www.attud.org	Association for the Treatment of Tobacco Use and Dependence. Organization of tobacco treatment providers

quit and confidence in quitting remains high, and his withdrawal and craving scores show a steady decline. The counselor tells Ben that he can call if he encounters any difficulties with his quitting, has any questions, or if he slips back to smoking.

Conclusions

Tobacco use produces the greatest health and economic burdens upon society of any addictive drug. Because tobacco use is legal and its adverse health consequences are usually delayed, research and treatment efforts have never been proportional to its burden. Nevertheless, recent decades have seen accelerated research progress in the assessment and treatment of nicotine dependence. An ongoing challenge for the field is the dissemination of evidence-based tobacco-related assessment and treatment options to the broader clinical community. In this chapter we attempted to capture the range of approaches to assessing and treating tobacco use. Table 13.3 provides some web-based resources for additional information. Although the literature is now expansive, there remain many unanswered questions. One gap that is revealed by our review is the disconnect between assessment and treatment. Ideally, assessment should inform treatment decisions, yet this only occurs today at a relatively superficial level (e.g., daily smoking rate determining NRT dosage, some tailoring of self-help materials). As the field continues to mature, we hope to see a greater integration of assessment and treatment.

Acknowledgments

Preparation of this chapter was supported by grants from the National Cancer Institute (R01CA94256), the National Institute on Alcohol Abuse and Alcoholism (R01AA011157), and the American Cancer Society (RSGPB CPPB-109035).

References

American Psychiatric Association (1980). *Diagnostic and Statistical Manual of Mental Disorders* (3rd ed.). Washington, DC: Author.

American Psychiatric Association (1994). *Diagnostic and Statistical Manual of Mental Disorders* (4th ed.). Washington, DC: Author.

American Psychiatric Association (1996). Practice guideline for the treatment of patients with nicotine dependence. American Psychiatric Association. *American Journal of Psychiatry, 153*, 1–31.

Arntzen, F. I. (1948). Some psychological aspects of nicotinism. *The American Journal of Psychology, 61*, 424–425.

Baker, T. B., Brandon, T. H., & Chassin, L. (2004). Motivational influences on cigarette smoking. *Annual Review of Psychology, 55*, 463–491.

Balfour, D. J., & Fagerstrom, K. O. (1996). Pharmacology of nicotine and its therapeutic use in smoking cessation and neurodegenerative disorders. *Pharmacology and Therapeutics, 72*, 51–81.

Bandura, A. (1977). *Social learning theory*. Englewood Cliffs, NJ: Prentice Hall.

Berrettini, W. H., & Lerman, C. E. (2005). Pharmacotherapy and pharmacogenetics of nicotine dependence. *American Journal of Psychiatry, 162*, 1441–1451.

Biener, L., & Abrams, D. B. (1991). Contemplation Ladder: Validation of a measure of readiness to consider smoking cessation. *Health Psychology, 10*, 360–365.

Bouton, M. E. (2002). Context, ambiguity, and unlearning: Sources of relapse after behavioral extinction. *Biological Psychiatry, 52*, 976–986.

Brandon, T. H., & Baker, T. B. (1991). The smoking consequences questionnaire: The subjective expected utility of smoking in college students. *Psychology Assessment, 3*, 484–491.

Brandon, T. H., Collins, B. N., Juliano, L. M., & Lazev, A. B. (2000). Preventing relapse among former smokers: A comparison of minimal interventions via telephone and mail. *Journal of Consulting & Clinical Psychology, 68*, 103–113.

Brandon, T. H., Meade, C. D., Herzog, T. A., Chirikos, T. N., Webb, M. S., & Cantor, A. B. (2004). Efficacy and cost-effectiveness of a minimal intervention to prevent smoking relapse: Dismantling the effects of content versus contact. *Journal of Consulting & Clinical Psychology, 72*, 797–808.

Brown, R. A., Burgess, E. S., Sales, S. D., Whiteley, J. A., Evans, D., & Miller, I. W. (1998). Reliability and validity of a smoking timeline follow-back interview. *Psychology of Addictive Behaviors, 12*, 101–112.

Cahill, K., Stead, L., & Lancaster, T. (2007). Nicotine receptor partial agonists for smoking cessation. *Cochrane Database of Systematic Reviews*, CD006103.

CDC (1999). *Best practices for comprehensive tobacco control programs*. US Department of Health and Human Services, Centers for Disease Control and Prevention, National Center for Chronic Disease Prevention and Health Promotion, Office on Smoking and Health: Atlanta, GA.

CDC (2002). Tobacco use among adults – United States, 2000. *Mortality and Morbidity Weekly Report, 51*, 642–645.

CDC (2005). Annual smoking-attributable mortality, years of potential life lost, and productivity losses – United States, 1997–2001. *Mortality and Morbidity Weekly Report, 54*, 625–628.

CDC (2007). Cigarette smoking among adults – United States, 2006. *Mortality and Morbidity Weekly Report, 56*, 1157–1161.

Cinciripini, P. M., Lapitsky, L. G., Seay, S., Wallfisch, A., Kitchens, K., & Van Vunakis, H. (1995). The effects of smoking schedules on cessation outcome: Can we improve on common methods of gradual and abrupt nicotine withdrawal? *Journal of Consulting & Clinical Psychology, 63*, 388–399.

Coe, J. W., Brooks, P. R., Vetelino, M. G., Wirtz, M. C., Arnold, E. P., Huang, J., et al. (2005). Varenicline: An alpha4beta2 nicotinic receptor partial agonist for smoking cessation. *Journal of Medicinal Chemistry, 48*, 3474–3477.

Collins, B. N., & Brandon, T. H. (2002). Effects of extinction context and retrieval cues on alcohol cue reactivity among nonalcoholic drinkers. *Journal of Consulting & Clinical Psychology, 70*, 390–397.

Compas, B. E., Haaga, D. A. F., Keefe, F. J., Leitenberg, H., & Williams, D. A. (1998). Sampling of empirically supported psychological treatments from health psychology: Smoking, chronic pain, cancer, and bulimia nervosa. *Journal of Consulting and Clinical Psychology, 66*, 89–112.

Conklin, C. A., & Tiffany, S. T. (2002). Applying extinction research and theory to cue-exposure addiction treatments. *Addiction, 97,* 155–167.

Copeland, A. L., Brandon, T. H., & Quinn, E. P. (1995). The Smoking Consequences Questionnaire - Adult: Measurement of smoking outcome expectancies of experienced smokers. *Psychological Assessment, 7,* 484–494.

Cox, L. S., Tiffany, S. T., & Christen, A. (2001). Evaluation of the brief questionnaire of smoking urges (QSU-brief) in laboratory and clinical settings. *Nicotine & Tobacco Research, 3,* 7–16.

Cromwell J., Bartosch, W. J., Fiore, M. C., Baker, T, & Hasselblad, V. (1997). Cost-effectiveness of the AHCPR guidelines for smoking. *Journal of the American Medical Association, 278,* 1759–1766.

Curry, S. J., Grothaus, L. C., & McBride, C. M. (1997). Reasons for quitting: Intrinsic and extrinsic motivation for smoking cessation in a population-based sample of smokers. *Addictive Behaviors, 22,* 727–739.

Curry, S. J., Wagner, E. H., & Grothaus, L. C. (1990). Intrinsic and extrinsic motivation for smoking cessation. *Journal of Consulting and Clinical Psychology, 58,* 310–316.

Dempsey, D. A., & Benowitz, N. L. (2001). Risks and benefits of nicotine to aid smoking cessation in pregnancy. *Drug Safety, 24,* 277–322.

Dwoskin, L. P., Rauhut, A. S., King-Pospisil, K. A., & Bardo, M. T. (2006). Review of the pharmacology and clinical profile of bupropion, an antidepressant and tobacco use cessation agent. *CNS Drug Reviews, 12,* 178–207.

Ellerbeck, E. F., Ahluwalia, J. S., Jolicoeur, D. G., Gladden, J., & Mosier, M.C. (2001). Direct observation of smoking cessation activities in primary care practice. *Journal of Family Practice, 50,* 688–693.

Etter, J. F., Le-Houezec, J., & Perneger, T. (2003). A self-administered questionnaire to measure dependence on cigarettes: The cigarette dependence scale. *Neuropsychopharmacology, 28,* 359–370.

Etter, J. F., & Stapleton, J. A. (2006). Nicotine replacement therapy for long-term smoking cessation: A meta-analysis. *Tobacco Control, 15,* 280–285.

Ezzati, M., & Lopez, A. D. (2003). Estimates of global mortality attributable to smoking in 2000. *Lancet, 362,* 847–852.

Fagerström, K. O. (1978). Measuring degree of physical dependence to tobacco smoking with reference to individualization of treatment. *Addictive Behaviors, 3,* 235–241.

Fiore, M. C., Jean, C. R., Baker, T. B., et al. (2008). *Treating tobacco use and dependence. 2008 Update. Clinical Practice Guideline.* Rockville, MD: US Department of Health and Human Services, Public Health Service. May, 2008.

Foulds, J. (2006). The neurobiological basis for partial agonist treatment of nicotine dependence: varenicline. *International Journal of Clinical Practice, 60,* 571–576.

Foulds, J., Steinberg, M. B., Williams, J. M., & Ziedonis, D. M. (2006). Developments in pharmacotherapy for tobacco dependence: Past, present and future. *Drug and Alcohol Review, 25,* 59–71.

Frishman, W. H., Mitta, W., Kupersmith, A., & Ky, T. (2006). Nicotine and non-nicotine smoking cessation pharmacotherapies. *Cardiology in Review, 14,* 57–73.

Gourlay, S. G., Stead, L. F., & Benowitz, N. L. (2004). Clonidine for smoking cessation. *Cochrane Database of Systematic Reviews,* CD000058.

Gwaltney, C. J., Shiffman, S., Norman, G. J., Paty, J. A., Kassel, J. D., Gyns, M., et al., (2001). Does smoking abstinence self-efficacy vary across situations?: Identifying context-specific within the Relapse Situation Efficacy Questionnaire. *Journal of Consulting and Clinical Psychology, 69,* 516–527.

Hajek, P., & Stead, L. F. (2001). Aversive smoking for smoking cessation. *Cochrane Database of Systematic Reviews, 3.*

Hajek, P., West, R., Foulds, J., Nilsson, F., Burrows, S., & Meadow, A. (1999). Randomized comparative trial of nicotine polacrilex, a transdermal patch, nasal spray, and an inhaler. *Archives of Internal Medicine, 159,* 2033–2038.

Hayford, K. E., Patten, C. A., Rummans, T. A., Schroeder, D. R., Offord, K. P., Croghan, I. T., et al. (1999). Efficacy of bupropion for smoking cessation in smokers with a former history of major depression or alcoholism. *British Journal of Psychiatry, 174,* 173–178.

Heatherton, T. F., Kozlowski, L. T., Frecker, R. C., & Fagerström, K. O. (1991). The Fagerström test for nicotine dependence: A revision of the Fagerström tolerance questionnaire. *British Journal of Addiction, 86,* 1119–1127.

Heatherton, T. F., Kozlowski, L. T., Frecker, R. C., Rickert, W., & Robinson, J. (1989). Measuring the heaviness of smoking: Using self-reported time to the first cigarette of the day and number of cigarettes smoked per day. *British Journal of Addiction, 84*, 791–799.

Heishman, S. J., Singleton, E. G., & Moolchan, E. T. (2003). Tobacco Craving Questionnaire: Reliability and validity of a new multifactorial instrument. *Nicotine & Tobacco Research, 5*, 645–654.

Hendricks, P. S., Ditre, J. W., Drobes, D. J., & Brandon, T. H. (2006). The early time course of smoking withdrawal effects. *Psychopharmacology, 187*, 385–396.

Henningfield, J. E. (1995). Nicotine medications for smoking cessation. *New England Journal of Medicine, 333*, 1196–1203.

Henningfield, J. E., Fant, R. V., Buchhalter, A. R., & Stitzer, M. L. (2005). Pharmacotherapy for nicotine dependence. *CA: A Cancer Journal for Clinicians, 55*, 281–299; quiz 322–283, 325.

Hughes, J. R. (1995). Combining behavioral therapy and pharmacotherapy for smoking cessation: An update. In L. S. Onken, J. D. Blaine, & J. J. Boren (Eds.), *Integrating behavior therapies with medication in the treatment of drug dependence: NIDA Research Monograph* (pp. 92–109). Monograph no. 150. Washington DC: US Government Printing Office.

Hughes, J. R. (2001). The evidence for hardening: Is the target hardening? *NCI Smoking and Tobacco Control Monograph.* Bethesda, MD: U.S. Department of Health and Human Services, National Institutes of Health, National Cancer Institute.

Hughes, J. R., Goldstein, M. G., Hurt, R. D., & Shiffman, S. (1999). Recent advances in the pharmacotherapy of smoking. *JAMA, 281*, 72–76.

Hughes, J. R., & Hatsukami, D. (1986). Signs and symptoms of tobacco withdrawal. *Archives of General Psychiatry, 43*, 289–294.

Hughes, J. R., Shiffman, S., Callas, P., & Zhang, J. (2003). A meta-analysis of the efficacy of over-the-counter nicotine replacement. *Tobacco Control, 12*, 21–27.

Hughes, J. R., Stead, L., & Lancaster, T. (2007). Antidepressants for smoking cessation. *Cochrane Database of Systematic Reviews, 1*, CD000031.

Irvin, J. E., & Brandon, T. H. (2000). The increasing recalcitrance of smokers in clinical trials. *Nicotine & Tobacco Research, 2*, 79–84.

Irvin, J. E., Bowers, C. A., Dunn, M. E., & Wang, M. C. (1999). Efficacy of relapse prevention: A meta-analytic review. *Journal of Consulting and Clinical Psychology, 67*, 563–570.

Irvin, J. E., Hendricks, P. S., & Brandon, T. H. (2003). The increasing recalcitrance of smokers in clinical trials II: Pharmacotherapy trials. *Nicotine & Tobacco Research, 5*, 27–35.

Jorenby, D. E., Hays, J. T., Rigotti, N. A., Azoulay, S., Watsky, E. J., Williams, K. E., et al. (2006). Efficacy of varenicline, an alpha4beta2 nicotinic acetylcholine receptor partial agonist, vs placebo or sustained-release bupropion for smoking cessation: A randomized controlled trial. *JAMA, 296*, 56–63.

Jorenby, D. E., Leischow, S. J., Nides, M. A., Rennard, S. I., Johnston, J. A., Hughes, A. R., et al. (1999). A controlled trial of sustained-release bupropion, a nicotine patch, or both for smoking cessation. *New England Journal of Medicine, 340*, 685–691.

Joseph, A. M., Norman, S. M., Ferry, L. H., Prochazka, A. V., Westman, E. C., Steele, B. G., et al. (1996). The safety of transdermal nicotine as an aid to smoking cessation in patients with cardiac disease. *New England Journal of Medicine, 335*, 1792–1798.

Keating, G. M., & Siddiqui, M. A. (2006). Varenicline: A review of its use as an aid to smoking cessation therapy. *CNS Drugs, 20*, 945–960.

Kessler, R. C., & Üstün, T. B. (2004). The world mental health (WMH) survey initiative version of the World Health Organization (WHO) composite international diagnostic interview (CIDI). *International Journal of Methods in Psychiatric Research, 13*, 93–121.

Killen, J. D., & Fortman, S. P. (1997). Craving is associated with smoking relapse: Findings from three prospective studies. *Experimental and Clinical Psychopharmacology, 5*, 137–142.

Lancaster, T., & Stead, L. F. (2004). Physician advice for smoking cessation. *Cochrane Database of Systematic Reviews, 4.*

Lancaster, T., & Stead, L. F. (2005). Self-help interventions for smoking cessation. *Cochrane Database of Systematic Reviews, 3.*

Lerman, C., Patterson, F., & Berrettini, W. (2005). Treating tobacco dependence: State of the science and new directions. *Journal of Clinical Oncology, 23*, 311–323.

Lichtenstein, E., Harris, D. E., Birchler, G. R., Wahl, J. M., & Schmahl, D. P. (1973). Comparison of rapid smoking, warm, smoky air, and attention placebo in the modification of smoking behavior. *Journal of Consulting and Clinical Psychology, 40*, 92–98.

Marlatt, G. A. (1985). Relapse prevention: Theoretical rationale and overview of the model. In G. A. Marlatt, & J. R. Gordon (Eds.), *Relapse prevention* (pp. 3–70). New York: Guilford Press.

Marlatt, G. A., & Gordon, J. R. (1985). *Relapse prevention*. New York: Guilford Press.

Munafò, M. R., Clark, T. G., Johnstone, E. C., Murphy, M. F. G., & Walton, R. T. (2004). The genetic basis for smoking behavior: A systematic review and meta-analysis. *Nicotine & Tobacco Research, 6*, 583–597.

Myers, M. G., MacPherson, L., McCarthy, D. M., & Brown, S. A. (2003). Constructing a short form of the Smoking Consequences Questionnaire with adolescents and young adults. *Psychological Assessment, 15*, 163–172.

Niaura, R., Rohsenow, D. J., Binkoff, J. A., Monti, P. M., Pedraza, M., & Abrams, D. B. (1988). Relevance of cue reactivity to understanding alcohol and smoking relapse. *Journal of Abnormal Psychology, 97*, 133–152.

O'Connell, K. A., Gerkovich, M. M., Cook, M. R., Shiffman, S., Hickcox, M., & Kakolewski, K. E. (1998). Coping in real time: Using ecological momentary assessment techniques to assess coping with the urge to smoke. *Research in Nursing and Health, 21*, 487–497.

Perkins, K. A., Conklin, C. A., & Levine, M. D. (2007). *Cognitive-behavioral therapy for smoking cessation: A practical guidebook to the most effective treatments.* New York: Routledge.

Phillips, K. M., & Brandon, T. H. (2004). Do psychologists adhere to the clinical practice guidelines for tobacco cessation? A survey of practitioners. *Professional Psychology: Research & Practice, 35*, 281–285.

Pierce, J. P., & Gilpin, E. A. (2002). Impact of over-the-counter sales on effectiveness of pharmaceutical aids for smoking cessation. *JAMA, 288*, 1260–1264.

Piper, M. E., Piasecki, T. M., Federman, E. B., Bolt, D. M, Smith, S. S., Fiore, M. C., & Baker, T. B. (2004). A multiple motives approach to tobacco dependence: The Wisconsin Inventory of Smoking Dependence Motives (WISDM-68). *Journal of Consulting and Clinical Psychology, 72*(2), 139–154.

Prochaska, J. O., DiClemente, C. C., & Norcross, J. C. (1992). In search of how people change: Applications to addictive behaviors. *American Psychologist, 47*, 1102–1114.

Prochazka, A. V. (2000). New developments in smoking cessation. *Chest, 117*, 169S–175S.

Robins, L. N. (1986). The development and characteristics of the NIMH Diagnostic Interview Schedule. In: M. M. Weissman, J. Myers, & C. Ross (Eds.), *Community surveys psychiatric disorders.* New Brunswick, NJ: Rutgers University Press.

Shiffman, S. (1988). Behavioral assessment. In D. Donovan & G. Marlatt (Eds.), *Assessment of addictive behavior* (pp. 139–199). New York: Guilford Press.

Shiffman S., & Jarvik, M. (1976). Trends in withdrawal symptoms in abstinence from cigarette smoking. *Psychopharmacologia, 50*, 35–39.

Shiffman, S., & Paty, J. (2006). Smoking patterns and dependence: Contrasting chippers and heavy smokers. *Journal of Abnormal Psychology, 115*, 509–523.

Shiffman, S., Rolf, C. N., Hellebusch, S. J., Gorsline, J., Gorodetzky, C. W., Chiang, Y. K., et al. (2002). Real-world efficacy of prescription and over-the-counter nicotine replacement therapy. *Addiction, 97*, 505–516.

Shiffman, S., Shadel, W. G., Niaura, R., Khayrallah, M. A., Jorenby, D. E., Ryan, C. F., & Ferguson, C. L. (2003). Efficacy of acute administration of nicotine gum in relief of cue-provoked cigarette craving. *Psychopharmacology, 166*, 343–350.

Shiffman, S., Waters, A. J., & Hickcox, M. (2004). The nicotine dependence syndrome scale: A multidimensional measure of nicotine dependence. *Nicotine & Tobacco Research, 6*, 327–348.

Silagy, C., Lancaster, T., Stead, L., Mant, D., & Fowler, G. (2004). Nicotine replacement therapy for smoking cessation. *Cochrane Database of Systematic Reviews*, CD000146.

Sobell, L. C., & Sobell, M. B. (1992). Timeline follow-back: A technique for assessing self-reported alcohol consumption. In: R. Z. Litten & J. P. Allen (Eds.), *Measuring alcohol consumption: Psychosocial and biochemical methods*, Totowa, NJ: Humana Press.

Stead, L. F., & Lancaster, T. (2005). Group behaviour therapy programs for smoking cessation. *Cochrane Database of Systematic Reviews, 2.*

Stead, L. F., Perera, R., & Lancaster, T. (2006). Telephone counseling for smoking cessation. *Cochrane Database of Systematic Reviews, 3.*

Stone, A. A., & Shiffman, S. (1994). Ecological momentary assessment (EMA) in behavioral medicine. *Annals of Behavioral Medicine, 16,* 199–202.

Swan, G. E., McAfee, T., Curry, S. J., Jack, L. M., Javitz, H., Dacey, S., et al. (2003). Effectiveness of bupropion sustained release for smoking cessation in a health care setting: A randomized trial. *Archives of Internal Medicine, 163,* 2337–2344.

Sweeney, C. T., Fant, R. V., Fagerstrom, K. O., McGovern, J. F., & Henningfield, J. E. (2001). Combination nicotine replacement therapy for smoking cessation: Rationale, efficacy and tolerability. *CNS Drugs, 15,* 453–467.

Tengs, T. O., Adams, M. E., Pliskin, J. S., Safran, D. G., Siegel, J. E., Weinstein, M. C., & Graham, J. D. (1995). *Risk Analysis, 16,* 369–390.

Tiffany, S. T., & Drobes, D. J. (1991). The development and initial validation of a questionnaire of smoking urges. *British Journal of Addiction, 86,* 1467–1476.

Uhl, G. R., Liu, Q., Drgon, T., Johnson, C., Walther, D., Rose, J. E., David, S. P., Niaura, R., & Lerman, C. (2008). Molecular genetics of successful smoking cessation: Convergent genome-wide association study results. *Archives of General Psychiatry, 65,* 683–693.

United States Public Health Service (1988). *The health consequences of smoking: Nicotine addiction. A report of the Surgeon General.* Washington, DC: U.S. Government Printing Office.

Velicer, W. F., DiClemente, C. C., Rossi, J. S., & Prochaska, J. O. (1990). Relapse situations and self-efficacy: An integrative model. *Addictive Behaviors, 15,* 271–283.

Velicer, W. F., Friedman, R. H., Fava, J. L., Gulliver, S. B., Keller, S., Sun, X., et al. (2006). Evaluating nicotine replacement therapy and stage-based therapies in a population-based effectiveness trial. *Journal of Consulting and Clinical Psychology, 74,* 1162–1172.

Warner, K. E., & Burns, D. M. (2003) Hardening and the hard-core smoker: Concepts, evidence, and implications. *Nicotine & Tobacco Research, 5,* 37–48.

Webb, M. S., Hendricks, P. S., & Brandon, T. H. (2007). Expectancy priming of smoking cessation messages enhances the placebo effect of tailored interventions. *Health Psychology, 26,* 598–609.

Webb, M. S., Simmons, V. N., & Brandon, T. H. (2005). Tailored interventions for motivating smoking cessation: Using placebo-tailoring to examine the influence of personalization and expectancies. *Health Psychology, 24,*179–188.

Wellman, R. J., DiFranza, J. R., Savageau, J. A., Godiwala, S., Friedman, K., & Hazelton, J. (2005). Measuring adults' loss of autonomy over nicotine use: The hooked on nicotine checklist. *Nicotine & Tobacco Research, 7,* 157–161.

Welsch, S. K., Smith, S. S., Jorenby, D. E., Wetter, D. W., Fiore, M. C., & Baker, T. B. (1999). Development and validation of the Wisconsin Smoking Withdrawal Scale. *Experimental and Clinical Psychopharmacology, 7,* 354–361.

Zhu, S.-H., Anderson, C. M., Tedeschi, G. J., Rosbrook, B., Johnson, C. E., Byrd, M., & Gutierrez-Terrell, E. (2002). Evidence of real-world effectiveness of a telephone quitline for smokers. *New England Journal of Medicine, 347,* 1087–1093.

14

Assessment and Treatment of Marijuana Use Disorders

Alison Looby and Mitch Earleywine

University at Albany

Contents

More people consume marijuana than any other illicit substance in the United States. Recent reports suggest that nearly 28% of adults aged 18 to 25 have used marijuana at least once in their lives, and 4.3% were daily users (Substance Abuse and Mental Health Services Administration [SAMHSA], 2005). Based on the 2003 National Household Survey on Drug Abuse, approximately 14.6 million individuals age 12 and above were past-month marijuana users and 3.1 million reported daily use (SAMHSA, 2003). Use is especially prominent among adolescents, who may be at the greatest risk for negative consequences. Among adolescents, marijuana use is more common than the use of all other illicit substances combined (Monitoring the Future

[MTF], 2001). Over the past several decades, marijuana use has risen in both adolescents and young adults. In 1965, only 1.8% of youths and 5% of young adults had tried marijuana, whereas in 2001 the rates had increased to nearly 22% and 54%, respectively (SAMHSA, 2003).

Although many marijuana users do not report experiencing problems, several studies have described a range of physical, social, psychological, and legal problems associated with its use (Agosti & Levin, 2004; Budney, Radonovich, Higgins, & Wong, 1998; Haas & Hendin, 1987). Marijuana is the primary substance mentioned in adolescent arrests, emergency room admissions, and autopsy reports (Bureau of Justice Statistics [BJS], 2000; SAMHSA, 2000a, 2000b). Additionally, approximately 9% of all marijuana users will meet the criteria for marijuana dependence during their lifetime (Anthony, Warner, & Kessler, 1994). Hall, Solowij, and Lemon (1994) indicate that the risk of dependence may be particularly strong, as high as 20–30%, for individuals who use marijuana on multiple occasions.

According to SAMHSA's Treatment Episode Data Set (TEDS), substance abuse treatment admission rates for marijuana as the primary substance of abuse has increased by 162% from 1992 to 2002 (SAMHSA, 2004). Thus, a large number of marijuana users are experiencing significant problems that warrant professional assistance.

Historical Conceptualization of Marijuana Use Disorders

The Emergence of Marijuana Use

Although marijuana has reportedly been used in the United States since the 1800s, it did not gain popularity until the 1960s (Earleywine, 2002). Incidence of use increased into the mid-1970s, dropped slightly in the early 1990s, and has been rising ever since (SAMHSA, 2000c). Historically, marijuana was not viewed as a drug of dependence due to the perceived absence of tolerance and withdrawal symptoms. By the late 1990s, however, there were twice as many new marijuana users per year than users of all other illicit drugs combined. Age of initiation of marijuana use has declined throughout the years, with the majority of new marijuana users since the mid-1970s being adolescents (Dennis, Babor, Roebuck, & Donaldson, 2002).

Although patients in treatment for substance dependence over the last few decades use marijuana more than other substances, researchers and practitioners have focused more attention on other drugs (Simpson et al., 1999). Research reveals that treatment for marijuana problems has proven difficult as this population tends to show the least amount of change compared with other substance abusers (Hser et al., 2001). Many problem users quit on their own (Price, Risk, & Spitznagel, 2001) and it is perhaps only the most difficult cases that reach treatment providers. In addition, few of the evaluated treatment programs that appear in the research literature used empirically supported and manual-guided treatments. These factors may all account for the lack of improvement seen among these individuals. These data, combined with increasing marijuana use and referrals to treatment centers, articulate the need for evidence-based treatments in the treatment of marijuana dependence.

Conceptualization of Marijuana Use Disorders

Originally, the *Diagnostic and Statistical Manual* (*DSM*) viewed psychiatric disorders from a psychodynamic perspective (e.g., a result of the personality's struggle to adjust to internal and external stressors). It was not until the publication of the *DSM–III* (American Psychiatric Association [APA], 1980) that researchers and clinicians made an effort to base psychiatric diagnoses on empirically supported clinical symptom patterns. In the *DSM–III*, substance dependence was conceptualized as symptoms of tolerance and withdrawal. Additionally, the diagnosis of marijuana dependence required a pattern of pathological use or impairment in social and occupational functioning. Pathological use required intoxication throughout the day and near-daily use for one month. However, the manual noted that the existence and clinical significance of tolerance to marijuana was controversial, and that there was not sufficient evidence for the existence of marijuana withdrawal. Consequently, a diagnosis of marijuana dependence according to the *DSM–III* was limited in validity and relied on frequency of use.

The revision of the *DSM–III* increased the diagnostic criteria for substance dependence to nine items, three of which had to be endorsed for a diagnosis of dependence (APA, 1987). The conceptualization of marijuana dependence was broadened to include information about the saliency of the drug in one's life, difficulty quitting or controlling use, and continued use despite problems. The *DSM–III–R*, however, continued to suggest that withdrawal symptoms likely did not apply to marijuana use. Although the frequency of use was no longer a criterion, this edition persisted in characterizing marijuana dependence by daily or near-daily use. It was not until the publication of the *DSM–IV* (APA, 1994) that frequency of use no longer suggested dependence. This approach is consistent with research demonstrating that only 24% of marijuana-dependent individuals reported daily use in 1998, and 26% reported less than weekly use (SAMHSA, 2000c). The *DSM–IV* and *DSM–IV–TR* (2000) require at least three of seven criteria for the dependence diagnosis. These editions allow for the specification of physiological dependence when tolerance and withdrawal appear. These latest versions assert that marijuana-associated withdrawal symptoms exist, but their clinical significance is uncertain. Thus, marijuana withdrawal is not included in the *DSM–IV–TR*.

The validity of marijuana withdrawal symptoms has generated considerable work. Research has largely confirmed the existence of marijuana withdrawal both in adults and in adolescents (Budney, Hughes, Moore, & Vandrey, 2004; Vandrey, Budney, Kamon, & Stanger, 2005). Treatment studies suggest that 50 to 95% of marijuana users report withdrawal symptoms (Copeland, Swift, & Rees, 2001a; Crowley, MacDonald, Whitmore, & Mikulich, 1998; Stephens, Babor, Kadden, Miller, & the Marijuana Treatment Project Research Group, 2002), and the magnitude and time-course of the symptoms are comparable to other withdrawal syndromes (Budney, Moore, Vandrey, & Hughes, 2003), particularly nicotine withdrawal (Vandrey, Budney, Moore, & Hughes, 2005). Thus, although the *DSM–IV–TR* questions the clinical significance of marijuana withdrawal, research indicates that the syndrome is indeed important. Based on this information, Budney (2006) has proposed that marijuana withdrawal disorder be included in the *DSM–V*. Common proposed marijuana withdrawal symptoms include anger or aggression, decreased appetite or weight loss, irritability, anxiety, restlessness, and sleep difficulties including strange dreams. Note that these symptoms do not parallel most stereotypes of drug withdrawal, as marijuana withdrawal lacks the severity observed in withdrawal from heroin or alcohol.

In addition to the marijuana withdrawal syndrome debate, several researchers question whether the *DSM* criteria for substance dependence are applicable and valid in diagnosing marijuana dependence. In general, data support a one-factor dependence syndrome across substances, and psychometric studies indicate that the *DSM* criteria appear to provide a reliable description of marijuana dependence across multiple cultures (Fiengold & Rounsaville, 1995; Morgenstern, Langenbucher, & Labouvie, 1994; Nelson, Rehm, Ustun, Grant, & Chatterji, 1999). Thus, the standard *DSM* dependence criteria perform as well for marijuana as they do for most other substance-dependence disorders. Additionally, there is evidence that the diagnostic criteria also pertain to adolescent users (Winters, Latimer, & Stinchfield, 1999). However, the threshold of three criteria for the diagnosis of marijuana dependence seems questionable inasmuch as its severity is typically less than that seen for other illicit substances. In fact, very few marijuana users endorse all seven dependence criteria (Feingold & Rounsaville, 1995; Nelson et al., 1999). Consequently, substance-specific cut-off scores for dependence severity might prove valuable for marijuana diagnoses.

Furthermore, the applicability of generic *DSM–IV* substance abuse criteria to marijuana is questionable. Although the diagnosis of abuse stipulates that a recurrent and maladaptive pattern of use causing significant impairment or distress is necessary, the meaning of this statement is left up to subjective clinical judgment. No empirical evidence has established quantity and severity guidelines to determine whether endorsement of an abuse criterion warrants a diagnosis. Because legal problems can lead to an abuse diagnosis, current policy and arrests may contribute to the rates of the diagnosis of abuse in peculiar ways (Earleywine, 2002). Despite this fact, the idea that users can abuse marijuana has considerable intuitive appeal. Even the National Organization for Reformation of Marijuana Laws (NORML), an organization devoted to ending marijuana prohibition, encourages those who choose to use to do so responsibly. They assert that marijuana can be detrimental when abused, but report difficulty in defining what constitutes abuse (Stroup, 1999). Thus, developing clear behavioral criteria for marijuana abuse and dependence necessitates more research attention.

Many critics of the *DSM* take issue with the diagnostic criteria for abuse and dependence. One particular area of concern involves the potential minimization of important substance-related problems that do not qualify for a diagnosis. Specifically, many marijuana users may meet one or two symptoms of dependence but no abuse symptoms, and accordingly will not be given a diagnosis of dependence. The term "diagnostic orphan" has been used to describe these individuals (Degenhardt, Lynskey, Coffey, & Patton, 2002), and this status may impede treatment availability. Approximately 6 to 23% of marijuana users report some difficulties associated with marijuana use (Earleywine, 2002), not all of whom meet the diagnostic criteria for dependence or abuse. Recent work suggests that focusing on abuse or dependence may prove less helpful than directing efforts toward minimizing substance-related problems (Marlatt, 1998). Thus, time may be better spent recognizing individual problems resulting from marijuana use to reduce the harm that marijuana may cause. Early intervention (e.g., before a diagnosis is actually present) may prove easier than waiting until problems increase in severity.

Contemporary Assessment of Marijuana Use Disorders

Both the assessment and the treatment of marijuana use disorders are challenging tasks. In addition to the problematic diagnostic issues, many users do not recognize problems that stem from marijuana consumption, leading them to lack the motivation to alter their use. Furthermore, clients may prove reluctant to discuss their use when clinicians do not know how to assess or recognize problems. Accurate and comprehensive assessment is a necessary and fundamental component for treatment planning in this population. Although assessing for marijuana abuse and dependence is certainly relevant, many other factors must also guide the treatment decisions and feedback that may motivate clients to change.

Assessing the Severity of Dependence

The most comprehensive method to assess for marijuana dependence requires interviews, such as the Structured Clinical Interview for *DSM–IV* Axis I Disorders (SCID; First, Spitzer, Gibbon, & Williams, 1996), the Composite International Diagnostic Interview (CIDI; World Health Organization, 1997), and, for adolescents, the Adolescent Diagnostic Interview (ADI; Winters & Henley, 1993). Many consider these interviews to be the gold standard in the diagnosis of substance use disorders as they show good inter-rater and test–retest reliability with trained interviewers. The number of dependence symptoms endorsed can serve as an index of severity and improvement following treatment. Although the validity of this approach has yet to be determined, decreases in the number of dependence symptoms appear to accompany reductions in marijuana use following treatment (Marijuana Treatment Project Research Group [MTPRG], 2004; Stephens, Roffman, & Curtin, 2000). This observation lends support to using dependence severity indices. However, other researchers assert that those with more severe forms of dependence report different symptoms compared to their peers classified with milder levels of dependence. Thus, simple counts of dependence symptoms may not be the optimal choice to assess treatment severity or treatment outcome (Andreatini, Galduroz, Ferri, & Formigoni, 1994).

The Severity of Dependence Scale (SDS; Gossop et al., 1995) helps address the need for an indicator of dependence severity. The SDS is a five-item scale that measures individuals' concerns about impaired control over substance use. High scorers likely also show marijuana dependence (Swift, Copeland, & Hall, 1998). This measure has good psychometric properties with adult marijuana users (Gossop et al., 1995; Swift et al., 1998) and scores have been shown to improve with treatment (Copeland, Swift, Roffman, & Stephens, 2001b). It also performs well with adolescents as a reliable and valid measure of severity of marijuana dependence (Martin, Copeland, Gates, & Gilmour, 2006). However, the cut-off score for marijuana dependence differs between adolescents and adults, and optimal identification of marijuana dependence requires a lower cut-off score than the score recommended for other drugs.

Consequently, although this measure provides a quick and easy way of gathering adequate diagnostic and severity information, practitioners and researchers may get more benefit from an instrument developed specifically for assessing marijuana use.

To that end, the Marijuana Screening Inventory (MSI; Alexander, 2003) focuses on troubles particularly relevant to marijuana. The MSI's 39 items survey both symptoms of dependence and associated problems, in an effort to identify problem users who do not meet the *DSM* criteria for a diagnosis. This self-report instrument has shown acceptable psychometric properties when used with adults (Alexander & Leung, 2006). It is the first validated substance-specific measure of marijuana dependence and severity and has utility as a screening tool. The utility of the MSI in treatment planning is not yet known, although it serves a useful function in measuring treatment outcome.

Although marijuana withdrawal remains controversial, it is important to assess for these symptoms as well given the recent support for this syndrome (Budney & Hughes, 2006). The Marijuana Withdrawal Symptom Checklist (Budney, Novy, & Hughes, 1999) is one such way to obtain this information. This measure includes 22 questions targeting affective and behavioral symptoms of marijuana withdrawal. Each symptom receives a severity rating, allowing for the assessment of the extent of withdrawal. Such information may help determine the severity of dependence and assist in treatment.

Assessing the Pattern of Use

Assessment of the frequency and quantity of marijuana consumption is essential to planning treatment and assessing its impact. However, estimates of the extent of use can prove difficult and cumbersome. No standard units of consumption exist for marijuana that are comparable to those established for legal drugs such as alcohol and nicotine. The quantity of use is affected by route of administration, preparation of the plant, and mechanism of delivery. Different plants show a wide range of potency, and joints/pipes range considerably in size. In addition, the subjective experience attained with any amount may vary substantially (Zimmer & Morgan, 1997).

There is currently limited evidence on the reliability and validity of self-reports detailing quantity consumed and frequency of marijuana use. Researchers have used several methods of gathering quantity of use data, such as inquiring about the amount of marijuana consumed per day or per week using various units of measurement (e.g., ounces, grams, joints, pipes, bowls; Stephens & Roffman, 2005). Similar single-item summary questions can be used to obtain frequency data. Another method of acquiring such information is to collect this information on a day-by-day basis using instruments such as the Timeline Follow-back (TLFB; Sobell & Sobell, 1992; Stephens et al., 2002) or self-monitoring approaches such as the daily diary. Although research suggests that the use of summary questions and the TLFB are valid ways of collecting frequency of use information among marijuana users (MTPRG, 2004; Stephens et al., 2000), evidence is not available regarding the use of these measures in obtaining estimates of quantity of use. It is important to note, however, that self-report accuracy may be influenced by many factors including social desirability, little interest in quitting, and lack of insight into problematic use (Babor, Brown, & Del Boca, 1990; Matt & Wilson, 1994). This is particularly true among adolescents (Buchan, Dennis, Tims, & Diamong, 2002). These findings demonstrate the advantages of using multiple sources of information in determining the extent of marijuana use, such as obtaining collateral confirmation or using urine drug screening tests.

Assessing Marijuana-Associated Problems

Numerous self-report questionnaires have been developed in order to assess problems associated with marijuana use. In addition to the defined dependence and abuse criteria, marijuana users may be experiencing social, occupational, legal, or health problems due to their drug use. Evaluations of these negative consequences are fundamental in examining the user's motivation for change. In addition, monitoring changes in associated problems may be valuable from a harm reduction standpoint, where complete abstinence is not the overarching goal.

The 19-item Marijuana Problem Scale (MPS; Stephens et al., 2000) was developed as an index of negative social, occupational, physical, and personal consequences resulting from marijuana use. The reliability and validity of this measure has not been reported, but it has been shown to be sensitive to treatment effects (MTPRG, 2004). A more comprehensive and global index of negative consequences has also been developed (Copeland et al., 2001a, 2001b), which was modeled after the psychometrically sound Alcohol Problems Questionnaire (Williams & Drummond, 1994). The Cannabis Problems Questionnaire (CPQ) contains 53 items and has proven to be reliable and valid in a population of adult marijuana users, as well as sensitive to treatment effects (Copeland, Gilmour, Gates, & Swift, 2005). The CPQ has also been adapted for use in an adolescent population (CPQ-A; Martin, Copeland, Gilmour, Gates, & Swift, 2006) and shows promise in detecting subdiagnostic marijuana-related problems among young people. Finally, the Addiction Severity Index (ASI; McLellan et al., 1992) has been used to asses the negative impact of marijuana use. The ASI has demonstrated validity and reliability across a variety of substances and objectively assesses problems and psychosocial functioning in numerous areas of life. An advantage of the ASI is that it does not necessitate the user to ascribe causation to the relationship between their marijuana use and their current problems. However, the ASI is a lengthy structured interview that must be administered by a trained clinician. Thus, practicality may preclude its use in clinical settings.

Assessing Readiness to Change

Assessing the client's level of readiness to change is very important in determining the best treatment for one's level of motivation. It is also useful to monitor whether the client's motivation increases throughout the treatment process. Many marijuana users may be in the precontemplation or contemplation stages prior to beginning treatment, which may necessitate the use of strategies such as motivational interviewing (see Chapter 28 for more information on this technique) before engaging in skills training. Several questionnaires have been developed that measure an individual's position on each dimension of the stages of change model. The University of Rhode Island Change Assessment (URICA; McConnaughy, Prochaska, & Velicer, 1983) is a 32-item questionnaire that identifies individuals in the precontemplation, contemplation, action, and maintenance stages. The Stages of Change Readiness and Treatment Eagerness Scale (SOCRATES; Miller & Tonigan, 1996) is another frequently used measure. This 20-item scale measures precontemplation, contemplation, determination, action, and maintenance. Finally, the Readiness to Change Questionnaire (RCQ; Rollnick, Heather, Gold, & Hall, 1992) contains 12 items that measure precontemplation, contemplation, and action. These instruments have been developed for use in populations of alcohol users, however, many researchers have modified the questions for use with marijuana users (i.e., Budney, Higgins, Radonovich, & Novy, 2000; Stephens et al., 2004).

Contemporary Treatment of Marijuana Use Disorders

Assessment of marijuana use and associated problems is a necessary precursor to treatment for several reasons. Most obvious is the importance of gathering information to make an informed treatment decision. Yet, assessment also serves the purpose of priming the individual for change and is an initial step in the onset of treatment implementation. Assessment requires clients to undergo a thorough history of their drug use and associated consequences, which may promote changes in awareness of their current situation and its impact on their lives. Without an initial assessment, many marijuana users may lack the motivation to engage in treatment.

Overview of Research Evidence

Treatment development and efficacy studies targeting marijuana dependence were first seen in the literature in the 1990s. The lack of research on the subject stemmed from the belief that marijuana use rarely occurred as a primary problem and did not produce a true dependence syndrome (McRae, Budney, & Brady, 2003). Data contrary to these beliefs appeared in the late 1980s, when media advertisements seeking adults who were concerned about their marijuana use managed to elicit responses from numerous marijuana-only users who declared interest in seeking treatment (Roffman & Barnhart, 1987). This prompted the emergence of treatments designed to specifically assist marijuana users in decreasing and/or terminating their use. The majority of interventions have been derived from empirically supported treatments for other substance use disorders, such as cognitive-behavioral therapy (CBT) and relapse prevention. Furthermore, brief interventions such as motivational interviewing (MI) have been of particular interest as a potential treatment for marijuana users due to the low motivation to change seen in this population (Budney et al., 1998). Changes in the concept of psychotherapy related to the interest in brief interventions include the approval and acceptance of time-limited goals, highlighting client strengths, use of behavioral modification techniques, and greater attention being paid to present rather than past precipitating circumstances (Bloom, 1992).

Treatment for Adult Marijuana Users   Research on treatment for marijuana use was initially evaluated in adult populations. The first controlled study to appear in the literature compared relapse-prevention techniques to a social support group (Stephens, Roffman, & Simpson, 1994). The two treatments highlighted different aspects of marijuana use. Relapse-prevention techniques are derived from the cognitive-behavioral model of treatment and focus on identifying feelings, thoughts, and situations that may increase the chance of using marijuana while planning alternative actions that do not include use of the drug. The social support group instead concentrated on identifying others who could assist them in maintaining abstinence. Both treatments used a group format and contained 10 sessions. Client improvement was seen for the 212 participants, regardless of the intervention. Both treatments were equally effective at minimizing marijuana problems, although the relapse-prevention group displayed an advantage in decreasing the frequency of marijuana use per day. Although abstinence was the goal of the treatment, only 14% of the participants remained abstinent for the entire year following treatment. This study suffered additional discouraging findings in that only one-third of the participants were considered improved at follow-up, participants increased their alcohol consumption, and 21% of the subjects did not complete the study. Nevertheless, these data suggest that some problem users are able to decrease their use with the assistance of brief relapse prevention and social support interventions. In addition, the improvement and retention rates seen in this study are comparable to those seen with other substances, lending support for the efficacy of these interventions.

Subsequently, researchers have suggested several changes that may improve treatment outcome based on the study by Stephens and colleagues including using individual therapy, increasing the number of sessions, and increasing levels of motivation. Stephens, Roffman, and Curtin (2000) implemented these techniques in a study comparing a 14-session cognitive-behavioral relapse-prevention group, a 2-session motivational interviewing condition, and a delayed-treatment control group (DTC). The enhanced relapse-prevention group was developed because the authors posited that the version used in the first study might not have been comprehensive enough to teach all of the skills needed to avoid relapse. Included were sessions focused on building motivation to change, handling high-risk situations, and conducting self-help sessions. The brief treatment was included due to recent evidence supporting the efficacy of brief interventions in the treatment of alcohol use disorders (Fleming, Barry, Manwell, Johnson, & London, 1997). Therapists provided individual feedback from a comprehensive assessment of the participant's marijuana use through motivational interviewing techniques and instructed the subjects on cognitive-behavioral techniques that could be used to abstain from use. Both active treatments resulted in greater reductions than the DTC, although no differences in outcome were observed between the active interventions. Unfortunately, at 16-month follow-up, the abstinence rates for both active treatments were found to be slightly less than 30%. However, this rate was significantly better than what was observed in the DTC group (9%) and was an improvement from the abstinence rates seen in their prior study. Retention rates were also slightly higher than those from the first study, as approximately 86% of the participants were retained.

Although this study did not find significant differences between the active treatments, these results contribute to the literature. Neither a cognitive-behavioral intervention nor motivational interviewing had been compared with an inactive treatment to determine efficacy in this population. These results indicated that the treatments were indeed useful in reducing marijuana use as the participants in the active treatment groups were significantly improved compared to their DTC group peers. Furthermore, the efficacy of the two-session intervention provided support for the utility of brief interventions in this population, and for the implementation of MI techniques.

Copeland et al. (2000b) expanded on the issue of optimal treatment duration by comparing a six-session intervention incorporating components of MI and relapse prevention to a one-session version of the longer intervention with a self-help book. Both interventions were additionally compared to a delayed-treatment control group. The aim of this study was to compare treatment length without confounding the results through different treatment modalities.

Consistent with the Stephens research group, no significant differences were seen between the active treatments, although both conditions were efficacious in reducing marijuana use compared to the control group. The interventions in this study were conducted in an individual format, offering support for brief, individual CBT interventions for marijuana use disorders.

Thus, treatments of varying lengths and modalities appear to be effective in treating marijuana users, although much room is left for improvement. However, two studies found support for one active intervention over another. The Stephens research group collaborated on a large multisite study, the Marijuana Treatment Project (Stephens et al., 2002). The aims of this study were (1) to evaluate the efficacy of two treatments of different durations in a more diverse population of marijuana users than had been previously studied, and (2) to improve on the methodology from prior research. Nine sessions of CBT including motivational enhancement therapy (MET) and case management components were evaluated against a two-session MET intervention and a delayed-treatment control. The nine-session intervention produced superior outcomes compared to the two-session and DTC groups with regard to the reduction of marijuana use at 15-month follow-up as well as decreases in symptoms of marijuana dependence and abuse (MTPRG, 2004). Although the MET intervention did not outperform the CBT group, participants in this condition did significantly decrease their marijuana use compared to the DTC group, again supporting the efficacy of brief motivational interventions.

Unlike in the previous studies, this more extensive CBT intervention produced superior outcomes compared to a brief intervention. Various explanations for this finding can be proposed. First, this was the only treatment to employ both individual CBT and MET rather than group therapy. Second, this study recruited a more ethnically and socioeconomically diverse sample and developed a manual-guided approach specifically intended to be utilized with diverse clientele. Early generations of evidence-based approaches often sought to minimize variability associated with therapists and treatment delivery. However, this approach allowed therapists the latitude to choose which modules to incorporate into treatment based on the individual needs of the participant (Steinberg et al., 2002). This may be particularly important when treating marijuana users, as individualized and marijuana-focused treatments may be necessary to successfully achieve abstinence or reduce use. Finally, although abstinence was promoted as the treatment goal, the interventions were not rigid in this regard. As greater improvements were observed for decreases in use and associated problems rather than for abstinence rates, many marijuana users may have responded to treatment primarily by cutting down rather than quitting entirely.

A second study comparing three active treatments found that a 14-session combination treatment of MET, behavioral coping skills, and voucher-based incentives resulted in greater levels of abstinence than 4 sessions of MET alone, or 14 sessions of MET plus behavioral coping skills (Budney et al., 2000). The theory behind the use of contingency management strategies asserts that voucher-based incentives are a strong reinforcer of abstinence behavior. During this period of abstinence, individuals are given the opportunity to step back from their use and evaluate the impact of this behavior on their lives. It is hoped that the client will also identify nondrug reinforcers that will serve as alternative behaviors to drug use once the contingency management intervention is no longer in place (see Chapter 26 for more information relevant to this topic). Although this is not a cost-effective strategy in clinical practice, these findings support the use of identifying alternative reinforcers in the client's life to replace drug-using behavior. However, participants in each group were not evaluated subsequent to extended periods of follow-up, so it is unclear whether these decreases in use were maintained. Furthermore, examination of the MET group and behaviorally enhanced MET conditions did not detect any meaningful differences in efficacy between the treatments, although both produced significant improvements on a number of outcome measures. Thus, this study offers support for a brief MET intervention, as no further improvement was seen with the addition of coping skills training or with extended treatment duration.

Treatment for Adolescent Marijuana Users   Once treatment efficacy was determined within adult samples, research on treating adolescent marijuana use became a priority, given the increasing rates of use in this age group. Prior to the early 2000s, treatment for adolescent marijuana users employed approaches that were developed for adults, which may be developmentally inappropriate for adolescents (Dennis, Dawud-Noursi, Muck, & McDermeit, 2002). The Cannabis Youth Treatment (CYT) study (Dennis et al., 2002) was designed as a multisite experiment to examine the cost-effectiveness and treatment efficacy of five manual-guided approaches for marijuana-dependent adolescents. One component of this study evaluated a combination MET/CBT intervention for either 5 or 12 sessions. This treatment was designed to resolve ambivalence around problematic use, increase motivation to change, teach basic skills for refusing marijuana, develop alternative activities, and recover from relapse. Second, the efficacy of a family support network was examined, which included 12 sessions of MET/CBT along with 6 parent education group meetings, based upon the assumption that family involvement is a necessary component in adolescent recovery. The final two approaches included Multidimensional Family Therapy, involving 12 to 15 group and individual sessions with the adolescent and parents in order to integrate substance use treatment into family therapy, and an Adolescent Community Reinforcement Approach, which incorporated elements of operant conditioning, skills training, and a social skills approach in 14 individual and group sessions with the adolescent and caregivers.

All five treatment conditions demonstrated significant reductions in marijuana use at 12-month follow-up (Dennis et al., 2004). Similar to data from adult populations, no single intervention appeared to be more efficacious than another. These results suggest that the more cost-effective interventions, such as the five-session CBT treatment, should be utilized with adolescents, particularly because the adolescents and their families found each treatment to be acceptable and worthwhile.

Given the findings from the CYT study, brief and cost-effective motivational interviewing interventions are being examined for use among adolescents. MI has been hypothesized to be particularly attractive to adolescents because it is nonconfrontational and does not force change (Lawendowski, 1998). A test of a single session of MI in adolescent drug users verified the efficacy of these techniques in reducing the use of a variety of substances, including marijuana (McCambridge & Strang, 2004).

Treatment for Nontreatment Seekers   Many adolescents and adults continue to use marijuana despite the fact that they are experiencing negative consequences. Explanations for this behavior include ambivalence about change, stigma associated with receiving treatment, and lack of insight regarding the role of marijuana use in contributing to these problems. Interventions have been designed to attract users who experience adverse consequences but are ambivalent about change and are unlikely to seek treatment. One such treatment, the Marijuana Check-Up (Doyle, Swan, Roffman, & Stephens, 2003), was specifically tailored to reach heavy marijuana users at an early stage of readiness to change (i.e., precontemplation or contemplation) and included an in-depth assessment interview as well as a personalized feedback session. Clients were provided with a single session of personalized information about their marijuana use compared to normative data in a nonjudgmental fashion consistent with motivational interviewing. Each participant was told that the project was not a treatment program and that there would be no pressure to change their marijuana use.

Data on the efficacy of this brief intervention have yet to be reported, however, the Marijuana Check-Up was successful in recruiting a large number of interested participants, the majority of whom were in early stages of readiness to change and reported near-daily use (Stephens et al., 2004). Interested participants were recruited from the same region and during the same time period as the Marijuana Treatment Project (2004) and were compared to determine whether the Check-Up attracted a population of users who differed from those who were actively seeking treatment. Those interested in the Check-Up tended to be younger, smoked less frequently, endorsed fewer marijuana-related problems, and reported lower readiness to change. Because these non-treatment-seeking participants reported fewer and less severe marijuana-associated problems, the Marijuana Check-Up could be a valuable early intervention for reducing marijuana problems before they become detrimental.

Similar programs have been evaluated for use among adolescents. The feasibility of a brief Adolescent Cannabis Check-Up (Martin, Copeland, & Swift, 2005) was assessed in young marijuana users who were not seeking treatment or making an effort to reduce their use. This intervention employed assessment and feedback sessions similar to those in the adult version, with an additional option of a single session of CBT for those users who were interested in exploring change. The Check-Up proved successful in recruiting and retaining adolescent marijuana users who were ambivalent about changing their use and provided encouraging findings regarding the feasibility of this intervention. Six months post-intervention, more than 75% of the participants reported voluntarily reducing their marijuana use, which resulted in fewer symptoms of dependence. As the Check-Up was reportedly valued by the participants, this study lends further support for the use of brief interventions utilizing MI techniques. However, a similar study employing a two-session MET intervention with non-treatment-seeking adolescents failed to find significant differences in the reduction of marijuana use between the treatment and control groups (Walker, Roffman, Stephens, Berghuis, & Kim, 2006). Nevertheless, participants in this study significantly reduced their level of use, demonstrating the promise of brief voluntary interventions among adolescents.

Many marijuana users quit their use without formal treatment. Researchers have examined quitting strategies used by those who have been successful in reducing or abstaining from use without professional help. The strategies fell into three main categories: changing one's environment/access to marijuana, seeking support from peers and family, and seeking medical help or attending self-help groups (Boyd et al., 2005). The first two strategies have been included in several of the treatments utilized for this population. Limited research, however, has examined the use of 12-step groups among marijuana users. Membership in 12-step facilitation groups enhances outcomes for alcoholics and data support the relative efficacy of this intervention as a strategy for minimizing alcohol problems compared with CBT and MET (Project MATCH, 1998). Thus, the effects of 12-step facilitation would likely generalize to those experiencing negative consequences from marijuana. Although few formal studies address success rates, members of Narcotics Anonymous and Marijuana Anonymous report successful abstinence from marijuana. The success of social support treatments implies that the supportive aspects of Marijuana Anonymous would help problem users. Hence, 12-step facilitation may be a valuable resource for marijuana users who are concerned with the stigma attached to seeking professional treatment, or if used in combination with an empirically supported intervention.

Additional Treatment Variables

Overall, many treatments are effective in reducing marijuana use and decreasing the associated symptoms of abuse and dependence. However, the failure of earlier clinical trials to identify differences in efficacy among treatments raises the possibility that the factors accounting for change may not be located in the specific procedures of a given treatment, but rather are associated with common elements of the treatment process. Outcome may be enhanced by combining elements from different approaches to meet the specific needs of marijuana users, such as integrating MI and CBT. Yet, it is debatable which aspects of particular treatments are specifically responsible for reductions in drug use.

Mechanisms of Action   CBT interventions have been shown to decrease the frequency of marijuana use, although research has not yet established the mechanisms of action by which this change occurs. Relapse-prevention techniques have been theorized to play a role in altering drug use behavior. A review of controlled clinical trials for a variety of substance use disorders concluded that relapse-prevention approaches were superior to no treatment, but were not performing better than other active treatments, especially for drugs such as cocaine and marijuana (Carroll, 1996). However, results from follow-up studies demonstrated that gains due to relapse-prevention techniques were sustained for significant periods of time. This finding was explained by concluding that clients are learning skills that they are using after completing treatment. Thus, the use of coping skills and other skills training techniques may be directly responsible for treatment outcome.

This assumption was rebuffed using data from the Marijuana Treatment Project (2004), in which the authors concluded that marijuana use outcome could not be accounted for by the use of coping skills (Litt, Kadden, Stephens, & MTPRG, 2005). Although the MET/CBT intervention included at least five sessions of coping skills training, it was no more effective in increasing the use of skills than the MET treatment, which did not include skills training. Instead, self-efficacy changes appeared to be influencing the reductions in substance use, as the MET/CBT condition was more successful at increasing self-efficacy, which in turn led to increased use of coping skills. It is unknown whether the increase in self-efficacy was due to the content of the MET/CBT intervention or to the increase in treatment duration. Consequently, mechanisms of coping skills treatments such as CBT may need to be reconceptualized and further explored. In addition, interventions designed to boost self-efficacy may further improve treatment outcomes for marijuana users.

Therapist Traits   The link between therapeutic alliance and client outcome has been well established. A strong working alliance, as defined by the quality and strength of the collaborative relationship between therapist and client, which includes a shared understanding of the goals of therapy, consistently predicts enhanced outcomes across a range of presenting problems and treatment approaches (Barber, Connolly, Crits-Christoph, Gladis, & Siqueland, 2000). Thus, therapist traits such as warmth, genuineness, empathy, and attention may be important common factors in treatment efficacy, regardless of the particular intervention applied (Luborsky, McLellan, Diguer, Woody, & Seligman, 1997; Luborsky, Singer, & Luborsky, 1975).

The creators of MI have stressed the importance of adhering to the spirit of the method and in establishing a collaborative relationship. Therapists should express empathy, acceptance, genuineness, and be nonjudgmental while administering this intervention (Rollnick & Miller, 1995). Nevertheless, deviations from MI techniques, such as confrontation and advising, have not been found to diminish treatment outcome as long as the clinician possesses basic interpersonal skills such as warmth and genuineness (Moyers, Miller, & Hendrickson, 2005). In fact, these inconsistent behaviors strengthened the therapeutic relationship in many instances. Thus, more so than the importance of implementing the best treatment, therapists should possess appropriate interpersonal skills and establish a positive alliance with the client.

Client Values   In addition to establishing a positive relationship between the client and therapist, many client characteristics and values may play an important role in enhancing treatment outcome. Levels of motivation and readiness to change may be pivotal in influencing treatment effects. Decisional balance interventions may be particularly useful in tipping the scales toward change for a client who reports problems associated with use but is not ready to alter behavior due to perceived advantages to maintaining their drug use. Moreover, clients may value a harm reduction approach to treatment rather than demanding abstinence. Users may wish to eliminate negative consequences by reducing their frequency or amount of use but desire to continue using recreationally. A focus on abstinence may deter many individuals from seeking or remaining in treatment.

Case Presentation

Dana, a 23-year-old African-American woman, presented to the Chemical Dependency Treatment Program at her local VA hospital. She was unwilling to participate in the inpatient program but agreed to weekly meetings to discuss general life stresses and marijuana use. An initial session was devoted to building rapport and assessing her life skills, social support, and marijuana-related symptoms.

In a semi-structured interview she endorsed only two symptoms of dependence: a great deal of time spent using, and reduced recreational activities. Dana used marijuana daily and reported being high at least six hours per day for the last two years. Her recreational activities were limited to watching TV during intoxication. She had at one time been more active in exercise and attendance at church events, but these had fallen off during the last two years. Based on current criteria she did not qualify for a diagnosis of dependence, but her involvement with marijuana was clearly extensive.

Dana initially endorsed only one symptom of marijuana abuse, but only one symptom is required for the diagnosis. She habitually drove her car while high, which would qualify as use in a hazardous circumstance. She had one traffic violation but no accidents in the last two years, and saw nothing wrong with her habit of driving after using marijuana. She did have one interaction with a police officer related to marijuana possession, which was actually the primary motivation for her to seek treatment. During the stop for her traffic violation, an officer had found her in possession of a small bag of marijuana. After a frightening exchange about the penalties for intention to distribute, she received a moving violation and was sent on her way. A single interaction related to possession seemed below the threshold for the abuse symptom that required recurrent drug-related legal problems, but it did offer further evidence of her involvement. Upon further query she agreed that her job performance might be less than optimal given her frequent use of the substance. Although her job performance was acceptable, she agreed that she was underachieving. Her current work as a cashier was not particularly demanding and seemed to take little advantage of her skills and abilities.

The remainder of this session provided a lesson in potential traps for clinicians who work with this population. It's embarrassing to admit that many minutes were wasted with an aside concerning how legal problems serve as a symptom of abuse and are intertwined with marijuana's status as an illicit substance. Dana was quite outspoken about many of her acquaintances who abused alcohol but did not risk legal problems. Discussions of the legal status of marijuana are often a variant of what Rollnick and Miller (1995) have called the blaming trap. The metamessage, particularly for users with legal problems, is that if marijuana policy changed, they would not have marijuana-related troubles. Comparable discussions of medical marijuana legislation can also derail a therapy session. Rollnick and Miller recommend many strategies for dealing with resistance of this sort. The most effective in this case involved shifting focus. After Dana finished expressing her outrage about marijuana's legal status, the simple statement, "Well, let's focus on you for now," helped move the discussion to her own use.

Due to time limitations, Dana could only complete one more assessment question, the Readiness To Change Ruler. She rated herself a 7 on the 10-point scale in response to the question of decreasing her marijuana use. When asked what it would take for her to move to an 8, she was unsure. She would not agree to a quit date but claimed she was willing to monitor use over the next week. The therapist explained a technique for her to record the time of day that she used, how she felt at the time, how much she used, and approximately how long she felt the effects of the drug. She also agreed to call the office if she needed to discuss any life problems related to marijuana or otherwise.

Six days later, Dana received a reminder call about her appointment and appeared punctually the following week. The second session began with a review of her self-monitoring, which revealed that during the week she only used after work, smoked approximately half a joint before dinner, and spent roughly three hours per day feeling the effects of the drug. She did get high three times per day on Saturday and Sunday, and stayed high for approximately nine hours on those days. The clinician asked if this level of use was typical and she said that it was not. For the previous two years she had used marijuana before work as well as after, and even occasionally on her lunch break. She claimed that she would have been embarrassed to return to a session and report this level of use, so she decided to only get high at the end of the day. Her experience of this new level of use was mixed. She said she found herself reluctant to head to work in the morning without using, and that the first day seemed to drag. On subsequent days she still found herself unenthusiastic about leaving for work without using, but that once she arrived at the workplace, it seemed tolerable. She claimed that people were nicer to her than she realized. This comment led to a discussion of marijuana-induced paranoia that Dana seemed to enjoy. She shared that she did not think that the clinician would know about that potential effect of marijuana, and seemed surprised.

The remainder of the session was devoted primarily to completing the decisional balance exercise. As part of this exercise, we recommend generating disadvantages to quitting before advantages to quitting. Clinical experience suggests that letting clients explore the disadvantages of quitting first allows us to end sessions on an optimistic note when they list the advantages of quitting later. Dana first detailed the disadvantages she thought she would experience if she quit using marijuana entirely. After she generated all of the disadvantages, she provided each with a weight of importance from 1 to 10. These included: she would be less happy (10), she would have less fun (9), she would enjoy sex less (6), she would find housework more difficult (6), her friends would grow suspicious of her (8), and she would be less creative in her work (6).

The experience of watching clients generate the disadvantages of a positive change can be awkward for any clinician, particularly when clients express beliefs that seem unlikely. For example, many users believe that marijuana enhances creativity despite evidence to the contrary (Bourassa & Vaugeois, 2001). It is tempting to try to challenge this belief as soon as a client generates it, but the strategy does not work well in the long run. If clients can generate all of their perceived disadvantages and advantages to quitting without interference, they seem more likely to generate longer lists that contain the most important items. In contrast, if a belief is challenged early in the process, clients might withhold reasons that are most important to them.

Dana could only think of two advantages to quitting her marijuana use, and gave them the following weights: She would have more money (6) and she would decrease her chances of legal problems (4). Given the number of advantages and disadvantages as well as their weights, it was clear why Dana was uninterested in quitting. A common strategy in this situation would require challenging each of the disadvantages in an effort to decrease their weights. This task seemed formidable, so the clinician chose an alternative strategy. Dana was asked to list the pros and cons of decreasing her use to only weekends. She did not see this approach as a reasonable option, but was willing to perform a decisional balance related to decreasing her use to three times per week.

The controversy surrounding an approach that focuses on decreasing consumption rather than demanding abstinence has grown quite heated (Marlatt, 2002). Many clinicians report that attempts to decrease consumption are doomed to failure because use will eventually return to levels associated with problems. Nevertheless, for clients who are unwilling to entertain an abstinence goal, a period that includes attempts at controlled use might provide valuable data. If the client shows an inability to control use despite a concerted attempt, the argument for an abstinence goal grows stronger. Dana appeared to understand the arguments against controlled use but felt that it was a goal she could support. A subsequent decisional balance led to comparable lists of advantages and disadvantages, but with different weights. The disadvantages to restricting use to three times per week included: she would be less happy (5), she would have less fun (5), she would enjoy sex less (3), she would find housework more difficult (4), her friends would grow suspicious of her (2), and she would be less creative in her work (3). The advantages of the change still included having more money (6) and decreasing the chances of legal problems (4). This arrangement did not improve the ratio of the number of advantages and disadvantages, but the average weights changed, bringing the means for the pros and cons closer.

Dana returned the following week and reported that it was difficult to give up her evening use during the week, but she had used only twice during the week and then each night on the weekend. The following week she used only three nights out of seven. She agreed that the process had gotten easier. She also noted that her sleep seemed better despite her previous belief that marijuana had helped her sleep. She was unwilling to decrease the frequency of use further, but agreed to a follow-up session in one month. A quick return to the Readiness Ruler revealed that Dana rated her motivation to keep use to only on three days per week was a 9 on the 10-point scale. One month later she had continued to use at most three times per week. One week she had only used twice because she was visiting family and did not want to bring marijuana with her. She agreed to a session two months later and returned to report that she had continued with this controlled use but was unwilling to consider further decreases. She was no longer driving after use, and seemed to experience few negative consequences. The number of hours she was intoxicated per day was now three hours on one weeknight and approximately five hours per day on the weekends. She no longer drove after using, suggesting that she would no longer qualify for an abuse diagnosis. She reported a return to exercising intermittently and a return to church attendance approximately twice per month. These improvements suggested a decrease in marijuana problems despite the continued use.

It is unclear if Dana would eventually return to problematic levels of use. The clinician was moving to a new location and suggested that Dana continue follow-up appointments at the treatment program. Although three months of controlled use might not qualify as a standard definition of treatment success, she appeared to no longer report symptoms of abuse or dependence. As controversial as it might sound, it appears that this decisional balance intervention helped a problem marijuana user move toward problem-free use.

Conclusions

Developments in the assessment and treatment of marijuana use disorders have been underway over the past decade. Individuals who experience negative consequences from marijuana have a number of imperfect but promising options for reducing and eliminating problems. Table 14.1 provides further information regarding resources for the assessment and treatment of marijuana use disorders. The majority of the existing measures and interventions have been adaptations of those utilized for other substances of abuse. Although empirical support has been established for many of these instruments, additional research is necessary to determine the best practice for this population. Further examination of the mechanisms

TABLE 14.1

Resources for the Assessment and Treatment of Marijuana Use Disorders

Resources

1. Marijuana Anonymous: www.marijuana-anonymous.org

2. National Organization for the Reform of Marijuana Laws [NORML]. (1996). *Principles of Responsible Cannabis Use.* Available from: http://www.norml.org/index.cfm?Group_ID=3417

3. Peele, S., & Brodsky, A. (2000). *Guidelines for sensible cannabis use.* Available from: http://www.peele.net/lib/guidelines. html

4. Rational Recovery Group: www.rational.org

5. Roffman, R., & Stephens, R. S. (Eds.) (2006). *Cannabis dependence: Its nature, consequences, and treatment.* New York: Cambridge University Press

of action for various interventions and of the valued components of treatment are warranted in order to meet the specific needs of marijuana users. Although no one treatment is perfect, many users are successful in decreasing their use of the drug and minimizing its negative effects.

References

Agosti, V., & Levin, F. R. (2004). Predictors of treatment contact among individuals with cannabis dependence. *American Journal of Drug and Alcohol Abuse, 30,* 121–127.

Alexander, D. (2003). A Marijuana Screening Inventory (Experimental Version): Description and preliminary psychometric properties. *The American Journal of Drug and Alcohol Abuse, 29,* 619–646.

Alexander, D., & Leung, P. (2006). The Marijuana Screening Inventory (MSI-X): Concurrent, convergent, and discriminant validity with multiple measures. *The American Journal of Drug and Alcohol Abuse, 32,* 351–378.

American Psychiatric Association. (1980). *Diagnostic and Statistical Manual of Mental Disorders* (3rd ed.). Washington, DC: Author.

American Psychiatric Association. (1987). *Diagnostic and Statistical Manual of Mental Disorders* (3rd ed., rev.). Washington, DC: Author.

American Psychiatric Association. (1994). *Diagnostic and Statistical Manual of Mental Disorders* (4th ed.). Washington, DC: Author.

American Psychiatric Association. (2000). Diagnostic and Statistical Manual of Mental Disorders (4th ed., text revision). Washington, DC: Author.

Andreatini, R., Galduroz, J. C. F., Ferri, C. P., & Formigoni, M. L. O. S. (1994). Alcohol dependence criteria in *DSM–III–R*: Presence of symptoms according to degree of severity. *Addiction, 89,* 1129–1134.

Anthony, J. C., Warner, L. A., & Kessler, R. C. (1994). Comparative epidemiology of dependence on tobacco, alcohol, controlled substances, and inhalants: Basic findings from the National Comorbidity Survey. *Experimental and Clinical Psychopharmacology, 2,* 244–268.

Babor, T. F., Brown, J., & Del Boca, F. K. (1990). Validity of self-reports in applied research on addictive behaviors: Fact or fiction? *Behavioral Assessment, 12,* 5–31.

Barber, J. P., Connolly, M. B., Crits-Christoph, P., Gladis, L., & Siqueland, L. (2000). Alliance predicts patients' outcome beyond in-treatment change in symptoms. *Journal of Consulting and Clinical Psychology, 68,* 1027–1032.

Bloom, B. L. (1992). Planned short-term psychotherapy: Current status and future challenges. *Applied and Preventive Psychology, 1,* 157–164.

Bourassa, M., & Vaugeois, P. (2001). Effects of marijuana use on divergent thinking. *Creativity Research Journal, 13*, 411–416.

Boyd, S. J., Tashkin, D. P., Huestis, M. A., Heishman, S. J., Dermand, J. C., Simmons, M. S., et al. (2005). Strategies for quitting among non-treatment seeking marijuana smokers. *The American Journal on Addictions, 14*, 35–42.

Buchan, B. J., Dennis, M. L., Tims, F. M., & Diamond, G. S. (2002). Cannabis use: Consistency and validity of self-report, on-site urine testing and laboratory testing. *Addiction, 97*, 98–108.

Budney, A. J. (2006). Are specific dependence criteria necessary for different substances: How can research on cannabis inform this issue? *Addiction, 101*, 125–133.

Budney, A. J., Higgins, S. T., Radonovich, K. J., & Novy, P. L. (2000). Adding voucher-based incentives to coping skills and motivational enhancement improves outcomes during treatment for marijuana dependence. *Journal of Consulting and Clinical Psychology, 68*, 1051–1061.

Budney, A. J., & Hughes, J. R. (2006). The cannabis withdrawal syndrome. *Current Opinions in Psychiatry, 19*, 233–238.

Budney, A. J., Hughes, J. R., Moore, B. A., & Vandrey, R. G. (2004). A review of the validity and significance of the cannabis withdrawal syndrome. *American Journal of Psychiatry, 161*, 1967–1977.

Budney, A. J., Moore, B. A., Vandrey, R. G., & Hughes, J. R. (2003). The time course and significance of cannabis withdrawal. *Journal of Abnormal Psychology, 112*, 393–402.

Budney, A. J., Novy, P., & Hughes, J. R. (1999). Marijuana withdrawal among adults seeking treatment for marijuana dependence. *Addiction, 94*, 1311–1322.

Budney, A. J., Radonovich, K. J., Higgins, S. T., & Wong, C. J. (1998). Adults seeking treatment for marijuana dependence: A comparison with cocaine-dependent treatment seekers. *Experimental and Clinical Psychopharmacology, 6*, 419–426.

Bureau of Justice Statistics. (2000). *Sourcebook of Criminal Justice Statistics 1999* (27th ed.). Washington, DC: US Department of Justice.

Carroll, K. M. (1996). Relapse prevention as a psychosocial treatment: A review of controlled clinical trials. *Experimental and Clinical Psychopharmacology, 4*, 46–54.

Copeland, J., Gilmour, S., Gates, P., & Swift, W. (2005). The Cannabis Problems Questionnaire: Factor structure, reliability, and validity. *Drug and Alcohol Dependence, 80*, 313–319.

Copeland, J., Swift, W., & Rees, V. (2001a). Clinical profile of participants in a brief intervention program for cannabis use disorder. *Journal of Substance Abuse Treatment, 20*, 45–52.

Copeland, J., Swift, W., Roffman, R., & Stephens, R. (2001b). A randomized controlled trial of brief cognitive-behavioral interventions for cannabis use disorder. *Journal of Substance Abuse Treatment, 21*, 55–64.

Crowley, T. J., MacDonald, M. J., Whitmore, E. A., & Mikulich, S. K. (1998). Cannabis dependence, withdrawal, and reinforcing effects among adolescents with conduct disorder symptoms and substance use disorders. *Drug and Alcohol Dependence, 50*, 27–37.

Degenhardt, L., Lynskey, M., Coffey, C., & Patton, G. (2002). 'Diagnostic orphans' among young adult cannabis users: Persons who report dependence symptoms but do not meet diagnostic criteria. *Drug and Alcohol Dependence, 67*, 205–212.

Dennis, M., Babor, T. F., Roebuck, C., & Donaldson, J. (2002). Changing the focus: The case for recognizing and treating cannabis use disorders. *Addiction, 97*, 4–15.

Dennis, M., Godley, S. H., Diamond, G., Tims, F. M., Babor, T., Donaldson, J., et al. (2004). The Cannabis Youth Treatment (CYT) Study: Main findings from two randomized trials. *Journal of Substance Abuse Treatment, 27*, 197–213.

Dennis, M., Titus, J. C., Diamond, G., Donaldson, J., Godley, S. H., Tims, F. M., et al. (2002). The Cannabis Youth Treatment (CYT) experiment: Rationale, study design and analysis plans. *Addiction, 97*, 16–34.

Dennis, M. L., Dawud-Noursi, S., Muck, R., & McDermeit, M. (2002). The need for developing and evaluating adolescent treatment models. In S. J. Stevens & A. R. Morral (Eds.), *Adolescent drug treatment: Theory and Implementation in Eleven National Projects*. Binghamton, NY: Haworth Press.

Doyle, A., Swan, M., Roffman, R., & Stephens, R. (2003). The Marijuana Check-Up: A brief intervention tailored for individuals in the contemplation stage. *Journal of Social Work Practice in the Addictions, 3*, 53–71.

Earleywine, M. (2002). *Understanding marijuana*. New York: Oxford University Press.

Feingold, A., & Rounsaville, B. (1995). Construct validity of the dependence syndrome as measured by *DSM–IV* for different psychoactive substances. *Addiction, 90*, 1661–1669.

First, M. B., Spitzer, R. L., Gibbon, M., & Williams, J. B. (1996). *Structured Clinical Interview for DSM-IV, Axis I Disorders – Patient Edition (SCID-I/P, Version 2.0)*. New York: Biometrics Research Department, New York State Psychiatric Institute.

Fleming, M. F., Barry, K. L., Manwell, L. B., Johnson, K., & London, R. (1997). Brief physician advice for problem drinkers. *Journal of the American Medical Association, 277*, 1039–1045.

Gossop, M., Darke, S., Griffiths, P., Hando, J., Powis, B., Hall, W., et al. (1995). The Severity of Dependence Scale (SDS): Psychometric properties of the SDS in English and Australian samples of heroin, cocaine and amphetamine users. *Addiction, 90*, 607–614.

Haas, A. P., & Hendin, H. (1987). The meaning of chronic marijuana use among adults: A psychosocial perspective. *Journal of Drug Issues, 17*, 333–348.

Hall, W., Solowij, N., & Lemon, J. (1994). *The health and psychological consequences of cannabis use* (National Drug Strategy Monograph Series No. 25). Canberra: Australian Government Publishing Service.

Hser, Y. L., Grella, C. E., Hubbard, R. L., Hsieh, S., Fletcher, B. W., Brown, B. S., et al. (2001). An evaluation of drug treatments for adolescents in 4 US cities. *Archives of General Psychiatry, 58*, 689–695.

Lawendowski, L. A. (1998). A motivational intervention for adolescent smokers. *Preventive Medicine, 27*, A39–A46.

Litt, M. D., Kadden, R. M., Stephens, R. S., & The Marijuana Treatment Project Research Group. (2005). Coping and self-efficacy in marijuana treatment: Results from the marijuana treatment project. *Journal of Consulting and Clinical Psychology, 73*, 1015–1025.

Luborsky, L., McLellan, A. T., Diguer, L., Woody, G., & Seligman, D. (1997). The psychotherapist matters: Comparison of outcomes across twenty-two therapists and seven patient samples. *Clinical Psychology: Science and Practice, 4*, 53–65.

Luborsky, L., Singer, B., & Luborsky, L. (1975). Comparative studies of psychotherapies: Is it true that 'everyone has won and all must have prizes'? *Archives of General Psychiatry, 32*, 995–1008.

Marijuana Treatment Project Research Group. (2004). Brief treatments for cannabis dependence: Findings from a randomized multisite trial. *Journal of Consulting and Clinical Psychology, 72*, 455–466.

Marlatt, A. (Ed.). (1998). *Harm reduction*. New York: Guilford.

Martin, G., Copeland, J., Gates, P., & Gilmour, S. (2006). The Severity of Dependence Scale (SDS) in an adolescent population of cannabis users: Reliability, validity and diagnostic cut-off. *Drug and Alcohol Dependence, 83*, 90–93.

Martin, G., Copeland, J., Gilmour, S., Gates, P., & Swift, W. (2006). The Adolescent Cannabis Problems Quesitonnaire (CPQ-A): Psychometric properties. *Addictive Behaviors, 31*, 2238–2248.

Matt, G. E., & Wilson, S. J. (1994). Describing the frequency of marijuana use: Fuzziness and context-dependent interpretation of frequency expressions. *Evaluation and Program Planning, 17*, 1106–1108.

McCambridge, J., & Strang, J. (2004). The efficacy of single-session motivational interviewing in reducing drug consumption and perceptions of drug-related risk and harm among young people: Results from a multi-site cluster randomized trial. *Addiction, 99*, 39–52.

McConnaughy, E. A., Prochaska, J. O., & Velicer, W. F. (1983). Stages of change in psychotherapy: Measurement and sample profiles. *Psychotherapy: Theory, Research and Practice, 20*, 368–375.

McLellan, A., Kushner, H., Metzger, D., Peters, R., Smith, I., Grissom, G., et al. (1992). The fifth edition of the Addiction Severity Index. *Journal of Substance Abuse Treatment, 9*, 199–213.

McRae, A. L., Budney, A. J., & Brady, K. T. (2003). Treatment of marijuana dependence: A review of the literature. *Journal of Substance Abuse Treatment, 24*, 369–376.

Miller, W. R. & Tonigan, J. S. (1996). Assessing drinkers' motivation for change: The Stages of Change Readiness and Treatment Eagerness Scale (SOCRATES). *Psychology of Addictive Behaviors, 10*, 81–89.

Monitoring the Future. (2001). Percent past-year drug and alcohol use among twelfth graders: 1975–2001. *Monitoring the Future*. Ann Arbor, MI: University of Michigan.

Morgenstern, J., Langenbucher, J., & Labouvie, E.W. (1994). The generalizability of the dependence syndrome across substances: An examination of some properties of the proposed *DSM–IV* criteria. *Addiction, 89*, 1105–1113.

Moyers, T. B., Miller, W. R., & Hendrickson, S. M. L. (2005). How does motivational interviewing work? Therapist interpersonal skill predicts client involvement within motivational interviewing sessions. *Journal of Consulting and Clinical Psychology, 73*, 590–598.

Nelson, C. B., Rehm, J., Ustun, T. B., Grant, B., & Chatterji, S. (1999). Factor structures for *DSM–IV* substance disorder criteria endorsed by alcohol, cannabis, cocaine and opiate users. Results from the WHO reliability and validity study. *Addiction, 94*, 843–855.

Price, R. K., Risk, N. K., & Spitznagel, E. L. (2001). Remission from drug abuse over a 25-year period: Patterns of remission and treatment use. *American Journal of Public Health, 91*, 1107–1113.

Project MATCH Research Group. (1998). Matching patients with alcohol disorders to treatments: Clinical implications from project MATCH. *Journal of Mental Health UK, 7*, 589–602.

Roberts, C. (1996). Data quality of the Drug Abuse Warning Network. *American Journal of Drug and Alcohol Abuse, 22*, 389–401.

Roffman, R. A., & Barnhart, R. (1987). Assessing need for marijuana dependence treatment through an anonymous telephone interview. *International Journal of the Addictions, 22*, 639–651.

Rollnick, S., Heather, N., Gold, R., & Hall, W. (1992). Development of a short "readiness to change" questionnaire for use in brief, opportunistic interventions among excessive drinkers. *British Journal of Addiction, 87*, 743–754.

Rollnick, S., & Miller, W. R. (1995). What is motivational interviewing? *Behavioural and Cognitive Psychotherapy, 23*, 325–334.

Simpson, D. D., Joe, G. W., Fletcher, B. W., Hubbard, R. L., & Anglin, M. D. (1999). A national evaluation of treatment outcomes for cocaine dependence. *Archives of General Psychiatry, 56*, 507–514.

Sobell, L. C., & Sobell, M. B. (1992). Timeline Follow-Back, a technique for assessing self-reported alcohol consumption. In R. Little & J.Allen (Eds.), *Measuring alcohol consumption* (pp. 41–72). Totowa, NJ: Humana.

Steinberg, K. L., Roffman, R. A., Carroll, K. M., Kabela, E., Kadden, R., Miller, M., et al. (2002). Tailoring cannabis dependence treatment for a diverse population. *Addiction, 97*, 135–142.

Stephens, R. S., Babor, T. F., Kadden, R. A., Miller, M., & the Marijuana Treatment Project Research Group. (2002). The Marijuana Treatment Project: Rationale, design, and participant characteristics. *Addiction, 97*, 109–124.

Stephens, R. S., & Roffman, R. A. (2005). Assessment of cannabis use disorders. In D. M. Donovan & G. A. Marlatt (Eds.), *Assessment of addictive behaviors* (2nd ed., pp. 248–273). New York: Guilford Press.

Stephens, R. S., Roffman, R. A., & Curtin, L. (2000). Comparison of extended versus brief treatments for marijuana use. *Journal of Consulting and Clinical Psychology, 68*, 898–908.

Stephens, R. S., Roffman, R. A., Fearer, S. A., Williams, C., Picciano, J. F., & Burke, R. S. (2004). The Marijuana Check-Up: Reaching users who are ambivalent about change. *Addiction, 99*, 1323–1332.

Stephens, R. S., Roffman, R. A., & Simpson, E. E. (1994). Treating adult marijuana dependence: A test of the relapse prevention model. *Journal of Consulting and Clinical Psychology, 62*, 92–99.

Stroup, R. (1999). Marijuana should be legalized for recreational and medical purposes. In W. Dudley (Ed.), *Marijuana: At issue. An opposing viewpoint series* (pp. 9–16). San Diego, CA: Greenhaven Press.

Substance Abuse and Mental Health Services Administration. (2000a). *Mid-Year 2000 Emergency Department Data From the Drug Abuse Warning Network (DAWN)* (Office of Applied Studies, DAWN Series D-17, DHHS Publication No. SMA 01-3502). Rockville, MD.

Substance Abuse and Mental Health Services Administration. (2000b). *End-Year 1999 Medical Examiner Data from the Drug Abuse Warning Network (DAWN)* (Office of Applied Studies, DAWN Series D-16, DHHS Publication No. SMA 01-3491). Rockville, MD.

Substance Abuse and Mental Health Services Administration. (2000c). *National Household Survey on Drug Abuse Main Findings, 1998* (Office of Applied Studies, Series H-11, DHHS Publication No. SMA 00-3381). Rockville, MD.

Substance Abuse and Mental Health Services Administration. (2003). *Results from the 2002 National Survey on Drug Use and Health: National Findings* (Office of Applied Studies, NHSDA Series H-22, DHHS Publication No. SMA 03–3836). Rockville, MD.

Substance Abuse and Mental Health Services Administration. (2004). *Treatment Episode Data Set (TEDS): 1992–2002. National Admissions to Substance Abuse Treatment Services* (Office of Applied Studies, DASIS series S-23, DHHS Publication No. SMA 04-3965). Rockville, MD.

Substance Abuse and Mental Health Services Administration. (2005). *Results from the 2004 National Survey on Drug Use and Health: National Findings* (Office of Applied Studies, NSDUH Series H-28, DHHS Publication No. SMA 05-4062). Rockville, MD.

Swift, W., Copeland, J., & Hall, W. (1998). Choosing a diagnostic cut-off for cannabis dependence. *Addiction, 93*, 1681–1692.

Vandrey, R., Budney, A. J., Kamon, J. L., & Stanger, C. (2005). Cannabis withdrawal in adolescent treatment seekers. *Drug and Alcohol Dependence, 78*, 205–210.

Vandrey, R. G., Budney, A. J., Moore, B. A., & Hughes, J. R. (2005). A cross-study comparison of cannabis and tobacco withdrawal. *American Journal of Addictions, 14*, 54–63.

Walker, D. D., Roffman, R. A., Stephens, R. S., Berghuis, J., & Kim, W. (2006). Motivational enhancement therapy for adolescent marijuana users: A preliminary randomized controlled trial. *Journal of Consulting and Clinical Psychology, 74*, 628–632.

Williams, B. T. R., & Drummond, D. C. (1994). The alcohol problems questionnaire: Reliability and validity. *Drug and Alcohol Dependence, 35*, 239–243.

Winters, K. C., & Henley, G. A. (1993). *Adolescent diagnostic interview schedule and manual.* Los Angeles: Western Psychological Services.

Winters, K. C., Latimer, W., & Stinchfield, R. D. (1999). The *DSM-IV* criteria for adolescent alcohol and cannabis use disorders. *Journal of Studies on Alcohol, 60*, 337–344.

World Health Organization. (1997). *Composite international diagnostic interview, Core Version 2.1, 12 Month Version.* Geneva: Author.

Zimmer, L. & Morgan, J. P. (1997). *Marijuana myths marijuana facts.* New York: Lindesmith Center.

15

Cocaine

Danielle Barry, Nancy M. Petry, and Sheila M. Alessi

University of Connecticut Health Center

Contents

Background and Historical Context

Cocaine can be administered in several ways. For most of its history, cocaine has been primarily sniffed or "snorted" in powder form or injected (Agar, 2003; Jonnes, 1996). During the 1970s, smoking cocaine became popular among some users because it allowed for more efficient absorption of the drug into the bloodstream, but early techniques for smoking cocaine were dangerous and used more product than sniffing and were thus not widespread (Johnson, Golub, & Dunlap, 2000). The development of crack cocaine made smoking a much more common means of administration. Crack cocaine is produced by cooking cocaine powder with baking soda, water, and often other adulterants. As the cooked mixture cools, it hardens into a resin that can be broken into pieces and smoked, which allows for a quicker, more intense high than intranasal administration (Agar, 2003). Throughout its existence, cocaine has also been injected by some users, alone or in combination with heroin in a mixture called a "speedball." In the early 1990s, some cocaine users began injecting crack cocaine after dissolving it in vinegar or lemon juice (Carlson, Falck, & Siegal, 2000).

Perceptions of cocaine have evolved as its availability and problems associated with its use have grown. First isolated from the *Erythroxylon coca* plant in the nineteenth century, cocaine was marketed in a number of patent medicines and beverages, and its stimulant properties were quickly appreciated. Recognition of its potential for addiction and concerns about its negative effects, however, led to legislation regulating and eventually prohibiting its use in the early twentieth century (Jonnes, 1996; Platt, 1997). Cocaine's popularity waned for many years, particularly as other stimulants such as amphetamines became available, but permissive attitudes toward drug use that emerged in the 1960s led to a resurgence of interest in cocaine (Platt, 1997). Throughout the 1970s and into the early 1980s, it was widely believed that cocaine use did not lead to dependence or addiction, in part because the dominant paradigm for drug dependence at that time included a physiological withdrawal reaction, a reaction not typically seen among individuals attempting to abstain from cocaine use (Agar, 2003; Gawin, 1991). In addition, prior to the emergence of crack cocaine in the 1980s, cocaine was an expensive drug, and the "typical" cocaine user portrayed in the media was young, well-educated, and financially successful, giving cocaine a glamorous image that masked public perception of its deleterious effects (Jonnes, 1996). When crack cocaine was introduced to the United States, it quickly gained popularity in economically disadvantaged areas, due to a combination of its potency, low price, and ease of production (Agar, 2003). The crack cocaine industry has been blamed for an increase in violent crime that occurred during the 1980s (Johnson et al., 2000), and it is now clear that cocaine is not a benign recreational drug.

Current Conceptualization

Cocaine has very potent reinforcing effects that lead to compulsive use and craving (Gawin, 1991). Cocaine's actions on mesolimbic dopamine pathways provide both positive and negative reinforcement of its continued use. The intense feeling of euphoria reported by cocaine users is positively reinforcing, making continued use more likely, and the amelioration of cocaine craving is negatively reinforcing because it removes an undesired state. Cocaine is also a powerful stimulus that quickly builds strong conditioned associations with cues to its procurement and use.

Between 10 and 17% of people who report lifetime use of cocaine will go on to develop cocaine abuse or dependence (Glantz, Conway, & Colliver, 2005). Five percent will develop dependence within two years of trying cocaine for the first time (O'Brien & Anthony, 2005).

Although cocaine use does not lead to physical dependence and withdrawal, abstinence after chronic use can be accompanied by a psychological withdrawal syndrome of dysphoria, agitation, inactivity, amotivation, and anhedonia (American Psychiatric Association, 2000).

Comorbidity of cocaine use disorders and other psychiatric and substance use disorders is common. Mood disorders and antisocial personality disorder are frequent comorbid diagnoses among individuals seeking treatment for cocaine use disorders (Rounsaville, 2004; Rutherford, Cacciola, & Alterman, 1999). It can be difficult to determine whether other psychiatric disorders predate and precipitate the onset of cocaine use, or if cocaine use contributes to other disorders. For example, cocaine's effects, including euphoria, high energy, and enhanced concentration, are in direct contrast to the symptoms of depression, and early abstinence following regular use of cocaine is often accompanied by dysphoric mood. Individuals who suffer from depression may thus be particularly vulnerable to cocaine's reinforcing effects. Careful interviewing to obtain an accurate chronology of symptom onset is therefore important when assessing individuals with comorbid cocaine use and psychiatric disorders (Rounsaville, 2004).

Many regular users of cocaine are also heavy alcohol drinkers (Martin et al., 1996), and rates of heroin use are elevated among cocaine users compared to the general population (Gossop, Manning, & Ridge, 2006). Alcohol and heroin may serve similar purposes when used with cocaine, reducing agitation or anxiety that can accompany prolonged cocaine use (Gossop et al., 2006). Cocaine use is common among patients in methadone maintenance programs (Condelli, Fairbank, Dennis, & Rachal, 1991). Despite its efficacy in reducing opioid use, methadone treatment appears to have little effect on levels of cocaine use, and concurrent use of cocaine is associated with greater attrition and poorer outcomes among individuals in methadone maintenance therapy (Williamson, Darke, Ross, & Teesson, 2006).

Assessment of Cocaine Use Disorders

Procedures for diagnosing *DSM–IV* cocaine abuse and dependence are similar to those used to diagnose other substance use disorders. A diagnosis of cocaine abuse requires one or more of four symptoms over a 12-month period. Specific symptoms include (1) failure to fulfill role obligations as a result of cocaine use, (2) recurrent use in potentially hazardous situations, (3) recurrent legal problems related to cocaine use, and (4) continued cocaine use in spite of persistent or recurrent use-related social or interpersonal problems (APA, 2000). A cocaine-dependence diagnosis requires that three or more of seven symptoms occur concurrently in the last 12 months. Symptoms of cocaine dependence include (1) tolerance (needing more cocaine to achieve a desired effect or feeling less effect with the usual dose); (2) withdrawal symptoms (two or more of the following: dysphoric mood, fatigue, vivid or unpleasant dreams, insomnia or hypersomnia, increased appetite, psychomotor retardation or agitation) when cocaine use is stopped for a few days or even hours; (3) using cocaine in larger amounts or over longer periods of time than intended; (4) persistent desire or unsuccessful attempts to reduce cocaine use; (5) spending a great deal of time obtaining, using, or recovering from cocaine use; (6) giving up or reducing other important activities because of cocaine use; and (7) continuing to use cocaine despite knowledge of physical or emotional problems caused or worsened by cocaine use (APA, 2000).

If an individual has ever met criteria for cocaine dependence, the diagnosis of cocaine abuse does not apply. Patients who currently meet diagnostic criteria for both abuse and dependence would receive a diagnosis of dependence. Those who formerly met criteria for dependence, but now exhibit only symptoms of abuse, would receive a diagnosis of *cocaine dependence in partial remission*. Remission would be characterized as *early* if cocaine-dependence criteria had been met within the past year, and *sustained* if not (APA, 2000). The most exhaustive instrument for obtaining accurate diagnosis of cocaine use disorders is the Structured Clinical Interview for *DSM–IV* Axis I Disorders (SCID; First, Spitzer, Gibbon, & Williams, 1996), a semi-structured interview with questions corresponding to each *DSM–IV* symptom criterion.

Obtaining detailed information about quantity and frequency of cocaine use is facilitated by the TimeLine Follow-Back Interview (TLFB; Sobell & Sobell, 1992). Originally designed to evaluate alcohol use, the TLFB is easily adapted for assessment of other substance use. The TLFB uses a calendar to orient patients to the time period of interest and help them reconstruct an accurate account of their drug and alcohol use during that period. The TLFB is particularly useful for detecting changes in patterns of use that may occur with treatment. For instance, a patient who has not been able to achieve sustained abstinence from cocaine may still show reductions in use quantity or frequency when assessed in this detailed manner. Because it uses significant events as memory cues for recall of use, the TLFB can also help clinicians identify events that trigger drug use (holidays, paydays, stressful events).

The Addiction Severity Index (ASI; McLellan et al., 1992) is s semi-structured interview that provides information, not only on the severity of drug and alcohol use, but on five other categories of problems often associated with substance use disorders (medical, employment/ support, family/social relationships, legal, psychiatric). The ASI allows clinicians to identify and address client needs and potential barriers or challenges to their goals of giving up or significantly reducing drug use. In addition to specific questions about problems in each category, the ASI allows the patient and the interviewer to rate severity of problems and need for services in each category.

Evidence-Based Treatments for Cocaine Use Disorders

The Drug Abuse Treatment Outcome Study (DATOS; Fletcher, Tims, & Brown, 1997) found that cocaine was the most common illegal drug used by individuals entering drug treatment programs (Simpson, Joe, Fletcher, Hubbard, & Anglin, 1999). As no pharmacotherapy has demonstrated consistently positive results in treating cocaine dependence (Higgins, Heil, & Lussier, 2004), treatment efforts have focused on psychotherapies. There are several promising behavioral treatments for cocaine use disorders, most of them adapted from effective treatments for alcohol abuse and dependence.

Cognitive-Behavioral Therapies

Cognitive-behavioral therapies (CBT) for cocaine addiction have been widely studied. CBT is based on social learning theory and the assumption that behavior is learned through a combination of classical conditioning, operant conditioning, and modeling (Carroll, 1998). When applied to cocaine use disorders, this model suggests that individuals first learn to use cocaine by observing other people using it. Once cocaine use is initiated, operant conditioning can occur as an individual experiences the pleasurable effects of cocaine and repeatedly uses it in order to re-create those effects and eliminate cravings. Classical conditioning contributes to dependence when cocaine use is repeatedly paired with environmental cues, such as certain people, locations, objects, times, situations, and feeling states. Over time, these cues trigger the craving for cocaine.

The first stage of CBT is a functional analysis, in which a patient's unique learning history and vulnerabilities that contribute to the current state of maladaptive cocaine use are identified, as well as strengths and resources that can be marshaled in the effort to reduce or discontinue cocaine use (Carroll, 1998). Subsequent to the functional analysis, CBT focuses on training patients in the skills they need to cope with the challenges of discontinuing cocaine use and dealing with the problems of life without the aid of cocaine. Specific skills include recognizing and coping with cravings, resisting offers of cocaine or pressure to use it, avoiding or planning ahead for situations that increase the risk of cocaine use, and problem solving. CBT is highly structured, personalized, and brief (usually 12 to 16 weeks) in duration (Carroll, 1998).

Studies comparing CBT to less structured treatments (e.g., interpersonal therapy, clinical management) show that treatment outcomes are generally comparable. However, in patients with severe cocaine dependence, CBT resulted in better outcomes, specifically greater likelihood of completing treatment and maintaining three or more weeks of continuous cocaine abstinence (Carroll et al., 1994b; Carroll, Rounsaville, & Gawin, 1991). CBT was associated with decreased or stable cocaine use in the year following treatment, regardless of dependence severity, whereas patients receiving the alternative treatment had returned to pretreatment levels of use (Carroll, 1994a). It therefore appears that the effects of CBT may be more enduring than other treatments despite comparable short-term efficacy.

Twelve-Step Facilitation Therapy (TSF)

Self-help groups that are based on the principles of Alcoholics Anonymous (AA) are a popular option for many individuals who want to stop using cocaine. These groups, which focus on completing 12 steps to recovery, are based on a model of addiction as a spiritual and medical disease. Twelve-Step Facilitation Therapy (TSF) is an individualized treatment, the main goal of which is to facilitate patients' active participation in 12-step groups (Nowinski, Baker, & Carroll, 1992). Patients are encouraged to accept the disease model, admit that they have lost control over substance use, and embrace the goal of abstinence. During treatment, TSF patients are expected to begin attending meetings with the intention of continuing in the fellowship indefinitely once treatment ends (Nowinski et al., 1992). TSF was developed for alcohol abuse and dependence, but it has been adapted for use with cocaine and other substance use disorders.

Like CBT, TSF has been associated with a continued modest reduction in cocaine use during the year following treatment completion compared to a slight increase in the frequency of cocaine use posttreatment in a comparison treatment (Carroll et al., 2000). Although TSF appeared to be somewhat less effective than CBT in helping urban crack cocaine users achieve four or more weeks of continuous cocaine abstinence (Maude-Griffin et al., 1998), patients who obtained low scores on a test of abstract reasoning were more likely to remain abstinent for four weeks in the TSF treatment and less likely in the CBT treatment. These findings suggest that patient characteristics can interact with characteristics of treatments in influencing outcomes. Nevertheless, similar to CBT, the beneficial effects of TSF are generally modest at best.

Individual Drug Counseling

The 12-step philosophy is also the foundation of Individual Drug Counseling (IDC; Crits-Christoph et al., 1997). Patients in IDC are encouraged to endorse the disease model of addiction, which views addiction as a chronic disease and recovery as a lifelong process. The importance of abstinence is strongly emphasized and patients are urged to attend 12-step groups such as AA, Narcotics Anonymous, and Cocaine Anonymous. Other problems, including unemployment, interpersonal problems, and illegal activities are addressed to the extent that they influence drug use (Mercer & Woody, 1999). Like CBT, IDC also provides patients with concrete behavioral strategies for recovery from cocaine addiction.

The National Institute on Drug Abuse Collaborative Cocaine Treatment Study found that adding IDC to group drug counseling for cocaine dependence led to greater and more rapid reductions in cocaine use compared to group drug treatment alone or in combination with cognitive or supportive-expressive therapies (Crits-Christoph et al., 1997). Because IDC includes aspects of both CBT (short-term focus, training in behavioral strategies) and TSF (disease model, participation in 12-step groups), this finding suggests that combining components of other modestly effective treatment approaches may provide additional benefits over the specific component treatments provided alone.

Motivational Enhancement Therapy

Levels of motivation to stop using can vary widely among cocaine users, even those seeking treatment. Motivational enhancement therapy (MET; Miller, Zweben, DiClemente, & Rychtarik, 1992) was designed to increase motivation to change in substance users ambivalent about the decision to stop using. MET begins with a thorough assessment of the patient's level of substance use relative to norms, consequences of use, and risks for further consequences. Two to four individual treatment sessions follow, during which the patient is given feedback on the assessment with the intent of generating discussion that will increase motivation and commitment to changing behavior. The therapist's role is not to convince the patient to stop using but to respond to the patient's statements in a way that will facilitate the growth of intrinsic motivation (Miller, 1996).

Benefits of providing individual MET prior to group substance abuse treatment were examined in a sample of cocaine abusers admitted to a partial hospital program (Rohsenow et al., 2004). Patients with low motivation to change prior to treatment were less likely to use cocaine in the year following treatment if they completed MET rather than the control treatment (meditation and relaxation training). The opposite was true for patients with high pretreatment motivation to change; they were more likely to use cocaine in the MET group.

Providing Motivational Interviewing (MI), the treatment upon which MET is based, prior to cocaine detoxification and a subsequent relapse prevention program did not increase overall completion rates for detoxification, but patients receiving MI were more likely to be abstinent from cocaine when they began the subsequent relapse prevention treatment (Stotts et al., 2001). Furthermore, among patients with low pretreatment motivation to change, those who received MI were more likely to complete detoxification. Together, these results suggest that MET and similar treatments designed to enhance motivation to change may be helpful for a specific subset of cocaine abusers who enter treatment with low motivation to change.

Other Approaches

Despite evidence supporting the efficacy of specific treatments and combinations of treatments and suggesting that efficacy can vary based on patient characteristics, most treatment programs in community settings are eclectic in nature, providing a mixture of individual and group counseling and self-help group involvement to all patients (Simpson et al., 1999). With several different treatments showing modest effectiveness, but none providing clearly superior outcomes, developing methods for enhancing existing treatments is an important area for exploration. Contingency management interventions have shown great promise in improving treatment outcomes.

Contingency Management Interventions

Contingency Management (CM) interventions are based on principles of operant conditioning. Drug use is conceptualized as an operant behavior that is maintained by the drug's reinforcing effects (Higgins, Budney, & Bickel, 1994a). Although negative consequences of drug use could be expected to reduce the likelihood of its being repeated, these consequences, such as incarceration, financial difficulties, or health problems, are typically remote from the time of use and not guaranteed to follow it, so their effect on behavior is relatively weak (Higgins et al., 1994a). CM therefore provides tangible incentives for reducing or abstaining from drug use. CM procedures involve identifying an appropriate target behavior (e.g., cocaine abstinence), obtaining objective evidence that the target behavior occurred (e.g., negative urine toxicology test), providing tangible incentives (e.g., voucher, prize) as soon as the target behavior is detected, and removing incentives when the target behavior does not occur.

CM is usually added to another treatment (behavioral, pharmacological) to improve outcomes. Early research on CM studied its efficacy in reducing drug use among patients receiving methadone maintenance treatment for opioid dependence. These studies demonstrated that providing supplemental methadone doses, take-home dosing, or cash rewards effectively reduced illegal drug use (Higgins, Stitzer, Bigelow, & Liebson, 1986; Stitzer, Bigelow, & Liebson, 1980). Although providing increasing methadone doses in response to negative urine drug screens and decreasing doses in response to positive screens were equally effective, patients who failed to reduce drug use were more likely to drop out of the study when doses were decreased, suggesting a relative benefit to reinforcement compared to punishment (Stitzer, Bickel, Bigelow,

& Liebson, 1986). The vast majority of CM approaches therefore provide rewards for positive behaviors rather than punishing undesired behaviors.

Voucher-Based Contingency Management

Voucher-based CM interventions have been extensively studied by Stephen Higgins and colleagues at the University of Vermont. These interventions typically provide vouchers worth a specific amount of money whenever a patient submits a urine sample negative for cocaine. The vouchers can be saved and exchanged for products of monetary value. An important component of a voucher program is that the value of vouchers earned increases with each consecutive instance of a desired behavior and voucher values are reset to an initially low value when a target behavior is not demonstrated, thus providing a powerful incentive to sustain abstinence over time (Roll, Higgins, & Badger, 1996).

Higgins and colleagues (1993) conducted a randomized study comparing a behavior therapy (community reinforcement) approach plus CM to 12-step-based drug counseling in 38 outpatients. Fifty-eight percent ($N = 11$) of patients assigned to CM and community reinforcement completed 24 weeks of treatment, compared to eleven percent ($N = 2$) of patients in 12-step counseling. Sixty-eight percent ($N = 13$) of patients receiving CM and community reinforcement achieved 8 weeks of continuous abstinence compared to eleven percent ($N = 2$) in the 12-step counseling group (Higgins et al., 1993). Group differences remained at 6, 9, and 12 month follow-up interviews, when patients who received CM and community reinforcement were more likely to report cocaine abstinence over the past 30 days and to submit cocaine-negative urine samples compared to patients who received 12-step counseling (Higgins et al., 1995).

In order to clarify the specific contribution of contingency management, Higgins and colleagues (1994b) next compared the community reinforcement approach alone to community reinforcement with voucher-based CM in a sample of 40 patients. There was a significant difference between groups in the proportion of patients who remained in treatment for 24 weeks, with 75% ($N = 15$) in the CM group and 40% ($N = 8$) of patients receiving community reinforcement alone completing treatment. Patients in the CM group achieved an average of 11.7 (± 2.0) weeks of continuous abstinence from cocaine, whereas patients in the comparison group achieved an average of 6.0 (± 1.0) weeks. The average duration of continuous cocaine abstinence was longer for the CM group compared to the control condition during the first 12 weeks of treatment when they received vouchers, as well as during the 12 weeks that followed when they no longer received vouchers, suggesting that the enhancement of early abstinence associated with reinforcement contributed to further abstinence when tangible reinforcements were no longer available (Higgins et al., 1994b). Subsequent research suggests that duration of initial abstinence during treatment is associated with sustained posttreatment abstinence (Higgins, Badger, & Budney, 2000).

A meta-analysis of 30 studies of voucher-based CM for substance use disorders demonstrated CM's superior efficacy to control treatments in facilitating abstinence (Lussier, Heil, Mongeon, Badger, & Higgins, 2006). Higher voucher value and more immediate delivery of vouchers after negative urine samples were associated with larger effect sizes. This meta-analysis included studies examining CM for a variety of drugs and alcohol, but the results are consistent with findings of specific studies in cocaine-using populations.

Prize-Based Contingency Management

Although they are effective in reducing drug use and increasing treatment retention, voucher-based CM interventions have not been widely adopted by community drug treatment programs, in part because they are too costly for many programs to implement as a standard component of treatment (Petry, 2000). Patients in some voucher-based CM studies can earn up to $1,200 worth of merchandise if all submitted urine specimens are negative for cocaine (Higgins et al., 1993, 1994b).

To address the issue of cost, we at the University of Connecticut Health Center (e.g., Petry, Martin, Cooney, & Kranzler, 2000) developed a prize-based CM intervention that provides intermittent tangible reinforcement for target behaviors such as cocaine abstinence. Patients in prize-based CM who provide evidence of abstinence or other target behaviors earn the opportunity to draw slips of paper that may be redeemable for prizes. In the typical prize CM program, patients draw slips from a bowl of 500. Half the slips have encouraging messages but do not result in prizes, and half the slips result in a prize. There are typically three prize magnitudes, "small" (worth about $1.00), "large" (worth about $20.00), and "jumbo" (worth about $100.00). The majority of the slips (e.g., 219) are associated with small prizes such as bus tokens and fast-food gift certificates, fewer (e.g., 30) are exchangeable for large prizes such as portable CD players or telephones, and one corresponds to a jumbo prize such as a DVD player or television. There is thus always an opportunity to earn something of high value, but overall earnings are relatively modest on average. Patients draw immediately after their negative drug tests are revealed, and prizes are kept on site so they can be provided immediately upon winning. In this way, the contingency between behavior and reinforcement is highlighted.

Prize-based CM provides tangible reinforcement on a variable ratio schedule, the reinforcement schedule that produces the highest rate of response and greatest resistance to extinction in experimental studies. Prize-based CM therefore has the potential to produce similar behavioral outcomes to voucher CM at a lower cost. Although the procedure involves an element of chance, raising concerns that it might promote gambling, examination of gambling behaviors among 803 patients participating in evaluations of CM in methadone and drug-free clinics found no differences in gambling behavior over time between patients assigned to prize-based CM and those assigned to standard care without CM (Petry et al., 2006).

Prize-based CM was first evaluated in a sample of 42 alcohol-dependent men participating in a Veterans Affairs outpatient substance abuse treatment program (Petry et al., 2000). Patients assigned to the CM condition earned the opportunity to draw for prizes when they submitted breath samples negative for alcohol. They earned additional draws for completing activities related to their treatment goals. Patients who received CM in addition to the standard treatment were significantly more likely than those receiving standard treatment alone to remain in treatment for the eight weeks of the study and to remain abstinent from alcohol for the duration of the study. CM patients were less likely than standard treatment patients to relapse to heavy alcohol use by the end of the study. The average value of prizes earned by each patient in the CM condition was $200.

A direct comparison of voucher- and prize-based CM interventions for cocaine- or opioid-dependent patients entering a community-based outpatient drug-free treatment program found both to be superior to standard treatment without CM (Petry, Alessi, Marx, Austin, & Tardiff,

2005a). Both CM interventions increased retention in treatment and duration of continuous abstinence from drugs relative to the standard treatment. Patients in standard treatment, voucher CM, and prize CM remained in treatment for 5.5 ± 3.6 weeks, 8.2 ± 3.8 weeks, and 9.3 ± 3.7 weeks, respectively. Although there were no statistically significant differences between the two CM groups, a trend toward longer duration of abstinence and retention in treatment in the prize CM group was noted. Patients receiving standard treatment achieved 4.6 (± 3.4) weeks of continuous abstinence from drugs and alcohol compared to 7.0 (± 4.2) weeks in voucher CM and 7.8 (± 4.2) weeks in prize CM. Only 8% ($N = 2$) of standard treatment patients remained abstinent for the duration of the study; 28% ($N = 15$) of patients in voucher CM and 45% ($N = 23$) in prize CM achieved 12 weeks of continuous abstinence. Although patients in the voucher CM condition had the opportunity to earn almost \$900 in vouchers, average earnings in this group were only \$335, compared with an overall value of prizes per patient in the prize CM condition of \$295.

Based on its positive results in controlled clinical studies, CM was selected by the National Institute on Drug Abuse Clinical Trials Network (CTN) for evaluation in community treatment settings (Petry et al., 2005b). The goal of the CTN is to transfer efficacious drug treatments from specialized research settings to community-based clinical settings. In the largest study of CM to date, 415 stimulant (cocaine, methamphetamine, or amphetamine) using patients were recruited from eight community clinics throughout the United States. The clinics were located primarily in urban settings, but suburban and rural settings were represented as well. All clinics provided psychosocial counseling as the platform treatment. As in other CM studies, patients were assigned to one of two groups, standard treatment or standard treatment plus prize CM, using a system of escalating draws for consecutive stimulant-free urine samples. The maximum number of draws available was 204, with average maximum expected earnings of about \$400 in prizes.

Patients who received CM plus standard treatment were more likely than patients receiving standard treatment alone to remain in treatment for the entire 12 weeks of the study (49%, $N = 102$, vs. 35%, $N = 72$). CM patients also attended more counseling sessions during the study period (19.2 ± 16.8) than standard care patients (15.7 ± 14.4). The longest duration of continuous verified abstinence from stimulants was significantly greater in the CM compared to the standard care group (8.6 ± 9.2 weeks vs. 5.2 ± 6.9 weeks), and CM patients were more likely than standard care patients to achieve twelve (19%, $N = 40$, vs. 5%, $N = 10$) weeks of continuous stimulant abstinence. The CTN study demonstrates that prize-based CM can improve treatment attendance and promote sustained abstinence in community-based drug free treatment settings.

Contingency Management for Cocaine Use in Methadone Clinics

Cocaine use is a significant problem in methadone maintenance clinics. Despite its efficacy in reducing illegal opioid use, methadone has little effect on rates of cocaine use, so many patients will continue to experience negative consequences of illicit drug use and maintain lifestyles that could increase their risk for opioid relapse, incarceration, and exposure to the human immunodeficiency virus (HIV) (Condelli et al., 1991). Both voucher- (Silverman et al., 1996, 1998) and prize-based (Petry & Martin, 2002) CM interventions have been successfully applied to reducing cocaine use in methadone maintenance patients.

The CTN evaluated the efficacy of a prize-based CM intervention for stimulant (cocaine, methamphetamine, or amphetamine) use in methadone maintenance clinics throughout the United States (Peirce et al., 2006). Methadone maintenance patients ($N = 389$) were assigned to one of two groups, usual care, consisting of daily methadone dosing and individual and group counseling, or usual care plus CM. Retention in the CTN study was comparable for the two groups as is common in CM studies conducted in methadone clinics. Patients in the two groups also attended a similar number of counseling sessions in the clinic during the course of the study. Patients in the CM condition were more likely than patients receiving standard care to submit stimulant-negative urine samples during the intervention period; 54% of submitted samples were negative for stimulants in the CM group compared to 39% of samples in the standard care group. The average longest duration of abstinence from stimulants was significantly greater in the CM compared to the standard care group (5.4 ± 7.9 consecutive visits vs. 2.3 ± 3.8 consecutive visits, respectively). Patients in the CM condition were 3 times as likely to achieve four or more weeks of continuous absence, 9 times as likely to achieve eight weeks, and 11 times as likely to achieve twelve weeks of continuous abstinence, and each of these odds ratios was significant.

Implementing Contingency Management Interventions in Community Settings

Research clearly supports the efficacy of contingency management interventions in enhancing treatment retention and reducing drug use. Early research on CM was conducted in clinics supported in whole or in part by research grants. Prize-based CM studies have been conducted in community-based clinics, but the CM interventions themselves have usually been implemented by trained research assistants rather than clinic staff. It is nevertheless likely that therapists and counselors could be trained to carry out formal CM procedures and encouraged to include them as components of routine drug treatment. Many aspects of CM for drug use disorders, including urine drug screening and reinforcements (e.g., snacks and coffee for those who attend treatment), are already part of routine treatment, although they are not used systematically and therefore their effect on outcomes may be somewhat diluted (Petry, 2000). In order to make CM widely available to patients, the next step is to study its efficacy when employed by community-based clinicians (Petry & Simcic, 2002), and research on this topic is currently underway.

One aspect of CM that could make it appealing to clinicians working in community-based settings is the ease with which it can be integrated into group treatment models commonly employed in drug treatment clinics. Petry, Martin, and Simic (2005) examined CM that reinforced abstinence from cocaine and attendance at group treatment sessions in a methadone clinic. Not only did patients assigned to CM submit more cocaine-negative urine samples and achieve longer durations of continuous abstinence than standard treatment patients, they also attended more group therapy sessions during the study, with CM patients attending an average of 6.6 ($\pm$ 4.0) and standard care patients attending an average of 3.0 ($\pm$ 0.5) sessions. The number of groups attended was associated with weeks of continuous cocaine abstinence in the CM group, suggesting that reinforcing attendance could improve abstinence-related outcomes. If this is the case, effective CM interventions could be feasible even in settings where regular urine drug screens are impractical. To further reduce time demands on clinic staff,

CM procedures can be effectively implemented in a group format, with patients drawing for prizes at the start of group sessions rather than individually following groups (Petry, Martin, & Finocche, 2001).

Prize-based CM can be a relatively inexpensive and efficacious addition to treatment for cocaine use disorders. Average cost per patient is less than $300, and some of the costs can be offset by soliciting donations from local merchants or philanthropists, and obtaining items on sale for less than their retail value. Restaurant gift certificates and movie passes are popular with patients in CM programs, and donations of these items may be relatively easy to solicit. Most prize CM interventions are associated with longer retention in treatment, and each additional week a patient remains in treatment could result in a substantial addition to reimbursement from public or private insurance providers, so the cost of prizes may also be offset by increased insurance reimbursement. If CM ultimately proves to be effective in reducing incarceration, emergency room visits, and transmission of infectious disease by lengthening cocaine abstinence and treatment retention, Federal and State funders may ultimately recognize its cost-effectiveness and support the modest costs of these procedures.

Case Presentation: Prize-Based Contingency Management for Cocaine Dependence

"Katie," a 29-year-old, divorced mother of two children, was admitted to the Intensive Outpatient Program of her local hospital, seeking treatment for cocaine dependence. Katie's major concern was with her use of crack cocaine. Her Intensive Outpatient Program (IOP) counselor referred her to the CM study being conducted at the clinic, and she met with the CM research assistant for an intake interview that included the SCID, TLFB, and ASI.

In response to the SCID, Katie endorsed two of four symptoms of *DSM–IV* cocaine abuse, including failure to fulfill major role obligations and continued use despite persistent and recurrent social or interpersonal problems. Specifically Katie related that she had sought treatment after using some money that her mother had given her to buy school supplies and clothes for her children to buy cocaine instead. Katie's children, aged 11 and 7, had been living with Katie's parents since Katie was arrested three years earlier for possession of cocaine and driving under the influence. Although those charges had been dropped because Katie's father had friends on the police force, Katie's parents insisted on taking custody of the children. Katie wanted to regain custody of her children, but she was unable to maintain a job or a suitable living situation because of her drug use. She reported that she was looking for a job, but finding it difficult because her telephone and cellular phone service had been discontinued for nonpayment. Her crack cocaine use and inability to support herself and her children led to frequent conflicts with her parents.

Katie also met *DSM–IV* criteria for cocaine dependence. She reported needing to increase her cocaine use to get the desired high and feeling depressed and fatigued when she stopped using. She stated that she had tried to stop using cocaine numerous times in the past, but despite attending Cocaine Anonymous (CA) meetings, she always went back to cocaine. She generally used more cocaine than she intended when she did use. She had lost several jobs because she failed to report for work, either after using cocaine or because she was seeking it.

Although the TLFB revealed that Katie had used an average of 2 grams of cocaine per day for the first two weeks of the month prior to the interview, she had not used cocaine in the past 16 days. She stated that spending money meant for her children on cocaine was a "new low" for her, and that she thought she had "hit bottom." She felt that something had to change. She started attending CA meetings again and entered the IOP program, where she was diagnosed with cocaine dependence.

Katie's responses to the ASI further characterized her history of crack cocaine use and revealed moderately severe problems related to employment and family/social relationships. Katie reported that she first smoked crack cocaine at age 16, and by age 18 she was using it at least three times a week. She reported that she had stopped using both times she was pregnant, but resumed use when faced with the stresses of caring for infants. Katie dropped out of high school in the 11th grade when she was pregnant with her first child. Although she had occasionally worked for brief periods of time, she quit or was fired from all her jobs within weeks, usually after failing to show up when scheduled. At the time of the interview, she received food stamps and a small amount of money each month from public assistance. Katie's ex-husband was also a crack cocaine user. He had moved out of state and lost contact with Katie and the children. Katie reported that she had difficulty making friends because she was very shy. She stated that one of the reasons she enjoyed using cocaine initially was because it made her feel more confident and outgoing, although she found it no longer had this effect. Katie's primary relationships were with her children and her parents, but she frequently quarreled with her parents and felt they had "given up" on her.

Katie was very interested in CM and consented to be in the study. She was scheduled to meet with the research assistant three times a week for the first three weeks, twice a week during weeks four through six, and once a week for weeks seven through twelve. Her first submitted urine specimen was negative for cocaine, and she earned one draw from the "fish-bowl." Her draw did not result in a prize, but the research assistant reminded her that if she stayed clean, the number of draws per negative sample would escalate and she would soon earn enough draws to win prizes with some regularity. At the second visit, she again submitted a negative sample and earned two draws, one of which resulted in a small prize. Katie chose a pack of gum, and expressed optimism about her chances of winning more prizes. At her third visit, however, Katie submitted a positive sample. The research assistant explained that he could not let her draw from the bowl, but praised her for coming in, and encouraged her to get back on track so she could again earn draws. Katie's fourth visit was equally disappointing; she submitted another positive sample, and became tearful as she talked about her feelings of depression and disappointment in herself. The research assistant asked if she was attending treatment at the IOP. Katie said she had skipped her groups this week because she felt too shy to speak up in front of the other patients. Because she didn't share her feelings in groups, other group members accused her of "being in denial." The RA encouraged her to talk to her counselor and the group leader about her problems participating in groups.

Katie missed her next session, but at the following scheduled visit she reported feeling more optimistic. She said she had spoken to the group leader, who had agreed to call on her occasionally so she didn't have to interrupt other more vocal group members. Katie's urine sample was negative for cocaine that day, so she drew from the fishbowl, and earned a large prize. As she looked through the cabinet where the prizes were stored, Katie noticed a cellular phone.

The research assistant explained that these phones did not require an account; they could be used with a phone card that she could also earn. "That could help me find a job," Katie said, "I'll take one of those." Over the next few visits, Katie remained cocaine-negative, and her number of draws escalated. Although most of her prizes were small, she earned occasional large prizes, which she used to buy phone cards for the cell phone. She reported that she had applied for a job at a fast-food restaurant, and given them her cell phone number. "The pay isn't great, but maybe I could make enough to buy Christmas presents for the kids this year." The research assistant suggested that Katie could also take her prizes in the form of gift cards and use those to buy Christmas gifts.

Katie continued to submit cocaine-negative urine samples throughout the 12 weeks of the study. She occasionally reported feeling discouraged and tempted to use, particularly after she was not hired by the fast-food restaurant. She had told her IOP counselor about her plan to use her CM winnings to buy Christmas presents for her children, and the counselor suggested she make a shopping list, keep it with her, and review it when she felt tempted to use. She said this had actually helped her avoid using, because she knew if she tested positive she would be reset back to one draw the next time she was positive and therefore fail to accumulate enough draws to win the gift cards she needed. She also stated that the CM sessions gave her an added incentive to attend the IOP.

Katie attended the IOP three days a week and attended CA and Narcotics Anonymous meetings two evenings a week. Her IOP counselor worked with her on developing coping skills and skills for refusing offers to use. She also employed cognitive behavioral techniques to help Katie combat negative thoughts about herself and take more credit for her achievements. Katie felt her biggest achievement in the IOP was making the decision to stop focusing on how she'd let her parents down and start working on regaining their trust.

By the end of the study, Katie had achieved 10 weeks of continuous cocaine abstinence, and earned enough gift cards to buy most of the items on her Christmas shopping list. She had also received one jumbo prize, a portable DVD player that the children could share. She was proud of her achievements, but also expressed anxiety that she would go back to using when she stopped earning draws.

Despite her fears, when Katie returned for a follow-up assessment three months after the end of treatment, she submitted a cocaine-negative urine specimen. She reported that she had slipped up and used cocaine on two occasions since finishing the study, but she remembered to use the skills she learned in the IOP to get back on track. "We had a great Christmas," she said, "Just seeing the kids' faces when they opened the presents, made me feel more committed to staying off crack. I try to think about that when I feel like using, how I managed to stay clean long enough to give them a nice Christmas." Katie had not yet found a job, and she admitted that applying for jobs and interviewing made her very anxious. She continued to attend CA meetings, and her counselor had offered to help her practice job interviews.

Overall, Katie's case provides an example of how CM can be combined with standard treatments for cocaine dependence. CM gave Katie tangible incentives to stay clean, which in turn increased her motivation to attend treatment and 12-step meetings. She was therefore able to take advantage of the benefits of the IOP treatment. By helping her stay clean, CM also helped to build her confidence and self-efficacy, which, combined with the skills she learned at the IOP, enabled her to rebound when she briefly relapsed after treatment and CM ended.

| **TABLE 15.1** |
| **Resources for Further Information on Cocaine** |

Cocaine Anonymous. www.ca.org

Website for CA World Services. Includes Cocaine Anonymous literature, meeting locator and list of upcoming events

National Institute on Drug Abuse. *Cocaine.* www.nida.nih.gov/drugpages/cocaine.html

  Contains links to manuals for several treatments mentioned in the chapter plus summary and detailed look at recent research findings, other NIDA publications

Petry, N. M., & Stitzer, M. L. (2002). *Contingency management: Using motivational incentives to improve drug abuse treatment.* (Yale University Psychotherapy Development Center, Training Series No. 6). West Haven, CT

  A manual outlining procedures for implementing prize-based contingency management in community-based drug treatment settings

SCID Web Page. www.scid4.org/

  Contains information on the Structured Clinical Interview for *DSM–IV* and instructions for ordering SCID materials

Treatment Research Institute. www.tresearch.org/resources/instruments.htm#manuals

  Contains links to Addiction Severity Index forms, manuals and information

Summary

Cocaine use disorders are recognized as a significant public health problem, and several empirically supported treatments have been developed (please refer to Table 15.1 above for additional resources). The efficacy of CM in improving retention in treatment and lengthening duration of cocaine abstinence has been repeatedly demonstrated, and prize-based procedures allow patients to receive the benefits of CM at a relatively low cost. CM can be combined with a variety of specific drug treatments, can be offered in individual and group formats, and can be applied to a range of target behaviors in addition to drug abstinence. Costs can be further reduced through creative marketing and solicitation of donations from the community or offset through insurance reimbursements. Given the high costs of cocaine use disorders to society, CM holds promise as a cost-effective method for promoting positive treatment outcomes.

Acknowledgment

The authors thank Stephen MacKinnon, Matthew Brennan, and Shanelle Carmichael for sharing their clinical experiences for use in the case presentation.

References

Agar, M. (2003). The story of crack: Towards a theory of illicit drug trends. *Addiction Research and Theory, 11,* 3–29.

American Psychiatric Association. (2000). *Diagnostic and statistical manual of mental disorders* (4th ed., text revision). Washington, DC: Author.

Carlson, R. G., Falck, R. S., & Siegal, H. A. (2000). Crack cocaine injection in the heartland: An ethnographic perspective. *Medical Anthropology, 18,* 305–323.

Carroll, K. M. (1998). *Therapy manuals for drug addiction: Manual 1. A cognitive-behavioral approach: Treating cocaine addiction.* (National Institute on Drug Abuse, NIH Publication No. 98-4308). Washington, DC: U.S. Department of Health and Human Services.

Carroll, K. M., Niche, C., Ball, S. A., McCance, E., Frankforter, T. L., & Rounsaville, B. J. (2000). One-year follow-up of disulfiram and psychotherapy for cocaine-alcohol users: Sustained effects of treatment. *Addiction, 95,* 1335–1349.

Carroll, K. M., Rounsaville, B. J., & Gawin, F. H. (1991). A comparative trial of psychotherapies for ambulatory cocaine abusers: Relapse prevention and interpersonal psychotherapy. *American Journal of Drug and Alcohol Abuse, 17,* 229–247.

Carroll, K. M., Rounsaville, B. J., Gordon, L. T., Nich, C., Jatlow, P. M., Bisighini, R. M., & Gawin, F. H. (1994a). Psychotherapy and pharmacotherapy for ambulatory cocaine abusers. *Archives of General Psychiatry, 51,* 177–187.

Carroll, K. M., Rounsaville, B. J., Nich, C., Gordon, L. T., Wirtz, P. W., & Gawin, F. H. (1994b). One year follow-up of psychotherapy and pharmacotherapy for cocaine dependence: Delayed emergence of psychotherapy effects. *Archives of General Psychiatry, 51,* 989–997.

Condelli, W. S., Fairbank, J. A., Dennis, M. L., & Rachal, J. V. (1991). Cocaine use by clients in methadone programs: Significance, scope, and behavioral interventions. *Journal of Substance Abuse Treatment, 8,* 203–212.

Crits-Christoph, P., Siqueland, L., Blaine, J., Frank. A., Luborsky, L., Onken, L. S., et al. (1997). The National Institute on Drug Abuse Collaborative Cocaine Treatment Study: Rationale and methods. *Archives of General Psychiatry, 54,* 691–694.

First, M. B., Spitzer, R. L., Gibbon, M., Williams, J. B. W. (1997). *Structured Clinical Interview for DSM-IV Axis I Disorders.* Washington, DC: American Psychiatric Press.

Fletcher, B. W., Tims, F. M., & Brown, B. S. (1997). Drug abuse treatment outcome study (DATOS): Treatment evaluation research in the United States. *Psychology of Addictive Behaviors, 11,* 216–229.

Gawin, F. H. (1991). Cocaine addiction: Psychology and neurophysiology. *Science, 251,* 1580–1586.

Glantz, M. D., Conway, K. P., & Colliver, J. D. (2005). Drug use heterogeneity and the search for subtypes. In Z. Sloboda (Ed.), *Epidemiology of drug abuse* (pp. 15–27). New York: Springer.

Gossop, M., Manning, V., & Ridge, G. (2006). Concurrent use of alcohol and cocaine: Differences in patterns of use and problems among users of crack cocaine and cocaine powder. *Alcohol & Alcoholism, 41,* 121–125.

Higgins, S. T., Badger, G. J., & Budney, A. J. (2000). Initial abstinence and success in achieving longer term cocaine abstinence. *Experimental and Clinical Psychopharmacology, 8,* 377–386.

Higgins, S. T., Budney, A. J., & Bickel, W. K. (1994a). Applying behavioral concepts and principles to the treatment of cocaine dependence. *Drug and Alcohol Dependence, 34,* 87–97.

Higgins, S. T., Budney, A. J., Bickel, W. K., Badger, G. J., Foerg, F. E., & Ogden, D. (1995). Outpatient behavioral treatment for cocaine dependence: One-year outcome. *Experimental and Clinical Psychopharmacology, 3,* 205–212.

Higgins, S. T., Budney, A. J., Bickel, W. K, Foerg, F. E., Donham, R., & Badger, G. J. (1994b). Incentives improve outcome in outpatient behavioral treatment of cocaine dependence. *Archives of General Psychiatry, 51,* 568–576.

Higgins, S. T., Budney, A. J., Bickel, W. K., Hughes, J. R., Foerg, F., & Badger, G. (1993). Achieving cocaine abstinence with a behavioral approach. *American Journal of Psychiatry, 150,* 763–769.

Higgins, S. T., Heil, S. H., & Lussier, J. P. (2004). Clinical implications of reinforcement as a determinant of substance use disorders. *Annual Review of Psychology, 55,* 431–461.

Higgins, S. T., Stitzer, M. L., Bigelow, G. E., & Liebson, I. A. (1986). Contingent methadone delivery: Effects on illicit-opiate use. *Drug and Alcohol Dependence, 17,* 311–322.

Johnson, B. D., Golub, A., & Dunlap, E. (2000). The rise and decline of hard drugs, drug markets, and violence in inner-city New York. In A. Blumstein & J. Wallman (Eds.), *The crime drop in America* (pp. 164–206). Cambridge: Cambridge University Press.

Jonnes, J. (1996). *Hep-cats, narcs, and pipe dreams: A history of America's romance with illegal drugs.* New York: Scribner.

Lussier, J. P., Heil, S. H., Mongeon, J. A., Badger, G. J., & Higgins, S. T. (2006). A meta-analysis of voucher-based reinforcement therapy for substance use disorders. *Addiction, 101,* 192–203.

Martin, C. S., Clifford, P. R., Maisto, S. A., Earleywine, M., Krisci, L., & Longabaugh, R. (1996). Polydrug use in an inpatient treatment sample of problem drinkers. *Alcoholism: Clinical and Experimental Research, 20,* 413–417.

Maude-Griffin, P. M., Hohenstein, J. M., Humfleet, G. L., Reilly, P. M., Tusel, D. J., & Hall, S. (1998). Superior efficacy of cognitive-behavioral therapy for urban crack cocaine abusers: Main and matching effects. *Journal of Consulting and Clinical Psychology, 66,* 832–837.

McLellan, A. T., Kushner, H., Metzger, D., Peters, R., Smith, I., Grissom, G., et al. (1992). The fifth edition of the Addiction Severity Index. *Journal of Substance Abuse Treatment, 9,* 199–213.

Mercer, D. E., & Woody, G. E. (1999). *Therapy manuals for drug addiction. An individual drug counseling approach to treat cocaine addiction: The Collaborative Cocaine Treatment Study Model.* (National Institute on Drug Abuse, NIH Publication No. 99-4380). Washington, DC: U.S. Department of Health and Human Services.

Miller, W. R. (1996). Motivational interviewing: Research, practice, and puzzles. *Addictive Behaviors, 21,* 835–842.

Miller, W. R., Zweben, A., DiClemente, C. C., & Rychtarik, R. G. (1992). *Motivational enhancement therapy manual: A clinical research guide for therapists treating individuals with alcohol abuse and dependence* (Vol. 2, Project MATCH Monograph Series). Rockville, MD: National Institute on Alcohol Abuse and Alcoholism.

Nowinski, J., Baker, S., & Carroll, K. (1992). *Twelve-Step facilitation therapy manual: A clinical research guide for therapists treating individuals with alcohol abuse and dependence* (Vol. 1, Project MATCH Monograph Series). Rockville, MD: National Institute on Alcohol Abuse and Alcoholism.

O'Brien, M. S., & Anthony, J. C. (2005). Risk of becoming cocaine dependent: Epidemiological estimates for the United States, 2000-2001. *Neuropsychopharmacology, 30,* 1006–1018.

Peirce, J. M., Petry, N. M., Stitzer, M. L., Blaine, J., Kellogg, S., Satterfield, F., et al. (2006). Effects of lower-cost incentives on stimulant abstinence in methadone maintenance treatment: A National Drug Abuse Treatment Clinical Trials Network study. *Archives of General Psychiatry, 63,* 201–208.

Petry, N. M. (2000). A comprehensive guide to the application of contingency management procedures in clinical settings. *Drug and Alcohol Dependence, 58,* 9–25.

Petry, N. M., Alessi, S. M., Marx, J., Austin, M., & Tardif, M. (2005a). Vouchers versus prizes: Contingency management treatment of substance abusers in community settings. *Journal of Consulting and Clinical Psychology, 73,* 1005–1014.

Petry, N. M., Kolodner, K. B., Li, R., Peirce, J. M., Roll, J. M., Stitzer, M. L., et al. (2006). Prize-based contingency management does not increase gambling. *Drug and Alcohol Dependence, 83,* 269–273.

Petry, N. M., & Martin, B. (2002). Low-cost contingency management for treating cocaine- and opioid-abusing methadone patients. *Journal of Consulting and Clinical Psychology, 70,* 398–405.

Petry, N. M., Martin, B., Cooney, J. L., & Kranzler, H. R. (2000). Give them prizes, and they will come: Contingency management for treatment of alcohol dependence. *Journal of Consulting and Clinical Psychology, 68,* 250–257.

Petry, N. M., Martin, B., & Finocche, C. (2001). Contingency management in group treatment: A demonstration project in an HIV drop-in center. *Journal of Substance Abuse Treatment,* 89–96.

Petry, N. M., Martin, B., & Simcic, F. (2005). Prize reinforcement contingency management for cocaine dependence: Integration with group therapy in a methadone clinic. *Journal of Consulting and Clinical Psychology, 73,* 354–359.

Petry, N. M., Peirce, J. M., Stitzer, M. L., Blaine, J., Roll, J. M., Cohen, A., et al. (2005b). Effect of prize-based incentives on outcomes in stimulant abusers in outpatient psychosocial treatment programs: A National Drug Abuse Treatment Clinical Trials Network study. *Archives of Clinical Psychiatry, 62,* 1148–1156.

Petry, N. M., & Simcic, F. (2002). Recent advances in the dissemination of contingency management techniques: Clinical and research perspectives. *Journal of Substance Abuse Treatment, 23,* 81–86.

Platt, J. J. (1997). *Cocaine addiction: Theory, research, and treatment.* Cambridge: Harvard University Press.

Rohsenow, D. J., Monti, P. M., Martin, R. A., Colby, S. M., Myers, M. G., Gulliver, S. B., et al. (2004). Motivational enhancement and coping skills training for cocaine abusers: Effects on substance use outcomes. *Addiction, 99,* 862–874.

Roll, J. M., Higgins, S. T., & Badger, G. J. (1996). An experimental comparison of three different schedules of reinforcement of drug abstinence using cigarette smoking as an exemplar. *Journal of Applied Behavior Analysis, 29,* 495–504.

Rounsaville, B. J. (2004). Treatment of cocaine dependence and depression. *Biological Psychiatry, 56,* 803–809.

Rutherford, M. J., Cacciola, J. S., & Alterman, A. I. (1999). Antisocial personality disorder and psychopathy in cocaine-dependent women. *American Journal of Psychiatry, 156,* 849–856.

Silverman, K., Higgins, S. T., Brooner, R. K., Montoya, I., Cone, E. J., Schuster, C. R., et al. (1996). Sustained cocaine abstinence in methadone maintenance patients through voucher-based reinforcement therapy. *Archives of General Psychiatry, 53,* 409–415.

Silverman, K., Wong, C. J., Umbricht-Schneiter, A., Montoya, I. D., Schuster, C. R., & Preston, K. L. (1998). Broad beneficial effects of cocaine abstinence reinforcement among methadone patients. *Journal of Consulting and Clinical Psychology, 66,* 811–824.

Simpson, D. D., Joe, G. W., Fletcher, B. W., Hubbard, R. L., & Anglin, D. (1999). A national evaluation of treatment outcomes for cocaine dependence. *Archives of General Psychiatry, 56,* 507–514.

Sobell, L. C., & Sobell, M. B. (1992). Timeline follow-back: A technique for assessing self-reported alcohol consumption. In R. Z. Litten & J. P. Allen (Eds.), *Measuring alcohol consumption: Psychosocial and biochemical methods* (pp. 41–72). Totowa, NJ: Humana Press.

Stitzer, M. L., Bickel, W. K., Bigelow, G. E., & Liebson, I. A. (1986). Effect of methadone dose contingencies on urinalysis test results of polydrug-abusing methadone-maintenance patients. *Drug and Alcohol Dependence, 18,* 341–348.

Stitzer, M. L., Bigelow, G. E., & Liebson, I. (1980). Reducing drug use among methadone maintenance clients: Contingent reinforcement for morphine-free urines. *Addictive Behaviors, 5,* 333–340.

Stotts, A. L., Schmitz, J. M., Rhoades, H. M., & Grabowski, J. (2001). Motivational interviewing with cocaine-dependent patients: A pilot study. *Journal of Consulting and Clinical Psychology, 69,* 858–862.

Substance Abuse and Mental Health Services Administration. (2006). *Results from the 2005 National Survey on Drug Use and Health: National findings* (Office of Applied Studies, NDSUH Series H-30, DHHS Publication No. SMA 06-4194). Rockville, MD.

Williamson, A., Darke, S., Ross, J., & Teesson, M. (2006). The effect of persistence of cocaine use on 12-month outcomes for the treatment of heroin dependence. *Drug and Alcohol Dependence, 81,* 293–300.

16

Evidence-Based Treatment of Amphetamine Dependence: Behavioral and Pharmacological Approaches

Craig R. Rush, Andrea R. Vansickel,
Joshua A. Lile, and William W. Stoops

University of Kentucky

Contents

Introduction

Amphetamine dependence in general, and methamphetamine in particular, is a significant public-health concern (Drug and Alcohol Services Information System [DASIS], 2004). In 2005, over 500,000 Americans age 12 or older reported current methamphetamine use

(National Survey on Drug Use and Health [NSDUH], 2006). Methamphetamine use was linked to approximately 73,400 emergency room visits in 2004 (Substance Abuse and Mental Health Administration [SAMHSA], 2006c). Methamphetamine dependence is associated with significant morbidity in that users often suffer from mental illness, malnutrition, tremors, heart and lung problems, and infection at injection sites as well as irregular periods and miscarriages in women (Hando, Topp, & Hall, 1997; Richards et al., 1999). Facial and ocular burns result from methamphetamine production accidents and account for up to 10% of admissions to burn-care units (Charukamnoetkanok & Wagoner, 2004). Methamphetamine use varies by region, with western states having higher per capita use (SAMHSA, 2006b). However, methamphetamine has been identified as a threat for the eastern United States suggesting that drug use and production may be spreading (National Drug Intelligence Center, 2006) (Table 16.1).

Historical Conceptualization of Amphetamine Dependence

Emergence of Amphetamine Use

Amphetamine isomers were first formulated from ephedrine in the late 1800s, but did not have a medical indication until the 1920s when they were used for bronchial dilation. After this, amphetamine isomers were commonly used to promote alertness, particularly in the military. Some historical anecdotes indicate that Japanese kamikaze pilots often used high doses of methamphetamine. After World War II, widespread use of amphetamine isomers resulted in the United States Food and Drug Administration outlawing nonprescription use. Illegal use of amphetamine isomers has cycled since that time (including the misuse of prescription compounds such as Dexedrine® [*d*-amphetamine] or Adderall® [mixed salts of *d*-and *l*-amphetamine]), but recently amphetamine abuse and dependence have increased as a result of the availability of manufactured methamphetamine.

TABLE 16.1
Resources for Amphetamine Use Disorders

1. Anonymous: www.Streetdrugs.org.
2. National Institute on Drug Abuse (NIDA): *NIDA InfoFacts: Methamphetamine*. www.nida. nih.gov/infofacts/methamphetamine.html.
3. National Institute on Drug Abuse (NIDA): NIDA Research Report: Methamphetamine: Abuse and Addiction. www.nida.nih.gov/ResearchReports/methamph/methamph.html.
4. McCain, M. J., Obert, J. L., Marinell-Casey, P., & Rawson, R. A. (2006). *Meth: The Basics*. Hazelden: City, Minnesota.
5. Johnson, D. (2005). *Meth: The Home-Cooked Menace*. Hazelden: Center City, Minnesota.
6. Rawson, R. A., Anglin, M. D., & Ling, W. (2002). Will the methamphetamine problem go away? *Journal of Addictive Disorders, 21*, 5–19.
7. Cretzmeyer, M., Sarrazin, M. V., Huber, D. L., Block, R. I., & Hall, J. A. (2003). Treatment of methamphetamine abuse: Research findings and clinical directions. *Journal of Substance Abuse Treatment, 24*, 267–277.
8. Lineberry, T. W., & Bostwick, J. M. (2006). Methamphetamine abuse: A perfect storm of complications. *Mayo Clinic Proceedings 81*, 77–84.

In the 1980s, methamphetamine was primarily smuggled into the country from Asia to Hawaii and from Mexico to California (Wermuth, 2000). However, more recently, methamphetamine has been manufactured and sold locally, using a simple but dangerous process called "pseudoephedrine reduction" (Wermuth, 2000). The directions for this process are commonly learned through books or Internet recipes (www.Steetdrugs.org). Methamphetamine can be manufactured using common household items including iodine, lye, anhydrous ammonia, and pseudoephedrine in small clandestine labs (Rawson, Anglin, & Ling, 2002; Wermuth, 2000). Although this practice of small lab production of methamphetamine remains common, the recent advent of "Superlabs" has been noted by the Department of Justice (NDIC, 2006).

Contemporary Assessment of Amphetamine Use Disorders

The diagnosis of methamphetamine abuse or dependence is made using comprehensive interviews such as the Structured Clinical Interview for *DSM–IV* (First, Spitzer, Gibbon, & Williams, 1996) to determine whether an individual meets various criteria. An individual is diagnosed with abuse of methamphetamine if he or she has a pattern of substance use that leads to clinically significant problems at least once during a 12-month period and does not meet criteria for methamphetamine dependence. An individual is diagnosed with dependence if he or she meets three of the following criteria during a 12-month period: becomes tolerant to the effects of the methamphetamine, has withdrawal following cessation of methamphetamine use, uses more methamphetamine longer than intended or takes more than intended, desires to cut down or has inability to cut down methamphetamine use, spends a great deal of time obtaining methamphetamine, misses important events to use methamphetamine, and continually uses methamphetamine despite knowledge of harm.

In 2005, approximately 20% of Americans that had used methamphetamine met *DSM–IV* criteria for stimulant abuse or dependence (NSDUH, 2006). In 2004, primary, secondary, or tertiary admissions for methamphetamine or amphetamine represented 12% of all substance abuse treatment admissions which is comparable to rates for cocaine (i.e., 14%; DASIS, 2006; SAMHSA, 2006a). Alarmingly, the dependence process may proceed more rapidly for methamphetamine than cocaine (Castro, Barrington, Walton, & Rawson, 2000). In this study, 39 regular users of methamphetamine, but not cocaine, were compared to 90 regular users of cocaine, but not methamphetamine. The period of time from initial to regular use, as well as entry into treatment, was significantly shorter for methamphetamine users.

Contemporary Treatment of Amphetamine Dependence

The epidemiological findings reviewed above underscore the need for effective treatment strategies for amphetamine dependence. Because the emergence of methamphetamine dependence as a public health concern is relatively recent, there is a paucity of studies that attempted to identify effective treatments. Cocaine dependence, by contrast, has been a significant public health concern for at least three decades and there is an extensive literature that attempted to identify effective treatments (for reviews, see Carroll, 2005; Carroll & Oksen, 2005;

de Lima, de Oliveira Soares, Reisser, & Farrell, 2002; Sofuoglu & Kosten, 2005). The successes and failures encountered while developing treatment strategies for cocaine dependence provide valuable information that can be used to guide the conduct of studies aimed at identifying effective treatments for methamphetamine dependence. The evidence-based literature on behavioral and pharmacological treatments for cocaine dependence is discussed when appropriate.

Behavioral Therapies for Amphetamine Dependence

Behavioral therapies are effective for reducing the use of illicit drugs, including amphetamine. The evidence-based literature on the behavioral treatments for amphetamine dependence reviewed below is not intended to be exhaustive inasmuch as such a review is beyond the scope of this chapter, and this topic has been comprehensively reviewed previously (Carroll, 2005; Carroll and Onken, 2005). Instead, the utility of contingency management or voucher-based reinforcement therapy for the treatment of amphetamine dependence is reviewed because these strategies appear to be effective for managing stimulant use disorders including methamphetamine. These strategies are heretofore referred to as contingency management for simplicity.

Contingency Management   Contingency management procedures are based on the principles of operant psychology (for a review, see Higgins, Heil, & Lussier, 2004). Briefly, contingency management procedures provide a reinforcer contingent upon a predetermined clinical response. The reinforcers are usually vouchers that are redeemable in the local community for material items. The predetermined clinical response is most often drug abstinence, which is verified via a drug-free biological specimen provided several times weekly. The reinforcer is withheld if the biological sample indicates recent drug use. The magnitude of the voucher increases with each successive drug-free urine sample. Contingency management is effective for initiating abstinence from drugs from diverse pharmacological classes including alcohol, cocaine, marijuana, nicotine, and opioids (e.g., Lussier, Heil, Mongeon, Badger, & Higgins, 2006). A recent meta-analysis suggests that contingency management procedures are effective for treating substance use disorders in general, and cocaine-use disorders in particular (Prendergast, Podus, Finney, Greenwell, & Roll, 2006).

In the seminal trial that demonstrated the efficacy of contingency management for establishing drug abstinence in cocaine dependent patients ($N = 13$), the voucher provided for the initial cocaine-free urine specimen was worth $1.50 (Higgins et al., 1991). Patients provided a urine specimen four times weekly that was tested for the presence of benzoylecgonine, a cocaine metabolite. The value of the voucher increased by $0.75 for each successive cocaine-free urine specimen. Participants also received $10.00 contingent on providing four consecutive cocaine-free urine specimens. If at any point during the trial the results of these tests indicated recent cocaine use, or the patient failed to provide a scheduled specimen, the voucher value was reset to $1.50. Patients could earn $1,038.00 if they abstained throughout this 12-week trial. Vouchers could be used to purchase items that counselors deemed consistent with the treatment goals. Patients ($N = 15$) in the control group received 12-step counseling. Patients in the contingency management group were retained in treatment significantly longer and achieved greater durations of continuous abstinence. Note that contingency management procedures are well accepted by patients (Higgins et al., 1991).

Contingency management principles were first utilized for the management of amphetamine dependence approximately 35 years ago (Boudin, 1972). In this report, a patient and therapist established a contingency contract that would result in the loss of $50 each time the patient reported using amphetamines or other drugs. This contingency was invoked only once during a three-month period. Although published as a case report involving a single patient and not particularly rigorous scientifically, this work provided the seminal evidence that contingency management procedures are effective for establishing and maintaining abstinence from amphetamines.

A large trial recently determined the efficacy of prize-based incentives for initiating abstinence from illicit stimulants and alcohol (Petry et al., 2005). Prize-based incentives are an innovative permutation of contingency management (e.g., Petry, Martin, Cooney, & Kranzler, 2000). Instead of receiving vouchers, when patients provided a drug-free urine specimen they drew 1–12 chips from a container that contained 500 chips. Each chip was marked with one of four options and the probability of drawing a particular option was fixed: (1) Good Job (250 chips or 50% probability); (2) Small Prize (worth approximately $1.00–$5.00; 209 chips or 41.8% probability); (3) Large Prize (worth approximately $20.00; 40 chips for 0.8% probability); or (4) Jumbo Prize (worth approximately $80.00–$100.00; 1 chip or 0.2% probability). Stimulant users (i.e., cocaine or methamphetamine) were randomly assigned to treatment as usual (N=222) or prize-based incentives plus treatment as usual (N=223). Methamphetamine, amphetamine, cocaine, and alcohol were the targeted drugs, and patients drew a chip when they had abstained from these drugs. The number of opportunities to draw a chip increased by one for each week that all samples indicated abstinence from the targeted drugs. Patients drew two additional chips each visit if they had also abstained from opioids and marijuana. Patients that abstained from all drugs for the entire 12-week trial drew a total of 204 chips. A single large prize was awarded after a patient initially achieved two weeks of abstinence. Patients assigned to the treatment-as-usual group received group therapy and some individual counseling as needed. Research staff also praised patients in the treatment-as-usual group when the urine samples indicated recent abstinence and encouraged them to discontinue using drugs when specimens were positive.

From this larger trial, data were extracted for 113 patients with methamphetamine use disorders (i.e., 51 had been assigned to prize-based incentives plus treatment as usual and 62 patients had been assigned to 12 weeks of treatment as usual; Roll et al., 2006). Patients assigned to these two conditions did not differ significantly on demographic characteristics. The results of this trial are marked in that patients assigned to prize-based incentives submitted significantly more urine samples that were negative for the target drugs. Patients assigned to prize-based incentives also achieved significantly longer periods of abstinence (4.6 versus 2.8 weeks). Significantly more patients receiving prize-based incentives were able to abstain for the duration of the trial (i.e., 17.6 versus 6.5%). The groups did not differ significantly in terms of treatment retention or counseling attendance, nor did they differ at follow-up (i.e., 3 and 6 months).

The results of this study are concordant with an extensive literature in which the efficacy of contingency management procedures has been demonstrated with other substance abuse disorders including cocaine dependence (Higgins, 2006). This concordance is important because studies conducted with abusers of drugs from diverse pharmacological classes provide a wealth of information that clinical researchers and practitioners can use to further refine these techniques and efficiently implement them for managing amphetamine dependence. Two examples warrant mentioning. First, the magnitude of the voucher affects abstinence (Higgins et al., 2007; Silverman, Chutuape, Bigelow, & Stitzer, 1999). In one trial, for example, 100 cocaine-dependent patients received high-value (i.e., maximum of $1,995.00 for 12-week trial; $N=50$) or low-value (i.e., maximum of $499.00 for 12-week trial; $N=50$) vouchers contingent on providing cocaine-free urines (Higgins et al., 2007). Patients assigned to the high-value voucher were retained in treatment for significantly longer (18.2 versus 14.6 weeks) and achieved significantly longer periods of abstinence (9.1 versus 4.7 weeks). Second, the reset contingency affects abstinence (Roll, Higgins, & Badger, 1996; Roll & Higgins, 2000).

In the more recent study, for example, 18 cigarette smokers participated in a within-subject trial in which three different conditions were tested (i.e., progressive increase in magnitude with a reset contingency, progressive increase in magnitude without a reset contingency, and fixed magnitude; Roll & Higgins, 2000). In the progressive–reset condition, participants received a $3.00 voucher for the first breath sample that indicated recent abstinence from smoking (i.e., carbon monoxide level ≤8 ppm). The value of the voucher increased by $0.50 across the five consecutive days that this schedule was in effect if the breath sample indicated continued abstinence. If a breath sample indicated recent smoking (i.e., carbon monoxide level >8 ppm), reinforcement was withheld and the value of the voucher returned to $3.00 for the next sample that indicated recent abstinence. In the progressive–no reset condition, the schedule was identical except for the reset component. In the fixed magnitude condition, participants received a voucher worth $9.80 for each breath sample that indicated recent abstinence. Significantly more participants initiated and sustained abstinence in the progressive–reset condition than either of the other two conditions.

The variables previously shown to affect abstinence with contingency management procedures for other forms of substance abuse have recently been extended to methamphetamine-dependent patients (Roll & Shoptaw, 2006; Roll et al., 2006). In one small trial, for example, 18 methamphetamine-dependent patients were randomly assigned to a progressively increasing schedule of voucher presentation with a reset contingency or an increasing schedule of voucher presentation without a reset contingency for 12 weeks (Roll & Shoptaw, 2006). Patients received a $2.50 voucher for the first urine sample that indicated recent abstinence from methamphetamine. The value of the voucher increased by $1.50 for consecutive samples that indicated recent abstinence. If a urine sample indicated recent methamphetamine use, reinforcement was withheld and the value of the voucher returned to $2.50 for the next sample that indicated abstinence. In the no-reset condition, the schedule was identical except there was not a reset component. Patients in the reset condition provided significantly more methamphetamine-free urines (i.e., 80 versus 38%) and achieved longer periods of continuous abstinence (i.e., 6.7 versus 2.8 weeks). These findings illustrate the similarities between methamphetamine-dependent patients and those with other substance abuse disorders.

Comparison of Contingency Management and Cognitive-Behavioral Therapies   Contingency management is effective for the management of methamphetamine use disorders. However, a number of other treatment interventions are effective in the management of substance-use disorders in general and stimulant-use disorders in particular (for reviews, see Carroll, 2005; Carroll & Onken, 2005). A large multisite, 16-week trial, for example, compared the efficacy of cognitive-behavioral therapy and treatment as usual for methamphetamine dependence (Rawson et al., 2004). Patients ($N=978$) were randomly assigned to receive treatment as usual or manual-driven cognitive-behavioral therapy. The cognitive-behavioral therapy sessions were delivered in combination with family education, social support, and individual counseling sessions. Treatment as usual was allowed to vary across each of the sites used in this trial in order to compare cognitive-behavioral therapy to treatments commonly used clinically. Across the eight sites, patients that received cognitive-behavioral therapy were retained in treatment longer, were more likely to complete, provided more methamphetamine-free urine samples, and had longer periods of continuous abstinence.

Because cognitive-behavioral therapy and contingency management are effective in the management of methamphetamine dependence, the relative efficacy of these treatment approaches is of considerable scientific and clinical interest. A recent report directly compared cognitive-behavioral therapy and contingency management for managing methamphetamine usage (Shoptaw et al., 2005). In a 16-week trial, 162 gay or bisexual men who were methamphetamine-dependent were randomly assigned to cognitive-behavioral therapy ($N=40$), contingency management ($N=42$), cognitive-behavioral therapy plus contingency management ($N=40$), or culturally tailored behavioral therapy ($N=40$). The cognitive-behavioral therapy group attended sessions thrice weekly. Cognitive-behavioral therapy was considered the standard of care condition. Patients in the contingency management group received a voucher worth $2.50 for the first urine specimen that indicated recent abstinence from methamphetamine and cocaine. The value of the voucher increased by $2.50 for each successive urine specimen that indicated abstinence from methamphetamine and cocaine. Patients also received a voucher worth $10.00 contingent on providing three consecutive urine specimens that indicated continued abstinence from methamphetamine and cocaine. Participants could earn $1,277.50 if they abstained throughout this 12-week trial. Patients in the cognitive-behavioral therapy plus contingency management received both forms of therapy. The culturally tailored behavioral therapy was designed to address drug-abuse treatment issues as well as reductions in behaviors associated with increased risk of HIV. At the end of treatment, patients assigned to contingency management procedures or cognitive-behavioral therapy plus contingency management procedures were retained in treatment significantly longer and achieved longer periods of continued abstinence than those assigned to cognitive-behavioral therapy. These group differences were no longer apparent at follow-up (i.e., 26 and 52 weeks). These results suggest that contingency management procedures may be especially effective for retaining methamphetamine-dependent patients in treatment and promoting abstinence.

Summary and Conclusions Behavioral therapies are effective for reducing the use of illicit drugs, including methamphetamine. Contingency management may be especially effective for retaining methamphetamine-dependent patients in treatment and initiating abstinence. The wealth of information available from the application of these strategies to the treatment of other forms of substance use disorders should allow clinical researchers and practitioners to further refine these techniques, efficiently implement them, and obtain maximal therapeutic benefit with methamphetamine-dependent patients.

Although contingency management procedures are effective for the management of substance use disorders in general and methamphetamine use disorders in particular, they are not without limitation. Cost, for example, is perhaps the most often-noted limitation associated with contingency management. In trials conducted with cocaine-dependent patients, those assigned to the contingency management condition can earn $1,000.00 to $2,000.00. For scientific purposes, patients assigned to the control condition often receive comparable payment, although the delivery of a voucher is not contingent on drug-free urine (e.g., Silverman et al., 1996). These costs may be prohibitive in many clinical situations. In response to this concern, investigators have developed prize-based incentive therapy, a low-cost permutation of contingency management (e.g., Petry et al., 2000). As described above, instead of receiving vouchers, when a patient provides a drug-free urine specimen he is allowed to draw a chip that may result in the presentation of a prize. In a seminal study, cocaine-dependent patients were randomly assigned to standard therapy or standard therapy plus prize-based incentives. Patients assigned to the standard therapy plus prize-based incentives drew a chip from a container with 250 chips each time they provided a cocaine- or opioid-free urine specimen. The prize-based incentive component was similar to the one described above (Petry et al., 2000). Patients assigned to standard therapy plus prize-based incentive therapy achieved significantly longer periods of continued abstinence. It is important to note that these patients earned an average of $137.00 worth of prizes. In the large trial described above designed to determine the efficacy of prize-based incentive therapy in stimulant abusers, patients assigned to the prize-based incentive condition earned $203.00 on average during the 12-week trial (Petry et al., 2005). In other words, in this trial, the cost was approximately $2.42 per day per patient. These findings indicate that a low-cost version of contingency management, prize-based incentive therapy, is economical and effective for initiating abstinence from stimulants.

Prize-based incentive therapy has raised concerns regarding increased gambling in patients assigned to this treatment condition. Prize-based incentive therapy involves an element of chance and substance use disorders are often comorbid with pathological gambling (e.g., Welte, Barnes, Wieczorek, Tidwell, & Parker, 2001). To address this concern, 803 stimulant users were randomly assigned to standard care (i.e., group counseling and twice weekly drug urine tests and breath samples) or standard care plus prize-based incentives (Petry et al., 2006). The prize-based incentives were similar to those described above (Petry et al., 2005). Patients were asked how many days they engaged in a gambling activity in the past month, including purchasing lottery tickets. The use of prize-based incentives did not negatively influence gambling behavior in that the frequency of gambling did not differ significantly across the treatment conditions.

Pharmacotherapies for Amphetamine Dependence

Although behavioral therapies in general, and contingency management procedures in particular, are effective for reducing methamphetamine use, improvement is still possible. As noted above, patients assigned to prize-based incentives plus treatment as usual or treatment as usual did not differ significantly in terms of treatment retention or counseling attendance at follow-up (i.e., 3 and 6 months; Roll et al., 2006). Considerable efforts have, therefore, been devoted to identifying a pharmacotherapy that might be used as an adjunct in the management of amphetamine dependence.

Identifying an effective pharmacotherapy for stimulant use disorders in general, and amphetamine dependence in particular, is an arduous process that requires the conduct of a multitude of controlled studies. Human laboratory studies are usually conducted initially to determine the safety and tolerability of a putative pharmacotherapy in combination with amphetamine. Safety and tolerability studies often include secondary outcome measures to determine whether the putative pharmacotherapy alters the behavioral effects of amphetamine (e.g., subjective effects). A putative pharmacotherapy that was well tolerated and altered at least some of the behavioral effects of amphetamine could then be tested in a clinical trial. Double-blind, placebo-controlled, randomized trials are the gold standard of clinical research. However, such trials are costly, time consuming, and labor intensive. Double-blind, placebo-controlled, randomized trials should be conducted only with the most promising medications for the management of amphetamine dependence.

Three approaches have been used to identify a putative pharmacotherapy for amphetamine dependence. The first approach focuses on identifying an "amphetamine antagonist." The premise of this approach is that patients treated with an antagonist would not experience the abuse-related effects of amphetamine (e.g., positive subjective effects such as euphoria). Drug-taking and drug-seeking behavior should then extinguish (for a review, see Gorelick, Gardner, & Xi, 2004). The second approach is agonist replacement therapy. As the name implies, a pharmacologically similar agent is substituted for amphetamine. The agonist replacement presumably would suppress withdrawal and produce tolerance to the reinforcing or positive subjective effects of amphetamine. Antagonist (i.e., mecamylamine and naltrexone) and agonist replacement (i.e., nicotine replacement products and methadone) therapies are effective for nicotine and opioid dependence, respectively (e.g., Ling, Rawson, & Compton, 1994; Rea, Bell, Young, & Mattick, 2004; Rose & Behm, 2004; Silagy, Lancaster, Stead, Mant, & Fowler, 2004). The third approach is to manage the symptoms of amphetamine withdrawal in an attempt to reduce the risk of relapse. Managing opioid withdrawal palliatively with clonidine and lofexidine has been shown to reduce the risk of relapse (Carnwath & Hardman, 1998).

Before reviewing the extant literature that tested these pharmacological strategies for the treatment of amphetamine dependence, a brief description of the neuropharmacology of amphetamines is provided as a reference for subsequent sections related to agonist and antagonist treatments. Abused stimulants produce their behavioral and physiological effects via interaction with monoamine transporters (dopamine [DA], serotonin [5-HT], and norepinephrine [NE]), although central dopamine systems are thought to play a prominent role in mediating the abuse-related effects of stimulants (reviewed in Johanson & Fischman, 1989; Seiden, Sabol, & Ricaurte, 1993). Based on in vitro studies, stimulants can be broadly categorized into two groups by their mechanism of action at these transporters. Cocaine and methylphenidate bind to monoamine transporters and prevent the reuptake of these monoamines into the presynaptic terminal, but are not themselves transported. Amphetamines, in contrast, act as substrates for monoamine transporters and are transported into the nerve terminal where they promote the release of monoamines into the synapse by preventing the accumulation of neurotransmitter in storage vesicles, and also by carrier-mediated exchange. Amphetamines also usually function as transporter blockers, although they are less potent at inhibiting reuptake compared to their ability to act as transporter substrates (Rothman et al., 2001).

Antagonist Therapy for Amphetamine Dependence

The neuropharmacology of amphetamines has prompted interest in compounds that directly or indirectly antagonize the effects of amphetamines on monoamine systems as putative pharmacotherapies. Compounds tested to date include atypical antipsychotics, γ-Aminobutyric-acid (GABA) agonists, opioid antagonists, and calcium channel blockers.

Atypical Antipsychotics Atypical antipsychotics are generally mixed DA/5-HT receptor antagonists and would be predicted to block the behavioral effects of amphetamine (e.g., Seeman, 2002). Risperidone (Risperdal®), for example, is a mixed D_2 and 5-HT_2 antagonist that is effective in the management of psychotic disorders (Grant & Fitton, 1994). Risperidone attenuates the behavioral effects of amphetamines under controlled laboratory conditions (Rush Stoops, Hays, Glaser, & Hays, 2003; Wachtel, Ortengren, & de Wit, 2002). However, the results of two double-blind, placebo-controlled clinical trials suggest risperidone is ineffective in the management of cocaine dependence (Grabowski et al., 2000; Grabowski, Shearer, Merrill, & Negus, 2004). In fact, risperidone may actually lower treatment retention (Grabowski et al., 2000). Risperidone-treated patients often mentioned side effects such as sedation, drowsiness, and fatigue as the reason for discontinuing their participation. These side effects were generally limited to the highest dose (8 mg/day).

Aripiprazole (Abilify®) is an atypical antipsychotic that is a partial agonist at D_2 receptors (Burris et al., 2002). Partial agonists are receptor ligands with high receptor affinity, but low intrinsic activity. Theoretically, these drugs would be expected to have the therapeutic advantages of both agonists and antagonists. Under conditions of low neurotransmitter activity, as is observed for DA and 5-HT during initial abstinence from chronic stimulant use (Parsons, Koob, & Weiss, 1995; Weiss, Markou, Lorang, & Koob, 1992), a partial agonist would produce some receptor stimulation and possibly function as an agonist replacement therapy. In contrast, a partial agonist would act as an antagonist when there are higher levels of neurotransmitter present in the synapse, as would occur following use of a stimulant during relapse. Aripiprazole also has significant affinity (<30 nM) for, and varying degrees of intrinsic efficacy at, the 5-HT_{1A}, 5-HT_{2A}, 5-HT_{2B}, and 5-HT_7 receptor subtypes (Shapiro et al., 2003).

Aripiprazole attenuates the behavioral effects of amphetamines under controlled laboratory conditions (reviewed in Stoops, 2006), however, a recently published double-blind, placebo-controlled trial failed to demonstrate efficacy of aripiprazole for the management of amphetamine dependence (Tiihonen et al., 2007). In this trial, amphetamine-dependent drug-injecting patients were randomly assigned to receive 15-mg/day aripiprazole ($N=19$) or placebo ($N=19$) for 20 weeks. The percentage of amphetamine-positive urine specimens was significantly higher in the aripiprazole-treated patients.

Although the results of this clinical trial were disappointing, several caveats warrant mentioning. First, the sample size was small. Second, only a single aripiprazole dose was tested.

Perhaps higher doses would reduce drug use. Alternatively, the dose tested may have produced unpleasant side effects and aripiprazole-treated patients continued to use amphetamine in an attempt to ameliorate them. In other words, perhaps lower doses would reduce drug use. Third, quantitative urine results were not obtained. Perhaps aripiprazole-treated patients significantly reduced daily drug use, but did not abstain completely. Considering these caveats along with the results of the human laboratory experiments, further research is needed to determine whether aripiprazole, or other dopamine and/or 5-HT receptor partial agonists, might be effective as adjuncts for amphetamine dependence.

GABA Agonists   Drugs that increase GABA activity, such as benzodiazepines which are $GABA_A$ positive modulators or γ-vinyl GABA, an irreversible GABA-transaminase inhibitor, are referred to here as GABA agonists for simplicity. Behavioral neuropharmacological studies suggest that central dopamine systems are under the inhibitory control of GABA systems. First, systemic injections of benzodiazepines (i.e., diazepam and midazolam) reduce the release of dopamine in the nucleus accumbens as measured by microdialysis (Finlay, Damsma, & Fibiger, 1992; Invernizzi, Pozzi, & Samanin, 1991). Second, lorazepam, another benzodiazepine, and γ-vinyl GABA, an irreversible GABA-transaminase inhibitor, attenuate stimulant-induced increases in dopamine levels in the striatum and nucleus accumbens (Dewey et al., 1997; Morgan & Dewey, 1998). Third, GABA agonists attenuate the effects of amphetamine under controlled laboratory conditions (e.g., Rush, Stoops, Wagner, Hays, & Glaser, 2004). Perhaps, then, GABA agonists may be useful as indirect antagonists in the management of amphetamine dependence.

We are aware of only a single double-blind, placebo-controlled trial in which GABA agonists were assessed for efficacy in the management of amphetamine dependence (Heinzerling et al., 2006). In this study, methamphetamine-dependent patients were randomly assigned to receive baclofen (20 mg TID; $N=25$), gabapentin (800 mg TID; $N=26$), or placebo ($N=37$) for 16 weeks. Baclofen is a $GABA_B$ receptor agonist that is used in the management of musculoskeletal disorders and gabapentin is an anticonvulsant that increases central GABA levels via the inhibition of GABA transaminase. Clinical assessments, drug urine testing, and psychosocial counseling were conducted thrice weekly. There were no statistically significant differences between the groups in terms of retention in treatment, medication adherence, clinic attendance, drug craving, or methamphetamine-negative urine samples. The effect of baclofen on methamphetamine-negative urine samples was, however, in the predicted direction (i.e., baclofen [50%] versus placebo [38%]). In an open label trial the efficacy of γ-vinyl GABA was determined for cocaine and methamphetamine dependence (Brodie, Figueroa, Laska, & Dewey, 2005). Participants were dependent on methamphetamine ($N=10$), cocaine ($N=3$), or both ($N=17$). The γ-vinyl GABA dose was titrated upward to a maintenance dose of 3 g/day. Eighteen of the participants completed the nine-week trial, 16 of whom tested negative for cocaine and methamphetamine during the final six weeks of the trial. These results suggest γ-vinyl GABA may be effective in the management of stimulant dependence, however, they must be viewed cautiously because of the use of an open-label design, which often produces false-positive results.

Nonetheless, as noted above, the effect of baclofen on methamphetamine-negative urine samples was in the predicted direction (i.e., baclofen > placebo). These results along with those observed with γ-vinyl GABA in an open-label trial suggest further research is needed to determine whether GABA agonists might be effective in the management of amphetamine dependence.

Opioid Antagonists	Neuroanatomical and neurochemical studies suggest that central dopamine and opioid systems interact. First, opioid receptors are found in the nucleus accumbens and ventral tegmental area (Finley, Maderdrut, & Petrusz, 1981; Khachaturian, Lewis, & Watson, 1983). Second, opioid agonists infused in the ventral tegmental area increase dopamine levels in the nucleus accumbens (Devine, Leone, & Wise, 1993; Spanagel, Herz, & Shippenberg, 1992). Third, naloxone, an opioid antagonist, attenuates amphetamine-induced increases in dopamine levels in both the nucleus accumbens and ventral tegmental area (Hooks, Jones, Justice, & Holtzman, 1992; Schad, Justice, & Holtzman, 1995). Fourth, opioid antagonists (e.g., naltrexone) attenuate the behavioral effects of amphetamine under controlled laboratory conditions (e.g., Jayaram-Lindstrom, Wennberg, Hurd, & Franck, 2004). These findings suggest that opioid antagonists may be useful in the management of amphetamine dependence.

We know of only a single open-label clinical trial in which the efficacy of naltrexone as a putative pharmacotherapy for amphetamine dependence was determined (Jayaram-Lindstrom, Wennberg, Beck, & Franck, 2005; Jayaram-Lindstrom et al., 2004). In this trial, 20 amphetamine-dependent patients were treated with naltrexone (50 mg/day) for 12 weeks (Jayaram-Lindstrom et al., 2005). Naltrexone was well tolerated by most patients. Amphetamine use (i.e., frequency and amount) and ratings of drug craving decreased significantly during treatment relative to baseline levels. Although these results suggest opioid antagonists may be effective in the management of amphetamine dependence, they must be viewed cautiously because of the use of an open-label design. Nonetheless, additional research is needed to determine whether opioid antagonists might be effective for treating amphetamine dependence.

Calcium Channel Blockers	As noted above, the dopamine-releasing effect of amphetamines is thought to play a prominent role in mediating their behavioral effects (Seiden et al., 1993). However, the influx of calcium through ion channels is necessary for the recruitment of dopamine-containing vesicles and their fusion with the synaptic membrane, which results in dopamine release into the synaptic cleft (Mills, Arsah, Ali, & Shockley, 1998). Perhaps, then, calcium-channel blockers might be effective in the management of amphetamine dependence. We know of only a single clinical trial in which the efficacy of a calcium-channel blocker was determined for amphetamine dependence. In this double-blind, placebo-controlled, randomized, eight-week trial, methamphetamine-dependent patients were maintained on 5-mg/day amlodipine ($N=26$), 10-mg/day amlodipine ($N=25$), or placebo ($N=26$; Batki et al., 2001). There were no significant between-group differences in terms of treatment retention, number of grams methamphetamine used, amount of money spent on methamphetamine, quality of methamphetamine-induced high or craving, or scores on the Addiction Severity Index. These findings are not surprising given that the results of human laboratory studies with calcium-channel blockers and amphetamine are mixed (e.g., Johnson, Roache, Bordnick, & Ait-Daoud, 1999; Johnson et al., 2005).

Agonist Therapy for Amphetamine Dependence

An alternative to the antagonist approach is agonist replacement therapy in which a pharmacologically similar agent is substituted for methamphetamine (reviewed in Grabowski et al., 2004; Shearer, Sherman, Wodak, & van Beek, 2002). Agonist replacement therapies are effective for nicotine and opioid dependence (e.g., Ling et al., 1994; Silagy et al., 2004), and the results of recent clinical trials suggest that a similar strategy may have utility for stimulant dependence (reviewed in Grabowski et al., 2004; Shearer et al., 2002).

d-Amphetamine   d-Amphetamine and methamphetamine are structurally related and produce a similar constellation of behavioral effects (e.g., Sevak et al., 2009; Seiden et al., 1993). We know of at least three published reports in which amphetamine-dependent patients treated with d-amphetamine were compared to untreated controls (Klee, Wright, Carnwath, & Merrill, 2001; McBride, Sullivan, Blewett, & Morgan, 1997; Shearer et al., 2001). The results of these studies are rather consistent in that amphetamine-treated patients improved to a greater extent than controls in terms of drug use, injecting behavior, dependence severity, and clinic attendance. In one study, for example, 63 amphetamine-dependent patients prescribed d-amphetamine (i.e., maximum 40 mg/day) were compared to 25 matched controls (McBride et al., 1997). There were statistically significant differences between the d-amphetamine-treated patients and controls in terms of illicit drug use and clinic attendance. Although encouraging, these findings need to be replicated using a double-blind, placebo-controlled design.

Methylphenidate   Methylphenidate is a prototypical stimulant that most notably inhibits dopamine reuptake, and produces amphetaminelike behavioral effects (Ritz, Lamb, Goldberg, & Kuhar, 1987; Sevak et al., 2009). A recently published double-blind, placebo-controlled clinical trial demonstrated that methylphenidate significantly reduces drug use in amphetamine-dependent patients (Tiihonen et al., 2007). In this trial, amphetamine-dependent patients who injected drugs were randomly assigned to receive 54 mg/day slow-release methylphenidate ($N = 17$) or placebo ($N = 19$) for 20 weeks. Methylphenidate-treated patients had significantly fewer amphetamine-positive urine specimens than placebo-treated patients. Although the sample size was small, these results suggest that agonist replacement therapy may be effective in treating amphetamine dependence.

Agonist replacement therapies may have some utility in treating amphetamine dependence, however, this strategy is controversial and may never gain widespread acceptance. Most notably, clinicians may be reluctant to use amphetamine derivatives to treat methamphetamine dependency because of their abuse potential. The viability of the agonist replacement approach for methamphetamine dependence may hinge on identifying novel agonist replacement therapies that have less abuse potential and are more acceptable to clinicians.

Bupropion   Bupropion is indicated for the treatment of depression and as a smoking cessation aid (e.g., Foley, Desanty, & Kast, 2006). Bupropion is a weak inhibitor of dopamine uptake that produces some stimulantlike behavioral effects (Foley et al., & Kast, 2006; Rush, Kollins, & Pazaglia, 1998). Note, however, that bupropion has less abuse potential than d-amphetamine or methylphenidate as measured by subjective ratings of drug liking (Rush et al., 1998). Bupropion also attenuates the behavioral effects of methamphetamine under controlled laboratory conditions (Newton et al., 2006). Bupropion, therefore, may be well suited as an agonist replacement therapy for methamphetamine dependence.

The results of a clinical trial further support the utility of bupropion for the management of methamphetamine dependence (Elkashef et al., 2006). In this double-blind trial, methamphetamine-dependent patients were randomly assigned to receive placebo ($N = 72$) or sustained-release bupropion (150 mg BID; $N = 79$). Clinical assessments, drug urine testing, and group therapy sessions were conducted thrice weekly. The drug urine tests were the primary outcome measure. The bupropion-treated patients provided fewer amphetamine-positive urine samples than the placebo-treated patients, although this effect did not attain significance according to traditional statistical standards ($p = 0.09$). Interestingly, secondary analyses revealed that relative to placebo, bupropion produced a statistically significant effect in patients that reported moderate drug use at intake. These data suggest that additional research is warranted to more fully determine the utility of bupropion as a putative pharmacotherapy for amphetamine dependence.

Managing Amphetamine Withdrawal

Amphetamine-dependent patients often experience withdrawal sequelae including dysphoric mood, fatigue, and changes in sleep (i.e., insomnia or hypersomnia; American Psychiatric Association, 2000 [DSM–IV–TR]) when drug use is discontinued. These symptoms are most severe during the first few days of abstinence, but may persist for longer periods (McGregor et al., 2005; Newton, Kalechstein, Duran, Vansluis, & Ling, 2004). Amelioration of these withdrawal symptoms might reduce the high rates of relapse observed in amphetamine-dependent patients (Tennant & Rawson, 1983).

Because dysphoric mood and depression are prominent symptoms of withdrawal that may contribute to relapse (Peck, Reback, Yang, Rotheram-Fuller, & Shoptaw, 2005), several antidepressants have been tested as putative pharmacotherapies for reducing amphetamine withdrawal and subsequent relapse. We know of three studies that explicitly examined the effects of an antidepressant on the severity of amphetamine withdrawal (Jittiwutikan, Srisurapanont, & Jarusuraisin, 1997; Kongsakon, Papadopoulos, & Saguansiritham, 2005; Srisurapanont, Jarusuraisin, & Jittiwutikan, 1999). Two randomized, double-blind, placebo-controlled trials evaluated amineptine, a dopamine agonist antidepressant, for the management of amphetamine withdrawal. In the first trial, amphetamine-dependent patients received 300-mg/day amineptine ($N = 15$) or placebo ($N = 15$) while hospitalized (Jittiwutikan et al., 1997). In the second study, amphetamine-dependent patients received 300-mg/day amineptine ($N = 21$) or placebo ($N = 22$) while hospitalized (Srisurapanont et al., 1999). The primary outcome measures were the Amphetamine Withdrawal Questionnaire (Srisurapanont et al., 1999), Questionnaire for Evaluating Cocaine Craving and Related Responses (Jittiwutikan et al., 1997), and Global Clinical Impression scale (Jittiwutikan et al., 1997; Srisurapanont et al., 1999). At the end of these two-week trials, amineptine-treated patients showed greater improvement on the Global Clinical Impression scale than their placebo-treated counterparts. Amineptine-treated patients also showed improvement on some aspects of the Questionnaire for Evaluating Cocaine Craving and Related Responses (e.g., sick feeling) relative to placebo-treated patients (Jittiwutikan et al., 1997). However, amineptine-treated patients did not differ from their placebo-treated counterparts on the Amphetamine Withdrawal Questionnaire (Srisurapanont et al., 1999). In the third trial, amphetamine-dependent patients received 15–30 mg mirtazapine ($N=9$), a 5-HT$_2$, 5-HT$_3$ serotonergic and α_2 noradrenergic antagonist, or placebo ($N=11$) for 14 days (Kongsakon et al., 2005). The primary outcome measures were the Amphetamine Withdrawal Questionnaire and the Montgomery and Åsberg Depression scale. Across the 14-day period, mirtazapine-treated patients improved significantly more than their placebo-treated counterparts as measured by total scores on the Amphetamine Withdrawal Questionnaire, but not the Montgomery and Åsberg Depression scale.

In addition to these studies that explicitly examined amphetamine withdrawal, we are aware of four double-blind, placebo-controlled trials in which an antidepressant was tested for efficacy, as measured by drug urine tests, in the management of amphetamine dependence (Galloway, Newmeyer, Knapp, Stalcup, & Smith, 1994, 1996; Piasecki, Steinagel, Thienhaus, & Kohlenberg, 2002; Shoptaw et al., 2006). In the first trial, 183 stimulant-dependent outpatients (i.e., cocaine [$N=151$]; methamphetamine [$N=32$]) were randomly assigned to receive 10 or 150 mg/day imipramine for 180 days (Galloway et al., 1994). In the second trial, methamphetamine-dependent outpatients were randomly assigned to receive either 10 ($N=10$) or 150 mg/day ($N=22$) imipramine for 180 days (Galloway et al., 1996). The low dose of imipramine was considered the control condition in these trials. In the third trial, 20 methamphetamine-dependent outpatients were randomly assigned to receive placebo or 20 mg/day paroxetine for at least five weeks (Piasecki et al., 2002). In the fourth trial, methamphetamine-dependent outpatients were randomly assigned to receive placebo ($N=55$) or 100 mg/day ($N=59$) sertraline for 12 weeks (Shoptaw et al., 2006). Imipramine, paroxetine, and sertraline inhibit the reuptake of serotonin and norepinephrine. These compounds were ineffective as measured by percent of drug-free urine samples. Neither imipramine nor sertraline significantly improved depressive symptoms as measured by the Beck Depression Inventory (Galloway et al., 1994, 1996; Shoptaw et al., 2006).

Finally, the effects of lisuride, a dopamine receptor agonist, on amphetamine withdrawal were determined in a single trial (Gillin, Pulvirenti, Withers, Golshan, & Koob, 1994). In this double-blind trial, hospitalized cocaine- or amphetamine-dependent patients received lisuride (4 mg/day, $N=10$) or placebo ($N=11$) for three weeks. The outcome measures included the Hamilton Rating Scale for Depression, Beck Depression Inventory, Profile of Mood States, Brief Psychiatric Rating Scale, and Craving Scale. Although all patients improved on these measures as a function of time, the lisuride- and placebo-treated patients did not improve differentially.

Summary and Conclusions

Direct and indirect dopamine antagonists from diverse pharmacological classes including atypical antipsychotics, GABA agonists, opioid antagonists, and calcium channel blockers, have been tested as putative pharmacotherapies for amphetamine dependence. These compounds have not demonstrated robust efficacy in double-blind, placebo-controlled clinical trials. The extant literature that tested direct and indirect dopamine antagonists for the treatment of amphetamine is reminiscent of the results of studies that employed a similar strategy for the management of cocaine dependence. Several direct and indirect dopamine antagonists from diverse pharmacological classes have been tested to determine their utility in the management of cocaine dependence, however, none has demonstrated robust efficacy (e.g., de Lima et al., 2002; Grabowski et al., 2004 for reviews). Research is needed to determine whether the antagonist approach may be effective in a subset of amphetamine-dependent patients (i.e., highly motivated patients).

Because dysphoric mood and depression are prominent symptoms of amphetamine withdrawal, several antidepressants have been tested as putative pharmacotherapies for reducing relapse. Although some of the compounds tested showed efficacy at reducing withdrawal symptoms in controlled environments (i.e., hospitals), none were effective in outpatient clinical trials that used percent of drug-free urine samples as the primary outcome measure. Interestingly, in many of the controlled studies and clinical trials, the medication under investigation did not significantly ameliorate the depressive symptoms as measured by the standardized clinical instruments (e.g., Beck Depression Inventory). The most parsimonious explanation for this observation is that insufficient doses were tested. Future studies are needed to determine if higher antidepressant doses might ameliorate the depressive symptoms experienced during amphetamine withdrawal, thereby reducing relapse as measured by drug-free urine samples.

The evidence-based literature suggests that agonist replacement therapy may be an effective strategy for the management of methamphetamine dependence. *d*-Amphetamine, methylphenidate, and bupropion have shown some efficacy in initial trials. Additional research, including clinical trials, is clearly needed to further determine the efficacy of agonist replacement therapies for the management of methamphetamine dependence. Most notably, additional research is needed to determine the efficacy of other novel agonist replacement therapies in the management of methamphetamine dependence. Modafinil (Provigil®), for example, is a novel stimulant indicated in the treatment of narcolepsy or excessive daytime sleepiness (e.g., Moldofsky, Broughton, & Hill, 2000). The behavioral effects of modafinil overlap to some extent with those of prototypical stimulants, but it has less abuse potential (e.g., Rush, Kelly, Hays, & Baker, & Wooten, 2002; Rush, Kelly, Hays, & Wooten, 2002). The results of a human laboratory experiment and a clinical trial suggest that modafinil is effective in managing cocaine dependence (Dackis et al., 2003, 2005). Modafinil might also be effective in the management of amphetamine-use disorders.

Finally, the availability of compounds (i.e., methylphenidate) that are clinically effective for reducing amphetamine use will now allow investigators to validate human laboratory models for screening putative pharmacotherapies. As noted above, double-blind, placebo-controlled trials, although the gold standard of clinical research, are costly, time consuming, and labor intensive. Identifying valid human laboratory models through a "reverse engineering" strategy will allow putative pharmacotherapies to be screened more rapidly and efficiently.

Case Presentation

Dave is a 23-year-old former methamphetamine (meth) user and cooker. Dave began using drugs at an early age, perhaps 15 or 16. He hung around with an older crowd (all approximately 15 years older than him) that he knew through an older brother. Meth was the first illicit drug Dave used, and it soon became his drug of choice. He had experiences with many other drugs, including marijuana, Ecstasy, cocaine, and heroin, but he always came back to meth. He described the high as ten times better than the best sex he ever had and would stay up for days at a time bingeing and cooking meth.

Dave started to cook meth shortly after he began to use it. Dave tried to cook meth unsuccessfully a couple of times before finally watching someone do it. After this lesson, he could cook meth anywhere. He described the process as a beautiful chemical reaction and noted the sky-blue color of the substrate. Cooking meth is dangerous: Dave has had anhydrous ammonia tanks blow holes in barns while he was cooking. He has also been shot at while trying to steal this ingredient but stealing anhydrous gave him a big rush, so he didn't mind the danger. While Dave was actively cooking, he maintained a job. Because of this he could use a lot of the meth he made, but still managed to be able to sell it, which he also saw as an addiction. He would also trade meth for sex and saw this as fair trade; women were only having sex with him for drugs, but he was only giving them drugs for sex. When Dave was cooking he would sell to anyone who wanted to buy, including friends, police officers, and affluent citizens. He did not care who he sold to; he described incidents in which parents could not afford coats for their children because they were buying meth from him. People still come to his girlfriend's house looking to buy, and he has to run them off. Dave would take meth via multiple routes of administration, but his primary method was smoking. He reported injecting it once, but feeling like he was going to die, so he never used that route again.

According to Dave, smoking meth "geeks" out the user and makes one extremely paranoid. Dave detailed another incident about meth use that nearly ended his life. One night, after being up for an extended period, he thought he saw someone in the woods. Taking a gun with him to investigate, he headed to check it out. Back at the house he had been in, a friend saw him and shot him in the back, not knowing who he was at the far distance. While actively cooking the drug, Dave invested in a camera surveillance system. He would stare at the camera screens for hours and look for any signs of trouble; usually anything he saw was a figment of his imagination. None of these incidents deterred Dave from using meth. It finally took the possibility of 20 years in jail for him to stop. He curtailed his use and manufacture of meth, but would still sell the drug. However, he would only meet people outside his home and would only sell to people who were alone. This was done in an effort to eliminate any temptation he had to use the drug. While he was using, Dave owned a house with his brother. After being arrested, he rented the house to an acquaintance. Unbeknownst to him, this man was letting meth cookers manufacture drugs in the house. Apparently, this was quite an extensive operation. The cookers would move in at midnight each night and clear out by seven each morning, just in time for Dave's daily eight o'clock inspection.

Dave no longer sells meth and avoids his friends who actively use and who do not respect that he is in recovery (i.e., friends who would use meth around him). He still experiences intense cravings and has vivid dreams about using meth. Even though his behavioral adaptations and the threat of jail have helped him to stop using, he expressed the desire for a medication to help him maintain his sobriety. He described how he will wake after such a vivid dream and be uncertain whether he had actually used or not. During our conversation, Dave mentioned several times that his heart was racing just talking about these things.

Dave's interview provided evidence of his methamphetamine dependence including spending a great deal of time to procure methamphetamine, continuing to use despite recurrent problems, and taking the substance over a prolonged period of time. Even though Dave is currently clean, it is apparent that he struggles every day to remain so.

Future Directions

The evidence-based literature suggests that contingency management and agonist replacement therapies may be effective strategies for treating methamphetamine dependence. Perhaps the most obvious extension of this work is to determine if combining these strategies produces unique clinical benefit. The results of two clinical trials with cocaine-dependent patients suggest that combining contingency management and a pharmacotherapy is more effective than either of the constituent strategies alone (Kosten et al., 2003; Poling et al., 2006). In the more recent trial, for example, cocaine-dependent patients were randomly assigned to one of four conditions: (1) contingency management plus placebo (N=25); (2) contingency management plus 300 mg/day bupropion (N=27); (3) voucher control plus placebo (N=24); or (4) voucher control plus 300 mg/day bupropion (N=30; Poling et al., 2006). Patients assigned to the contingency management group received a $3.00 voucher for their first drug-free urine (cocaine or opioids). The value of the voucher increased by $1.00 for each subsequent drug-free urine specimen to a maximum of $15.00. Patients assigned to a voucher control group received a $3.00 voucher for each urine specimen, regardless of the results. These patients also received $1.00 if they provided three samples in a week. Patients assigned to voucher-based reinforcement therapy plus 300 mg/day bupropion reduced their cocaine use during the 25-week trial relative to the third week. This effect was most evident during weeks 3–13, but was discernible for weeks 14–25. Cocaine use increased during weeks 3–13 in patients assigned to contingency management plus placebo, but then decreased during weeks 14–25. Patients assigned to the voucher control groups did not show improvement by the end of the trial.

These findings are especially provocative because, as reviewed above, bupropion-treated patients provided fewer amphetamine-positive urine samples than the placebo-treated patients, although this effect did not attain significance according to traditional statistical standards (Elkashef et al., 2006). Future studies are clearly needed to determine if combining contingency management and bupropion might significantly reduce drug use in methamphetamine-dependent patients.

Contingency management may also be useful for increasing compliance with pharmacological treatments. Although several direct and indirect dopamine antagonists from diverse pharmacological classes have been tested to determine their utility in the management of methamphetamine or cocaine dependence, none has demonstrated efficacy (e.g., de Lima et al., 2002; Grabowski et al., 2004 for reviews). Poor compliance is a limitation of antagonist therapy (Grabowski et al., 2004). Contingency management has been used to increase compliance with the dosing regimen with antagonists (i.e., naltrexone) for other forms of substance abuse disorders (i.e., opioids; Preston et al., 1999). In this study, opioid-dependent patients were randomly assigned to one of three groups: contingency management (i.e., vouchers contingent on ingesting scheduled naltrexone doses, N = 19); noncontingent (i.e., vouchers delivered on an unpredictable schedule independent of ingesting scheduled naltrexone doses, $N=19$); and no voucher ($N=20$). Patients in the contingency management group were retained in treatment longer and ingested more naltrexone doses than either of the other groups. Whether similar results might be observed with putative antagonists for methamphetamine is unknown.

In conclusion, the evidence-based literature suggests that contingency management and agonist replacement therapies may be effective strategies for treating methamphetamine dependence. Contingency management may be especially effective for retaining methamphetamine-dependent patients in treatment and promoting abstinence. d-Amphetamine, methylphenidate, and bupropion have shown some efficacy in initial trials. The wealth of information available from the application of these strategies to cocaine dependence should allow clinical researchers and practitioners to further refine these techniques, efficiently implement them for managing methamphetamine dependence, and achieve maximal clinical benefit.

References

American Psychiatric Association. (2000). *Diagnostic and statistical manual of mental disorders* (4th ed., text revision). Washington, DC: Author.

Batki, S. L., Moon, J., Delucchi, K., Hersch, D., Bradley, M., Aguillon-Doms, C., et al. (2001). Amlodipine treatment of methamphetamine dependence, a controlled outpatient trial: Preliminary Analysis. *Drug and Alcohol Dependence, 63*, S12.

Boudin, H. M. (1972). Contingency contracting as a therapeutic tool in the deceleration of amphetamine use. *Behavior Therapy, 3*, 604–608.

Brodie, J. D., Figueroa, E., Laska, E. M., & Dewey, S. L. (2005). Safety and efficacy of gamma-vinyl GABA (GVG) for the treatment of methamphetamine and/or cocaine addiction. *Synapse, 55*, 122–125.

Burris, K. D., Molski, T. F., Xu, C., Ryan, E., Tottori, K., Kikuchi, T., et al. (2002). Aripiprazole, a novel antipsychotic, is a high-affinity partial agonist at human dopamine D2 receptors. *Journal of Pharmacology and Experimental Therapeutics, 302*, 381–389.

Carnwath, T., & Hardman, J. (1998). Randomised double-blind comparison of lofexidine and clonidine in the out-patient treatment of opiate withdrawal. *Drug and Alcohol Dependence, 50*, 251–254.

Carroll, K. M. (2005). Recent advances in the psychotherapy of addictive disorders. *Current Psychiatry Reports, 7*, 329–336.

Carroll, K. M., & Onken, L. S. (2005). Behavioral therapies for drug abuse. *American Journal of Psychiatry, 162*, 1452–1460.

Castro, G. F., Barrington, E. H., Walton, M. A., & Rawson, R. A. (2000). Cocaine and methamphetamine: Differential addiction rates. *Psychology of Addictive Behaviors, 14*, 390–396.

Charukamnoetkanok, P., & Wagoner, M. D. (2004). Facial and ocular injuries associated with methamphetamine production accidents. *American Journal of Ophthalmology, 138*, 875–876.

Dackis, C. A., Kampman, K. M., Lynch, K. G., Pettinati, H. M., & O'Brien, C. P. (2005). A double-blind, placebo-controlled trial of modafinil for cocaine dependence. *Neuropsychopharmacology, 30*, 205–211.

Dackis, C. A., Lynch, K. G., Yu, E., Samaha, F. F., Kampman, K. M., Cornish, J. W., et al. (2003). Modafinil and cocaine: A double-blind, placebo-controlled drug interaction study. *Drug and Alcohol Dependence, 70*, 29–37.

de Lima, M. S., de Oliveira Soares, B. G., Reisser, A. A., & Farrell, M. (2002). Pharmacological treatment of cocaine dependence: A systematic review. *Addiction, 97*, 931–949.

Devine, D. P., Leone, P., & Wise, R. A. (1993). Mesolimbic dopamine neurotransmission is increased by administration of mu-opioid receptor antagonists. *European Journal of Pharmacology, 243*, 55–64.

Dewey, S. L., Chaurasia, C. S., Chen, C. E., Volkow, N. D., Clarkson, F. A., Porter, S. P., et al. (1997). GABAergic attenuation of cocaine-induced dopamine release and locomotor activity. *Synapse, 25,* 393–398.

Drug and Alcohol Services Information System (2004). *The DASIS Report: Primary methamphetamine/amphetamine treatment admissions increase: 1992–2002.* Office of Applied Studies. Retrieved January, 12, 2007, from http://www.oas.samhsa.gov/2k4/methTX/methTX.htm.

Drug and Alcohol Services Information System (2006). *The DASIS Report: Methamphetamine/amphetamine treatment admissions in urban and rural areas: 2004.* Office of Applied Studies. Retrieved January, 12, 2007, from http://www.oas.samhsa.gov/2k6/methRuralTX/methRuralTX.htm.

Elkashef, A. M., Rawson, R. A., Smith, E., Anderson, A., Kahn, R., Pierce, V., et al. (2006). *Bupropion for the treatment of methamphetamine dependence.* Paper presented at the annual meeting of the College on Problems of Drug Dependence, Scottsdale, AZ.

Finley, J. C., Maderdrut, J. L., & Petrusz, P. (1981). The immunocytochemical localization of enkephalin in the central nervous system of the rat. *Journal of Comparative Neurology, 198,* 541–565.

Finlay, J. M., Damsma, G., & Fibiger, H. C. (1992). Benzodiazepine-induced decreases in extracellular concentrations of dopamine in the nucleus accumbens after acute and repeated administration. *Psychopharmacology (Berl), 106,* 202–208.

First, M.B., Spitzer, R.L., Gibbon, M., & Williams, J.B. (1996). *Structured Clinical Interview for DSM–IV, Axis I Disordersó Patient Edition (SCID-I/P, Version 2.0).* New York: Biometrics Research Department, New York State Psychiatric Institute.

Foley, K. F., DeSanty, K. P., & Kast, R. E. (2006). Bupropion: Pharmacology and therapeutic applications. *Expert Review of Neurotherapeutics, 6,* 1249–1265.

Galloway, G. P., Newmeyer, J., Knapp, T., Stalcup, S. A., & Smith, D. (1994). Imipramine for the treatment of cocaine and methamphetamine dependence. *Journal of Addictive Diseases 13,* 201–216.

Galloway, G. P., Newmeyer, J., Knapp, T., Stalcup, S. A., & Smith, D. (1996). A controlled trial of imipramine for the treatment of methamphetamine dependence. *Journal of Substance Abuse Treatment, 13,* 493–497.

Gillin, J. C., Pulvirenti, L., Withers, N., Golshan, S., & Koob, G. (1994). The effects of lisuride on mood and sleep during acute withdrawal in stimulant abusers: A preliminary report. *Biological Psychiatry, 35,* 843–849.

Gorelick, D. A., Gardner, E. L., & Xi, Z. X. (2004). Agents in development for the management of cocaine abuse. *Drugs, 64,* 1547–1573.

Grabowski, J., Rhoades, H., Silverman, P., Schmitz, J. M., Stotts, A., Creson, D., et al. (2000). Risperidone for the treatment of cocaine dependence: Randomized, double-blind trial. *Journal of Clinical Psychopharmacology, 20,* 305–310.

Grabowski, J., Shearer, J., Merrill, J., & Negus, S. S. (2004). Agonist-like, replacement pharmacotherapy for stimulant abuse and dependence. *Addictive Behaviors, 29,* 1439–1464.

Grant, S., & Fitton, A. (1994). Risperidone. A review of its pharmacology and therapeutic potential in the treatment of schizophrenia. *Drugs, 48,* 253–273.

Hando, J., Topp, L., & Hall, W. (1997). Amphetamine-related harms and treatment preferences of regular amphetamine users in Sydney, Australia. *Drug and Alcohol Dependence, 46,* 105–113.

Heinzerling, K. G., Shoptaw, S., Peck, J. A., Yang, X., Liu, J., Roll, J., et al. (2006). Randomized, placebo-controlled trial of baclofen and gabapentin for the treatment of methamphetamine dependence. *Drug and Alcohol Dependence, 85,* 177–184.

Higgins, S. T. (2006). Extending contingency management to the treatment of methamphetamine use disorders. *American Journal of Psychiatry, 163,* 1870–1872.

Higgins, S. T., Delaney, D. D., Budney, A. J., Bickel, W. K., Hughes, J. R., Foerg, F., et al. (1991). A behavioral approach to achieving initial cocaine abstinence. *American Journal of Psychiatry, 148,* 1218–1224.

Higgins, S. T, Heil, S. H., Dantona, R., Donham, R., Matthews, M., & Badger, G. J. (2007). Effects of varying the monetary value of voucher-based incentives on abstinence achieved during and following treatment among cocaine-dependent outpatients. *Addiction, 102,* 271–281.

Higgins, S. T., Heil, S. H., & Lussier, J. P. (2004). Clinical implications of reinforcement as a determinant of substance use disorders. *Annual Review of Psychology, 55,* 431–461.

Hooks, M. S., Jones, D. N., Justice, J. B., Jr., & Holtzman, S. G. (1992). Naloxone reduces amphetamine-induced stimulation of locomotor activity and in vivo dopamine release in the striatum and nucleus accumbens. *Pharmacology Biochemistry and Behavior, 42,* 765–770.

Invernizzi, R., Pozzi, L., & Samanin, R. (1991). Release of dopamine is reduced by diazepam more in the nucleus accumbens than in the caudate nucleus of conscious rats. *Neuropharmacology, 30,* 575–578.

Jayaram-Lindstrom, N., Wennberg, P., Beck, O., & Franck, J. (2005). An open clinical trial of naltrexone for amphetamine dependence: Compliance and tolerability. *Nordic Journal of Psychiatry, 59,* 167–171.

Jayaram-Lindstrom, N., Wennberg, P., Hurd, Y. L., & Franck, J. (2004). Effects of naltrexone on the subjective response to amphetamine in healthy volunteers. *Journal of Clinical Psychopharmacology, 24,* 665–669.

Jittiwutikan, J., Srisurapanont, M., & Jarusuraisin, N. (1997). Amineptine in the treatment of amphetamine withdrawal: A placebo-controlled, randomised, double-blind study. *Journal of the Medical Association of Thailand, 80,* 587–592.

Johanson, C. E., & Fischman, M. W. (1989). The pharmacology of cocaine related to its abuse. *Pharmacological Reviews, 41,* 3–52.

Johnson, B. A., Roache, J. D., Ait-Daoud, N., Wallace, C., Wells, L., Dawes, M., et al. (2005). Effects of isradipine, a dihydropyridine-class calcium-channel antagonist, on d-methamphetamine's subjective and reinforcing effects. *International Journal of Neuropsychopharmacology, 8,* 203–213.

Johnson, B. A., Roache, J. D., Bordnick, P. S., & Ait-Daoud, N. (1999). Isradipine, a dihydropyridine-class calcium channel antagonist, attenuates some of d-methamphetamine's positive subjective effects: A preliminary study. *Psychopharmacology (Berl), 144,* 295–300.

Khachaturian, H., Lewis, M. E., & Watson, S. J. (1983). Enkephalin systems in diencephalon and brainstem of the rat. *Journal of Comparative Neurology, 220,* 310–320.

Klee, H., Wright, S., Carnwath, T., & Merrill, J. (2001). The role of substitute therapy in the treatment of problem amphetamine use. *Drug and Alcohol Review, 20,* 417–429.

Kongsakon, R., Papadopoulos, K. I., & Saguansiritham, R. (2005). Mirtazapine in amphetamine detoxification: A placebo-controlled pilot study. *International Clinical Psychopharmacology, 20,* 253–256.

Kosten, T., Oliveto, A., Feingold, A., Poling, J., Sevarino, K., McCance-Katz, E., et al. (2003). Desipramine and contingency management for cocaine and opiate dependence in buprenorphine maintained patients. *Drug and Alcohol Dependence, 70,* 315–325.

Ling, W., Rawson, R. A., & Compton, M. A. (1994). Substitution pharmacotherapies for opioid addiction: From methadone to LAAM and buprenorphine. *Journal of Psychoactive Drugs, 26,* 119–128.

Lussier, J. P., Heil, S. H., Mongeon, J. A., Badger, G. J., & Higgins, S. T. (2006). A meta-analysis of voucher-based reinforcement therapy for substance use disorders. *Addiction, 101,* 192–203.

McBride, A. J., Sullivan, G., Blewett, A. E., & Morgan, S. (1997). Amphetamine prescribing as a harm reduction measure: A preliminary study. *Addiction Research, 5,* 95–112.

McGregor, C., Srisurapanont, M., Jittiwutikarn, J., Laobhripatr, S., Wongtan, T., & White, J. M. (2005). The nature, time course and severity of methamphetamine withdrawal. *Addiction, 100,* 1320–1329.

Mills, K., Arsah, T. A., Ali, S. F., & Shockley, D. C. (1998). Calcium channel antagonist isradipine attenuates cocaine-induced motor activity in rats: correlation with brain monoamine levels. *Annals of the New York Academy of Sciences, 844,* 201–207.

Moldofsky, H., Broughton, R. J., & Hill, J. D. (2000). A randomized trial of the long-term, continued efficacy and safety of modafinil in narcolepsy. *Sleep Medicine Reviews, 1,* 109–116.

Morgan, A. E., & Dewey, S. L. (1998). Effects of pharmacologic increases in brain GABA levels on cocaine-induced changes in extracellular dopamine. *Synapse, 28,* 60–65.

National Drug Intelligence Center (2006). *National drug threat assessement 2007.* U.S. Department of Justice. Retrieved January, 12, 2007, from http://www.usdoj.gov/ndic/pubs21/21137/index.htm.

National Survey on Drug Use and Health (2006). *Results from the 2005 National Survey on Drug Use and Health: National findings.* Office of Applied Studies. Retrieved January, 12, 2007, from http://www.oas.samhsa.gov/NSDUH/2k5NSDUH/2k5results.htm.

Newton, T. F., Kalechstein, A. D., Duran, S., Vansluis, N., & Ling, W. (2004). Methamphetamine abstinence syndrome: Preliminary findings. *American Journal of Addiction, 13*, 248–255.

Newton, T. F., Roache, J. D., De La Garza, R., 2nd, Fong, T., Wallace, C. L., Li S. H., et al. (2006). Bupropion reduces methamphetamine-induced subjective effects and cue-induced craving. *Neuropsychopharmacology, 31*, 1537–1544.

Parsons, L. H., Koob, G. F., & Weiss, F. (1995). Serotonin dysfunction in the nucleus accumbens of rats during withdrawal after unlimited access to intravenous cocaine. *Journal of Pharmacological and Experimental Therapeutics, 274*, 1182–1191.

Peck, J. A., Reback, C. J., Yang, X., Rotheram-Fuller, E., & Shoptaw, S. (2005). Sustained reductions in drug use and depression symptoms from treatment for drug abuse in methamphetamine-dependent gay and bisexual men. *Journal of Urban Health, 82*, 1100–1108.

Petry, N. M., Kolodner, K. B., Li, R., Peirce, J. M., Roll, J. M., Stitzer, M. L., et al. (2006). Prize-based contingency management does not increase gambling. *Drug and Alcohol Dependence, 83*, 269–273.

Petry, N. M., Martin, B., Cooney, J. L., & Kranzler, H. R. (2000). Give them prizes, and they will come: Contingency management for treatment of alcohol dependence. *Journal of Consulting and Clinical Psychology, 68*, 250–257.

Petry, N. M., Peirce, J. M., Stitzer, M. L., Blaine, J., Roll, J. M., Cohen, A., et al. (2005). Effect of prize-based incentives on outcomes in stimulant abusers in outpatient psychosocial treatment programs: A national drug abuse treatment clinical trials network study. *Archives of General Psychiatry, 62*, 1148–1156.

Piasecki, M. P., Steinagel, G. M., Thienhaus, O. J., & Kohlenberg, B. S. (2002). An exploratory study: The use of paroxetine for methamphetamine craving. *Journal of Psychoactive Drugs, 34*, 301–304.

Poling, J., Oliveto, A., Petry, N., Sofuoglu, M., Gonsai, K., Gonzalez, G., et al. (2006). Six-month trial of bupropion with contingency management for cocaine dependence in a methadone-maintained population. *Archives of General Psychiatry, 63*, 219–228.

Prendergast, M., Podus, D., Finney, J., Greenwell, L., & Roll, J. (2006). Contingency management for treatment of substance use disorders: A meta-analysis. *Addiction, 101*, 1546–1560.

Preston, K. L., Silverman, K., Umbricht, A., DeJesus, A., Montoya, I. D., & Schuster, C. R. (1999). Improvement in naltrexone treatment compliance with contingency management. *Drug and Alcohol Dependence, 54*, 127–135.

Rawson, R. A., Anglin, M. D., & Ling, W. (2002). Will the methamphetamine problem go away? *Journal of Addictive Diseases, 21*, 61–74.

Rawson, R. A., Marinelli-Casey, P., Anglin, M. D., Dickow, A., Frazier, Y., Gallagher, C., et al. (2004). A multi-site comparison of psychosocial approaches for the treatment of methamphetamine dependence. *Addiction, 99*, 708–717.

Rea, F., Bell, J. R., Young, M. R., & Mattick, R. P. (2004). A randomised, controlled trial of low dose naltrexone for the treatment of opioid dependence. *Drug and Alcohol Dependence, 75*, 79–88.

Richards, J. R., Bretz, S. W., Johnson, E. B., Turnipseed, S. D., Brofeldt, B. T., Derlet, R. W. (1999). Methamphetamine abuse and emergency department utilization. *Western Journal of Medicine, 170*, 198–202.

Ritz, M. C., Lamb, R. J., Goldberg, S. R., & Kuhar, M. J. (1987). Cocaine receptors on dopamine transporters are related to self-administration of cocaine. *Science, 237*, 1219–1223.

Roll, J. M., & Higgins, S. T. (2000). A within-subject comparison of three different schedules of reinforcement of drug abstinence using cigarette smoking as an exemplar. *Drug and Alcohol Dependence, 58*, 103–109.

Roll, J. M., Higgins, S. T., & Badger, G. J. (1996). An experimental comparison of three different schedules of reinforcement of drug abstinence using cigarette smoking as an exemplar. *Journal of Applied Behavior Analysis, 29*, 495–505.

Roll, J. M., Petry, N. M., Stitzer, M. L., Brecht, M. L., Peirce, J. M., McCann, M. J., et al. (2006). Contingency management for the treatment of methamphetamine use disorders. *American Journal of Psychiatry, 163*, 1993–1999.

Roll, J. M., & Shoptaw, S. (2006). Contingency management: Schedule effects. *Psychiatry Research, 144*, 91–93.

Rose, J. E., & Behm, F. M. (2004). Extinguishing the rewarding value of smoke cues: Pharmacological and behavioral treatments. *Nicotine and Tobacco Research,* 6, 523–532.

Rothman, R. B., Baumann, M. H., Dersch, C. M., Romero, D. V., Rice, K. C., Carroll, F. I., et al. (2001). Amphetamine-type central nervous system stimulants release norepinephrine more potently than they release dopamine and serotonin. *Synapse, 39,* 32–41.

Rush, C. R., Kelly, T. H., Hays, L. R., Baker, R. W., & Wooten, A. F. (2002). Acute behavioral and physiological effects of modafinil in drug abusers. *Behavioural Pharmacology, 13,* 105–115.

Rush, C. R., Kelly, T. H., Hays, L. R., & Wooten, A. F. (2002). Discriminative-stimulus effects of modafinil in cocaine-trained humans. *Drug and Alcohol Dependence, 67,* 311–322.

Rush, C. R., Kollins, S. H., & Pazzaglia, P. J. (1998). Discriminative-stimulus and participant-rated effects of methylphenidate, bupropion, and triazolam in d-amphetamine-trained humans. *Experimental Clinical Psychopharmacology, 6,* 32–44.

Rush, C. R., Stoops, W. W., Hays, L. R., Glaser, P. E., & Hays, L. S. (2003). Risperidone attenuates the discriminative-stimulus effects of d-amphetamine in humans. *Journal of Pharmacology and Experimental Therapeutics, 306,* 195–204.

Rush, C. R., Stoops, W. W., Wagner, F. P., Hays, L. R., & Glaser, P. E. (2004). Alprazolam attenuates the behavioral effects of d-amphetamine in humans. *Journal of Clinical Psychopharmacology, 24,* 410–420.

Schad, C. A., Justice, J. B., Jr., & Holtzman, S. G. (1995). Naloxone reduces the neurochemical and behavioral effects of amphetamine but not those of cocaine. *European Journal of Pharmacology, 275,* 9–16.

Seeman, P. (2002). Atypical antipsychotics: Mechanism of action. *Canadian Journal of Psychiatry, 47,* 27–38.

Seiden, L. S., Sabol, K. E., & Ricaurte, G. A. (1993). Amphetamine: Effects on catecholamine systems and behavior. *Annual Review of Pharmacology and Toxicology, 33,* 639–677.

Sevak, R. J., Stoops, W. W., Hays, L. R., & Rush, C. R. (2009). Discriminative stimulus and subject-rated effects of methamphetamine, d-amphetamine, methylphenidate, and triazolam in methamphetamine-trained humans. *Journal of Pharmacology and Experimental Therapeutics, 328,* 1007–1018.

Shapiro, D. A., Renock, S., Arrington, E., Chiodo, L. A., Liu, L. X., Sibley, D. R., et al. (2003). Aripiprazole, a novel atypical antipsychotic drug with a unique and robust pharmacology. *Neuropsychopharmacology, 28,* 1400–1411.

Shearer, J., Sherman, J., Wodak, A., & van Beek, I. (2002). Substitution therapy for amphetamine users. *Drug and Alcohol Review, 21,* 179–185.

Shearer, J., Wodak, A., Mattick, R. P., van Beek, I., Lewis, J., Hall, W., et al. (2001). Pilot randomized controlled study of dexamphetamine substitution for amphetamine dependence. *Addiction, 96,* 1289–1296.

Shoptaw, S., Huber, A., Peck, J., Yang, X., Liu, J., Jeff, D., et al. (2006). Randomized, placebo-controlled trial of sertraline and contingency management for the treatment of methamphetamine dependence. *Drug and Alcohol Dependence, 85,* 12–18.

Shoptaw, S., Reback, C. J., Peck, J. A., Yang, X., Rotheram-Fuller, E., Larkins, S., et al. (2005). Behavioral treatment approaches for methamphetamine dependence and HIV-related sexual risk behaviors among urban gay and bisexual men. *Drug and Alcohol Dependence, 78,* 125–134.

Silagy, C., Lancaster, T., Stead, L., Mant, D., & Fowler, G. (2004). Nicotine replacement therapy for smoking cessation. *Cochrane Database System Reviews:* CD000146.

Silverman, K., Chutuape, M. A., Bigelow, G. E., & Stitzer, M. L. (1999). Voucher-based reinforcement of cocaine abstinence in treatment-resistant methadone patients: Effects of reinforcement magnitude. *Psychopharmacology (Berl), 146,* 128–138.

Silverman, K., Higgins, S. T., Brooner, R. K., Montoya, I. D., Cone, E. J., Schuster, C. R., et al. (1996). Sustained cocaine abstinence in methadone maintenance patients through voucher-based reinforcement therapy. *Archives of General Psychiatry, 53,* 409–415.

Sofuoglu, M., & Kosten, T. R. (2005). Novel approaches to the treatment of cocaine addiction. *CNS Drugs, 19,* 13–25.

Spanagel, R., Herz, A., & Shippenberg, T. S. (1992). Opposing tonically active endogenous opioid systems modulate the mesolimbic dopaminergic pathway. *Proceedings of the National Academy of Sciences of the United States of America, 89,* 2046–2050.

Srisurapanont, M., Jarusuraisin, N., & Jittiwutikan, J. (1999). Amphetamine withdrawal: II. A placebo-controlled, randomised, double-blind study of amineptine treatment. *Australian and New Zealand Journal of Psychiatry, 33,* 94–98.

Stoops, W. W. (2006). Aripiprazole as a potential pharmacotherapy for stimulant dependence: Human laboratory studies with d-amphetamine. *Experimental Clinical Psychopharmacology, 14,* 413–421.

Substance Abuse and Mental Health Services Administration (2006a). Office of Applied Studies. *Treatment Episode Data Set (TEDS). Highlights-2004. National admissions to substance abuse treatment services,* DASIS Series: S-31, DHHS Publication No. (SMA) 06-4140, Rockville, MD.

Substance Abuse and Mental Health Services Administration (2006b). *The NSDUH Report: State estimates of past year methamphetamine use.* Office of Applied Studies. Retrieved January, 12, 2007, from http://www.oas.samhsa.gov/2k6/stateMeth/stateMeth.htm.

Substance Abuse and Mental Health Services Administration (2006c) Office of Applied Studies. *Drug abuse warning network, 2004 national estimates of drug-related emergency department visits.* DAWN Series D-28, DHHS Publication No. (SMA) 06-4143, Rockville, MD.

Tennant, F. S., Jr., & Rawson, R. A. (1983). Cocaine and amphetamine dependence treated with desipramine. *NIDA Research Monograph, 43,* 351–355.

Tiihonen, J., Kuoppasalmi, K., Fohr, J., Tuomola, P., Kuikanmaki, O., Vorma, H., et al. (2007). A comparison of aripiprazole, methylphenidate, and placebo for amphetamine dependence. *American Journal of Psychiatry, 164,* 160–162.

Wachtel, S. R., Ortengren, A., & de Wit, H. (2002). The effects of acute haloperidol or risperidone on subjective responses to methamphetamine in healthy volunteers. *Drug and Alcohol Dependence, 68,* 23–33.

Weiss, F., Markou, A., Lorang, M. T., & Koob, G. F. (1992). Basal extracellular dopamine levels in the nucleus accumbens are decreased during cocaine withdrawal after unlimited-access self-administration. *Brain Research, 593,* 314–318.

Welte, J., Barnes, G., Wieczorek, W., Tidwell, M. C., & Parker, J. (2001). Alcohol and gambling pathology among U.S. adults: Prevalence, demographic patterns and comorbidity. *Journal of Studies on Alcohol, 62,* 706–712.

Wermuth, L. (2000). Methamphetamine use: Hazards and social influences. *Journal of Drug Education, 30,* 423–433.

17

Heroin and Other Opioids

Lisa A. Marsch

National Development and Research Institutes

Warren K. Bickel

University of Arkansas for Medical Sciences

Contents

Introduction to Heroin and Other Opioids

Opioids (sometimes referred to as "opioid analgesics" or "narcotics") are a class of drugs that relieve pain, and are chemically related to opium, a substance collected from the poppy plant. Opioids include both nonsynthetic opiates, such as heroin (diacetylmorphine), which is processed from morphine, as well as synthetic substances, such as codeine, hydromorphone (Dilaudid), fentanyl, hydrocodone (Vicodin), oxycodone (Percocet, OxyContin), propoxyphene (Darvon), and merperidone (Demerol). Opioids act by binding to specific proteins in the brain, spinal cord, and gastrointestinal tract, called opioid receptors. Although several types of opioid receptors exist (e.g., mu, kappa, and delta), opioids largely produce their analgesic (pain-relieving) and reinforcing effects via activation of the mu-opioid receptor (Jaffe & Jaffe, 2004).

Heroin

The opiate, heroin, is an illegal, highly addictive drug which produces the most rapid effect of all opioids. Heroin is often sold as a white or brownish powder or as a black substance known as "black tar heroin". In the United States, the purity of heroin has greatly increased in recent years (Drug Enforcement Administration, 2003), which allows for it to be used via an intranasal route ("snorting"); however, heroin may be also be injected or smoked. Heroin, despite its route of administration, has a high addictive potential. Intravenous injection produces the most rapid rise in brain levels of heroin and the greatest intensity and most rapid onset of euphoria accompanied by a warm flushing sensation (the "rush", which is typically felt within 7–8 seconds after injection). The euphoric sensation after intramuscular injection of heroin typically occurs within 5–8 minutes. After sniffing or smoking heroin, the peak euphoric effects are experienced within about 10–15 minutes. This initial pleasurable sensation is then followed by a longer-lasting altered state (the "high"). Individuals in this state generally alternate between a wakeful and drowsy state (the "nod"; Jaffe & Martin, 1975).

Recreational use of heroin is associated with significant mortality and morbidity. Although purer heroin is increasingly available, it is still typically "cut" with other substances such as starch, sugar, or quinine. These additives can result in clogged blood vessels, which may cause infection in vital organs. Also, because both the purity and contents of heroin can vary widely, individuals who use it are at risk of overdose or death. Chronic heroin users may develop abscesses, cellulitis, infection of the heart lining and valves, and liver disease. They may also experience pulmonary complications (e.g., pneumonia) from poor health conditions and from heroin's depressing effect on respiration. Heroin users are at significant risk of infectious diseases including the Human Immunodeficiency Virus (HIV), hepatitis, and tuberculosis (Hagan, Thiede, & Des Jarlais, 2005; Santibanez et al., 2006), largely due to injection drug use.

Approximately 3.1 million household residents in the United States reported having used heroin in their lifetime, and 398,000 reported heroin use in the last year (SAMHSA, 2005a). In addition, more countries, including many areas in Eastern Europe and Asia, are reporting increases in heroin use than are reporting stability or declines in use in the recent past (Aceijas, Stimson, Hickman, & Rhodes, 2004; United Nations International Drug Control Programme Report, 2003).

Nonheroin Opioids

Prescription opioids are potent and effective pain relievers when provided to individuals with acute and chronic pain conditions (Savage, 2003). If taken as prescribed, opioids can often manage pain effectively and safely. However, prescription opioids have significant abuse and addictive potential, and thus serious health liabilities, when used for nonmedical reasons.

As with heroin, other opioids can produce euphoria, drowsiness, and, if taken in sufficient quantities, can depress breathing, possibly leading to overdose and death.

Among the abused opioids in the United States are OxyContin, which is a controlled release form of oxycodone hydrochloride that promotes nearly instant euphoria when crushed before consumption (often intranasally) and Vicodin (hydrocodone and acetaminophen). About 32 million household residents in the United States reported abuse of an opioid medication in their lifetime, and over 11 million reported abuse of an opioid medication in the last year. Unfortunately, recreational use of prescription opioids (use without a prescription) is a significant and growing public health concern. For example, the incidence of opioid analgesic abuse increased from 628,000 initiates in 1990 to 2.5 million initiates in 2004 (SAMHSA, 2005a). The financial societal cost of untreated opioid dependence in the United States is estimated to be $20 billion annually (Levine, Reif, Lee, Ritter, & Horgan, 2004).

Abuse and Dependence on Opioids

Opioid abuse is generally characterized by a pattern of use that leads to problems in fulfilling responsibilities and obligations in one's life, social or interpersonal problems with others, risking physical harm, or experiencing legal problems as a result of opioid use within a 12-month period. Opioid abuse is diagnosed using the *Diagnostic and Statistical Manual of Mental Disorders*, fourth edition (*DSM–IV*; American Psychiatric Association, 2000).

Opioid dependence (also diagnosed using the *DSM–IV*), frequently referred to as "opioid addiction", reflects a progression in one's opioid use beyond a diagnosis of opioid abuse. Opioid dependence often includes physical dependence on opioids. One such aspect of physical dependence is "tolerance" to the effects of opioids, which is experienced by the user as a need to consume larger amounts of opioids to achieve the same drug effect. Additionally, individuals who are physically dependent on opioids will experience a painful "withdrawal" syndrome if they abruptly discontinue their opioid use. Individuals in withdrawal from opioids experience severe flulike symptoms, including restlessness, muscle aches, joint and bone pain, cold flashes, lacrimation, insomnia, diarrhea, and vomiting. The onset and duration of withdrawal symptoms are directly related to the rate at which an opioid drug is cleared from the opioid receptors. Withdrawal symptoms may start to emerge within a few hours after the last opioid use (to coincide with the duration of action of short-acting opioids of abuse), often peak with 48–72 hours after the last opioid use and may last for 5–7 days. In addition, protracted withdrawal symptoms, consisting of dysphoria, mood instability, and low feelings of self-worth, may last for several weeks to months after the acute withdrawal phase. Avoidance of withdrawal symptoms is a significant contributing factor to continued opioid use among opioid-dependent individuals (Jaffe & Jaffe, 2004; Jaffe & Martin, 1975).

The loss of control of opioid use is the hallmark characteristic of opioid dependence and the primary feature that differentiates opioid dependence from opioid abuse. This phenomenon also distinguishes the diagnosis of opioid addiction from the physical dependence a person who chronically consumes prescribed opioid medications for treatment of pain experiences as a result of chronic exposure to opioids. This loss of control phenomenon often includes continued opioid use despite negative consequences, a persistent desire or unsuccessful efforts to cut down or discontinue use, spending a considerable amount of time obtaining opioids or recovering from their effects, and continuing to use despite awareness of a physical and/or psychological problem with opioids (American Psychiatric Asssociation, 2000).

Opioid dependence is a chronic, relapsing medical disorder. Dependence is currently considered to be caused by a combination of environmental, genetic, and drug-induced factors. Despite the initial cause of opioid use, the neurobiological basis of opioid dependence is generally well established. Opioids, like many substances of abuse, cause a series of neuroadaptations in various neuronal circuits in the brain involved in motivation, memory, control, and disinhibition, resulting in an increased and long-lasting reward value associated with the drug and environmental cues associated with it, and a decreased reward value associated with natural reinforcers encountered in everyday life events (Volkow, Fowler, & Wang, 2004).

Treatment of Opioid Dependence

Decades of scientific research and clinical experience demonstrate that opioid dependence is a chronic medical disorder that can be effectively treated with a combination of medication and psychosocial services. Each such component of evidence-based treatment for opioid dependence is described in this section.

Psychosocial Interventions

Treatment for opioid dependence has been shown to be most effective when pharmacotherapy is provided along with science-based psychosocial interventions. Indeed, psychiatric comorbidity, including personality disorders, depression, anxiety, family dysfunction, unemployment, legal problems, and other behavioral problems (e.g., drug and sex-related HIV risk behavior) are highly prevalent among opioid-dependent individuals (e.g., Brooner, King, Kidorf, Schmidt, & Bigelow, 1997; Institute of Medicine, 1995). The provision of employment, family counseling, psychiatric services, and patient education services (e.g., HIV/AIDS and hepatitis education, relapse prevention skills training, prosocial life skills training) as part of treatment is often critical for treatment to be maximally effective. In a striking demonstration of the role of psychosocial interventions offered during maintenance treatment with methadone medication (described in more detail in the next section), patients were randomly assigned to receive (1) methadone medication only at doses of 60 mg or higher with no other services, (2) the same doses of methadone plus counseling, or (3) the same doses of methadone plus counseling and onsite medical/psychiatric, employment, and family therapy (McLellan, Arndt, Metzger, Woody, & O'Brien, 1993). Results indicated that 69%, 41%, and 19% of patients in each of these three conditions had unremitting use of opiates or cocaine, respectively, demonstrating convincingly that the quantity and quality of psychotherapeutic interventions markedly affect patient outcomes in methadone maintenance treatment.

These findings have been replicated in numerous clinical studies demonstrating that patients in treatment for opioid dependence who are provided with a range of psychosocial interventions of demonstrated efficacy are significantly more likely to remain in treatment and to experience markedly greater reductions in drug use than those who receive the standard drug counseling typically offered in Opiate Treatment Programs (OTPs; e.g., Condelli & Dunteman, 1993; Glass, 1993; O'Brien, Woody, & McLellan, 1995; Rounsaville, Glazer, Wilber, Weissman, & Kleber, 1983). This finding has been shown to be especially true for opioid-dependent patients with psychiatric disorders, as this subpopulation of patients generally experiences poor outcomes from standard substance abuse counseling alone. Approximately 60–85% of patients in OTPs have psychiatric disorders, furthering underscoring the critical importance of providing effective psychotherapeutic interventions to this group (O'Brien et al., 1995; Woody, McLellan, Luborsky, & O'Brien, 1990).

Several efficacious approaches to offering psychosocial treatment to opioid-dependent individuals exist and include the provision of cognitive-behavioral therapy and the Community-Reinforcement Approach (CRA) (e.g., Abbott,Weller, Delaney, & Moore, 1998; Mayet, Farrell, Ferri, Amato, & Davoli, 2005). These behavioral interventions are designed to increase patients' ability to cope with life stressors and modify their thoughts, expectancies, and behaviors to help them discontinue illicit opioid use. Additionally, behavioral contingency management procedures (sometimes called "motivational incentives" procedures) have been shown to reliably improve outcomes during treatment for opioid dependence. These procedures typically involve the provision of scheduled nonpharmacological consequences (e.g., "points" that can be exchanged for items that encourage healthy living) or pharmacologically based privileges (e.g., take-home methadone) contingent on opiate-free urine samples (e.g., Bickel, Amass, Higgins, Badger, & Esch, 1997; Griffith, Rowan-Szal, Roark, & Simpson, 2000).

Pharmacotherapy

Several medications have been shown to be effective as pharmacotherapeutic agents for the treatment of opioid dependence. The most effective medications for the treatment of opioid dependence are long-acting opioid medications, sometimes referred to as "opioid-substitution therapy". Long-acting opioid medications address the neurobiological dysregulation of opioid-dependent individuals by stabilizing their brain neurochemistry and preventing withdrawal symptoms (e.g., Leshner, 1998). Also, due to the affinity (binding) of these opioid medications to the same opioid receptors as short-acting opioids of abuse, as well as their cross-tolerance (tolerance to a pharmacologically similar substance), these medications can block the effects of other opioids an individual may self-administer (e.g., heroin). This blockade effect functions as an additional deterrent to continued illicit opioid use (Dole, 1988; Dole, Nyswander, & Kreek, 1966; Jasinski, Pevnick, & Griffith, 1978; Ling, Charuvastra, Kaim, & Klett, 1976).

Methadone

Methadone hydrochloride is a synthetic opioid medication that has been used in the treatment of opioid dependence since the mid-1960s and is the most widely used pharmacotherapy for opioid dependence (Ball & Ross, 1991; Dole et al., 1966; Dole & Nyswander, 1965). Methadone is considered a full mu-opioid agonist, meaning that it largely exerts its action at the mu-opioid receptor site and can produce maximal response at these receptors (e.g., higher doses of methadone produce greater physiological and subjective effects). Methadone is a long-acting opioid that can stablize the brain neurochemistry of an opioid-dependent individual and block the effects of other opioids when administered every 24 hours. When used for the treatment of opioid dependence, methadone is typically administered orally as a liquid solution (SAMHSA TIP 43, 2005b).

Methadone treatment for opioid dependence in the United States is provided in designated OTPs. OTPs were previously approved and monitored by the Food and Drug Administration (FDA) but are now governed by the Substance Abuse and Mental Health Services Administration, Department of Health and Human Services (SAMHSA, 2001). In this regulatory model, OTPs are required to comply with appropriate certification requirements and federal opioid treatment standards, with a strong emphasis on adherence to best-practice guidelines and accreditation standards developed by SAMHSA-approved accreditation bodies. SAMHSA retains oversight of a program's accreditation and individual states can regulate OTPs under the federal regulations.

Methadone treatment may include either medication-assisted withdrawal (sometimes referred to as "detoxification") or maintenance treatment. In the former model, opioid-dependent individuals are typically initially stabilized on methadone and then the medication dose is reduced to assist the individual in becoming opioid-free. Methadone-assisted withdrawal may occur in an inpatient (hospital-based setting) or outpatient setting at OTPs. Unfortunately, as a chronic disorder, rates of relapse to opioid use are typically quite high after discontinuation of agonist treatment among opioid-dependent adults (Ball & Ross, 1991; Paraherakis, Charnet, Palacious-Boix, & Gill, 2000), and thus long-term maintenance treatment is considered the standard of care in the treatment of opioid dependence. In methadone maintenance treatment, opioid-dependent individuals are given escalating doses of methadone, typically starting at about 20–40 mg and then increased over a period of days to weeks until a "steady state" is achieved (meaning the level of medication in a person's blood remains fairly steady because the drug's rate of intake equals the rate of its breakdown and excretion; SAMHSA TIP 43, 2005b). Continued methadone dosing is then typically offered under observation at OTPs 6–7 days per week, although patients can receive "take-home" doses of methadone after a period of stabilization (SAMHSA, 2001).

A substantive scientific literature has demonstrated that methadone treatment is most effective when adequate clinical doses of the medication (ranging from 80–120 mg daily) are provided (e.g., D'Aunno & Vaughn, 1992; Donny, Walsh, Bigelow, Eissenberg, & Stitzer, 2002; Strain, Bigelow, Liebson, & Stitzer, 1999). These findings have been incorporated into policies and guidelines regarding methadone dosing in the treatment of opioid dependence. For example, the National Institutes of Health (NIH) Policy Statement on effective medical treatment of opiate addiction has called for widespread use of sufficiently high therapeutic doses of methadone (NIH, 1997). In addition, in their most recent *Federal Register* outlining regulations regarding the use of opioid drugs in the treatment of opiate addiction, the Department of Health and Human Services (DHHS) removed the requirement that physicians in opioid treatment programs need to justify all methadone doses above 100 mg (SAMHSA, 2001).

In order to be eligible for methadone maintenance treatment, an individual must meet *DSM–IV* criteria for opioid dependence and have used opioids for at least one year. Exceptions to these admission criteria may exist, however, in cases where previously dependent individuals are recently released from an incarcerated setting (due to high expected relapse rates), or cases of pregnant women for whom a relapse to opioid abuse or dependence is a concern. Individuals presenting for methadone treatment who are also alcohol- and/or sedative-dependent, and whose dependence may be concerning due to central nervous system depression which may cause serious adverse events during methadone treatment, may be required to successfully detoxify from these other substances prior to methadone treatment. Individuals under the age of 18 are rarely offered methadone treatment and, when they are, they are typically only considered after having at least two documented, unsuccessful attempts at short-term detoxification or drug-free treatment (21 CFR, Part 291).

Methadone treatment has repeatedly been shown to be safe and effective in the treatment of opioid dependence and to significantly reduce mortality and morbidity. Specifically, methadone maintenance treatment produces marked reductions in illicit opioid use, criminal activity, and behavior that may place one at risk for infection with HIV, hepatitis, or other infectious diseases (e.g., Ball & Ross, 1991; Marsch, 1998; Strain, Stitzer, Liebson, & Bigelow, 1993). Over 1,000 opioid treatment programs provide methadone treatment to over 227,000 individuals in the United States (SAMHSA, 2004a).

Levomethadyl Acetate (LAAM)

Levomethadyl Acetate, LAAM also a full mu-opioid agonist, was approved by the Food and Drug Administration as a pharmacotherapeutic agent for the treatment of opioid dependence in 1993. LAAM is a longer-acting medication relative to methadone and, unlike methadone which has to be administered daily, LAAM can be effectively administered thrice weekly (Ling et al., 1976). LAAM was shown to be equally efficacious to methadone in the treatment of opioid dependence (Johnson et al., 2000). However, LAAM was recently withdrawn from the U.S. market by its manufacturer, largely in light of a postmarketing surveillance report of its association with a prolonged QT interval as measured by electrocardiogram (EKG) readings of the electrical activity of one's heartbeat and several reports of torsades de pointes, a life-threatening ventricular arrhythmia (abnormal rhythm in the lower chambers of the heart; Kreek & Vocci, 2002).

Buprenorphine

Buprenorphine is a partial mu-opioid agonist, which was FDA-approved as a treatment for opioid dependence in 2002. As a partial agonist, buprenorphine has been demonstrated to have a ceiling effect on its agonist activity, such that increases in dose will increase the medication's physiological and subjective effects only to a certain level, after which time further increases in dose produce no additional effects (Bickel & Amass, 1995; Lewis, 1985; Kenakin, 1987; Walsh, Preston, Bigelow, & Stitzer, 1995). Note that, by this mechanism, buprenorphine is less likely than full agonists, such as methadone, to cause major respiratory depression (Cowan, Doxey, & Harry, 1977). This property of buprenorphine greatly increases its safety profile and limits its abuse liability as well as the possibility of overdose (Walsh, Preston, Stitzer, Cone, & Bigelow, 1994). In addition, due to buprenorphine's high affinity for, and slow dissociation from, the mu-opioid receptor, discontinuation of buprenorphine administration has been shown to result in reduced withdrawal symptomatology relative to that which typically results after discontinuation of full agonist administration. Buprenorphine can also block the effect of other opioids one may self-administer (Eissenberg et al., 1997; Jasinski et al., 1978; Rance & Dickens, 1978).

Unlike methadone which must be provided to patients in a designated OTPs in the United States, buprenorphine may be provided to opioid-dependent patients by qualified physicians in both OTPs as well as in an office-based setting (although methadone is also offered in office-based settings in some other countries; Fiellin & O'Connor, 2002). Treatment of opioid dependence in an office-based setting (allowed by the Drug Addiction Treatment Act of 2000) greatly expands access to treatment of opioid dependence and shifts the treatment of opioid-dependence into mainstream medical care. In order to prescribe buprenorphine, physicians must obtain the appropriate certification by completing the appropriate 8-hour training, or have board certification in addiction psychiatry from the Addiction Board of Medical Specialties, addiction certification from the American Society of Addiction Medicine, board certification in addiction medicine from the American Osteopathic Association, or other appropriate training and experience (see www.buprenorphine.samhsa.gov for details).

Like methadone, buprenorphine is largely used for the treatment of opioid dependence among adults and is offered in both medication-assisted withdrawal and maintenance treatment paradigms (SAMHSA TIP 40, 2004b). Recent evidence suggests that it may also be safe and efficacious in treating opioid-dependent adolescents (Marsch et al., 2005a) and opioid-dependent pregnant women (Jones et al., 2005), although it is not approved for these indications at this time.

When used for the treatment of opioid dependence, buprenorphine is administered sublingually in tablet form. Patients can receive a prescription for up to a month's supply of the medication at a time. Clinically effective doses of buprenorphine typically range from 4–36 mg daily, with average doses of 16 mg daily (SAMHSA TIP 40, 2004b). The medication is placed under the tongue and absorbed via the membranes in the mouth. It has poor oral bioavailability and is thus absorbed poorly if consumed orally. Two formulations of buprenorphine are available for the treatment of opioid dependence. The sublingual formulation of buprenorphine (Subutex; Reckitt Benkiser) is currently approved for use in 44 countries (Carrieri et al., 2006). In addition, a sublingual formulation of buprenorphine and naloxone (in a 4:1 ratio) is available (Suboxone; Reckitt Benkiser). Naloxone is a pure opioid antagonist, which binds to the mu-opioid receptor and thus prevents other opioids from binding to the receptor. Naloxone was added to this formulation to create a more abuse-resistant version of the medication. Specifically, if taken sublingually as intended, Suboxone has comparable safety, efficacy, and bioavailability to Subutex (e.g., Strain, Moody, Stoller, Walsh, & Bigelow, 2004). However, if one were to inject the tablet, the bioavailability of naloxone would theoretically be greater than that of buprenorphine and thus the individual would experience opioid withdrawal symptoms, thus creating a deterrent to injection of the medication.

Numerous studies and clinical experiences have highlighted the effectiveness of buprenorphine and generally shown that, when equi-effective doses of buprenorphine, LAAM, or methadone medications are provided, their effectiveness in the treatment of opioid dependence is comparable. Like methadone, buprenorphine has been shown to significantly reduce illicit opioid use, criminal activity, and behavior that may place one at risk for HIV, hepatitis, and other infectious diseases (e.g., Johnson, Jaffe, & Fudala, 1992; Johnson et al., 2000; Ling et al., 1998; Marsch, Bickel, Badger, & Jacobs, 2005b). Due to the ceiling on buprenorphine's agonist activity, several reports suggest that it may be less effective than the full agonist, methadone, in the treatment of individuals with very high levels of opioid dependence and greater tolerance to the effects of opioids (Fiellin, Friedland, & Gourevitch, 2006); however, mixed evidence exists (Marsch et al., 2005c). Both buprenorphine and methadone are included in the World Health Organization's (WHO) List of Essential Medicines (WHO, 2006).

Naltrexone

Naltrexone is a mu-opioid antagonist, which was FDA-approved in 1984. As an opioid antagonist, naltrexone binds to the mu-opioid receptor and prevents receptor activation by other opioids. Naltrexone is consumed orally, with a dose of 50 mg blocking other opioids from the mu-receptor for approximately 24 hours. Thus, if an individual chooses to self-administer an opioid drug, she or he cannot experience any reinforcing effects from that drug while naltrexone is actively exerting its effect.

Prior research has demonstrated that transferring opioid-dependent adults to treatment with naltrexone after treatment with an opioid agonist (e.g., Kosten, Morgan, & Kleber, 1992; Umbricht et al., 1999) can function to markedly increase the efficacy of the intervention relative to conditions where no naltrexone is provided. However, although naltrexone seems to be an ideal medication for preventing relapse to opioid use (e.g., Ginzburg, 1985; Leavitt, 2002), naltrexone treatment frequently results in poor treatment compliance in studies with opioid-dependent adults, because it lacks morphinelike effects and thereby requires highly motivated patients for treatment success (Kleber, 1985; Kosten & Kleber, 1984; Preston et al., 1999; Rothenberg et al., 2002). Indeed, generally only 10–15% of opioid-dependent adults are willing to take naltrexone (Rounsaville, 1995). However, compliance with naltrexone can be enhanced when patients receive a monetary voucher incentive contingent on naltrexone tablet ingestion (e.g., Grabowski, O'Brien, Greenstein, & Ternes, 1979; Preston et al., 1999). Specifically, patients receiving incentives contingent on compliance with naltrexone treatment remain in treatment longer, and have more continuous weeks of abstinence from opioids (Carroll, Sinha, Nich, Babuscio, & Rounsaville, 2002; Preston et al., 1999; Rothenberg et al., 2002). Such incentives may target naltrexone's weakness, including the high attrition and poor compliance often associated with naltrexone treatment (Carroll et al., 2002). Despite the limited utility of naltrexone in opioid-dependent adults to date, recent research suggests it may be acceptable and potentially efficacious in the treatment of opioid-dependent adolescents after a medication-assisted taper (Marsch et al., 2005a).

Case Presentation

"Sarah," a 34-year-old female, presented for treatment for her opioid use at an outpatient substance abuse treatment program affiliated with her local hospital. When completing a detailed substance abuse history with an intake worker at this program, Sarah reported that she had been using opioids for about 10 years. She reported that her opioid use had started with pain pills, particularly OxyContin and Percocet, which she had used for about 1 year before she started snorting heroin. She had been introduced to opioids by her older boyfriend at the time, who was an active user and who was a small-time dealer who "copped" drugs largely to support his own habit. On an average day during the period that she used opioid pain pills, Sarah typically used between 80–120 mg of OxyContin daily, which she crushed and snorted. As she continued to regularly use opioid pain pills during that year, Sarah reported that she had to increase the amount of pills she was using to obtain the same effect and to stave off withdrawal symptoms. She then transitioned to snorting heroin, which she found to be a less expensive habit to maintain at the time. Sarah snorted approximately 2–5 bags of heroin daily for about 8 months and then gradually increased her use up to about 7–9 bags of heroin daily over the next 1.5 years. At this time, a friend of hers showed her how to inject heroin to achieve a more rapid effect of the drug. She had been injecting heroin for about 6.5 years at the time of this treatment entry and was reporting injecting between 10–12 bags of heroin daily on average (although sometimes she still used opioid pain pills to prevent withdrawal when heroin was unavailable to her). She also reported use of cocaine, which she injected along with heroin about 12–15 days per month on average. Sarah reported having gone to four opioid inpatient detoxification programs in the past several years but always relapsed to opioid use after each program. She had also participated in Narcotics Anonymous (NA) support groups at several points during her use, and typically immediately after her detoxification attempts. She had been diagnosed with hepatitis C about five years ago (which she thinks she contracted from sharing drug injection equipment with other users) and had been arrested several times for drug possession, shoplifting, and prostitution, in which she engaged to support her drug habit. She was currently on probation and was at significant risk of losing custody of her young children (aged 5 and 6), which she reported as the main factor motivating her to stop her opioid use.

According to the *DSM–IV*, Sarah met criteria for opioid dependence, including criteria for physical dependence on opioids and withdrawal when discontinuing her opioid use. She also met criteria related to having lost control of her opioid use, including having given up important activities in her life because of her opioid use, having used despite numerous negative consequences, and having used for a much longer period of time than she ever intended. An evaluation of her psychiatric status revealed that she also met criteria for major depressive disorder and posttraumatic stress disorder as a result of both trauma she had experienced as a child and in an abusive relationship with a former boyfriend.

Upon entering the treatment program, Sarah expressed interest in trying the "new medication," buprenorphine. A few acquaintances of hers had told her about their experience taking buprenorphine and how you can feel "really good" when taking it, but not "doped up." She wanted to participate in treatment for a much longer period of time than she had previously, because she felt that she needed ongoing support to help in her recovery. Based on the array of clinical data collected about Sarah, it was determined that Sarah was eligible for treatment with buprenorphine and was scheduled for an outpatient "induction." Due to the partial agonist pharmacological profile of buprenorphine, it was explained to Sarah that she needed to take her first dose of buprenorphine on a day she had not used heroin and when she was experiencing mild to moderate opioid withdrawal (as measured by the Clinical Opiate Withdrawal Scale or COWS and Subjective Opiate Withdrawal Scale or SOWS; see SAMHSA TIP 40, 2004b). On her initial day of buprenorphine treatment, she was initially administered a dose of 4 mg of sublingual buprenorphine, followed by an additional 4 mg dose 2 hours later (for a total of 8 mg on the first day). Sarah's daily maintenance dose was then gradually increased to 16 mg daily, at which point her withdrawal symptoms appeared well controlled and she reported feeling stable. She also reported improved mood and reduced cravings for heroin.

Sarah was also offered the opportunity to participate in both group and individual substance abuse counseling sessions at the substance abuse treatment program, referred to an onsite psychiatrist for her depression and related psychiatric issues, and referred to a liver specialist for a more thorough assessment and possible treatment of her hepatitis C. At this time, Sarah has been an active participant in buprenorphine maintenance treatment for 5 months, has not used other opioids for about 75% of that time, and has only used cocaine on a few occasions since entering treatment. She feels stable but, like many opioid-dependent individuals in treatment, is interested in continuing her buprenorphine treatment participation indefinitely to prevent relapsing to heroin use.

Concluding Comments

As reviewed in this chapter, opioid dependence is a chronic relapsing disorder associated with significant mortality and morbidity. Dependence is currently considered to be caused by a combination of environmental, genetic, and drug-induced factors. Fortunately, however, opioid dependence is a medical disorder that has a well-established neurobiological basis and can be effectively treated with a combination of pharmacological and psychosocial interventions. Several medications, including the full mu-opioid agonist, methadone, and the partial opioid agonist, buprenorphine, have been shown to be exceptionally effective in the treatment of opioid dependence. (Table 17.1 provides a summary of additional resources for the assessment and treatment of opioid dependence.)

The combination of pharmacotherapy to effectively manage withdrawal symptoms and decrease the rewarding value of opioids, along with psychosocial interventions that promote an increase in alternative rewarding behaviors and strengthen inhibitory control, appears to promote the most positive treatment outcomes among opioid-dependent individuals. That is, the pharmacotherapy may stabilize brain dysregulation due to opioid dependence, allowing

---

TABLE 17.1
Additional Resources for the Assessment and Treatment of Opioid Dependence

E. C. Strain & M. L. Stitzer (Eds.) (2006). *The Treatment of Opioid Dependence*. Baltimore, MD: Johns Hopkins University Press.

Center for Substance Abuse Treatment, Substance Abuse and Mental Health Services Administration. Available online at: http://csat.samhsa.gov.

Substance Abuse and Mental Health Services Administration (SAMHSA), Office of Applied Studies. (2004). *Clinical Guidelines for the Use of Bupenorphine in the Treatment of Opioid Addiction. TIP 40*. Rockville, MD: Substance Abuse and Mental Health Services Administration, Office of Applied Studies. Available online at: http://www.ncbi.nlm.nih.gov/books/bv.fcgi?rid=hstat5.chapter.72248.

Substance Abuse and Mental Health Services Administration (SAMHSA). (2005). *Medication-assisted treatment for opioid addiction in opioid treatment programs. A treatment improvement protocol. TIP 43*. Rockville, MD: Substance Abuse and Mental Health Services Administration, Office of Applied Studies. Available online at: http://www.ncbi.nlm.nih.gov/books/bv.fcgi?rid=hstat5.chapter.82676.

Methadone Treatment Programs by State. Available online at: http://dpt2.samhsa.gov/treatment/directory.aspx.

Buprenorphine Treatment Physician Locator by State. Available online at: http://buprenorphine.samhsa.gov/bwns_locator/index.html.

individuals to engage in therapeutic activities to learn new skills and behaviors that do not involve drug use and which are critical to successfully discontinuing opioid use. Indeed, opioid-dependent individuals frequently present for treatment with an array of clinically meaningful issues including high levels of risk behavior and high levels of psychiatric problems. A comprehensive treatment program that addresses this broad clinical profile has the greatest likelihood of producing optimal treatment outcomes among this clinical population.

Acknowledgments

The preparation of this chapter was supported by National Institute on Drug Abuse (NIDA) Grants # R01DA021818, R01DA018297, R01DA12997 & R42DA14727.

References

Abbott, P. J., Weller, S. B., Delaney, H. D., & Moore, B. A. (1998). Community reinforcement approach in the treatment of opiate addicts. *American Journal of Drug and Alcohol Abuse, 24,* 17–30.

Aceijas, C., Stimson, G. V., Hickman, M., & Rhodes, T. (2004). Global overview of injecting drug use and HIV infection among injecting drug users. *AIDS, 18,* 2295–303.

American Psychiatric Association (2000). *Diagnostic and statistical manual of mental disorders* (4th ed.), Text Revision (*DSM–IV–TR*).Washington, DC: Author.

Ball, J. C., & Ross, A. (1991). *The effectiveness of methadone maintenance treatment: Patients, programs, services and outcome.* New York: Springer-Verlag.

Bickel, W. K., & Amass, L. A. (1995). Buprenorphine treatment of opioid dependence. A review. *Experimental and Clinical Psychopharmacology, 3,* 477–489.

Bickel, W. K., Amass, L., Higgins, S. T., Badger, G. J., & Esch, R. A. (1997). Effects of adding behavioral treatment to opioid detoxification with buprenorphine. *Journal of Consulting and Clinical Psychology, 65,* 803–810.

Brooner, R. K., King, V. L., Kidorf, M., Schmidt, C. W., & Bigelow, G. E. (1997). Psychiatric and substance use comorbidity among treatment-seeking opioid abusers. *Archives of General Psychiatry, 54,* 71–80.

Carrieri, M. P., Amass, L., Lucas, G. M., Vlahov, D., Wodak, A., & Woody, G. E. (2006). Buprenorphine use: The international experience. *Clinical Infectious Diseases, 43* (Suppl. 4), S197–S215.

Carroll, K. M., Sinha, R., Nich, C., Babuscio, T., & Rounsaville, B. J. (2002). Contingency management to enhance naltrexone treatment of opioid dependence: A randomized, clinical trial of reinforcement magnitude. *Experimental and Clinical Psychopharmacology, 10,* 54–63.

Condelli, W. S., & Dunteman, G. H. (1993). Exposure to methadone programs and heroin use. *American Journal of Drug and Alcohol Abuse, 19,* 65–78.

Cowan, A., Doxey, J. C., & Harry, E. J. R. (1977). The animal pharmacology of buprenorphine: An oripavine analgesic agent. *British Journal of Pharmacology, 60,* 547–554.

D'Aunno, T., & Vaughn, T. E. (1992). Variations in methadone treatment practices. Results from a national study. *Journal of the American Medical Association, 267,* 253–258.

Dole, V. P. (1988). Implications of methadone maintenance for theories of narcotic addiction. *Journal of the American Medical Association, 260,* 3025–3029.

Dole, V. P., & Nyswander, M. E. (1965). A medical treatment for diacetyl morphine (heroin) addiction: A clinical trial with methadone hydrochloride. *Journal of the American Medical Association, 193,* 646–650.

Dole, V. P., Nyswander, M. E., & Kreek, M. J. (1966). Narcotic blockade. *Archives of Internal Medicine, 118,* 304–309.

Donny, E. C., Walsh, S. L., Bigelow, G. E., Eissenberg, T., & Stitzer, M. L. (2002). High-dose methadone produces superior opioid blockade and comparable withdrawal suppression to lower doses in opioid-dependent humans. *Psychopharmacology, 161,* 202–212.

Drug Enforcement Administration (DEA, 2003). *Illegal drug price and purity report.* U.S. Department of Justice. http://www.usdoj.gov/dea/pubs/intel/02058/02058.pdf. Accessed on June 1, 2007.

Eissenberg, T., Johnson, R. E., Bigelow, G. E., Walsh, S. L., Liebson, I. A., Strain, E. C., et al. (1997). Controlled opioid withdrawal evaluation during 72 h dose omission in buprenorphine-maintained patients. *Drug and Alcohol Dependence, 45,* 81–91.

Fiellin, D. A., Friedland, G. H., & Gourevitch, M. N. (2006). Opioid dependence: Rationale for and efficacy of existing and new treatments. *Clinical Infectious Diseases, 43,* S173–S177.

Fiellin, D. A., & O'Connor, P. G. (2002). New federal initiatives to enhance the medical treatment of opioid dependence. *Annals of Internal Medicine, 137,* 688–692.

Ginzburg, H. M. (1985). Naltrexone: Its clinical utility. *Advances in Alcohol and Substance Abuse, 5,* 83–101.

Glass, R. M. (1993). Methadone maintenance. New research on a controversial treatment. *Journal of the American Medical Association, 269,* 1995–1996.

Grabowski, J., O'Brien, C. P., Greenstein, R., & Ternes, J. (1979). Effects of contingent payment on compliance with a naltrexone regimen. *American Journal of Drug and Alcohol Abuse, 6,* 355–365.

Griffith, J. D., Rowan-Szal, G. A., Roark, R. R., & Simpson, D. D. (2000). Contingency management in outpatient methadone treatment: A meta-analysis. *Drug and Alcohol Dependence, 58,* 55–66.

Hagan, H., Thiede, H., & Des Jarlais, D. C. (2005). HIV/hepatitis C virus co-infection in drug users: Risk behavior and prevention. *AIDS,* Suppl. 3, *19,* S199, 207.

Institute of Medicine, Rettig, R. A., & Yarmolinsky, A. (Eds.). (1995). *Federal regulations of methadone treatment.* Washington, DC: National Academy Press.

Jaffe, J. H. & Jaffe, A. B. (2004). Neurobiology of opioids. In M. Galanter & H. D. Kleber (Eds.), *Textbook of substance abuse treatment* (pp. 17–30). Washington, DC: American Psychiatric.

Jaffe, J. H., & Martin, W. R. (1975). Narcotic analgesics and antagonists. In L. S. Goodman & A. Gilman (Eds.), *The pharmacological basis of therapeutics* (pp. 245–324). New York: Macmillan.

Jasinski, D. R., Pevnick, J. S., & Griffith, J. D. (1978). Human pharmacology and abuse potential of the analgesic buprenorphine: A potential agent for treating narcotic addiction. *Archives of General Psychiatry, 35,* 501–516.

Johnson, R. E., Chutuape, M. A., Strain, E. C., Walsh, S. L., Stitzer, M. L., & Bigelow, G. E. (2000). A comparison of levomethadyl acetate, buprenorphine, and methadone for opioid dependence. *New England Journal of Medicine, 343,* 1290–1297.

Johnson, R. E., Jaffe, J. H., & Fudala, P. J. (1992). A controlled trial of buprenorphine treatment for opioid dependence. *Journal of the American Medical Association, 267,* 2750–2755.

Jones, H. E., Johnson, R. E., Jasinski, D. R., O'Grady, K. E., Chisholm, C. A., Choo, R. E., et al. (2005). Buprenorphine versus methadone in the treatment of pregnant opioid-dependent patients: Effects on the neonatal abstinence syndrome. *Drug and Alcohol Dependence, 79,* 1–10.

Kenakin, T. (1987). Agonists, partial agonists, antagonists, inverse agonists and agonists/antagonists. *Trends in Pharmacological Sciences, 8,* 423–426.

Kleber, H. D. (1985). Naltrexone. *Journal of Substance Abuse Treatment, 2,* 117–122.

Kosten, T. R., & Kleber, H. D. (1984). Strategies to improve compliance with narcotic antagonists. *American Journal of Drug and Alcohol Abuse, 10,* 249–266.

Kosten, T. R., Morgan, C., & Kleber, H. D. (1992). Phase II clinical trials of buprenorphine: Detoxification and induction onto naltrexone. *NIDA Research Monograph, 121,* 101–119.

Kreek, M. J., & Vocci, F. J. (2002). History and current status of opioid maintenance treatments: Blending conference session. *Journal of Substance Abuse Treatment, 23,* 93–105.

Leavitt, S. B. (2002). Naltrexone in the prevention of opioid relapse. *Addiction Treatment Forum. August,* 1–6.

Leshner, A. I. (1998). Addiction is a brain disease, and it matters. *Science, 278,* 45–47.

Levine, H. J., Reif, S., Lee, M. T., Ritter, G. A., & Horgan, C. M. (2004). *Alcohol and Drugs Services Study (ADSS). The national treatment system: Outpatient methadone facilities.* Rockville, MD: Substance Abuse and Mental Health Services Administration, Office of Applied Studies.

Lewis, J. W. (1985). Buprenorphine. *Drug and Alcohol Dependence, 14,* 363–372.

Ling, W., Charuvastra, C., Collins, J.F., Batki, S., Brown, L. S., Jr., Kintaudi, P., et al. (1998). Buprenorphine maintenance treatment of opiate dependence: A multicenter, randomized clinical trial. *Addiction, 93,* 475–478.

Ling, W., Charuvastra, V. C., Kaim, S. C., & Klett, C. J. (1976). Methadyl acetate and methadone as maintenance treatments for heroin addicts. A veterans administration cooperative study. *Archives of General Psychiatry, 33,* 709–720.

Marsch, L. A. (1998). The efficacy of methadone maintenance interventions in reducing illicit opiate use, HIV risk behavior and criminality: A meta-analysis. *Addiction, 93,* 515–532.

Marsch, L. A., Bickel, W. K., Badger, G. J., & Jacobs, E. A. (2005b). Buprenorphine treatment for opioid dependence: The relative efficacy of daily, twice and thrice weekly dosing. *Drug and Alcohol Dependence, 77,* 195–204.

Marsch, L. A., Bickel, W. K., Badger, G. J., Stothart, M. E., Quesnel, K. J., Stanger, C., et al. (2005a). Comparison of pharmacological treatments for opioid dependent adolescents: A randomized, controlled trial. *Archives of General Psychiatry, 62,* 1157–1164.

Marsch, L. A., Chutuape, M. A., Mudric, T., Strain, E. C., Bigelow, G. E., & Johnson, R. E. (2005c). Predictors of outcome in LAAM, buprenorphine and methadone treatment for opioid dependence. *Experimental and Clinical Psychopharmacology, 13,* 293–302.

Mayet, S., Farrell, M., Ferri, M., Amato, L., & Davoli, M. *Psychosocial treatment for opiate abuse and dependence. Cochrane Databse System Review.* http://www.mrw.interscience.wiley.com/cochrane/clsysrev/articles/CD004330/frame.html. Accessed on June 1, 2007.

McLellan, A. T., Arndt, I. O., Metzger, D. S., Woody, G. E., & O'Brien, C. P. (1993). The effects of psychosocial services in substance abuse treatment. *Journal of the American Medical Association, 269,* 1953–1959.

National Institutes of Health. (1997). *Effective medical treatment of opiate addiction. NIH Consensus Statement Online. 1997 November 17–19.* Retrieved September 15, 2005, from http://consensus.nih.gov/1997/1998TreatOpiateAddiction108html.htm.

O'Brien, C. P., Woody, G. E., & McLellan, A. T. (1995). Enhancing the effectiveness of methadone using psychotherapeutic interventions. *NIDA Research Monograph, 150,* 5–18.

Paraherakis, A., Charnet, D. A., Palacious-Boix, J., & Gill, K. (2000). An abstinence-oriented program for substance use disorders: Poorer outcome associated with opiate dependence. *Canadian Journal of Psychiatry, 45,* 927–931.

Preston, K. L., Silverman, K., Umbricht, A., DeJesus, A., Montoya, I. D., & Schuster, C. R. (1999). Improvement in naltrexone treatment compliance with contingency management. *Drug and Alcohol Dependence, 54,* 127–135.

Rance, M. J., & Dickens, J. N. (1978). The influence of drug-receptor kinetics on the pharmacological and pharmaco-kinetic profiles of buprenorphine. In J. M. Van Ree & L. Pereniums (Eds.), *Characteristics and functions of opioids* (pp. 65–66). Amsterdam: Elsevier/North-Holland Biomedical Press, 65–66.

Rothenberg, J. L., Sullivan, M. A., Church, S. H., Seracini, A., Collins, E., Kleber, H. D., et al. (2002). Behavioral naltrexone therapy: An integrated treatment for opiate dependence. *Journal of Substance Abuse Treatment, 23,* 351–360.

Rounsaville, B. J. (1995). Can psychotherapy rescue naltrexone treatment in opioid addiction? *NIDA Research Monograph, 159,* 37–52.

Rounsaville, B. J., Glazer, W., Wilber, C. H., Weissman, M. M., & Kleber, H. D. (1983). Short-term interpersonal psychotherapy in methadone-maintained opiate addicts. *Archives of General Psychiatry, 40,* 629–636.

Santibanez, S. S., Garfein, R. S., Swartzendruber, A., Purcell, D. W., Paxton, L. A., & Greenberg, A. E. (2006). Update and overview of practial epidemiological aspects of HIV/AIDS among injection drug users in the United States. *Journal of Urban Health, 83,* 86–100.

Savage, S. R. (2003). Opioid medications in the management of pain. In A. W. Graham, T. K. Schultz, M. F. Mayo-Smith, R. K. Ries, & B. B. Wilford (Eds.), *Principles of addiction medicine* (pp. 1451–1463). Chevy Chase, MD: American Society of Addiction Medicine.

Strain, E. C., Bigelow, G. E., Liebson, I. A., & Stitzer, M. L. (1999). Moderate- vs high-dose methadone in the treatment of opioid dependence: A randomized trial. *Journal of the American Medical Association, 281,* 1000–1005.

Strain, E. C., Moody, D. E., Stoller, K. B., Walsh, S. L., & Bigelow, G. E. (2004). Relative bioavailability of different buprenorphine formulations under chronic dosing conditions. *Drug and Alcohol Dependence, 74,* 37–43.

Strain, E. C., Stitzer, M. L., Liebson, I. A., & Bigelow, G. E. (1993). Dose-response effects of metha-done in the treatment of opioid dependence. *Annals of Internal Medicine, 119,* 23–27.

Substance Abuse and Mental Health Services Administration (SAMHSA). (2001). *Federal Register. Opioid drugs in maintenance and detoxification treatment of opiate addiction; Final rule.* (Volume 66, Issue 11, 42 CFR Part 8). Rockville, MD: Department of Health and Human Services.

Substance Abuse and Mental Health Services Administration (SAMHSA), Office of Applied Studies. (2004a). *National survey of substance treatment services (N-SSATS): 2003. Data on substance abuse treatment facilities, DASIS Series: S-24.* (DHHS Publication No. SMA 04-3966). Rockville, MD: Author.

Substance Abuse and Mental Health Services Administration (SAMHSA), Office of Applied Studies. (2004b). *Clinical guidelines for the use of bupenorphine in the treatment of opioid addiction. TIP 40.* Rockville, MD: Substance Abuse and Mental Health Services Administration, Office of Applied Studies.

Substance Abuse and Mental Health Services Administration (SAMHSA). (2005a). *2004 National Survey on Drug Use and Health. Available online at: http://www.oas.samhsa.gov/NSDUH.htm#NSDUHinfo.* Rockville, MD: Substance Abuse and Mental Health Services Administration, Office of Applied Studies.

Substance Abuse and Mental Health Services Administration (SAMHSA). (2005b). *Medication-assisted treatment for opioid addiction in opioid treatment programs. A treatment improvement protocol. TIP 43.* Rockville, MD: Substance Abuse and Mental Health Services Administration, Office of Applied Studies.

Umbricht, A., Montoya, I. D., Hoover, D. R., Demuth, K. L., Chiang, C. T., & Preston, K. L. (1999). Naltrexone shortened opioid detoxification with buprenorphine. *Drug and Alcohol Dependence, 56,* 181–190.

United Nations International Drug Control Programme Report. (2003). http://www.unodc.org/unodc/index.html. Accessed on June 1, 2007.

Volkow, N. D., Fowler, J. S., & Wang, G. (2004). The addicted human brain viewed in the light of imaging studies: Brain circuits and treatment strategies. *Neuropharmacology, 47,* 3–13.

Walsh, S. L., Preston, K. L., Bigelow, G. E., & Stitzer, M. L. (1995). Acute administration of buprenor-phine in humans: Partial agonist and blockade effects. *The Journal of Pharmacology and Experimental Therapeutics, 274,* 361–372.

Walsh, S. L., Preston, K. L., Stitzer, M. L., Cone, E. J., & Bigelow, G. E. (1994). Clinical pharmacology of buprenorphine: Ceiling effects at high doses. *Clinical Pharmacology and Therapeutics, 55,* 569–580.

WHO (2006). *WHO essential medicines library.* http://mednet3.who.int/EMLib/. Accessed on June 1, 2007.

Woody, G. E., McLellan, A. T., Luborsky, L., & O'Brien, C. P. (1990). Psychotherapy and counseling for methadone-maintained opiate addicts: Results of research studies. *NIDA Research Monograph, 104,* 9–23.

18

Inhalants

William D. Crano, Sarah A. Ting, and Vanessa Hemovich

Claremont Graduate University

Contents

Historical Overview and Prevalence

Inhalants are breathable chemical vapors that produce psychoactive or mind-altering effects (National Institute on Drug Abuse: NIDA, 2006). In their administration, inhalants differ from other commonly abused substances in that they are vapors that must be inhaled to have their effect. In the past, other substances that could be inhaled, such as marijuana, cocaine, heroin, and methamphetamines were grouped in the general inhalant category. Today, researchers exclude these drugs from the definition, and restrict inhalants to include any volatile chemical substance that is deliberately inhaled, sniffed, or sprayed directly into the nose or mouth for the purpose of achieving intoxication. Inhalants can have profound physical and psychological effects. Medical consequences associated with this class of drugs are severe; furthermore, the typical inhalant user is a child or young adolescent who knows relatively little of the toxicity associated with inhalant use. The problems caused by inhalants are real, and apparently growing, in a sector of the population that is extremely vulnerable to the depredations that use of these drugs can bring about. Accordingly, in this chapter we focus primarily on the effects and treatment of inhalant use in the young. In addition, we consider treatment alternatives for inhalant users, and explore treatment strategies that may prove useful in the future.

Classification

Inhalants may be classified as volatile solvents, aerosols, gases, or nitrates (Balster, 1998; Brouette & Anton, 2001; NIDA, 2006). Volatile solvents include art or industrial supply solvents, paint thinners, gasoline, and glue. Aerosols include spray paints, vegetable sprays, fabric protectors, and hair and deodorant sprays. Gases are found in butane lighters, propane tanks, whipping cream dispensers, and nitrous oxide. Nitrates include cyclohexyl, butyl, and amyl nitrate. They are sometimes, although rarely, used for legitimate medical purposes. Nitrous oxide or "laughing gas" is a commonly abused gaseous inhalant substance. In addition to being a prescription anesthetic, nitrous oxide is found in whipped cream dispensers and cooking sprays. Abuse of nitrous oxides has been found to cause deactivation of certain areas of the brain, including the posterior cingulate and regions of the hippocampus (Gyulai et al., 1996) that primarily regulate emotion, memory, and spatial orientation. Other nitrates or "poppers" are inhaled almost exclusively among populations of gay and bisexual men to enhance sexual pleasure. Nitrates induce muscle relaxation by dilating blood vessels throughout the body. They produce feelings of euphoria, floating sensations, vertigo, increased skin sensitivity, and muscle relaxation (Campagna, Miller, & Forman, 2003; Newell, Spitz, & Wilson, 1988; Ridenour, 2005). Inhalation triggers a sudden drop in blood pressure, fainting, mutation at the chromosomal level, hypotension, respiratory failure, and restricted blood flow by way of arteriolar dilation and cardiovascular collapse, which can lead to anoxemia and death.

Mechanisms and Toxicology of Use

Inhalants are commonly found in thousands of commercial and household products. In addition to affording relatively easy access, these products are inexpensive and can be purchased legally. The diverse nature of substances that can be inhaled to induce psychoactive effects creates a multitude of possible pharmacological and physiological consequences. Inhalation involves sniffing substances directly, emptying or spraying a substance into a bag and inhaling the fumes ("bagging"), or soaking a rag with the substance and inhaling the fumes through the mouth ("huffing"). Duration of an inhalant high can range from a few minutes to several hours.

Although a wide range of inhalants may create similar intoxication effects, the psychophysiological consequences of these different chemical compounds vary greatly.

Because volatile solvents are highly soluble, they enter the bloodstream quickly to induce a rapid onset of intoxication, which may present as slurred speech, disorientation, and hallucinations. These substances are absorbed quickly in the lungs and deposited in organs and tissues of high lipid or fatty contents such as the kidneys, liver, and adrenal glands. Inhaled substances remain in the body for extended periods of time (NIDA, 2005). Their absorption into the fatty tissues renders detoxification difficult and lengthy, and the slow release of toxins into the bloodstream often inhibits remarkable withdrawal symptoms (Fornazarri, 1988).

Inhalant use can trigger a multitude of detrimental health consequences, which include chronic coughing, wheezing, hallucinations, hearing loss, organ failure, suppression of the immune system, bone marrow deficiency, cardiac morbidity, vomiting, and death by suffocation or asphyxia (Anderson & Loomis, 2003; Anthony, Warner, & Kessler, 1994; Bowen & Balster, 1999; Filley, Heaton, & Rosenberg, 1990; Ridenour, 2005). Chronic toluene abuse has been linked to cerebral and brainstem atrophy and reduced white matter in periventricular portions of the brain (Aydin et al., 2002; Caldemeyer, Pascuzzi, Moran, & Smith, 1993; Meadows & Verghese, 1996; Rosenberg et al., 1988; Yamanouchi et al., 1995). Rosenberg, Grigsby, Dreisbach, Busenbark, and Grigsby (2002) found that even after controlling for age, education, and ethnicity, chronic inhalant users demonstrated greater levels of cognitive impairment and less effective working memories than chronic cocaine users. Even a single session of inhalant use can result in what is known as sudden sniffing death, which occurs as a result of ventricular fibrillation and heart failure (Bass, 1970; NIDA, 2006). Cardiac fibrosis, hypoxia, and arrhythmia also are common outcomes of persistent volatile solvent inhalation (Shepard, 1989).

Trends and Statistics

Older children and young adolescents represent the modal inhalant user. The rapid onset and relatively short-term high produced by inhalants, accompanied by their ready accessibility, are attractive features for youthful users. The number of youth engaging in inhalant use remains troublesome. After marijuana, inhalants are one of the most widely used drugs of choice among youth. Nearly 4.7 million adolescents reported lifetime inhalant use in 2005 (PDFA, 2005). According to the PDFA (2004), inhalant use has increased 44% among 6th graders (from 18 to 26%) and by 18% among 8th graders (from 22 to 26%). Among 8th graders in particular, inhalant use rose significantly, from 7.7% in 2002 to 9.6% in 2004 (Johnston et al., 2004). Today, 8.3% of 8th graders, 6.6% of 10th graders, and 3.7% of 12th graders report having used inhalants at least once in their lifetime (Johnston et al., 2008). Unlike the development of other drug use trajectories, inhalant use typically declines as users grow older and expanding social networks facilitate access to other illicit substances. It is common for youthful inhalant users to transition as rapidly as they can to marijuana and other illicit substances (Bennett, Walters, Miller, & Woodall, 2000; Wu & Howard, 2007; Young, Longstaffe, & Tenenbein, 1999). Indeed, Siegel, Alvaro, Patel, and Crano (2008a) found that older adolescents considered inhalants a "kid's drug" to be used only if other, more grown-up drugs (e.g., marijuana) were unobtainable. Inhalant users generally were demeaned as immature and unable to obtain "real" drugs. SAMHSA (2004) reports that the most commonly used inhalants used by adolescent are glue, shoe polish, and toluene (30.3%). Nitrous oxide (24.9%), gasoline or lighter fluid (24.9%), and spray paint (23.4%) also were common.

Age of usage onset appears to have an important relation with later substance use. Youth who reported inhalant use at 13–14 years of age were six times more likely to develop inhalant-dependence problems than youth who reported adoption at ages 15–17 (Wu, Pilowsky, & Schlenger, 2004). Early onset of inhalant use also has been linked to future hard drug and alcohol abuse, as well as later dependence in adulthood (Bennett, Walters, Miller, & Woodall, 2000; Dinwiddie, Reich, & Cloninger, 1991b; Schutz, Chilcoat, & Anthony, 1994; Soderberg, 1998; Storr, Westergaard, & Anthony, 2005; Wu & Howard, 2007; Young et al., 1999). Sharpening these findings, Johnson, Schutz, Anthony, and Ensminger (1995) discovered that individuals who reported inhalant use in early adolescence were nine times more likely than noninhalant users to have initiated heroin use as adults.

Among various racial and ethnic groups in the United States, research suggests greater prevalence rates for inhalant use among Native American and Hispanic American adolescents (Bachman et al., 1991; Compton et al., 1994; Gfellner & Hundleby, 1995; Mackesey-Amiti & Fendrich, 1999; Mosher, Rotolo, Phillips, Krupski, & Stark, 2004; Neumark, Delva, & Anthony, 1998). Various sociocultural factors may play a role with regard to inhalant use in these groups. Researchers postulate that marginalized ethnic groups experiencing low socioeconomic status or poverty are particularly susceptible to inhalants (Dinwiddie, 1994). Rural or reservation-based Native American youth engage in inhalant use more often than their Native American peers in urban settings (Howard, Walker, Walker, Cottler, & Compton, 1999), and Ramirez et al. (2004) found rural adolescents five times more likely to have used inhalants in the past 30 days than their urban counterparts. Native American inhalant users also are more likely than Native American nonusers to come from impoverished families (Howard et al., 1999).

Other prominent risk factors for inhalant use include dysfunctional family environment, low socioeconomic status, low academic achievement, and chronic absenteeism from school (Compton et al., 1994; Dinwiddie, 1994; Howard & Jenson, 1999; Kozel et al., 1995; Oetting & Webb, 1992; Pagare, Meena, Singh, & Saha, 2004; Sakai et al., 2004). Participation in deviant or delinquent acts also predicts inhalant abuse (Wu et al., 2004). Research suggests that incarcerated adolescents are more likely to use inhalants before other illicit substances (Young et al., 1999). Unlike other drugs, affiliation with drug-using peer groups does not always act as a precursor for future inhalant use (Mosher et al., 2004). Inhalant use often is depicted as a solitary activity that takes place in the home, in the absence of peers, although McGarvey and colleagues (1999) found that adolescents may use inhalants with other drug-using peers and in other social contexts. A number of psychological factors also appear strongly associated with inhalant use. Controlling for age, race, and gender, inhalant users often are more likely than nonusers to exhibit antisocial personality disorder (Compton et al., 1994), and to report greater feelings of hopelessness and episodes of major depression, low self-esteem, and feelings of alienation and suicide (Dinwiddie, Reich, & Cloninger, 1991a; Edeh, 1989; Howard & Jenson, 1999; Kelder, Orpinas, & McReynolds, 2001; Mackesey-Amiti & Fendrich, 1999; Swadi, 1996).

Despite ongoing research, causal interpretation of many of these relationships remains uncertain. For instance, it is not clear if inhalant use impairs learning and leads to poorer academic achievement (Oetting & Webb, 1992), or if doing poorly in school leads to inhalant use

(Dinwiddie, 1994; Howard & Jenson, 1999). Similarly, it is not clear if delinquency predicts inhalant use (Wu et al., 2004), or if inhalant use predicts delinquency (Mosher et al., 2004).

Although inhalants are associated with serious health consequences and even death, users remain largely unaware of the dangers of sniffing toxic chemicals to get high. Public knowledge regarding the risks of inhalant use also is lacking, and parents continue to underestimate the likelihood that their child may be in danger of initiating use. Establishing effective inhalant prevention and treatment programs remains largely undeveloped. Although much has been learned about inhalants, relatively few preventative strategies are available to deter youth from initiating experimentation with these substances (but see Crano et al., 2007; Crano, Gilbert, Alvaro, & Siegel, 2008a).

Guidelines for Assessing and Treating Inhalant Abuse

Recognizing Inhalant Abuse

The first step in treating inhalant abuse is to recognize the signs of use. Teenagers who use inhalants may have chapped faces or lips; paint stains on their faces, hands, or clothes; a chemical odor on their breath; or bloodshot eyes. Empty spray paint or solvent containers and chemical-soaked rags or clothing are other indicants of inhalant use. Common symptoms of inhalant use include a drunk and disordered appearance, slurred speech, nausea, loss of appetite, lack of coordination, and irritability. Inhalant users often complain of persistent headaches, dizziness, memory loss, sleep disorders, or vision problems. Their work in school is subpar, and attendance often suffers as well.

Assessment

Classifying the Inhalant User and Abuser   Although several sociological, psychological, and ethnographic similarities have been found among inhalant abusers, a universally accepted classification system has not yet evolved (Texas Commission on Alcohol and Drug Abuse; TCADA, 1997). Regardless, prior to treatment, it is necessary to recognize that inhalant abusers, specifically volatile solvent abusers, usually suffer from many psychological and social problems in addition to chemical abuse (Oetting & Webb, 1992). One useful system classes users into one of three categories: (1) young inhalant users, (2) polydrug users, and (3) inhalant-dependent adults (Oetting, Edwards, & Beauvais, 1988). Individuals qualify as young inhalant users if they are less than 14 years old and use inhalants over an extended period of weeks or months. The polydrug user category requires additional clarification before definitive assignment. This is a unique category that often is confounded with the multidrug user (TCADA, 1997). A *multidrug* user is an individual who consumes several different drugs at the same time; a *polydrug* user uses several drugs, often in consecutive order, but only one at a time (TCADA, 1997). Polydrug users tend to be older adolescents between the ages of 14 and 18 who use a variety of drugs, including inhalants. For those classed as inhalant-dependent adults, inhalants are the drug of choice. Inhalant-dependent adults often are alcohol or drug users who cannot afford these substances, and use inhalants as an inexpensive alternative. Nearly continuous inhalant use characterizes the inhalant-dependent adult.

It is not sufficient to distinguish drug users from nonusers (Fishbein, Hall-Jamieson, Zimmer, von Haeften, & Nabi, 2002; Fishbein et al., 2002; Siegel, Alvaro, & Burgoon, 2003). A distinction must be made between those abusing inhalants, those who have used inhalants once or twice, and those who may have experimented with inhalants for a brief period (Jumper-Thurman & Beauvais, 1992). In addition to the user and nonuser categorization, Crano et al. (2007; Crano, Siegel, Alvaro, Lac, & Hemovich, 2008b) categorized nonusers as resolute or vulnerable, and showed that these classifications have implications for drug use intentions and actual use.

Three primary determinants of intention are identified by Fishbein's (2000) model: (1) attitude toward performing a behavior, (2) perceived norms concerning performance of the behavior, and (3) self-efficacy with respect to performance. To understand why people do or do not hold a given intention (or perform a given behavior), it is important first to determine the degree to which that intention (or behavior) is under attitudinal, normative, or self-efficacy control. According to Fishbein's (2000) model, a behavior is most likely to occur if the individual has a strong intention to perform the behavior, has the necessary skills and abilities, and there are no contextual or other constraints preventing the behavior's performance. The primary implication of this model is that interventions should vary depending on respondents' intentions. For example, an intervention for an individual who intends to engage in a behavior but is unable to do so should be different from an intervention directed at someone who has little or no intention to perform the specified behavior (Crano, Siegel, Alvaro, & Patel, 2007).

Physical and Psychological Assessment   Although physical examinations are routine in most substance abuse treatment intake procedures, medical examinations hold particular importance for inhalant abusers (Jumper-Thurman & Beauvais, 1992; Sharp & Rosenberg, 1991). Physical damage among users is common, particularly in cases of chronic solvent use, and can impede treatment progress if not diagnosed properly (Hormes, Filley, & Rosenberg, 1986; Nicholi, 1983; Rosenberg & Sharp, 1992). During physical examination, several medical complications must be assessed. Problems of (1) central nervous system damage, (2) renal and hepatic abnormalities, (3) lead poisoning, (4) cardiac arrhythmia, (5) pulmonary distress, and (6) nutritional deficiencies must be determined before adequate diagnosis and treatment can proceed.

Neurological impairment often is detected in inhalant abusers during treatment intake (Jumper-Thurman & Beauvais, 1992), but it is difficult to know whether these problems existed prior to inhalant use. It is critical to determine before beginning treatment whether patients have cognitive deficiencies that may impede treatment or contribute to disruptive behavior. Reidel et al. (1995) recommend the Halstead–Reitan Neuropsychological Test Battery (HRNTB; Reitan, 1959) to assess cognitive impairment. The HRNTB assesses the likelihood of brain damage while offering a comprehensive view of a patient's individual functions. It consists of a fixed set of eight tests used to evaluate brain and nervous system functioning in persons aged 15 years and older. Children's versions are available (the Reitan Indiana Neuro-psychological Test Battery for ages 5–8 and the Halstead Neuropsychological Test Battery for Older Children, aged 9–14). The HRNTB typically is used to evaluate children with suspected brain damage.

The battery provides useful information regarding the cause of damage, which part of the brain was damaged, whether damage occurred during childhood development, and whether the damage is progressing, staying the same, or ameliorating. Information regarding severity of impairment and areas of personal strengths can be used to develop rehabilitation or care plans. The purpose of the battery is to provide the clinician with a database for inferring the nature, location, and extent of structural changes in the brain that may explain the pattern of intact and impaired functions derived from the measures and qualitative information obtained. The present battery consists of 10 tests that have been shown empirically to discriminate best between those with normal cognitive functioning and patients with documented cortical damage. Through this battery, a Neurocognitive Deficit Score (NDS; Reitan & Wolfson, 1988) is determined for each patient. The HRNTB has been normed for children (ages 14 and younger) and adults (15 years and older). The NDS reflects the extent of each patient's neurocognitive impairment. To chart progress in treatment, the NDS is assessed at some point near intake and again at discharge. The difference between intake and discharge NDS scores allows for assessment of change in neurocognitive functioning.

This assessment should be administered two weeks following treatment intake to determine neurocognitive impairment and to facilitate formulating a specific neurocognitive rehabilitation program. Testing should be repeated in several months as well as at discharge to assess progress. To date, there is no conclusive evidence that neurological damage from inhalant abuse can be reversed, but reports from treatment professionals indicate that dramatic improvement in functioning can occur over the course of several weeks' treatment (Reidel et al., 1995).

Neurocognitive rehabilitation may seem daunting; however, Reidel and his colleagues found that their inhalant-specific treatment program, the Reitan Evaluation of Hemispheric Abilities and Brain Improvement Training (REHABIT; Reitan & Senac, 1983) was effective as a treatment for inhalant abusers classified as neurocognitively impaired or nonimpaired. Impaired functioning is characterized by disturbance in consciousness involving reduced clarity of awareness of the environment, changes in cognition including alteration in attention, disorganized thinking, disturbed psychomotor activity, and an abnormal sleep–wake cycle (APA, 2000). This change in consciousness is associated with cognitive abnormalities that may include memory impairment, disorientation, or language disturbance such as inability to name objects or to write, or the development of perceptual disturbances, which may include misinterpretations, illusions, or hallucinations. As impairment covers a wide range of potential barriers, the guiding principle of REHABIT is that remediation should focus on, and target, specific areas of deficit, rather than creating broad strategies to compensate for general neurological impairments. Specific areas of deficit are determined by the results of the HRNTB.

REHABIT is organized along five tracks (A–E) of neurocognitive remediation, which include two tracks (A–B) of remediation activities for basic and higher-level language-based function, two tracks (D–E) of remediation activities for basic and higher-level visual–spatial and visual–motor function, and a central track (C) involving remediation activities that involve logic, reasoning, and problem solving that are not highly dependent on language or visual–spatial skills.

Track A involves developing cognitive abilities in the area of verbal, language, and academic competence. These include preliminary reading skills, such as vocabulary building, practice with word beginnings and endings, reading comprehension, handwriting, and improving auditory verbal comprehension skills. Individuals who have difficulties in academic subject matter or have neuropsychological evaluations indicating learning disabilities should receive specific training with the auditory verbal comprehension materials in Track A (Reitan, 1992).

Track B also is focused on verbal and language content; however, the material is more difficult than Track A's, necessitating greater proficiency in complex abstraction and reasoning abilities. Exercises in this section require the individual to associate pictorial representations with numerical or verbal symbols.

Track C is the central feature of REHABIT. It is concerned with basic abilities in abstraction and reasoning, and is designed to establish a link between verbal and language skills (left cerebral hemisphere) and spatial/manipulative abilities (right cerebral hemisphere). Little emphasis is placed on task content. Reitan (1992) emphasizes that rebuilding basic brain functioning during this phase is an important prerequisite for training specific skills. The REHABIT process acknowledges that until the individual develops ample abstraction and reasoning ability, in addition to the capacity to understand complex situations, the prognosis for successful training of basic academic skills is dismal.

Track D reflects right hemisphere functioning. It involves visual–spatial, tactile–spatial, and sequential tasks. Materials in this track emphasize development of skills in naming, counting, sorting, grouping, and recall. To address the visual–spatial aspect, exercises require perception of the stimulus material through central processing and expression of a response.

Track E focuses on providing basic experiences related to spatial relationships. Tasks include learning to draw various shapes, acknowledging spatial relationships (e.g., over and under), solving puzzles, developing visual–motor skills, directionality, and memory and concentration. More advanced aspects of Track E address training in visual perception of details. These exercises allow for an evaluation of the individual's problem-solving skills, as well as integration of procedures to help the client complete tasks more efficiently.

Social Groups and Treatment

Beyond biological considerations, assessment of family stability, structure, and dynamics must be a major component of any adolescent inhalant abuse treatment program. Treatment providers need to recognize that alcohol and other drug abuse are common for siblings and parents of inhalant abusers (Jumper-Thurman & Beauvais, 1992). Poor communication, sadness, and physical, emotional, and psychological abuse also are common occurrences in the home. Treatment should focus on therapeutic intervention with the family by providing drug education, parenting, and social bonding skills.

In addition, exploring peer group dynamics is important as peers are consistently implicated as a powerful influence in adolescent drug use (Oetting & Beauvais, 1986). This is particularly relevant for adolescent inhalant abusers because their peer groups tend to be deviant, increasing the likelihood of positive social influences toward inhalant use (Crano et al., 2008a; Oetting & Webb, 1992). For younger children, sniffing and huffing often occurs in groups.

Assessment should consider the norms and structure of the peer group to develop treatment goals that help users break negative peer group bonds and replace them with more positive peer groups (Jumper-Thurman & Beauvais, 1992). Best results are derived from understanding what initially attracted the inhalant abuser to the peer group (Leal, Mejia, Gomez, & Salinas, 1978).

Diagnosis

Inhalant abusers share common characteristics that may help identify them as users. Special attention should be directed toward the signs and symptoms commonly associated with persons who abuse inhalants. Assessment should include inquiry about other drugs of abuse and a family history of drug and alcohol use or addiction. The diagnostic criteria are based solely on the history and a very high index of suspicion. Referencing the *DSM–IV* criteria is integral for accurately identifying, assessing, and diagnosing inhalant abuse (American Psychiatric Association, 2000).

Treatment

Inhalant abusers are considered a hidden population primarily because they do not actively seek treatment. The most effective referral strategies involve communication between providers to offer the most comprehensive treatments (Jumper-Thurman, Plested, & Beauvais, 1995). However, treatment for inhalant abuse raises myriad issues. Many substance abuse treatment providers believe that there is no hope for inhalant abusers and often are reluctant to accept them into treatment (Jumper-Thurman et al., 1995). This extreme pessimism is not supported by the evidence. Inhalant abusers do respond to treatment, albeit more slowly than other substance users, emphasizing the need for setting realistic expectations to prevent burnout by staff. Adolescents entering treatment often are angry and apprehensive about the treatment environment and anxious about being separated from family and friends. Inhalant abusers often are impaired cognitively, and this prevents them from taking part effectively in academic and treatment sessions. Accordingly, initial interventions should be very brief (15 to 30 minutes), informal, and concrete. Walking and talking sessions may facilitate development of rapport and encourage interaction. The inhalant abuser's attention span and complexity of thinking are greatly reduced in the early stages of treatment. Thus, cognition should be continually assessed to determine changing levels of functioning. The "typical" 28-day current treatment stay is far too short to realistically expect change. One reason for this is the prolonged period inhalants persist in the body. Treatment time is uncertain and typically requires months, not weeks. The White Buffalo Youth Inhalant Treatment Centre in Saskatchewan, Canada, one of the few facilities in North America dedicated to treatment of young inhalant abusers, describes itself as a six-month residential inhalant abuse treatment program for adolescents. Intensive aftercare and follow-up are essential to rebuild life skills and reintegrate the client with school, family, and community. Consistent with Fiorentine and Anglin's (1996) research, Reidel et al. (1995) suggest that inhalant abuse programs allow a minimum stay of 90–120 days to observe effects of substance abuse treatment (see also Dell, Dell, & Hopkins, 2005).

Detoxification   Because chemicals are stored in the fatty tissues of the body, the inhalant abuser may experience residual effects of inhalant use for quite some time. These effects could include altered affect and dullness of intellectual functioning. The inhalant detoxification period requires several weeks, not days, which is more than that allotted for other drugs. The current suggested timeframe to prepare sufficiently for treatment is, at minimum, four weeks. Not allowing sufficient time for detoxification often limits the client's capacity to engage in the various therapeutic phases of treatment (Jumper-Thurman et al., 1995). During the detoxification process, the focus should be on providing the patient with basic care: nutrition, exercise, sleep, and a calm environment. Group session attendance should be encouraged, but participation should not be required. Informal engagement in the treatment program will provide the client an opportunity to become acquainted with the staff, in addition to becoming familiarized with treatment procedures. Treatment programs should be prepared to engage the inhalant abuser in an extended period of supportive care marked by abstinence from inhalants. Nonconfrontation and an emphasis on basic life skills are recommended. Action therapies involving art, music, drumming, dance, and activities that require hand–eye coordination may be beneficial. Recreational activities that encourage multisensory action also may facilitate recovery.

Peer Advocates   Feedback from patients and providers indicates that upon treatment admission, adolescent inhalant abusers are distant and hard to reach, yet anxious to bond to a peer group (Jumper-Thurman et al., 1995). With this in mind, some facilities have used "peer patient advocate" systems, which pair a "peer" who is further along in the treatment process with the incoming adolescent client. Although reported as effective by adolescents in treatment, there must be close staff monitoring of the peer–patient relationship.

Many health programs, specifically those focused on issues regarding sexual health (e.g., condom use, HIV/STD testing), encourage the integration of peer advocates into the intervention regimen (Mosena, Ely, Ho, & Ruch-Ross, 2004). The Peer Advocates for Health (PAH) program employs male adolescents as educators in a program to increase condom use among adolescent African-American males. An eight-week training session is required during the summer to bolster knowledge on the topic, instill confidence, and create a network among the peer advocates (Mosena et al., 2004). Rational behavior models suggest that changes in knowledge are necessary, but not sufficient, to change behavior (Glanz, Lewis, & Rimer, 1997). These frameworks suggest that changes in attitudes, skill levels, and self-efficacy also must occur. Peer advocates provide a unique and seemingly effective way to encourage behavior change leading to an attenuation of destructive health decisions.

Family Involvement   Family involvement is a key component to retaining and effectively treating those who are abusing inhalants (Mason, 1979). Management programs targeting inhalant abusers are included in the maintenance program guidelines for parents on how to improve listening skills, provide ample affection, and support activities such as sports (Smart, 1986). Research indicates that children and adolescents model the behavior of their siblings and parents (Gfroerer, 1987). Therefore, parents of recovering inhalant abusers provide a good example by avoiding cigarette, alcohol, and other drug use.

Community Involvement   In a clinical review of inhalants, Brouette and Anton (2001) stressed that although treatment of inhalant use is important, the growing challenge of inhalant abuse is better viewed as a public health issue. To improve prevention and intervention responses, community members, family, and friends must be made aware of the prevalence and dangers of inhalant use. Community-based programs should be tailored to the needs of the community. For example, prevention efforts for gasoline sniffing in Canada will differ from glue sniffing prevention efforts for Hispanics in Arizona (Smart, 1986).

Prevention

Treatment is an integral part of reducing inhalant abuse; however, efforts to "stop the addiction before it starts" should not be discounted. Prevention efforts including legal, community, and school-based education programs have been implemented to prevent initiation of inhalant use (Smart, 1986). For instance, the city of Winnipeg passed a bylaw that prohibited the sale of solvents to anyone under the age of 18 and required the removal of glue, paint thinner, and other solvents from open shelves where they could be stolen easily. Although enforcement officials reported that the laws were useful, they often are viewed as ineffective because minors can access solvents and inhalants in their own homes. Other considerations designed to prevent solvent use focus on implementing chemical inhibitors to reduce or eliminate the intoxicating effects of inhalants (e.g., Fernandez, 1978; Lee, Schiffer, & Dewey, 2004; Wega, 1978). However, these additives also affected individuals not intending to use the substances for purposes of intoxication, resulting in falling sales, and eventually the removal of denaturants in these products (Fernandez, 1978).

Another effective prevention method is education, yet there are relatively low levels of community concern about inhalant abuse (Crano et al., 2007; Smart, 1986). Often, inhalant use is not seen as a problem even in communities in which abuse is prevalent, because only 10–12% of youth are involved. However, considering the dangers of inhalants and the difficulty of treating inhalant abusers, user numbers alone should not be a determining factor for community involvement. Responsible adults must support prevention efforts in their communities, and the first step in the process may involve persuading other adults of the necessity of such programs.

Case Presentation

Alex is a 12-year-old male, currently in the sixth grade. He is a good student with an A average and no negative behavior reports from his teachers. Over the past six months, however, his parents report that he has become withdrawn and irritable. His relationship with his parents has suffered, in part because his attendance in school has fallen off. His usual happy demeanor has been replaced by a somewhat depressed and aggressive comportment. Mood swings have become common. His parents attributed these changes to his unhappiness about their impending divorce, and to the fact that Alex's best friend had moved across country. Furthermore, they viewed these changes as somewhat expected, as other parents of adolescents had reported similar behaviors. Around the time of these noteworthy changes, Alex began complaining of frequent headaches, and his parents noticed that his nose was often irritated and runny. They attributed this to allergies. After his friend moved, Alex dropped out of all clubs and extracurricular activities, claiming that he was "too busy to be bothered." His parents noted a significant increase in interest in art projects, however, and recalled his frequent need for paints, solvents, markers, and correction fluid.

Three weeks ago, Alex was found unconscious in the backyard. A fuel container for a butane cigarette lighter and a plastic bag were found next to him. There also were several bottles of correction fluid in his pocket. Paramedics examined him and noticed that his face and lips were slightly chapped, there were remnants of correction fluid on his hands, and a chemical odor on his breath. At the advice of the attending physicians, Alex's parents immediately transferred him to a substance abuse treatment facility upon his release from the hospital. Prior to admission, a clinician there assessed Alex and diagnosed him as inhalant dependent. The therapist based this diagnosis on the *DSM–IV* criteria noting behavioral changes observed by Alex's parents, his poor attendance at school, and his depressive symptoms. In addition, the therapist noted Alex's report of a marked increase in inhalant tolerance, his withdrawal from activities he had enjoyed previously, and Alex's admission that he had been rendered unconscious more than once by inhalant use. As inhalants affect a wide range of physiological functions, the clinician immediately referred Alex for medical examinations and neurological testing in a residential treatment facility. Several weeks were allotted for sufficient detoxification; afterward, the HRNTB was administered. As no evidence of cognitive impairment or brain damage was evident, Alex was allowed to attend group therapy sessions. He was not required to participate.

Initially recalcitrant, Alex's gradual integration into group therapy helped the therapist determine that he was ready to advance through the various stages of treatment. In addition to group therapy, Alex received individual and family counseling. Over the course of his treatment, Alex befriended James, a peer counselor who was nearing discharge from the treatment facility.

After two months of relatively intensive treatment, Alex returned home to relative normalcy. He appears to have suffered no permanent damage from his inhalant abuse. He is intact cognitively and his grades are improving steadily. His coordination, speech, and motivation level appear to match his preinhalant status. His circle of friends has grown, and he expresses a positive outlook. Alex's treatment coordinator calls weekly, as does his friend James, who has become an "older brother" for Alex. His parents now devote extra time to Alex, even though their marriage has ended. He appears to enjoy the company of both parents. The outlook for Alex is positive. He appears to have weathered the storm.

This case could have had a variety of different and almost inevitably less positive outcomes. Alex's inhalant use could have caused substantial neurological damage. If this had occurred, his recovery to normalcy, if it occurred, surely would have been delayed significantly. Alex might have proved resistant to treatment. Again, this behavior would have resulted in a more negative prognosis. Prior to his admission, Alex might have developed a group of friends whose common bond was inhalant use. Returning to this group upon discharge would have proved extremely risky. All of these factors are noted to provide a sense of the precariousness of inhalant use, once it is initiated, and to emphasize the point that has underscored all of this presentation, namely that prevention rather than its cure is the indicated and more certain option.

Conclusions

Not all substances are created equal. Inhalant abuse treatment requires many unique considerations. Current inhalant abuse treatment practices involve adapting strategies from other substance abuse treatment programs. However, due to interruptions in their thought processes, inhalant abusers tend to have diminished reasoning skills and less resistance than alcoholics and other drug abusers (Fornazzari, 1988). Furthermore, the extended detoxification time needed, the array of neurological impairments that inhalant abusers present, and the social and psychological problems they face, suggest a need for inhalant abusers to be treated separately from other drug abusers. Retention is a concern for every type of substance abuse treatment, but it is even more critical for inhalant abusers as they experience higher dropout and expulsion rates than any other type of drug abuser (Mason, 1979). Recreational or activity therapy is useful in maintaining interest in a treatment program. Going to the homes of abusers to engage them in treatment also has proved effective (Mason, 1979).

Those involved in treating the inhalant abuser need to be aware of all aspects of inhalant abuse. There is a definite need to educate intake and assessment staff on the dangers and complexity of inhalants. One problem specific to inhalant treatment is the frustration of the treatment staff over the slow rate of recovery exhibited by the abuser. Proper training and education on the progression and effects of the disorder will help staff develop reasonable expectations and maintain morale. Before contemplating involvement in inhalant abuse treatment, one must be prepared to work with individuals who have a greater breadth and depth of personal and social problems (Jumper-Thurman & Beauvais, 1992). Treatment generally is long-term, with several weeks required for detoxification alone. Creating a comprehensive treatment plan that attacks the diversity of problems presented by inhalant-abusing patients facilitates the treatment process for practitioner and patient.

In summarizing findings from an inhalant abuse treatment program created to treat rural inhalant-abusing youth in South Dakota, Reidel et al. (1995) emphasized the importance of increasing awareness and educating health care professionals about inhalant abuse. Reidel and his colleagues made several suggestions on how to stimulate systemwide prevention efforts. These recommendations include an advisory board in which each level of service delivery is represented (e.g., treatment providers, administrators, medical professionals). Educating professionals about inhalants could be done via workshops specific to inhalant-related topics at local, national, and international events. Educational videos could be designed and distributed to educate and inform professionals across the region on the dangers and signs of inhalant abuse, and using media sources for news releases and awareness campaigns could become a priority. Admittedly, these suggestions merely scratch the surface of possibilities; the important point is that local, regional, and national networks are needed to ameliorate the lack of knowledge of inhalants, their etiology, outcomes, and treatments. Meanwhile, to learn more about inhalant prevention, the scope of the problem, and resources for assistance, we suggest the following sources.

Alliance for Consumer Education
website: www.inhalants.org.

American Council for Drug Education
1.488.DRUG
http://www.acde.org.

National Inhalant Prevention Coalition (NIPC)
website: http://www.inhalants.org/guidelines.htm
Telephone: 800-269-4237.

National Institute on Drug Abuse
website: www.nida.nih.gov.

National Clearinghouse for Alcohol and Drug Information
1.800.SAY.NOTO
http://ncadi.samhsa.gov.

Office of Applied Statistics
website: www.oas.samhsa.gov.

White Buffalo Youth Inhalant Treatment Centre
website: www.addictionresourceguide.com/listings/white.html.

Acknowledgments

Preparation of this chapter was facilitated by a grant R01-DA015957-03 from the National Institute on Drug Abuse to the first author, which we gratefully acknowledge. The contents of this chapter are solely the responsibility of the authors and do not necessarily reflect the views of the National Institute on Drug Abuse.

References

American Psychiatric Association (APA). (2000). *Diagnostic and statistical manual of mental disorders–Text revision.* (4th ed., pp. 257–264). Washington, DC: Author.
Anderson, C. E., & Loomis, G. A. (2003). Recognition and prevention of inhalant abuse. *American Family Physician, 68,* 869–874.
Anthony, J. C., Warner, L. A., & Kessler, R. C. (1994). Comparative epidemiology of dependence on tobacco, alcohol. Controlled substances, and inhalants: Basic findings from the National Comorbidity Study. *Experimental and Clinical Psychopathology, 2,* 244–268.
Aydin, K., Sencer, S., Demir, T., Ogel, K., Tunaci, A., & Minareci, O. (2002). Cranial MR findings in chronic toluene abuse by inhalation. *American Journal of Neuroradiology, 23,* 1173–1179.
Bachman, J. G., Wallace, J. M., O'Malley, P. M., Johnston, L. D., Kurth, C. L., & Neighbors, H. W. (1991). Racial and ethnic differences in smoking, drinking, and illicit drug use among American high school seniors. *American Journal of Public Health, 81,* 372–377.

Balster, R. L. (1998). Neural basis of inhalant use. *Drug and Alcohol Dependence, 51,* 207–214.

Bass, M. (1970). Sudden sniffing death. *Journal of the American Medical Association, 212,* 2075–2079.

Bennett, M. E., Walters, S. T., Miller, J. H., & Woodall, W. G. (2000). Relationship of early inhalant use to substance use in college students. *Journal of Substance Abuse, 12,* 227–240.

Bowen, S. E., & Balster, R. L. (1999). Deaths associated with inhalant abuse in Virginia from 1987 to 1996. *Drug and Alcohol Dependence, 53,* 239–245.

Brouette, T., & Anton, R. (2001). Clinical review of inhalants. *The American Journal on Addictions, 10,* 79–94.

Caldemeyer, K. S., Pascuzzi, R. M., Moran, C. C., & Smith, R. R. (1993). Toluene abuse causing reduced MR signal intensity in the brain. *American Journal of Roentgenology, 161,* 1259–1261.

Campagna, J. A., Miller, K. W., & Forman, S. A. (2003). Mechanisms of actions of inhaled anesthetics. *New England Journal of Medicine, 348,* 2110–2125.

Compton, W. M., Cottler, L. B., Dinwiddie, S. H., Spitznagel, E. L., Mager, D. E., & Asmus, G. (1994). Inhalant use: Characteristics and predictors. *The American Journal on Addictions, 3,* 263–272.

Crano, W. D., Gilbert, C., Alvaro, E. M., & Siegel, J. (2008a). Factors that discriminate inhalant intenders and nonintenders in at-risk and not at-risk samples of early adolescents. *Addictive Behaviors.*

Crano, W. D., Siegel, J. T., Alvaro, E. M., Lac, A., & Hemovich, V. (2008b). The at-risk marijuana nonuser: Expanding the standard distinction. *Prevention Science.*

Crano, W. D., Siegel, J. T., Alvaro, E. M., & Patel, N. M. (2007). Overcoming adolescents' resistance to anti-inhalant appeals. *Psychology of Addictive Behaviors, 21,* 516–524.

Dell, C. A., Dell, D. E., & Hopkins, C. (2005). Resiliency and holistic inhalant abuse treatment. *Journal of Aboriginal Health, March,* 1–12.

Dinwiddie, S. H. (1994). Abuse of inhalants: A review. *Addiction, 89,* 925–939.

Dinwiddie, S. H., Reich, T., & Cloninger, C. R. (1991a). Solvent use as a precursor to intravenous drug use. *Comparative Psychiatry, 32,* 133–140.

Dinwiddie, S. H., Reich, T., & Cloninger, C. R. (1991b). The relationship of solvent use to other substance use. *American Journal of Drug and Alcohol Use, 17,* 173–186.

Edeh, J. (1989). Volatile substance abuse in relation to alcohol and illicit drugs: Psychosocial perspectives. *Human Toxicology, 8,* 313–317.

Fernandez, J. (1978). Solvents – An industrial perspective. In A. Gabe & J. Kurys (Eds.), *Solvents, adhesives, and aerosols* (pp. 1–26). Toronto: Addiction Research Foundation.

Filley, C. M., Heaton, R. K., & Rosenberg, N. L. (1990). White matter dementia in chronic toluene abuse. *Neurology, 40,* 532–534.

Fiorentine, R., & Anglin, M. (1996). More is better: Counseling participation and the effectiveness of outpatient drug treatment. *Journal of Substance Abuse Treatment, 13,* 341–348.

Fishbein, M. (2000). The role of theory in HIV prevention. *AIDS Care, 12,* 273–278.

Fishbein, M., Cappella, J., Hornik, R., Sayeed, S., Yzer, M., & Ahern, R. K. (2002). The role of theory in developing effective anti-drug public service announcements. In W. D. Crano, & M. Burgoon (Eds.), *Mass media and drug prevention: Classic and contemporary theories and research* (pp. 89–117). Mahwah, NJ: Erlbaum.

Fishbein, M., Hall-Jamieson, K., Zimmer, E., von Haeften, I., & Nabi, R. (2002). Avoiding the boomerang: Testing the relative effectiveness of antidrug public service announcements before a national campaign. *American Journal of Public Health, 92,* 238–245.

Fornazzari, L. (1988). Clinical recognition and management of solvent abusers. *Internal Medicine for the Specialist, 9,* 99–109.

Fredlund, E. (1993). *Volatile substance abuse among the Kickapoo people in the Eagle Pass, Texas area, 1993* (pp. 1–30). Austin: Texas Commission on Alcohol and Drug Abuse, November.

Gfellner, B. M., & Hundleby, J. D. (1995). Patterns of drug use among Native and White adolescents: 1990–1993. *Canadian Journal of Public Health, 86,* 95–97.

Gfroerer, J. (1987). Correlation between drug use by teenagers and drug use by older family members. *American Journal of Drug and Alcohol Abuse, 13,* 95–108.

Glanz, K., Lewis, F. M., & Rimer. B. K. (1997). *Health behavior and health education: Theory, research and practice.* San Francisco: Jossey-Bass.

Gyulai, F. E., Firestone, L. L., Mintun, M. A., & Winter, P. M. (1996). In vivo imaging of human limbic responses to nitrous oxide inhalation. *Anesthesia & Analgesia, 83,* 291–298.

Hormes, J., Filley, C., & Rosenberg, N. (1986). Neurologic sequelae of chronic solvent vapor abuse. *Neurology, 36,* 698–702.

Howard, M. O., & Jenson, J. M. (1999). Inhalant use among antisocial youth: Prevalence and correlates. *Addictive Behaviors, 24,* 59–74.

Howard, M. O., Walker, R. D., Walker, P. S., Cottler, L. B., & Compton, W. M. (1999). Inhalant use among urban American Indian youth. *Addiction, 94,* 83–95.

Johnson, E. O., Schutz, C. G., Anthony, J. C., & Ensminger, M. E. (1995). Inhalants to heroin: A prospective analysis from adolescence to adulthood. *Drug and Alcohol Dependence, 40,* 159–164.

Johnston, L. D., O'Malley, P. M., & Bachman, J. G. (2001). *Monitoring the Future national survey results on drug use, 1975–2000: Secondary school students* (NIH Publication No. 01-4924). Rockville, MD: National Institute on Drug Abuse.

Johnston, L. D., O'Malley, P. M., Bachman, J. G., & Schulenberg, J. E. (2004). *Overall teen drug use continues gradual decline; But use of inhalants rises.* Retrieved October 9, 2006, from www.monitoringthefuture.org, accessed October 15, 2006.

Johnston, L. D., O'Malley, P. M., Bachman, J. G., & Schulenberg, J. E. (2008). *Monitoring the Future national results on adolescent drug use: Overview of key findings, 2007* (NIH Publication No. 08-6418). Bethesda, MD: National Institute on Drug Abuse.

Jumper-Thurman, P., & Beauvais, F. (1992). *Treatment of volatile solvent abusers* (National Institute on Drug Abuse [NIDA] Research Monograph 129). Washington, DC: U.S. Government Printing Office.

Jumper-Thurman, P., Plested, B., & Beauvais, F. (1995). *Treatment strategies of volatile solvent abusers in the United States* (National Institute on Drug Abuse [NIDA] Research Monograph 148). Washington, DC: U.S. Government Printing Office.

Kelder, S., Orpinas, P., & McReynolds, L. (2000). Depression and substance use in minority middle-school students. *American Journal of Public Health, 91,* 761–766.

Kozel, N., Sloboda, Z., & De la Rosa, M. (1995). *Epidemiology of inhalant abuse: An international perspective* (NIH Publication No. 95-3831). Rockville, MD: National Institute on Drug Abuse.

Leal, H., Mejia, L., Gomez, L., & Salinas de Valle, O. (1978). Naturalistic study on the phenomenon of inhalant use in a group of children in Mexico City. In: C. W. Sharp & L. T. Carroll (Eds.) *Voluntary inhalation of industrial solvents.* Rockville, MD: National Institute on Drug Abuse.

Lee, D. E., Schiffer, W. K., & Dewey, S. L. (2004). Gamma-vinyl GABA (vigabatrin) blocks the expression of toluene-induced conditioned place preference (CPP). *Synapse, 54,* 183–185.

Macksey-Amiti, M. E., & Fendrich, M. (1999). Inhalant use and delinquent behavior among adolescents: A comparison of inhalant users and other drug users. *Addiction, 94,* 555–564.

Mason, T. (1979). *Inhalant use and treatment* (National Institute on Drug Abuse [NIDA] Research Monograph Series). Washington, DC: U.S. Government Printing Office.

McGarvey, E. L., Clavet, G. J., Mason, W., & Waite, D. (1999). Adolescent inhalant use: Environments of use. *American Journal of Drug and Alcohol Abuse, 25,* 731–741.

Meadows, R., & Verghese, A. (1996). Medical complications of glue sniffing. *Southern Medical Journal, 89,* 455–462.

Mosena, P., Ely, J., Ho, J., & Ruch-Ross, H. (2004). Peer advocates for health: A community-based program to improve reproductive health knowledge and lifestyle choices among adolescent males. *International Journal of Men's Health, 3,* 221–240.

Mosher, C., Rotolo, T., Phillips, D., Krupski, A., & Stark, K. D. (2004). Minority adolescents and substance use risk/protective factors: A focus on inhalant use. *Adolescence, 39,* 489–502.

National Clearinghouse for Alcohol and Drug Information (NCADI). (2000). *Strengthening Substance Abuse Treatment Services for Adolescents.* Retrieved on November 10, 2006, from http://www.recoverymonth.gov/2000/chat2.htm.

National Inhalant Prevention Coalition. (nd.). *Inhalants.* Retrieved on February 8, 2007, from http://www.inhalants.org/guidelines.htm.

National Institute on Drug Abuse (2005). *Research Report: Inhalant Abuse.* Retrieved May 25, 2008, from http://www.drugabuse.gov/PDF/RRInhalants.pdf.

National Institute on Drug Abuse (2006). *NIDA Infofacts: Inhalants*. Retrieved October 31, 2006, from http://www.drugabuse.gov/infofacts/inhalants.html.

Neumark, Y. D., Delva, J., & Anthony, J. C. (1998). The epidemiology of adolescent inhalant drug involvement. *Archives of Pediatrics and Adolescent Medicine, 152,* 781–786.

Newell, G. R., Spitz, M. R., & Wilson, M. B. (1988). *Nitrate inhalants: Historical perspective* (Research Monograph No. 83). Washington, DC: National Institute on Drug Abuse.

Nicholi, A. (1983). The inhalants: An overview. *Psychosomatics, 24,* 914–921.

Oetting, E., & Beauvais, F. (1986). Peer cluster theory: Drugs and the adolescent. *Journal of Counseling & Development, 65,* 17–22.

Oetting, E., Edwards, R., & Beauvais, F. (1988). *Social and psychological factors underlying inhalant abuse* (National Institute on Drug Abuse [NIDA] Research Monograph 85). Washington, DC: U.S. Government Printing Office.

Oetting, E., & Webb, J. (1992). *Psychosocial characteristics and their links with inhalants: A research agenda* (National Institute on Drug Abuse [NIDA] Research Monograph 129). Washington, DC: U.S. Government Printing Office.

Office of Applied Studies. (2001). *Trends in initiation of substance use.* Retrieved on February 1, 2007 from http://www.oas.samhsa.gov/nhsda/2k1nhsda/vol1/chapter5.htm#5.inh.

Office of Applied Studies. (2003). *Results from the 2002 National Survey on Drug Use and Health: National findings* (DHHS Publication No. SMA 03–3836, NHSDA Series H–22). Rockville, MD.

Pagare, D., Meena, G., Singh, M., & Saha, R. (2004). Risk factors of substance use among street children from Delhi. *Indian Pediatrics, 41,* 221–225.

Partnership for a Drug Free America. (2004). *More pre-teens abusing inhalants.* Retrieved on October 9, 2006, from http://www.drugfree.org/Portal/About/NewsReleases/More_Pre_Teens_AbusingInhalants.

Partnership for a Drug Free America. (2005). *The Partnership Attitude Tracking Study.* Retrieved on November 3, 2006, from http://www.drugfree.org/Files/Full_Teen_Report.

Ramirez, J. R., Crano, W. D., Quist, R., Burgoon, M., Alvaro, E. M., & Grandpre, J. (2004). Acculturation, familism, parental monitoring, and knowledge as predictors of marijuana and inhalant use in adolescents. *Psychology of Addictive Behaviors, 18,* 3–11.

Reidel, S., Hebert, T., & Byrd, P. (1995). *Inhalant abuse: Confronting the growing challenge* (Technical Assistance Publication Series No. 17). Rockville, MD: Center for Substance Abuse Treatment.

Reitan, R. M. (1959). *Manual for administration of Neuropsychological Test Batteries for Adults and Children.* Tucson, AZ: Neuropsychological Press.

Reitan, R. M. (1992). *Trail making test: Manual for administration and scoring.* Tucson, AZ: Neuropsychological Press.

Reitan, R. M., & Senac, D. A. (1983). *The efficacy of the REHABIT technique in remediation of brain injured people.* Paper presented at the meeting of the American Psychological Association, Anaheim, CA.

Reitan, R. M. & Wolfson, D. (1988). The Halstead–Reitan neuropsychological test battery and REHABIT: A model for integrating evaluation and remediation of cognitive impairment. *Cognitive Rehabilitation, 6,* 10–17.

Ridenour, T. (2005). Inhalants: Not to be taken lightly anymore. *Current Opinion in Psychiatry, 18,* 243–247.

Rosenberg, N. L., Grigsby, J., Dreisbach, J., Busenbark, D., & Grigsby, P. (2002). Neuropsychologic impairment and MRI abnormalities associated with chronic solvent abuse. *Journal of Toxicology: Clinical Toxicology, 40,* 21–34.

Rosenberg, N. L., Kleinschmidt-DeMasters, B. K., Davis, K. A., Dreisbach, J. N., Hormes, J. T., & Filley, C. M. (1988). Toluene abuse causes diffuse central nervous system white matter changes. *Annals of Neurology, 23,* 611–614.

Rosenberg, N. L., & Sharp, C. (1992). *Solvent toxicity: A neurological focus* (National Institute on Drug Abuse [NIDA] Research Monograph 129). Washington DC: U.S. Government Printing Office.

Sakai, J. T., Hall, S. K., Mikulich-Gilbertson, S. K., & Crowley, T. J. (2004). Inhalant use, abuse, and dependence among adolescent patients: Commonly comorbid problems. *Journal of American Academy of Child and Adolescent psychiatry, 43,* 1080–1088.

Schutz, C. G., Chilcoat, H. D., & Anthony, J. C. (1994). Breach of privacy in surveys on adolescent drug use: A methodological inquiry. *International Journal of Methods in Psychiatric Research, 4*, 183–188.

Sharp, C., & Rosenberg, N. (1991). Volatile substances. In J. Lowinson, P. Ruiz, R. Millman, & J. Langrod (Eds.), *Substance Abuse – A Comprehensive Textbook* (2nd ed., pp. 303–327). Baltimore: Williams & Wilkins.

Shepard, R. T. (1989). Mechanism of sudden death associated with volatile substance abuse. *Human Toxicology, 8*, 287–2291.

Siegel, J. T., Alvaro, E. M., & Burgoon, M. (2003). Perceptions of the at-risk nonsmoker: Are potential intervention topics being overlooked? *Journal of Adolescent Health, 33*, 458–461.

Siegel, J. T., Alvaro, E. M., Patel, N., Crano, & W. D. (in press) "…you would probably want to do it. Cause that's what made them popular": Exploring perceptions of inhalant utility among young adolescent non-users and occasional users. *Substance Use and Misuse*.

Smart, R. (1986). Solvent use in North America: Aspects of epidemiology, prevention and treatment. *Journal of Psychoactive Drugs, 18*, 87–96.

Soderberg, L. S. (1998). Immunomodulation by nitrate inhalants may predispose abusers to AIDS and Kaposi's sarcoma. *Journal of Neuroimmunology, 83*, 157–161.

Storr, C. L., Westergaard, R., & Anthony, J. C. (2005). Early onset inhalant use and risk for opiate initiation by young adulthood. *Drug and Alcohol Dependence, 78*, 253–261.

Substance Abuse and Mental Health Services Administration. (2004). *NSDUH report: Characteristics of recent adolescent inhalant initiates* (Office of Applied Studies, NSDUH Series H-28, DHHS Publication No. SMA 05-4062). Rockville, MD: Substance Abuse and Mental Health Services Administration.

Substance Abuse and Mental Health Services Administration. (2005). *Overview of findings from the 2004 National Survey on Drug Use and Health* (Office of Applied Studies, NSDUH Series H-27, DHHS Publication No. SMA 05-4061). Rockville, MD.

Swadi, H. (1996). Psychiatric symptoms in adolescents who abuse volatile substances. *Addiction Research, 4*, 1–9.

Texas Commission on Alcohol and Drug Abuse. (1997). *Understanding inhalant users: An overview for parents, educators, and clinicians*. Retrieved on October 16, 2006, from http://www.tcada.state.tx.us/research/populations/inhale97.pdf.

Wega, J. (1978). Aerosol product safety. In A. Gabe & J. Kurys (Eds.), *Solvents, adhesives, and aerosols*. (pp. 27–33) Toronto: Addiction Research Foundation.

Wu, L. T., & Howard, M. O. (2007). Is inhalant use a risk factor for heroin and injection drug use among adolescents in the United States? *Addictive Behaviors, 32*, 265–281.

Wu, L. T., Pilowsky, D. J., & Schlenger, W. E. (2004). Inhalant abuse and dependence among adolescents in the United States. *Journal of the American Academy of Child and Adolescent Psychiatry, 43*, 1206–1214.

Yamanouchi, N., Okada, S., Kodama. K., Hirai, S., Sekine, H., Murakami, A., et al. (1995). White matter changes caused by chronic solvent abuse. *American Journal of Neuroradiology, 16*, 1643–1649.

Young, S. J., Longstaffe, S., & Tenenbein, M. (1999). Inhalant abuse and the abuse of other drugs. *American Journal of Drug and Alcohol Abuse, 25*, 371–375.

19

Hallucinogens

Joji Suzuki and John H. Halpern
Harvard Medical School

Torsten Passie
Hannover Medical School

Pedro E. Huertas
Harvard Medical School

Contents

Overview of Hallucinogen Use

Historical Issues

Psychoactive substances derived from plant materials have been used ritualistically for millennia (Schultes, Hofmann, & Rätsch, 2001). Simultaneous developments during the second half of the twentieth century in the biology of the mind and in synthetic organic chemistry have recast natural and synthetic intoxicants in a new biological and clinical light (Nichols, 2004). These chemicals, referred to improperly as "hallucinogens," alter psychoneurobiological behavior in ways both subtle and overt. The term *hallucinogen* implies an induction of hallucinations well known within clinical psychiatry, but this is not the case with most of the substances in question and some of them (i.e., entactogens such as MDMA) do not induce major sensory alterations. The terms *psychotomimetics* (psychosis-mimicking) or *psychedelics* have also been used. "Psychotomimetic" is not in common usage now, because, much as with "hallucinogen," these substances are not primarily psychotogenic, whether mimicking or otherwise, although these drugs can exacerbate or contribute to worsening the mental health of those vulnerable to a formal thought disorder. "Psychedelic" may be the most commonly used lay term for hallucinogens and used to be an accepted alternate descriptor in the scientific literature. The psychiatrist Humphrey Osmond (1957) first offered this term meaning "mind manifesting" and called it "clear, euphonious and uncontaminated by other associations" (which apparently did weigh down the term by the end of the 1960s).

Hallucinogens were primarily used for thousands of years for religious and shamanic purposes. Evidence suggests that Soma of the 3500-year-old Hindu–Aryan Rig Veda (Smith, 2000), and the Kykeon of ancient Greece's Eleusinian Mysteries (Wasson, Ruck, & Hofmann, 1978) may have been botanical hallucinogens. Prehistoric rock art in the Tassili n'Ajjer mountains in Algeria dating from 5000 to 7000 years ago often includes one of a bee-like shaman covered with mushrooms that may have been hallucinogenic (as *Psilocybe cubensis* and related subspecies can be preserved in honey or are sometimes eaten together (Bogusz et al., 1998)) (see Figure 19.1). Hallucinogens played a prominent role in the cultures of Mesoamerican peoples. Indeed, ayahuasca remains an important spiritual medicine of many native peoples of the Amazon Basin (Schultes et al., 2001). The plant *Tabernanthe iboga*, containing the hallucinogen ibogaine, is used in ceremonies of Central African hunter-gatherers (Mbenga Pygmies) and is the sacrament of the West-Central African religion of Bwiti, practiced primarily in Gabon, Cameroon, and Congo (Pope, 1969; Samorini, 1995). The peyote cactus (*Lophophora williamsii*), containing the hallucinogen mescaline, has been venerated for over 3000 years by the Huichol and Tarahumara ethnic groups of

FIGURE 19.1
The Bee-Faced Mushroom Shaman of Tassili-n-Ajjer.

(a)   (b)

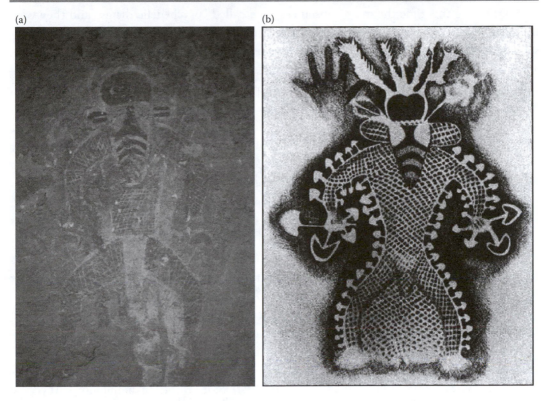

Sources. (a) Reprinted with permission of the photographer, Andras Zboray, www.tassili.net. (b) Drawing by Kathleen Harrison based on the photography of Henri Lhote (1959). The Search for the Tassili Frescoes: The Story of the Prehistoric Rock Paintings of the Sahara. New York: E. P. Dutton,. Reprinted with permission of the artist.

northern Mexico (Schaefer & Furst, 1998) and is the sacrament of the Native American Church (NAC) in the United States and Canada (the NAC is the largest faith among native peoples of North America with some 400,000 adherents; Stewart, 1987). Harvested peyote was recovered from an archeological dig in Texas with radiocarbon dating estimating the specimens to 3780 to 3660 BC (El-Seedi, DeSmet, Beck, Possnert, & Bruhn, 2005). The Spanish Inquisition prohibited the use of peyote, holding some 90 trials from 1614 to 1779 (Stewart, 1987), and Native use was not clearly protected in the United States until the American Indian Religious Freedom Act Amendments of 1994.

In 1938, the Swiss chemist Albert Hofmann synthesized lysergic acid diethylamide (LSD), the 25th compound in a chemical research series to evaluate ergot alkaloid derivatives for analeptics and circulatory and respiratory stimulants. He accidentally exposed himself to LSD in 1943 and three days later on April 19 intentionally ingested LSD (250 mcg. p.o.). Hofmann had a fully hallucinogenic experience. Following his experience and research, hallucinogens became a force of intense interest in psychiatric research and stimulated the discovery of the neurotransmitter systems and their functions in the brain.

Over 10,000 subjects from 1950 to the mid-1960s received LSD (and other hallucinogens) in controlled research settings, resulting in more than 1,000 clinical papers, dozens of books, and six international conferences on psychedelic therapy (Cohen, 1960; Malleson, 1971; Passie, 1997). During this time the main substances were called "psychedelic drugs" and they were used for enhancing creativity (Stafford & Golightly, 1969; Masters & Houston, 1966), de-schematizing of perceptual processes (cf. Schneider, Leweke, Sternemann, Weber, & Emrich, 1966), induction of "experimental psychotic states" (cf. Hollister, 1972), education of psychiatric staff through temporary self-experience of quasi-psychotic states (Beringer, 1927; Grof, 1980), and experimental exploration of religious and mystical experiences (Pahnke, 1963; Griffiths, Richards, McCann, & Jesse, 2006). Another important application was *psycholytic* therapy, where lower dosages (of LSD or psilocybin) were used to induce a dreamlike state with affective and sensory activation to access unconscious material for therapeutic processing in psychoanalytic settings. The American concept of psychedelic therapy used the induction of mystical experiences by high doses for transformation of personality traits (cf. Abramson, 1967; Passie, 1997). These therapeutic approaches were left alone not for reasons of dangers (cf. Cohen, 1960; Malleson, 1971) or inefficacy, but because of criminalization of the substances. Since the 1990s there has been renewal of interest in these therapeutic applications (Winkelman & Roberts, 2007). This is due in part to the specific therapeutic potential of the entactogenic substances such as MDMA and MDE (cf. Holland, 2001).

By the late 1960s LSD was synthesized in underground laboratories and widely distributed for introspective, spiritual, and recreational purposes by laymen. Because of specific historical circumstances, LSD became a lightning rod for the social upheaval of that era, and was "blamed" for catalyzing the antiwar movement, the civil rights movement, women's liberation, and environmentalism (Dyck, 2005; Grob, 1994). Since this time, hallucinogens became readily accessible to Western populations. In these mostly less-structured, "permissive" settings, inexperienced use of these compounds for often careless experimentation, relaxation, thrill-seeking, or other "recreational" purposes (with street doses of LSD typically of 250 mcg or more in the 1960s), resulted not rarely in indirect medical (ex., physical accidents) and/or psychological emergencies (ex., brief psychotic reactions and suicidality) causing emergency room visits (Schwartz, 1995). Thus, devoid of their ritualistic use and traditional contexts, hallucinogens can and do often become drugs of abuse (Halpern, 2004).

An important differentiation which has to be considered here is that there are four major clusters of substances which may be called hallucinogens: (1) the classical hallucinogens (ex., mescaline, psilocybin, LSD, dimethyltryptamine), (2) the entactogenic phenethylamines (MDA, MDMA, MDE, MBDB), (3) the anticholinergic hallucinogens (atropine, hyoscyamine, scopolamine), and (4) miscellaneous hallucinogens (N_2O, ketamine, salvinorin A). This chapter deals mainly with substances of the first two clusters, but mentions the other substances where appropriate or necessary. One reason for this is the less common use and abuse of substances from the other two clusters.

Current Conceptualization

The federal government's Substance Abuse and Mental Health Services Administration's (SAMHSA) National Household Survey on Drug Abuse (NHSDUH) estimates that in year

2006 of Americans aged 12 or older close to 4 million used hallucinogens that year with 1.1 million trying one for the first time ever, and some 35.3 million Americans have tried one at least once in their lifetime (SAMHSA, 2007a). 380,000 Americans age 12 or over are estimated to meet *DSM–IV* criteria for hallucinogen abuse or dependence in 2006 (out of a total of 23.6 million persons classified with any substance abuse or dependence that year; SAMHSA, 2007a). SAMHSA's Drug Abuse Warning Network (DAWN) data for 2005 estimates 16,408 emergency room visits for the entire United States involved a hallucinogen (not including PCP: 7535) with 10,752 for the entactogen MDMA and less than 1,900 for the classical hallucinogen LSD (out of a total of 1.45 million drug-related visits; SAMHSA, 2007b).

Among high school students, the Monitoring the Future data have shown a continuous decline since the late 1990s in the lifetime, annual, and past month use of hallucinogens (Johnston, Bachman, & O'Malley, 2006). In 2006, 8.3% of U.S. 12th graders reported lifetime use of hallucinogens, a drop from 15.1% in 1997 (Johnston et al., 2006).

Far more people are currently ingesting hallucinogens with far fewer acute medical complications than in the supposed heyday of the 1960s. This may be due to the decrease in average street dose of LSD (typically now 50–100 mcg per "hit") and/or due to increased general awareness of respect for mental preparation ("set") and attention to a conducive environment ("setting"; Zinberg, 1986). The calculation of several hundred thousand hallucinogen users in the NHSDUH reporting seeking treatment for hallucinogen use is due to broad inclusion of any type of treatment at all.

Taken together, these numbers indicate that the prevalence of hallucinogen use still is lower compared to other substances of abuse and is significantly lower in morbidity and mortality. The prevalence of the various hallucinogen related disorders is not known.

Although not often encountered now in the emergency room or outpatient office, hallucinogens have remained a force within certain subcultures (e.g., the musical tours of the Grateful Dead band, some large rock music festivals, and other events such as the "Rainbow Gatherings" and "Burning Man" festivals). With the advent of the Internet, formerly "underground" information on hallucinogens became easily available. Because vast amounts of information are posted to the Internet (see www.erowid.org in particular), the Internet has also become an important source for the purchase and distribution of ethnobotanical hallucinogens not yet regulated by governments (Halpern & Pope, 2001).

Rarely noted, many botanical sources of hallucinogenic and/or dissociative compounds exist. Most parts of the United States, and the Americas, have such plants growing indigenously, yet little is known about the extent of their use and abuse (Halpern, 2004).

The typical hallucinogen user is male and of college age (Wright, Sathe, & Spagnola, 2007). Most adolescents in different cultures typically go through a period of experimentation with altered states of consciousness during their search for identity (Grob & Dobkin de Rios, 1992). Not only for this reason, hallucinogen use is typically time-limited. Hallucinogens are not physiologically reinforcing and the profound nature of the experience of altered perception and sense of self may be sometimes terrifying to the user. For example, recent popular press reports on the use/abuse of the plant *Salvia divinorum* increased experimentation in young people as a consequence of hype (Halpern, 2004). *S. divinorum* contains the kappa-opiate agonist salvinorin A which has a brief hallucinogenlike intoxication when smoked or chewed (Roth et al., 2002). The dissociativeness and intensity of the experience with salvinorin A is far more disturbing than recreational: one survey of 32 users noted that 66% stated they would not like to ingest it repeatedly (González, Riba, Bouso, Gómez-Jarabo, & Barbanoj, 2006).

There are important subpopulations of users, as well. One is the adolescent experimenting with different drugs and other risky behaviors in a search for identity who abandons hallucinogen use after a few uses. Then there are the "hippie underground" users (psychedelic "psychonauts") whose life and lifestyle appear to revolve around hallucinogen use or about the dissemination of information about such use. Another, less-numbered, population of particular concern for psychiatrists, are those individuals with dual diagnoses: hallucinogen abusers who also have major psychiatric illness. These are the individuals most likely to present for psychiatric help and their drug use, in general, may be kindling their psychiatric condition or worsening it. Then there are individuals who have sincere religious conviction that their use of hallucinogens is sacramental. The term "entheogen" means "to generate God within" and is now commonly used among those who ingest hallucinogens with this purpose (Ruck, Bigwood, Staples, Ott, & Wasson, 1979). In recent years, seekers of spiritual meaning have sought out "entheogen tours" to the Amazon, for example (De Rios, 1994; 2006; Halpern & Pope, 2001; Winkelman, 2005). There are also legitimate religions existing with hallucinogenic sacraments, and such use is literally the "nondrug sacramental use" rather than the seeking of a drug high. In addition to Native American members of the NAC, some non-Native U.S. citizens have joined religions originating from Brazil that are syncretic, combining elements of Christianity and Native beliefs. These religions include the Santo Daime, the União do Vegetal (UDV), and the Barquinha (Labate & Araujo, 2004). The UDV's right to sacramental ayahuasca has been reviewed in federal court and the U.S. Supreme Court in a unanimous decision sided with the UDV against the federal government, which seeks to deny such religious expression.

Current Concepts

Basic Pharmacology   Table 19.1 lists the more common hallucinogens. As can be seen from the list, the various hallucinogens are wide ranging in dosage and duration. The major hallucinogens exert their effects by sympathomimetic actions on the CNS. This activation may be due to their agonistic properties on different neurotransmitter-modulated brain systems that are serotonergic, adrenergic, and dopaminergic. The serotonergic system appears to be specifically stimulated. It consists of approximately 40,000 neurons, mainly located in the dorsal raphe nucleus of the mid-brain. This tiny population of neurons maintains a widely distributed network throughout the brain which modulates nearly every kind of brain activity.

Despite their heterogeneity, most of the classical hallucinogens appear to exert their major pharmacologic action through their agonist effect on $5\text{-HT}_{2a/c}$ receptors (Nichols, 2004). Hallucinogens have high affinity for 5-HT receptors (González-Maeso & Sealfon, 2006; Roth, Willins, Kristiansen, & Kroeze, 1998), and genetic or pharmacologic inactivation of 5-HT_{2a} receptors blocks behavioral effects in preclinical models as well as subjective effects in humans (Fiorella, Helsley, Lorrain, Rabin, & Winter, 1995; González-Maeso et al., 2003; Vollenweider, Wollenweider-Scherpenhuyzen, Babler, Vogel, & Hell, 1998). Yet why do only some 5-HT_{2a} agonists induce hallucinogenic effects whereas others do not? One group has reported that hallucinogenic 5-HT_{2a} agonists differ from nonhallucinogenic 5-HT_{2a} agonists

TABLE 19.1
Common Hallucinogens (Partial List)

Class	Chemical Name	Common or Street Name	Source	Dosage	Route	Duration of Action	Major Neurobiological Target	Notes
Indole-alkylamines	Lysergic acid diethylamide	LSD, Acid, Blotter	Synthesis	50–200 μg	PO	8–14 hrs	5-HT$_{2a}$ partial agonist	Distributed on small squares of blotting paper, drops of liquid, gel-caps, small pills.
	Psilocybin	Magic mushrooms, Shrooms	*Psilocybe cubensis*, Psilocybe azurescens, & many other subspecies	10–50 mg, 1–5 g dried mushroom; quite variable.	PO	4–8 hrs	5-HT$_{2a}$ partial agonist	Psilocybin is converted in the body to psilocin, the actual active hallucinogen. Continued shamanic use in Mexico. Bruising of mushroom turns blue.
	Dimethyl-tryptamine	DMT, Yopo, Cohoba	Psychotria viridis, Anadenanthera peregrina, Mimosa hostilis, and many other natural sources, also by synthesis	5–40 mg	Smoked, inhaled snuff	30–60 mins	5-HT$_{2a}$ partial agonist	Continued Amazonian shamanic use
	Dimethyl-tryptamine + monoamine oxidase inhibitors (harmala beta-carbolines)	Ayahuasca, Yaje, Hoasca, Daime, "Vine of the soul"	Psychotria viridis (DMT) + Banisteropsis caapi (MAOI)	Variable	PO	2–4 hrs	5-HT$_{2a}$ partial agonist	Brewed as a tea; religious sacrament
	Ibogaine	Ibogaine	Tabernathe iboga	200–300 mg	PO	12+ hrs	likely 5-HT$_{2a}$ partial agonist	Religious sacrament; long-acting metabolites may contribute to purported anti-opiate withdrawal benefits.

(*Continued*)

TABLE 19.1
(Continued)

Class	Chemical Name	Common or Street Name	Source	Dosage	Route	Duration of Action	Major Neurobiological Target	Notes
Phenyl-alkylamines	3,4,5-trimethoxyphenyl ethylamine	Mescaline, Peyote, San Pedro	*Lophophora williamsii*, Echinopsis panachoi, other cacti; also by synthesis	200–500mg, 10–20 g or 5–10 dried peyote buttons, 1kg fresh E. pachanoi	PO	6–12 hrs	$5-HT_{2a}$ partial agonist	Religious sacrament
Entactogenic Phenyl-alkylamine	3,4-methylenedioxy-methamphetamine	MDMA, Ecstacy, X, XTC, Rolls, Molly	Synthesis	80–150 mg	PO	4–6 hrs	5–HT release & depletion	Mildly hallucinogenic at high doses
	3,4-methylenedioxy-amphetamine	MDA, Love drug, Adam	Synthesis	75–160 mg	PO	4–8 hrs	5–HT release & depletion	
	4-bromo-2,5-dimethoxy-phenethylamine	2C-B, Nexus	Synthesis	5–30 mg	PO	4–8 hrs	Unknown	
	4-chloro-2,5-dimethoxyamphetamine	DOC	Synthesis	1–5 mg	PO	4–8 hrs	Unknown	Has been found on blotting paper
	4-methyl-2,5-dimethoxy-amphetamine	DOM, STP	Synthesis	1–10 mg	PO	14–20 hrs	Unknown	Higher doses used in the 1960s resulted in many ER visits then
Dissociative	Ketamine	Ketamine, Special K, Vitamin K, K hole	Synthesis	25–50 mg (IM), 50–100 mg (PO or snorted)	IM, PO, snorted	1–2 hrs (IM), 1–4 hrs (PO)	NMDA antagonist	Subanesthetic dose: Lost sense of time, space, verbal skills, balance, drooling
	Dextromethorphan	DXM, Robo, DM	Synthesis	100–600 mg	PO	4–8 hrs	NMDA antagonist	
	Phencyclidine	PCP, Angel dust	Synthesis	3–10 mg	PO	8–24 hrs	NMDA antagonist	

				Dose	Route	Duration	Mechanism	Notes
Other	Salvinorin A	Salvia, Sally D, Diviner's sage	Salvia divinorum	250–750 mg (smoked), 2–10 g dried leaves (PO)	Smoked, PO	30–60 mins (Smoked), 1–3hrs (PO)	Kappa-opioid selective agonist	Atypical hallucinogen; no longer found in the wild
	Scopolamine & Atropine	Datura, Jimson weed, loco weed, Thorn apple, Angel's trumpet, belladonna, deadly nightshade	Datura stramonium, Atropa belladonna, many related species	Highly variable	PO	12–48 hrs	Competitive muscarinic acetylcholine antagonist	Plants of the Solanaceae family contain various ratios of scopolamine to atropine; blurred vision
	Muscimol (5-(aminomethyl)-3-isoxazolol)	Fly agaric, Amanita	Amanita muscaria, Amanita pantherina	1–30 g dried mushrooms	PO	5–10 hrs	$GABA_A$ agonist Glutamate	Shamanic use in eastern Siberia; over 600 species of agarics; easy to misidentify. Some are extremely poisonous such as "death cap" A. phalloides; mushrooms also contain ibotenic acid – as it dries/ages decarboxylation of ibotenic acid creates muscimol.

in their regulation of signaling and physiology by also involving pertussis toxin-sensitive heterotrimeric $G_{i/o}$ proteins and the Src tyrosine kinase proteins, both of which are intrinsic to $5\text{-}HT_{2a}$ receptor-expressing cortical pyramidal neurons (González-Maeso et al., 2007). $5\text{-}HT_{2a}$ receptors are most abundant in layer V pyramidal neurons (Lopez-Gimenez, Vilaro, Palacios, & Mengod, 2001). González-Maeso and colleagues (2007) hypothesize that hallucinogenic $5\text{-}HT_{2a}$ agonists "may perturb the normal gating functions of layer V cortex," disrupting cognition and sensory processing of this "output" cortex layer (Sapienza, Talbi, Jacquemin, & Albe-Fessard, 1981), and, thereby, induce expression of effects characteristic to hallucinogens. Tolerance to the effects of hallucinogens develops rapidly, due to receptor downregulation, and repeated administration will lead to markedly diminished effects within several days (Nichols, 2004).

On the neurobiological level it is still not clear if there is a specific pattern of alterations of brain functioning involved. Neurometabolic studies to date point to activation of frontal regions, the (para-)limbic structures and the right hemisphere (Gouzoulis-Mayfrank et al., 1999; Hermle et al., 1992; Riba et al., 2006; Vollenweider et al., 1997).

The entactogenic substances such as MDA and MDMA differ from the classical hallucinogens in that they appear to exert their effects by inducing a marked release of serotonin from serotonin-containing neurons and dopamine release from dopamine-containing neurons (Vollenweider, 2001). Their neurometabolic actions show minor deactivation of cortical regions and limbic activation and deactivation of the left amygdala (Gamma, Buck, Bethold, Liechti, & Vollenweider, 2000; Gouzoulis-Mayfrank et al., 1999). The latter may be responsible for their most prominent effect: the decrease of emotional tension and anxiety.

Psychological and Biological Effects   Intoxication with hallucinogens, commonly referred to as "tripping," may induce some physiologic effects and a wide variety of behavioral, emotional, and cognitive effects (Table 19.2; Halpern, 2003; Hollister, 1984). The visual imagery experienced are typically not true hallucinations but illusions, such as the perception of geometric patterns or scenic dreamlike visions appearing before closed eyes, perception of movement in stationary objects, and synesthesias. Contents of these visual as well as most emotional phenomena typically reflect the psychodynamics of the user (Leuner, 1962; Grof, 1975). Colors may appear intensified, and altered human and animal forms may appear in the visual field (Ungerleider & Pechnick, 1999). Hallucinogens activate affectivity and may cause significant changes of mood, where users may change from euphoria to depression or anxiety or vice versa (Tacke & Ebert, 2005). In some cases psychotic-like reactions may also be experienced. In short, the psychological effects of hallucinogens are highly variable and strongly influenced by the individual's mindset and setting (Zinberg, 1986). The "set" refers to the user's psychological state at the time of the ingestion, as well as beliefs, intentions for use, prior experiences, and expectations. The "setting" refers to the user's physical and social setting.

Toxicity of LSD, psilocybin, and other classical hallucinogens is very low. Overdosing is possible in respect to psychological reactions, but no case of lethal overdose is known, and there is no evidence of long-term toxicity (Halpern & Pope, 1999). A recent review of the harmful consequences of drugs of abuse found that the classical (and by far, the most used) hallucinogen LSD is near the bottom in a ranking of risk to users and society (Nutt, King, Saulsbury, & Blakemore, 2007).

TABLE 19.2
Hallucinogenic Effects

Hallucinogen[a] Intoxication may include a Cluster of the Following

Physical Effects[b]	Psychological Effects
Regular (mild to very mild):	Intensification of affectivity with euphoria, anxiety, depression, and/or
tachycardia, palpitations, hypertension or	cathartic expressions
hypotension, diaphoresis, hyperthermia,	Dreamlike state
motor incoordination, tremors, hyperreflexia,	Sensory activation with illusions, pseudo-hallucinations,[c] hallucinations,
altered neuroendocrine functioning.	and synesthesias
	Altered experience of time and space
Regular (mild to strong):	Altered body image
mydriasis, arousal, insomnia	Psychological lability
	Increased suggestibility
Occasional:	Acute neuropsychological/cognitive impairments with loosening of
Nausea, vomiting, diarrhea, blurred vision,	associations, inability for goal-directed thinking, memory disturbances
nystagmus, piloerection, salivation	Paranoid/suicidal ideation
	Impaired judgment
	Megalomania, impulsivity, odd behavior
	Lassitude, indifference, detachment
	psychosomatic complaints
	derealization, depersonalization
	mystical experiences
	sense of profound discovery/healing

[a]   Indolealkylamine and phenylalkylamine hallucinogens only (Table 19.1).

[b]   Some effects are reactionary to psychological content (ex., increased heart rate and nausea due to anxiety), and complaints can be dependent on factors such as mindset, setting, dose, and supervision. Intoxicated individuals may also deny physical impairment and/or claim increased energy, sharpened mental acuity, and improved sensory perception.

[c]   A subject experiencing "pseudo-hallucinations" retains the capacity to recognize that these "novel" experiences are transient and drug induced, as opposed to true hallucinations in which no such discernment is possible.

Hallucinogen Use Disorders   As in other substance use disorders, both hallucinogen abuse and hallucinogen dependence are recognized in the *DSM–IV*. Both abuse and dependence are characterized by patterns of compulsive and repeated drug use despite the knowledge of significant harm caused by the substance use. Hallucinogen use only very rarely leads to the development of classic dependence syndromes as seen with opiates or alcohol. A more typical pattern is for users to experiment with a few doses of a hallucinogen and then discontinue use (Hillebrand, Olszewksi, & Sedefov, 2006). As a class, the hallucinogens lack significant direct effect on the dopamine system, and studies to date have failed to train animals to self-administer these compounds (Nichols, 2004). However, the *DSM–IV–TR* (American Psychiatric Association, 2000) does allow for the diagnosis of both abuse and dependence of hallucinogens. Users do not experience withdrawal symptoms as seen with other substances of abuse, and so this symptom is not a criterion in diagnosing hallucinogen dependence. Note that tolerance rapidly increases, in general, when hallucinogens are used with frequency.

Hallucinogen-Induced Disorders   Similar to other substances of abuse, the *DSM–IV* allows for the diagnosis of numerous substance-induced disorders. They include: hallucinogen intoxication, hallucinogen persisting perception disorder (HPPD), and hallucinogen-induced psychotic, mood, anxiety, delirium, or not otherwise specified (NOS) disorder. These disorders arise in the context of substance use and may manifest during intoxication, withdrawal, or long after the drug has been ingested and the acute effects have subsided (American Psychiatric Association, 2000). The diagnosis of a hallucinogen-induced psychotic/mood/anxiety/delirium disorder is made only if the symptoms are in excess of what is expected from intoxication or withdrawal (American Psychiatric Association, 2000).

For the current *DSM–IV–TR*, the substance-induced disorders are categorized into three groups based on temporal relation to ingestion (American Psychiatric Association, 2000). The modifier "Onset during intoxication" is added when the symptoms appear during intoxication that is more severe than what is normally expected from the ingestion. An example in this setting includes severe hallucinations and delusions above and beyond what is normally expected in hallucinogen intoxication. The next modifier, "Onset during withdrawal," is given when the symptoms appear during the withdrawal phase, and does not apply to hallucinogens. The third category of substance-induced persisting disorders is substance-induced persisting dementia, substance-induced persisting amnestic disorder, and HPPD (American Psychiatric Association, 2000). The HPPD diagnosis is a specific diagnosis of re-experiencing some visual perceptual symptoms intermittently after cessation of drug use. Persisting psychotic symptoms following hallucinogen ingestion, however, are very rare and differentiated from HPPD, and a protracted psychotic reaction may warrant a diagnosis of psychosis NOS.

Assessment and Treatment

Hallucinogen Intoxication   **DSM–IV–TR Criteria 292.89**

Hallucinogen Intoxication

A. Recent use of hallucinogen.
B. Clinically significant maladaptive behavior or psychological changes (e.g., marked anxiety or depression, ideas of reference, fear of losing one's mind, paranoid ideation, impaired judgment, or impaired social or occupational function) that developed during or shortly after, hallucinogen use.
C. Perceptual changes occurring in a state of full wakefulness and alertness (e.g., subjective intensification of perceptions, depersonalization, derealization, illusions, hallucinations, synesthesias) that developed during, or shortly after, hallucinogen use.
D. Two (or more) of the following signs, developing during, or shortly after, hallucinogen use:

   (1) pupillary dilatation
   (2) tachycardia
   (3) sweating
   (4) palpitations
   (5) blurring vision

(6) tremors

(7) incoordination

E. The symptoms are not due to a general medical condition or are not better accounted for by another mental disorder.

Reprinted with permission from the *Diagnostic and Statistical Manual of Mental Disorders*, (Fourth Edition, Text Revision). Copyright 2000, American Psychiatric Association.

Assessment   Patients will present for treatment most often because he or she is experiencing a panic and/or depressive reaction, commonly referred to as a "bad trip." The panic and/or depressive reaction can begin any time after the onset of effects and may include marked anxiety or fears of "going insane" (Strassman, 1984). There may be also paranoid ideation, feelings of being manipulated, or being in a situation without any escape. The acute syndrome of hallucinogen intoxication should be suspected when a patient (or his friends) reports recent ingestion of a hallucinogen and presents with a characteristic constellation of sympathomimetic findings with a clear sensorium. Because laboratory testing is generally not available in most acute settings, obtaining an accurate history and clinical examination is critical in establishing this diagnosis. Street drugs often contain various substances, therefore the actual identity of the offending substance ingested may not be known. However, the hallucinogens typically produce similar effects, which should be carefully assessed. Signs and symptoms of hallucinogen intoxication are reviewed in the previous section (see Table 19.2). Physical examination will also provide important clues that can help support the diagnosis of hallucinogen intoxication (in particular, widely dilated pupils that do not rapidly/tightly constrict to accommodate bright light). As indicated previously, various hallucinogens have varying duration of action; that is, LSD's effects can last 8–12 hours whereas psilocybin's extends for 4–6 hours. Nevertheless, the acute reaction typically lasts less than 12–24 hours, and reactions lasting longer will require further investigation to rule out other etiologies.

Differential Diagnosis   Because polysubstance ingestion is very common, history should be sought on whether other substances were consumed in combination. Urine toxicology should also be performed, but tests for specific hallucinogens are special-ordered and typically will not have results for a few days. Anticholinergic intoxication should be considered in patients with a suggestive history (e.g., ingestion of jimson weed [datura]) with findings of hyperthermia, delirium, dry mouth, urinary retention, headache, and blurred vision. Delirium due to alcohol, sedative, or hypnotic withdrawal will present with sympathomimetic findings, but will also present with confusion, seizures, tremors, and visual, auditory, or tactile hallucinations. Stimulant psychosis, a psychosis in the setting of a clear sensorium induced by chronic stimulant use, will present with paranoid delusions and visual or auditory hallucinations and may report cumpulsive fascination with and performance of complex, stereotyped repetitive behaviors known as "punding" (Ellinwood, King, & Lee, 1998). PCP, ketamine, or dextromethorphan ("DXM") intoxication may present with signs and symptoms similar to that of hallucinogen intoxication, but may be distinguished by the presence of additional symptoms, including ataxia, horizontal nystagmus, rage, erythema, amnesia, and dry skin (Giannini, Loiselle, & Price, 1984). DXM intoxication will also produce a distinctive, plodding "zombielike" gait abnormality (Boyer, 2004). In addition, PCP overdose can prolong the toxic effects to three days owing to its long half-life (Abraham, McCann, & Ricaurte, 2002).

If mood, anxiety, and psychotic symptoms warrant independent clinical investigation, then hallucinogen-induced mood, anxiety, or psychotic disorder, respectively, should be considered. Psychiatric diagnoses including affective psychoses, schizophrenia, anxiety, and dissociative disorders can also present with varying degrees of acute dysphoria, depersonalization, and hallucinations. Medical causes of perceptual disturbances and mental status change should be ruled out, including medication reaction, metabolic disturbances, infections, dementia, strokes, seizures, CNS tumors, and Charles Bonnet syndrome. A careful history and physical, collateral information from family and friends, where appropriate, and laboratory data, will all be needed in ruling out such diagnoses.

Treatment   The "talk down" (more accurately the "talk through") is usually the only intervention indicated in these situations (Tayler, Maurer, & Tinklenberg, 1970). This consists of keeping the patient in a low-stimulus environment (i.e., a quiet space with dimmed lights and minimal distractions) and providing emotional support. Arrange for a reliable sitter (a non-intoxicated family member or friend) to look after the patient. The sitter can help keep the patient calm and oriented by providing a sympathetic presence. In addition, provide reassurance to the patient that the experience is generally nonhazardous, drug-induced, and time-limited, which will resolve with full recovery. The patient should not be left alone until the effects of the drug wear off (Tacke & Ebert, 2005). As mentioned earlier, the acute reaction typically lasts less than 12–24 hours.

Because hallucinogens are rapidly absorbed in the GI tract, unless the ingestion occurred within 30 minutes of presentation, gastric lavage is unlikely to be effective in removing the substances. The anxiety, depressive, and paranoid state of the patient will invariably worsen if gastric lavage is forcefully attempted and should be avoided.

If severe agitation does not respond to redirection and concerns for safety for the patient and/or others remain, benzodiazepines are quite effective in reducing anxiety and panic (Abraham et al., 2002). Many authorities recommend diazepam or lorazepam, PO if possible, but IM and IV are also effective (Dribben & Wood, 2006). Avoid physical restraints if possible and limit the use of neuroleptics because paradoxical effects have been reported with chlorpromazine (Strassman, 1984) and HPPD symptoms have been reported to worsen after receiving phenothiazines (Abraham, 1983; Schwarz, 1968) and 5-HT2a antagonists such as risperidal (Abraham & Mamen, 1996; Morehead, 1997). Although there are no controlled trials that have examined the efficacy of antipsychotics in this setting, haloperidol may be considered in rare cases of severely agitated patients who require further interventions after benzodiazepines have not proven sufficient. Great caution must be exercised, however, because neuroleptics lower the seizure threshold and may also induce hypotension (Tacke & Ebert, 2005).

Once the acute symptoms subside, patients are usually able to go home accompanied by a family member or friend (Strassman, 1984). It is important to advise patients that subsequent ingestion of hallucinogens may precipitate similar reactions. If symptoms persist for longer than 24 hours or there are accompanying severe mood or psychotic symptoms that warrant independent clinical attention, hospitalization may be considered (Strassman, 1995).

Hallucinogen Abuse and Dependence   ***DSM–IV–TR* Criteria. 305.30**

Hallucinogen Abuse

A. A maladaptive pattern of hallucinogen use leading to clinically significant impairment or distress, as manifested by one (or more) of the following, occurring within a 12-month period:

   (1) recurrent hallucinogen use resulting in a failure to fulfill major role obligations at work, school, or home (e.g., repeated absences or poor work performance related to the substance use; substance-related absences, suspensions, or expulsions from school; neglect of children or household)
   (2) recurrent hallucinogen use in situations in which it is physically hazardous
   (3) recurrent hallucinogen-related legal problems
   (4) continued hallucinogen use despite having persistent or recurrent social or interpersonal problems caused or exacerbated by the effects of the substance

B. The symptoms have never met the criteria for Substance Dependence for this class of substance.

Reprinted and modified with permission from the *Diagnostic and Statistical Manual of Mental Disorders*, Fourth Edition, Text Revision. Copyright 2000 American Psychiatric Association.

Assessment

Because hallucinogen ingestion is the central component of hallucinogen abuse and dependence, evaluation and treatment should proceed similarly to that in patients diagnosed with hallucinogen intoxication. The diagnosis of hallucinogen abuse should be considered when patients report using hallucinogens despite evidence and knowledge of harm as a result of this substance use. The more significant diagnosis of dependence should be considered when the pattern of use appears to be out of control, such as using larger amounts than intended or the inability to cut down the use (American Psychiatric Association, 2000).

As mentioned previously, the overall rates of abuse and dependence are thought to be low compared to other substances (Johnston et al., 2006; Wright et al., 2007). Based on data from the U.S. NHSDUH from 2000 and 2001, which included MDMA and PCP in the definition of hallucinogen, hallucinogen dependence is estimated at 2% in recent-onset users (first use within 24 months of survey) and 5% in past-onset users (first use 24+ months, last use within 12 months), with relative risk of dependence apparently greater in users with very early age of onset of hallucinogen use (10–11 yo; Stone, O'Brien, De La Torre, & Anthony, 2007). In clinical settings, patients often present as polysubstance users, therefore a complete history is always needed to assess for other drug use.

Differential Diagnosis

Because polydrug use is common, the differential must always contain other substance use or substance-induced disorders. In addition, a significant portion of illicit drugs that are sold as LSD (or some other hallucinogen) may contain other substances such as amphetamines or PCP (Tacke & Ebert, 2005). Therefore the diagnosis of amphetamine or phencyclidine abuse and dependence should be included in the differential. Alcohol appears to be a commonly abused comorbid drug and should also be assessed carefully in this population (El-Mallakh, Halpern, & Abraham, 2008). Schizophrenia, schizophreniform disorder, bipolar disorder, and schizoaffective disorder should also be ruled out in these patients, by assessing the longitudinal course of the symptom constellation and their temporal relation to hallucinogen ingestion.

Treatment

There are no controlled trials that have examined the treatment of hallucinogen abuse or dependence. However, general principles that apply to other substances of abuse should be employed in treating these patients (El-Mallakh et al., 2008). Motivational interviewing, detoxification, relapse prevention, intensive outpatient counseling, and family therapies are examples of interventions that need to be individualized for each particular patient. As with other addiction issues, involvement with AA or NA or other self-help groups should be encouraged.

Because polysubstance abuse and dependence are common, treatment should also target other substance abuse and dependence that are thought to be contributing to the disturbances. Furthermore, treatment should be provided with a dual diagnosis approach, and any underlying psychiatric disorder should be treated concurrently. No controlled trials have been conducted to evaluate the efficacy of pharmacotherapies.

Hallucinogen Persisting Perception Disorder   **DSM–IV–TR Criteria. 292.89**

Hallucinogen Persisting Perception Disorder (Flashbacks)

A. The reexperiencing, following cessation of use of a hallucinogen, of one or more of the perceptual symptoms that were experienced while intoxicated with the hallucinogen (e.g., geometric hallucinations, false perception of movement in the peripheral visual fields, flashes of color, intensified colors, trails of images of moving objects, positive afterimages, halos around objects, macropsia, and micropsia).

B. The symptoms in Criterion A cause clinically significant distress or impairment in social, occupational, or other important areas of functioning.

C. The symptoms are not due to a general medical condition (e.g., anatomical lesions and infections of the brain, visual epilepsies) and are not better accounted for by another mental disorder (e.g., delirium, dementia, schizophrenia) or hypnopompic hallucinations.

Reprinted with permission from the *Diagnostic and Statistical Manual of Mental Disorders*, Fourth Edition, Text Revision. Copyright 2000 American Psychiatric Association.

Assessment

The diagnosis of HPPD has to be differentiated into two kinds of phenomena. The international ICD-10 gives only evidence for the re-emergence of fragments, scenarios, and/or altered states of consciousness and mood such as those experienced during the hallucinogen intoxication. This implies a re-experience ("flashback") of the altered state of mood and consciousness as experienced during the initial intoxication. These "flashbacks," as they are often nonspecifically called, may (in some rare cases) occur intermittently over weeks, months, or years after the actual intoxication. Some people intentionally try to induce these re-experiences (with specific music/surroundings) and call them "free trips." Flashback episodes are very short-lived (usually seconds), but may extend longer if induced by ingestion of cannabis. There is no documented case in the literature of a flashback leading to danger or suicide (Holland, 2004). Holland (2004) discussed critically 15 different models to explain flashback phenomena. There seems to be no monocausal model, but the individual case may fit more than one of these models, which implies a complex multicausal origin.

The HPPD phenomena as described by Abraham et al. (2002) and specified in the *DSM–IV* are nearly all visual in nature (including flashes of color, geometric images, and afterimages of moving objects ("trails;" El-Mallakh et al., 2008), and appear to be a continous phenomenon starting in the days to weeks after the consumption of a hallucinogen.

Patients may also report that these perceptual changes are triggered by intoxication from other substances, although strictly speaking the *DSM–IV* diagnostic criteria require that the patient not be intoxicated with other substances (Halpern & Pope, 2003). As such, urine tox screens should be performed to assess for the presence of other substances.

Differential Diagnosis

Hallucinogen-induced psychotic disorder should be considered in patients experiencing significant psychotic symptoms shortly after their use of hallucinogens, but currently the *DSM–IV* does not provide a diagnosis for hallucinogen-induced persistent psychotic symptoms that are not intermittent in nature. However, the literature suggests that prolonged post-LSD psychosis does rarely occur, and appears more likely to be reported in patients with schizophrenia (Strassman, 1984). Psychotic disorders, including schizophrenia and bipolar disorder, should be ruled out by carefully assessing the history. Medical causes of intermittent perceptual disturbances should be considered as well, including medication reaction, metabolic disturbances, migraines, temporal lobe epilepsy, ocular diseases, strokes, or tumors.

Treatment

Episodes of derealization in combination with visual disturbances may trigger anxious fears of "brain damage" in the HPPD individual. Simple reassurance that their symptoms do not reflect brain damage and that the complained symptoms typically resolve over more time, can prove tremendously effective. A variety of treatments has been reported to aid in reducing the symptoms as well as the distress associated with HPPD in several case series, including the use of benzodiazepines, clonidine, haloperidol, olanzapine, carbamazepine, psychotherapy, behavior modifications, and the use of sunglasses (Halpern and Pope, 2003). Some interventions have been reported to worsen the symptoms, including risperidone (Abraham & Mamen, 1996), phenothiazines (Abraham, 1983), and SSRIs (Markel, Lee, Holmes, & Domino, 1994). Clearly, avoiding further hallucinogen use is recommended. In addition, other substances, particularly marijuana, may also trigger HPPD symptoms. Avoiding their use is an important element of treatment. Treatment should take into account the need for symptom relief, which needs to be balanced with the concern for benzodiazepine abuse and dependence, as polysubstance abuse and dependence is common in this patient population (El-Mallakh et al., 2008).

Hallucinogen-Induced Psychotic Disorder   **DSM–IV–TR Criteria**

Substance-Induced Psychotic Disorder

A. Prominent hallucinations or delusions, Note: Do not include hallucinations if the person has insight that they are substance induced.
B. There is evidence from the history, physical examination, or laboratory findings of either (1) or (2)

   (1) the symptoms in Criterion A developed during or within a month of substance intoxication or withdrawal
   (2) substance use is etiologically related to the disturbance

C. The disturbance is not better accounted for by a psychotic disorder that is not substance induced. Evidence that the symptoms are better accounted for by a psychotic disorder that is not substance induced might include the following: the symptoms precede the onset of the substance use (or medication use); the symptoms persist for a substantial period of time (e.g., about a month) after the cessation of acute withdrawal or severe intoxication or are substantially in excess of what would be expected given the type or amount of the substance used or the duration of use; or there is other evidence that suggests the existence of an independent non-substance-induced psychotic disorder (e.g., a history of recurrent nonsubstance related episodes).
D. The disturbance does not occur exclusively during the course of delirium.

Note: This diagnosis should be made instead of a diagnosis of substance intoxication or substance withdrawal only when the symptoms are in excess of those usually associated with the intoxication or withdrawal syndrome and when the symptoms are sufficiently severe to warrant independent clinical attention.

Code specific substance-induced psychotic disorder.

   292.11 amphetamine (or amphetamine-like substance), with delusions;
   292.12 amphetamine (or amphetamine-like substance), with hallucinations;

292.11 hallucinogen, with delusions;

292.12 hallucinogen, with hallucinations.

Specify:

With onset during intoxication: if criteria are met for intoxication with the substance and the symptoms develop during the intoxication syndrome.

With onset during withdrawal: if criteria are met for withdrawal from the substance and the symptoms develop during, or shortly after, a withdrawal syndrome.

Reprinted with permission from the *Diagnostic and Statistical Manual of Mental Disorders*, Fourth Edition, Text Revision. Copyright 2000 American Psychiatric Association.

Assessment

Hallucinogen-induced psychotic disorder should be considered in patients with recent ingestion of a hallucinogen who also present with marked psychotic symptoms, often lacking in insight that the symptoms are caused by the substance. Although this reaction may be a more severe form of the "bad trip," the diagnosis is made in the setting where a patient's psychotic symptoms are more severe than what would be expected from hallucinogen intoxication. The *DSM–IV* allows for modifiers to indicate whether hallucinations or delusions are prominent features (American Psychiatric Association, 2000). The psychotic reaction usually ends once the effects of the drug wear off.

Differential Diagnosis

The differential diagnosis for hallucinogen-induced psychotic disorder should include those diagnoses that are considered in any acute psychosis. Because toxicology screens do not routinely test for hallucinogens, a thorough history and physical exam is critical. As usual in these settings, collateral information from families and friends will aid in narrowing the possible diagnoses. As has been repeatedly noted so far, evaluating for other substances of abuse is also very important considering the frequency in which they are ingested. Formal thought disorders and affective psychoses should be considered and relevant historical information should be sought. Etiologies for delirium need to be evaluated, including infections, medication reactions, metabolic disturbances, CNS tumors, stroke, and head injuries. Finally, a distinction should be made with HPPD, which represents re-experiencing of the perceptual disturbances of the hallucinogen intoxication (see above).

Treatment

No controlled trials exist that have evaluated the efficacy of specific pharmacological intervention for hallucinogen-induced psychotic disorder. Procedures for the treatment of hallucinogen intoxication should be followed in those who have recently ingested hallucinogens, and underlying etiologies for psychosis should be investigated. Although rare, the patient may require hospitalization as the prolonged reaction can persist for days or weeks.

Case Presentations

Brief Psychotic Reaction Post-hallucinogen Abuse

A 25-year-old female graduate student was brought to the emergency room by her friends because of their concerns that she was having a "bad trip." She reportedly took several "pills" at a dance party earlier that evening, given to her approximately 14 hours prior to arrival. Her friends confirm they each had taken what they thought was LSD. The friends began noticing diminishing effects from the drug after about 6–8 hours of intoxication, but the patient was found to still be "tripping hard." The friends reported the patient experienced increasing anxiety and paranoid ideation that worsened overnight. Because her symptoms persisted for over 12 hours, and concerned that she was having a psychotic break, the friends brought her to the hospital for evaluation.

The patient's history was remarkable for a major depressive episode five years ago but with no history indicative of a psychotic illness. Her depression had been treated with an SSRI for about six months, but since that time she had not been on any medications and had no reported recurrences of depression. She was not taking any other over-the-counter or herbal medications. She admitted to regular use of alcohol and infrequent use of various drugs, including cannabis, psilocybin mushrooms, and cocaine, primarily at rock concerts. She admitted to prior LSD use in such settings but had not experienced any similar severe reactions as the one resulting in her presentation to the emergency room. She was living with roommates near her school and reported moderate stress related to her schoolwork. Her judgment and insight were limited.

On examination, the patient was a thin female, appeared her stated age, alert and oriented, cooperative, poor eye contact, visibly agitated, and pacing the exam room, without any ataxia. Her speech was occasionally unintelligible, but otherwise was of normal volume and rate with no slurring. Her affect was anxious and labile. Her thought process was at times tangential. She reported that various objects were sending her messages but was unable to elaborate on their content. She appeared to be intermittently responding to internal stimuli. She denied any suicidal or homicidal ideation. Her physical exam was remarkable for dilated pupils, mild tachycardia, and hypertension. Laboratory tests were within normal limits, and her urine toxicology screen was negative for tested drugs of abuse.

She was diagnosed with presumed hallucinogen-induced psychotic disorder and she was monitored in a quiet and dimly lit room in the ED, accompanied by her friends. She readily accepted lorazepam 2 mg PO to help with her anxiety. This patient was reassured that her state was likely induced by her drug ingestion and would be time-limited. Within one hour of the lorazepam administration, patient reported feeling much less anxious. Four hours later she reported feeling somewhat embarrassed about the situation, but very much close to her usual self. She no longer reported receiving special messages, and confides she was terrified she had been "going insane." Her vitals were stable. She was discharged home with a follow-up appointment with her psychiatrist. She was encouraged to maintain sobriety and to avoid ingesting hallucinogens in the future due to the potential risk of precipitating similar reactions.

Acute Toxic Psychosis

A 28-year-old male was brought to the emergency room by the police after he was found wandering naked through the streets. The police reported that calls were made to 911 after the patient was seen walking through the street oblivious to the oncoming traffic, yelling comments at passersby. When the police arrived, the patient was agitated, confused, and appeared to be interacting with people he was hallucinating. Other than reporting he was "burning up" and "very thirsty," he was unable to provide any history. He was bleeding from both hands around his knuckles. He also had what appeared to be numerous superficial lacerations and contusions on his torso and legs. With some difficulty the EMTs were able to bring the patient to the hospital for evaluation. In the emergency room, the patient was unable to relate a coherent history, and no identifying information could be found. Current medications, past medical and psychiatric history, and other information were therefore unavailable.

On exam, the patient was a thin male, alert but oriented to person only, disheveled, agitated, and restless. No tremors or myoclonus were noted. He was actively responding to internal stimulation. Memory was grossly impaired. His speech was variable in volume and rate, often mumbling words that were difficult to discern. His affect was moderately anxious and fearful, at times grimacing as if in pain. His thought process was markedly disorganized. He was experiencing auditory and visual hallucinations. No suicidal or homicidal ideation was reported. His judgment and insight were markedly impaired. His vitals were moderately elevated but afebrile. His physical exam showed numerous superficial lacerations on his upper body and both legs. His skin felt dry, warm, and diffusely erythematous. Mucous membranes were dry. Pupils were equally dilated. Heart and lung exams were unremarkable except for tachycardia. Minimal bowel sounds and palpation revealed mild tenderness in the suprapubic region. No focal neurological deficits were observed. Laboratory tests were within normal limits, and urine toxicology screen was negative. Gastric lavage was performed. His bladder distention indicated urinary retention, and the patient tolerated the placement of a urinary catheter.

He was admitted for presumed anticholinergic delirium. Vitals were monitored, and IV hydration was given. His condition steadily improved during the next 24 hours, and he was soon able to confirm that he did in fact ingest some jimsonweed seeds to "see what it would be like." He had no recollection of the events since the ingestion, except that he recalled encountering monsters and other frightening beings. Retrograde amnesia spanned a period of approximately 36 hours. He reported that he would never take datura again and was discharged in stable condition to follow up with his PCP.

Resources for More Information

To know more about the assessment and treatment of hallucinogen substance use disorders is to primarily become familiar with the sources of information about hallucinogen use. The largest repository on the Internet is www.erowid.org. This website contains thousands of "trip reports" on most every known hallucinogen identified. This website also provides detailed information on basic chemistry, synthesis, pharmacology, and social/legal issues. It must be stressed, however, that websites like erowid contain a wide range of quality and accuracy of information, and much of it is oriented from the perspective of and for drug users. A simple Internet search will also present many other websites offering information on how to identify and forage for botanical hallucinogens. Still other websites sell hallucinogens, most typically "ethnobotanicals" that are unregulated. Awareness of such websites will increase the credibility of those health care providers who wish to have a frank discussion about hallucinogen drug use/abuse and to do otherwise may extend the collusion of silence in the doctor's office where if we don't ask, the user will not tell. Finally, legitimate research of hallucinogens is expanding and the two most active not-for-profits that fund such research maintain detailed websites on their progress: The Multidisciplinary Association for Psychedelic Studies (www.MAPS.org) and the much smaller Heffter Research Institute (www.Heffter.org).

References

Abraham, H. D. (1983). Visual phenomenology of the LSD flashback. *Archives of General Psychiatry, 40,* 884–889.

Abraham, H. D., & Mamen, A. (1996). LSD-like panic from risperidone in post-LSD visual disorder. *Journal of Clinical Psychopharmacology, 16,* 228–231.

Abraham, H. D., McCann, U. D., & Ricaurte, G. A. (2002). Psychedelic drugs. In K. L. Davis, D. Charney, J. T. Coyle, & C. Nemeroff (Eds.), *Neuropsychopharmacology: The fifth generation of progress* (pp. 1545–1556). Philadelphia: Lippincott Williams & Wilkins.

Abramson, H. A. (Ed.). (1967). *The use of psychotherapy and alcoholism.* Indianapolis: Bobbs Merrill.

American Psychiatric Association. (2000). *Diagnostic criteria from DSM-IV-TR.*, Washington, DC: American Psychiatric Press.

Beringer, K. (1927). *Der Meskalinrausch.* Berlin: Julius Springer.

Bogusz, M. J., Maier, R. D., Schäfer, A., & Erkens, M. (1998). Honey with psilocybe mushrooms: A revival of a very old preparation on the drug market? *International Journal of Legal Medicine, 111,* 147–150.

Boyer, E. W. (2004). Dextromethorphan abuse. *Pediatric Emergency Care, 20,* 858–963.

Cohen, S. (1960). Lysergic acid diethylamide: Side effects and complications. *Journal of Nervous and Mental Disease, 130,* 30–40.

De Rios, M. D. (1994). Drug tourism in the Amazon. *Anthropology of Consciousness, 5,* 16–19.

De Rios, M. D. (2006). Mea culpa: Drug tourism and the anthropologist's responsibility. *Anthropology News, 47,* 20.

Dribben, B., & Wood, A. (2006). Toxicity, hallucinogens—LSD. eMedicine article topic #2809 (www.emedicine.com).

Dyck, E. (2005). Flashback: Psychiatric experimentation with LSD in historical perspective. *Canadian Journal of Psychiatry, 50,* 381–388.

Ellinwood, E. H., King, G. R., & Lee, T. H. (1998). Chronic amphetamine use and abuse. In S. J. Watson (Eds.) *Psychopharmacology: The fourth generation of progress* – CD-ROM. Philadelphia: Lippincott Williams & Wilkins.

El-Mallakh, R. S., Halpern, J. H., & Abraham, H. D. (2008). Substance abuse: Hallucinogen- and MDMA-related disorders (Chapter 60). In A. Tasman, M. Maj, M. B. First, J. Kay, & J. A. Lieberman (Eds.), *Psychiatry* (3rd ed., pp. 1100–1126). London: John Wiley & Sons.

El-Seedi, H. R., De Smet, P. A., Beck, O., Possnert, G., & Bruhn, J. G. (2005). Prehistoric peyote use: Alkaloid analysis and radiocarbon dating of archaeological specimens of Lophophora from Texas, *Journal of Ethnopharmacology, 101,* 238–242.

Fiorella, D., Helsley, S., Lorrain, D. S., Rabin, R. A., & Winter, J. C. (1995). The role of the 5-HT2A and 5-HT2C receptors in the stimulus effects of hallucinogenic drugs. III: The mechanistic basis for supersensitivity to the LSD stimulus following serotonin depletion. *Psychopharmacology (Berl), 121,* 364–372.

Gamma, A., Buck, A., Berthold, T., Liechti, M. E., & Vollenweider, F. X. (2000). 3,4-Methylene-dioxymethamphetamine (MDMA) modulates cortical and limbic brain activity as measured by [H(2)(15)O]-PET in healthy humans. *Neuropsychopharmacology, 23,* 388–395.

Giannini, A. J., Loiselle, R. H., & Price, W. A. (1984). Antidotal strategies in phencyclidine intoxication. *International Journal of Psychiatry in Medicine, 4,* 513–518.

González, D., Riba, J., Bouso, J. C., Gómez-Jarabo, G., & Barbanoj, M. J. (2006). Pattern of use and subjective effects of Salvia divinorum among recreational users. *Drug and Alcohol Dependence, 85,* 157–162.

González-Maeso, J., & Sealfon, S. (2006). Hormone signaling via G protein-coupled receptors. In DeGoot L. C. & Jameson J. L. (Eds.), *Endocrinology* (pp. 177–203). Amsterdam: Elsevier.

González-Maeso, J., Weisstaub, N. V., Zhou, M., Chan, P., Ivic, L., Ang, R., et al. (2007). Hallucinogens recruit specific cortical 5-HT$_{2a}$ receptor-mediated signaling pathways to affect behavior. *Neuron, 53,* 439–452.

González-Maeso, J., Yuen, T., Ebersole, B. J., Wurmbach, E., Lira, A., Zhou, M., et al. (2003). Transcriptome fingerprints distinguish hallucinogenic and nonhallucinogenic 5-hydroxytryptamine 2A receptor agonist effects in mouse somatosensory cortex. *Journal of Neuroscience, 23,* 8836–8843.

Gouzoulis-Mayfrank, E., Schreckenberger, M., Sabri, O., Arning, C., Thelen, B., Spitzer, M., et al. (1999). Neurometabolic effects of psilocybin, 3,4-methylenedioxyethylamphetamine (MDE) and d-methamphetamine in healthy volunteers. *Neuropsychopharmacology, 20,* 565–581.

Griffiths, R. R., Richards, W. A., McCann, U., & Jesse, R. (2006). Psilocybin can occasion mystical-type experiences having substantial and sustained personal meaning and spiritual significance. *Psychopharmacology (Berl), 187,* 268–283.

Grob, C., & Dobkin de Rios, M. (1992). Adolescent drug use in cross-cultural perspective. *Journal of Drug Issues, 22,* 121–138.

Grob, C. S. (1994). Psychiatric research with hallucinogens: What have we learned? Yearbook *Ethnomed, 3,* 91–112.

Grof, S. (1975). *Realms of the human unconsciousness.* New York: Viking.

Grof, S. (1980). *LSD psychotherapy.* Pomona, CA: Hunter House.

Halpern, J. H. (2003). Hallucinogens: An update. *Current Psychiatry Reports, 5,* 347–354.

Halpern, J. H. (2004). Hallucinogens and dissociative agents naturally growing in the United States. *Pharmacology and Therapeutics, 102,* 131–138.

Halpern, J. H., & Pope, H. G., Jr. (1999). Do hallucinogens cause residual neuropsychological toxicity? *Drug and Alcohol Dependence, 53,* 247–256.

Halpern, J. H., & Pope, H. G., Jr. (2001). Hallucinogens on the Internet: A vast new source of underground drug information. *American Journal of Psychiatry, 158,* 48–483.

Halpern, J. H., & Pope, H. G., Jr. (2003). Hallucinogen persisting perception disorder: What do we know after 50 years? *Drug and Alcohol Dependence, 69,* 109–119.

Hermle, L., Funfgeld, M., Oepen, G., Botsch, H., Borchardt, D., Gouzoulis, E., et al. (1992). Mescaline-induced psychopathological, neuropsychological, and neurometabolic effects in normal subjects: experimental psychosis as a tool for psychiatric research. *Biological Psychiatry, 32,* 976–991.

Hillebrand, J., Olszewksi, D., & Sedefov, R. (2006). *Hallucinogenic mushrooms: An emerging trend case study.* Lisbon: European Monitoring Centre for Drugs and Drug Addiction.

Holland, D. (2004). Flashback-Phänomene als Nachwirkung von Halluzinogeneinnahme. Hannover: Hannover Medical School Dissertation.

Holland, J. (Ed.). (2001). *Ecstasy: The complete guide.* Rochester, VT: Park Street Press.

Hollister, L. E. (1972). *Formularbeginn chemical psychoses.* Springfield, IL: C.C. Thomas.

Hollister, L. E. (1984). Effects of hallucinogens in humans. In B. L. Jacobs (Ed.), *Hallucinogens: Neurochemical, behavioral, and clinical perspectives* (pp. 19–33). New York: Raven Press.

Johnston, L. D., Bachman, J. G., & O'Malley, P. M. (2006). *Monitoring the Future: Questionnaire responses from the nation's high school seniors, 2005.* Ann Arbor, MI: Institute for Social Research.

Labate, B. C., & Araujo, W. S. (Eds.). (2004). *O Uso Ritual da Ayahuasca* (2nd ed.). Campinas, Brazil: Mercado de Letras.

Leuner, H. (1962). *Die experimentelle psychose* Berlin: Julius Springer.

Lopez-Gimenez, J. F., Vilaro, M. T., Palacios, J. M., & Mengod, G. (2001). Mapping of 5-HT2A receptors and their mRNA in monkey brain: [3H]MDL100,907 autoradiography and in situ hybridization studies. *Journal of Comparative Neurology, 429,* 571–589.

Malleson, N. (1971). Acute adverse reactions to LSD in clinical and experimental use in the United Kingdom. *British Journal of Psychiatry, 118,* 229–230.

Markel, H., Lee, A., Holmes, R. D., & Domino, E. F. (1994). LSD flashback syndrome exacerbated by selective serotonin reuptake inhibitor antidepressants in adolescents. *Journal of Pediatrics, 125,* 817–819.

Masters, R. E. L., & Houston, J. (1966). *The varieties of psychedelic experience.* New York: Holt.

Morehead, D. B. (1997). Exacerbation of hallucinogen-persisting perception disorder with risperidone. *Journal of Clinical Psychopharmacology, 17,* 327–328.

Nichols, D. E. (2004). Hallucinogens. *Pharmacological Therapeutics, 101,* 131–181.

Nutt, D., King, L. A., Saulsbury, W., & Blakemore, C. (2007). Development of a rational scale to assess the harm of drugs of potential misuse. *Lancet, 369,* 1047–1063.

O'Brien, C. P. (2005). Drug addiction and drug abuse (Chapter 23). In L. Brunton, J. Lazo, & K. Parker (Eds.), *Goodman & Gillman's The Pharmacological Basis of Therapeutics*, (11th ed., pp. 607–628). New York: McGraw-Hill.

Osmond, H. (1957). A review of the clinical effects of psychotomimetic agents. *Annals of New York Academy of Sciences, 66,* 418–434.

Pahnke, W. N. (1963). Drugs and mysticism: An analysis of the relationship between psychedelic drugs and the mystical consciousness. Harvard University Dissertation, Cambridge, MA.

Passie, T. (1997). *Psycholytic and psychedelic therapy research: A complete international bibliography 1931-1995.* Hannover: Laurentius.

Pope, H. G., Jr. (1969). Tabernanthe iboga: An African narcotic plant of social importance. *Economic Botany, 23,* 174–184.

Riba, J., Romero, S., Grasa, E., Mena, E., Carrio, I., & Barbanoj, M. J. (2006). Increased frontal and paralimbic activation following ayahuasca, the pan-Amazonian inebriant. *Psychopharmacology, 186,* 93–98.

Roth, B. L., Baner, K., Westkaemper, R., Siebert, D., Rice, K. C., Steinberg, S., et al. (2002). Salvinorin A: A potent naturally occurring nonnitrogenous kappa opiod selective agonist. *Proceedings of the National Academy of Sciences, 99,* 11934–11939.

Roth, B. L., Willins, D. L., Kristiansen, K., & Kroeze, W. K. (1998). 5-Hydroxytryptamine2-family receptors (5-hydroxytryptamine2A, 5-hydroxytryptamine2B, 5-hydroxytryptamine2C): Where structure meets function. *Pharmacological Therapeutics, 79,* 231–257.

Ruck, C. A. P., Bigwood, J., Staples, D., Ott, J., & Wasson, G. (1979). Entheogens. *Journal of Psychedelic Drugs, 11,* 145–146.

Samorini, G. (1995). The Bwiti religion and the psychoactive plant Tabernanthe iboga (Equatorial Africa). *Integration, 5,* 105–114.

SAMHSA, Office of Applied Studies (2007a). *Results from the 2006 National Survey on Drug Use and Health: National Findings.* NSDUH Series H-32, DHHS Publication No. SMA 07-4293, Rockville, MD.

SAMHSA, Office of Applied Studies (2007b). *Drug Abuse Warning Network, 2005: National Estimates of Drug-Related Emergency Department Visits.* DAWN Series D-29, DHHS Publication No. SMA 07-4256, Rockville, MD.

Sapienza, S., Talbi, B., Jacquemin, J., & Albe-Fessard, D. (1981). Relationship between input and output of cells in motor and somatosensory cortices of the chronic awake rat. A study using glass micropipettes. *Experimental Brain Research, 43,* 47–56.

Schaefer, S. B., & Furst, P. T. (Eds.). (1998). *People of the peyote: Huichol Indian history, religion and survival.* Albuquerque: University of New Mexico Press.

Schneider, U., Leweke, F. M., Sternemann, U., Weber, M. M., & Emrich, H. M. (1966). Visual 3D illusion: A systems-theoretical approach to psychosis. *European Archives of Psychiatry and Clinical Neuroscience, 246,* 256–260.

Schultes, R. E., Hofmann. A., & Rätsch, C. (2001). *Plants of the gods: Their sacred, healing and hallucinogenic powers* (2nd ed.). Rochester, VT: Inner Traditions.

Schwarz, C. J. (1968). The complications of LSD: A review of the literature. *Journal of Nervous and Mental Disorders, 146,* 174–186.

Schwartz, R. H. (1995). LSD. Its rise, fall, and renewed popularity among high school students. *Pediatrics Clinics of North America, 42,* 403–413.

Smith, H. (2000). *Cleansing the doors of perception: The religious significance of entheogenic plants and chemicals.* New York: Penguin Putnam.

Stafford, P. G., & Golightly, B. H. (1969). *LSD in action.* London: Sidgwick & Jackson.

Stewart, O. (1987). *Peyote religion: A history.* Norman: University of Oklahoma Press.

Stone, A. L., O'Brien, M. S., De La Torre, A., & Anthony, J. C. (2007). Who is becoming hallucinogen dependent soon after hallucinogen use starts? *Drug and Alcohol Dependence, 87,*153–163.

Strassman, R. J. (1984). Adverse reactions for psychedelic drugs: A review of the literature. *Journal of Nervous and Mental Disorders, 172,* 577–595.

Strassman, R. J. (1995). Hallucinogenic drugs in psychiatric research and treatment: Perspectives and prospects. *Journal of Nervous and Mental Disorders, 183,* 127–138.

Tacke, U., & Ebert, M. H. (2005). Hallucinogens and phencyclidine. In H. R. Kranzler & D. A. Ciraulo (Eds.), *Clinical manual of addiction psychopharmacology* (pp. 211–241).Washington, DC: American Psychiatric.

Taylor, R. L., Maurer, J. I., & Tinklenberg, J. R. (1970). Management of "bad trips" in an evolving drug scene. *Journal of American Medical Association, 213,* 422–425.

Ungerleider, J. T., & Pechnick, R. N. (1999). Hallucinogens. In M. Galanter & H. D. Kleber (Eds.). *Textbook of substance abuse treatment* (pp. 195–203). Washington, DC: American Psychiatric.

Vollenweider, F. X. (2001). Brain mechanisms of hallucinogens and entactogens. *Dialogues in Clinical Neuroscience, 3,* 265–279.

Vollenweider, F. X., Leenders, K. L., Scharfetter, C., Maguire, P., Stadelmann, O., & Angst, J. (1997). Positron emission tomography and fluorodeoxyglucose studies of metabolic hyperfrontality and psychopathology in the psilocybin model of psychosis. *Neuropsychopharmacology, 16,* 357–372.

Vollenweider, F. X., Vollenweider-Scherpenhuyzen, M. F., Babler, A., Vogel, H., & Hell, D. (1998). Psilocybin induces schizophrenia-like psychosis in humans via a serotonin-2 agonist action. *Neuroreport, 9,* 3897–3902.

Wasson, R. G., Ruck, C. A. P., & Hofmann, A. (1978). *The road to Eleusis: Unveiling the secret of the mysteries* (1st ed.). New York: Harcourt Brace Jovanovich.

Winkelman, M. (2005). Drug tourism of spiritual healing? Ayahuasca seekers in Amazonia. *Journal of Psychoactive Drugs, 37,* 209–218.

Winkelman, M. J., & Roberts, T. B. (Eds.). (2007). *Psychedelic medicine: New evidence for hallucinogenic substances as treatments.* Westport, CT: Praeger.

Wright, D., Sathe, N., & Spagnola, K. (2007). *State estimates of substance use from the 2004-2005 National Surveys on Drug Use and Health* (DHHS Publication No. SMA 07-4235, NSDUH Series H-31). Rockville, MD: Substance Abuse and Mental Health Services Administration, Office of Applied Studies.

Zinberg, N. E. (1986). *Drug, set, and setting: The basis for controlled intoxicant use.* New Haven, CT: Yale University Press.

20

Club Drugs: An Overview

John J. Echeverry and Christopher D. Nettles

The George Washington University

Contents

> My skin feels warm and tingly . . . all I want is to touch and be touched in a never ending mutual caress that makes me feel wanted and sexy. And I hate when the sensation ends and I feel alone, distant, and sort of dead inside. Makes me want to use . . . again.

Club drugs are the epitome of incongruence. Pleasure and sorrow, fun and desolation, fulfillment and wanting are some of the typical effects on users, not unlike most of the so-called recreational drugs. The above quote comes from a regular user of Ecstasy, one of the most common club drugs in the United States. After several years of using various club drugs, alone or in combination with other drugs, the user felt trapped by the temporary feelings of elation and physical pleasure felt while using, and also trapped by the inability to stop regular use, not necessarily because of a physical craving, but out of a desire to re-experience the pleasure he felt while under the influence. This is not an atypical scenario.

This chapter presents an overview of some of the most common club drugs used in this country, and includes information on available treatments for club drug abusers. It covers what club drugs are; what they are called in the streets; what their effects are on the user's behavior, emotions, mental functioning, and body; evidence-based information on treatments available for club drug abuse; the importance of culture and context to our understanding of these substances and their use; which subpopulations are most at risk; and current and future research trends. This chapter also includes a list of resources for information on this complex group of drugs. The text is in the form of questions and answers that cover some of the most salient aspects of club drug use. Technical matters such as the physiological, neurobiological, and genetic aspects of drug abuse are covered in much greater detail in other chapters of this and other books.

What is a Club Drug?

A club drug is a controlled substance or chemical that is typically used by young people at bars, dance clubs, and all-night dancing parties called *raves, trances, sex,* or *circuit parties.* These drugs are also known as party drugs, rave drugs, designer drugs, and synthetic drugs. The term designer drug, in particular, refers to a drug available in the illegal market that is a chemical analog of another psychoactive drug.

Which are the Most Common Club Drugs?

There are several drugs that are considered club or designer drugs, but the typical list includes: Ecstasy, Rohypnol, ketamine, GHB, crystal methamphetamine, and poppers. Table 20.1 shows the club drugs discussed in this chapter, along with other terms by which each drug is known, including street names. As with most drugs, some of the street names are regional or even local.

Some include in their list of club drugs substances such as cocaine in its various forms, LSD, and alcohol. Users and abusers of some club drugs also have their specific names. Those who abuse Ecstasy may be called *E-tards* or *peepers*, and abusers of crystal meth are called *cranksters*, *speed freaks*, or *tweakers*.

TABLE 20.1
Common Club Drugs

Drug Name	Also Known As	Street Names
Ecstasy	MDMA; 3-4 methylenedyoxymethamphetamine	XTC; Adam; hug drug; beans; love drug; go; happy pill; disco biscuit; and E!
Rohypnol	Flunitrazepam	The date rape drug; rophies; roofies; roach; forget-me pill; rope; and Mexican valium
Ketamine	Ketamine hydrochloride	K; Special "K"; vitamin K; Kit Kat; Keller; super C; super acid; jet; and cat valium
Crystal meth	Crystal methamphetamine	Meth; tina; chalk; speed; ice; crystal; tweek; bling bling; and poor man's coke
GHB	Gamma hydroxybutyrate	Liquid Ecstasy; Georgia home boy; easy lay; vita-G; grievous bodily harm; great hormones at bedtime; goop; max; and soap
Poppers	Volatile or inhaled nitrites; Amyl nitrite; Isobutyl nitrite	Aimes; aimies; ames; amys; boppers; locker room; Viagra in a bottle; and pearls

Sources. http://ncadistore.samhsa.gov/catalog/facts.aspx?topic=13&h=drugs; http://www.drugabuse.gov/infofacts/metham phetamine.html; http://www.whitehousedrugpolicy.gov/streetterms/.

Which are the Populations at Risk for Club Drug Use?

As is the case for most illicit drugs consumed in the United States, adolescents and young adults constitute the largest at-risk group for club drug use. College students, women, and gay, bisexual, and other men who have sex with men are also vulnerable groups.

Ecstasy

What is Ecstasy?

Ecstasy, or MDMA, is a mind-altering or psychoactive compound with properties that resemble those of hallucinogens (such as mescaline) and amphetamines (NIDA, 2008a). Its chemical structure, 3,4-methylenedyoxymethamphetamine, is similar to that of methamphetamine, which is known to cause brain damage. Ecstasy has been available in the United States for decades, and is traditionally manufactured in small clandestine labs in Europe (mainly in the Netherlands, Belgium, and Luxembourg), Canada, and Asia. This drug typically comes in tablet form. The tablets may contain MDMA alone, or in combination with other substances such as caffeine, codeine, acetaminophen, ketamine, or methamphetamine.

Each tablet may cost between $15 and $50 on the street, but this cost may experience up and down fluctuations depending on drug availability, demand, and location.

How Prevalent is Ecstasy Use?

There have been some studies on Ecstasy use in national samples, such as a study on college students by Strote, Lee, and Wechsler (2002), in which they found a last-year prevalence of use of 4.7%. Monitoring the Future (MTF), found that 11% of 12th graders reported having used Ecstasy at some point (Johnston, O'Malley, & Bachman, 2001). However, two more recent statistics suggest that Ecstasy use may be on the decline. A SAMHSA report (2003) shows a substantial decline in the number of Ecstasy-related emergency room admissions, and The University of Maryland Center for Substance Abuse Research (CESAR) reported that 0.8% of U.S. household residents over the age of 12 stated having used Ecstasy in 2005. CESAR (2004) has also reported a dramatic decline in first-time use of Ecstasy, from 1.8 million in 2001 to 1.1 million in 2002, and the National Survey on Drug Use and Health (NSDUH) found an even more dramatic decline in past year use among persons aged 12 or older, from 3.2 million in 2002 to 2.1 million in 2003 (NSDUH Report, 2005).

What are the Effects of Ecstasy on the Person?

There is a widespread belief that Ecstasy increases openness and trust among people, therefore, decreasing barriers in interpersonal relations. Users report a sense of increased energy and wakefulness, euphoria, excitement, and heightened sexual pleasure (Novoa, Ompad, Wu, Vlahov, & Galea, 2005), and talkativeness, tolerance, calmness, and self-assurance (Camí & Farré, 1996). However, users may also experience a number of adverse effects that include physical/physiological problems, and psychological difficulties. A user may experience increases in heart rate and blood pressure, sleep problems, muscle tension, bruxism (involuntary teeth clenching), nausea, sweating or chills, blurred vision, and fainting. In high doses, Ecstasy affects the body's ability to regulate temperature. Likewise, the user can experience confusion, paranoia, severe anxiety, detachment, and depression. These issues can occur during use and even days or weeks thereafter (NIDA, 2008a).

For some users, Ecstasy is intrinsically linked to sexual activity. These include gay and bisexual women, gay, bisexual, and other men who have sex with men (MSM). Emotional closeness and sexual arousal, as well as frequent risky sexual behavior (defined as engaging in sex without a condom) were found in a sample of Ecstasy users (McElrath, 2005). Novoa et al. (2005) found that in a sample of drug users, Ecstasy use predicted early sexual activity (before age 14), and having two or more partners in the preceding two months.

Who are the Typical Users of Ecstasy?

Ecstasy is available virtually everywhere in the United States. Adolescents, college students, and young adults of both sexes seem to be the most likely users. Moreover, recent studies suggest that users of Ecstasy are also very likely to use other drugs. The most recent NSDUH found that more than 90% of Ecstasy users used other illegal drugs, whereas less than 14% of nonusers did (2005). Lesbian and bisexual women may be an at-risk group, as well as men who have sex with men. McErlath (2005) found that gay and bisexual women use Ecstasy as a "sexual aid." Although Ecstasy may have been primarily used by Whites, its use may be spreading among ethnic and racial minorities in this country.

Is there a Treatment for Ecstasy Abuse?

Harm reduction seems to be the only intervention for Ecstasy abuse that appears in the literature. Regulating Ecstasy use and therefore reducing its potential for neurocognitive and neurophysiological changes and damage falls more in the realm of prevention than on a specific intervention (Baggott, 2002; Panagopoulos & Ricciardelli, 2005). It may indeed be the case that interventions that have been used to address abuse and addiction to other drugs are useful for Ecstasy abuse. These interventions may include individual, family, and group psychotherapy; 12-step programs, and support groups. Moreover, because Ecstasy-only abuse is unlikely, a more general approach may be efficacious.

What are the Current Behavioral Research Trends on Ecstasy?

Much attention is being paid to the connection between Ecstasy use and risky sexual behavior, particularly because many users consume Ecstasy as a tool for enhanced sex. This combination of Ecstasy use and sex without adequate protection may have potentially dire consequences to communities of users, such as MSM and gay and bisexual women, among whom the risk of contracting a sexually transmitted infection such as HIV may be high. Some researchers are beginning to note a shift of Ecstasy use from raves and similar contexts such as clubs to other venues, including private homes, and increasing use in groups such as heroin and cocaine users

(Novoa et al., 2005), whereas other data indicate a possible decrease in the overall number of new users, which for some may suggest that consumption is becoming experimental (occasional or one-time) rather than a matter of addiction (Camí & Farré, 1996; CESAR, 2006). Much more research is needed to elucidate further the physiological, cognitive, emotional, and behavioral consequences of Ecstasy abuse.

Rohypnol

What is Rohypnol?

Rohypnol is the trade name for flunitrazepam, which belongs to a class of drugs called benzodiazepines. Its street names include *roach, roofies, Mexican Valium,* and *rophies*. Its original medical use was as a preoperative anesthetic, and for sedation and treatment of insomnia (Maxwell, 2005b). It typically comes in the form of pills.

How Prevalent is Rohypnol Use?

Rohypnol is not widely used compared to some other club drugs, and some recent studies suggest a decline in use among high school students, particularly 10th graders, among whom lifetime use declined from 2.0% in 1998 to 0.8% in 2006 (NIDA, 2008b).

What are the Effects of Rohypnol on the Person?

Rohypnol severely affects short-term memory, making its users unable to remember events that occurred while using the drug. It also may incapacitate users, making them unable to resist assaults, including sexual abuse. For this reason, it is sometimes known as the *date rape drug*, along with some of the other club drugs, including ketamine and GHB. Furthermore, when mixed with alcohol, Rohypnol may prove to be lethal. Confusion, dizziness, and occasional aggressive behavior may also occur among users. As abuse peaked several years ago, in October 1996, Congress enacted the Drug-Induced Rape Prevention and Punishment Act of 1996, with the purpose of increasing federal penalties for the use of any controlled substance in the context of sexual assaults (NIDA, 2008b).

Who are the Typical Users of Rohypnol?

Teenagers and young adults are the typical Rohypnol users, particularly those who attend raves or are frequently part of the club, rave, and trance scenes. It is also commonly used among college students. Heroin and cocaine addicts are also typical users, particularly because it decreases the "crash" among the latter.

Is there a Treatment for Rohypnol Abuse?

As it appears that Rohypnol is used in combination with other drugs and alcohol, and that some of its users may be in the criminal justice system. Treatment may typically consist of the "treatment as usual" concept (TAU): outpatient services including regular Narcotics Anonymous (NA) meetings, group therapy, and individual psychotherapy to address issues such as a conduct disorder, when present.

What are the Current Behavioral Research Trends on Rohypnol?

Although Rohypnol does not appear to be the focus of much behavioral research in the United States, an overview of the existing recent literature suggests that some research is being conducted on the adverse effects of the drug, its connection with juvenile delinquency, and on the dangers of its combination with alcohol and other substances of abuse.

Ketamine

What is Ketamine?

Ketamine is an anesthetic that has been used for humans and animals—especially cats and monkeys—in the United States since the early 1970s. Most of the current use is for veterinary medicine purposes (NIDA, 2008b). Ketamine is also known as a dissociative anesthetic because it distorts an individual's perceptions of sound and sight, and produces feelings of detachment. It can be snorted or injected, and is known also by its street names of *Special K, K, Kit-Kat,* and *Vitamin K.* It is marketed as Ketalar by Parke-Davis for human medical use in the United States (Porrata, 2006).

How Prevalent is Ketamine Use?

According to the 2006 findings from the Monitoring the Future Survey (MTF), 1.0% of 10th graders and 1.4% of 12th graders reported using ketamine that year in the United States (NIDA, 2008b). It can be injected, taken in tablets, or inhaled in powder form. Ketamine users typically use other drugs, such as heroin, marijuana, cocaine, and alcohol. Unlike crystal methamphetamine, for example, it is not easily manufactured, inasmuch as its production requires multistep sophisticated procedures.

What are the Effects of Ketamine on the Person?

The effects of ketamine depend on the dosage used. Some doses may cause hallucinations and dreamlike states, and higher doses may cause depression, potentially fatal respiratory problems, amnesia, insomnia, slurred speech, and high blood pressure (NIDA, 2008b). Flashbacks from ketamine use are common (Porrata, 2006). A dose is called a "bump" and users are referred to as "K-heads" (Porrata, 2006).

Despite some of the pleasant effects of ketamine, many users of other club drugs dislike this particular drug and would not ingest Ecstasy pills, for example, if they knew it contained traces of ketamine, which is not uncommon. Johnston et al. (2006) reported that over 57% of Ecstasy users using kits to test the purity of their Ecstasy pills, would not use these pills if they found it contained ketamine.

Who are the Typical Users of Ketamine?

Young people who participate regularly in the rave party scene appear to be the most common users of ketamine, either by itself, but more typically in combination with GHB and MDMA (Ecstasy). Similar to other club drugs, its use appears to be more prevalent among adolescents and young adults, including those who are part of Gay, Lesbian, Bisexual and Transgender (GLBT) communities. Frequent use of ketamine among gay and bisexual males who attend circuit parties in some large cities has been found to be associated with unsafe sex practices (Mattison, Ross, Wolfsan, & Franklin, 2001). Because of its effect of amnesia, it is sometimes given to unsuspecting individuals who then become vulnerable to sexual assault, as in the case of Rohypnol, another so-called "date rape drug."

Ketamine injectors were found to participate in polydrug-using events in the New York City area (Lankenau & Clatts, 2005). The sequence of drug use, types or combinations of drugs used, and the modes of administration were found to vary, adding an additional layer of complexity to ketamine use and abuse.

Is there a Treatment for Ketamine Abuse?

There is no specific treatment for ketamine abuse. Abusers are typically treated using the same methods used for abusers of other club drugs, as seen above, while paying particular attention to dangerous overdose effects such as respiratory distress, hallucinations, and paranoid ideation. Most ketamine abusers who seek treatment do so because of overdoses, wanting detoxification, or because of unpleasant and unexpected reactions to the drug. Specific treatment strategies used for polydrug users who include ketamine in their drug using behavior may be helpful.

What are the Current Behavioral Research Trends on Ketamine?

A brief review of the literature on ketamine suggests that much of the research focus on this drug appears to be on its benefits rather than on its deleterious effects. Some studies have found that ketamine may be the medication of choice for treatment-resistant major depression (Berman, et al., 2000; Khamsi, 2006; Zárate, et al., 2006), and for pain treatment. Much research is needed to learn more about the long-term effects of ketamine use, its potential for psychological and physical dependence, and its emergence as a drug of choice among polydrug-using ketamine intravenous and intramuscular injectors.

Gamma Hydroxybutyrate (GHB)

What is GHB?

Gamma hydroxybutyrate (GHB) is a central nervous system depressant that was widely available in health food stores until the early 1990s because of its fat reduction and muscle-building properties. Eventually it became a substance of abuse because of its euphoric and sedative effects (NIDA, 2008b). In high doses it provides anesthetic effects. Some of its street names include *Georgia Home Boy*, *liquid Ecstasy*, *G*, *Juice*, *Fantasy*, and *soap*. It typically comes in powder form, which is then mixed with juice or a type of beverage that hides its salty taste. GHB is a fatty acid that is found naturally in humans, but there is scant information on what levels are normal and in what parts of the body GHB tends to concentrate.

How Prevalent is GHB Use?

According to NIDA's 2008a MTF survey, 0.7% of 10th graders and 1.1% of 12th graders that year reported using GHB. Although in global numbers GHB is not widely used, its use is high among certain subgroups, as detailed below. Its availability in gyms, some health food stores, over the Internet, on the street, at raves, nightclubs, and gay male circuit parties is well known. Like Rohypnol and alcohol, it is known as a date rape drug.

What are the Effects of GHB on the Person?

Seizures and coma are relatively common among GHB users, and the effects may be exacerbated by combining it with other drugs or alcohol, in which case may lead to breathing difficulties and unconsciousness. A salient characteristic of GHB is that it may produce serious withdrawal symptoms that include sweating, insomnia, anxiety, and tremors (McDaniel & Miotto, 2001). Its abuse has been linked to overdoses, poisonings, sexual assaults, and deaths (NIDA, 2008b). Some of the effects considered positive by users include euphoria, increased libido, and increased ability to socialize. It is not known if prolonged GHB use causes permanent physical harm.

Who are the Typical Users of GHB?

According to the information contained in the best known website on GHB, www.project. ghb.org, there are several subgroups of typical GHB users. These subgroups include all ages, ethnicities, and sexual orientations, such as frequent travelers who think of it as a safe sleep aid; those who attend rave or circuit parties; members of GLBT communities who perceive GHB as a recreational drug; sexual predators who may want to take sexual advantage of others who are under the influence of the drug; and bodybuilders, who have been among the main subgroups of GHB users from the beginning, due to the drug's apparent ability to improve athletic performance and build muscle.

Is there a Treatment for GHB Abuse?

Treatment for GHB abuse typically consists of detoxification, medication for any comorbid condition such as depression, and 12-step meetings. Some studies suggest that most substance abuse treatment providers lack sufficient information and knowledge to recognize GHB dependence and symptoms, and are particularly concerned about gay and bisexual male users who may also be HIV-positive, because of the implications of mixing GHB and antiretrovirals (Maxwell, 2005a).

What are the Current Behavioral Research Trends on GHB?

Research on GHB use appears to focus on the frequency and dangers of overdosing, the difficulties assessing what doses are dangerous and for whom, the risks of combining GHB with other drugs or alcohol, contextual factors associated with its use, such as polydrug use, use and abuse among young bodybuilders, and the difficulty in quickly treating severe withdrawal reactions.

Crystal Methamphetamine

What is Crystal Methamphetamine?

Crystal methamphetamine, also known as *speed, glass, crank,* or *tina,* is an extremely addictive central nervous system stimulant producing intoxication through stimulation of dopamine and norepinephrine receptors in the brain (Covey, 2007; NIDA, 2008b). Methamphetamine is synthetically derived from ephedrine or pseudoephedrine, an ingredient in many decongestants (Anglin, Burke, Perrochet, Stamper & Dawud-Noursi, 2000; Barker & Antia, 2006; Puder, Kagan & Morgan, 1988). It sometimes resembles small shards of glass, shiny blue-white "rocks," or an odorless, white powder (Covey, 2007; NIDA, 2008b). Methamphetamine can be snorted intranasally, smoked (Beebe & Walley, 1995; Harris, et al., 2003), injected intravenously (Maglione, Chao, & Anglin, 1998), taken orally (Kim, Oyler, Moolchan, Cone & Huestis, 2004), and inserted into the anus (called *booty bumping*; Wiener, Hexdall, McStay, Nelson, & Hoffman, 2004).

How Prevalent is Crystal Methamphetamine Use?

In the 1980s methamphetamine use in the United States was mainly limited to the West Coast (Anglin, et al., 2000; Derlet & Heischober, 1990). In recent years, however, crystal methamphetamine use has spread through much of the United States. It has been compared to an epidemic, spreading from the West to the Southwest and then to the rest of the country (NIDA, 2008a; Rawson, Anglin, & Ling, 2002). The 2005 NSDUH estimates that 10.4 million Americans aged 12 or older used methamphetamine at least once in their lifetimes for nonmedical reasons or 4.3% of the U.S. population in that age group. Those reporting use in the preceding year were approximately 1.3 million or 0.5% of the population aged 12 or older and the number of past month methamphetamine users was 512,000 or 0.2% (SAMHSA, 2006).

What are the Effects of Crystal Methamphetamine on the Person?

Crystal methamphetamine increases arousal by boosting levels of norepinephrine and dopamine in the central nervous system. As with other stimulants, crystal methamphetamine heightens alertness while suppressing appetite and fatigue. Physical effects include increased heart rate, increased blood pressure, and hyperthermia. At high doses, it causes euphoria and exhilaration. Prolonged use or very high doses can cause agitation, paranoia, and symptoms similar to psychosis (Covey, 2007; NIDA, 2008b). Long-term abuse is also associated with a condition called "meth mouth" where there is severe tooth decay at the gum line (Richards & Brofeldt, 2000). Recent literature also points to increased need and urgency for sex, the ability to have sex over extended timeframes, and inorgasmia (Parsons & Bimbi, 2006; Semple, Zians, Grant, & Patterson, 2006.). The sexual compulsivity combined with reduced inhibitions is thought to increase the likelihood that intercourse will occur without condom use, therefore increasing the chances of sexually transmitted infections and HIV exposure (Bogart et al., 2005; Colfax & Guzman, 2006; Semple, Patterson, & Grant, 2004).

Who are the Typical Users of Crystal Methamphetamine?

Crystal methamphetamine use has been documented in both urban and rural communities (Booth, Leukefeld, Falck, Wang & Carlson, 2006; Wu, Pilowsky, Wechsberg, & Schlenger, 2004). Although use is most prevalent in Caucasian heterosexual and GLBT communities, there is evidence of increasing use among African-American and Hispanic populations (Brecht, Greenwell & Anglin, 2005; Díaz, Heckert, & Sánchez, 2005; Green & Halkitis, 2006; Wohl, et al. 2002).

Is there a Treatment for Methamphetamine Abuse?

There is growing evidence for several approaches to treatment for methamphetamine abuse. Treatment approaches include cognitive-behavioral therapy (CBT), contingency management, and harm reduction strategies. One recent study points to the efficacy of combining contingency management and cognitive-behavioral approaches (Shoptaw et al., 2005). Harm reduction strategies are also important approaches to reducing the harm associated with methamphetamine use and abuse (Tatarsky, 2003).

What are the Current Behavioral Research Trends on Crystal Methamphetamine?

Research on crystal methamphetamine is continuing at a very rapid pace. A recent search of Google Scholar produced over 1,000 articles published during 2007 with the word "methamphetamine" in the article. Behavioral research is expanding at a rapid pace on evidence-based treatments, associated high-risk sexual behavior, use among men who have sex with men, among rural populations, among youth, and among minorities in the United States. Understanding the behavioral and neurological effects associated with long-term use of crystal methamphetamine is of vital importance.

Poppers

What are Poppers?

Poppers are one of the street names for various nitrites, compounds that are inhaled directly for recreational purposes. The most common poppers are amyl, butyl and isobutyl nitrites.

Some times they are sold legally as air fresheners or video head cleaners, although this latter use is quickly disappearing thanks to advances in technology. Poppers have been around for a long time, but their use became rampant with the sexual freedom of the disco scene of the 1980s, particularly in clubs and bars and among homosexual and bisexual men to enhance sexual pleasure. In the 1990s and even today, poppers have been popular in the rave scene. *Locker room*, *Viagra in a bottle*, *Rush, Liquid Gold*, and *amyes*, are some of the other street names for poppers. Names may change from place to place.

How Prevalent is Poppers Use?

As with most of the other club drugs described here, it is somewhat difficult to estimate accurately how prevalent popper use is, in part because it may disappear for long periods and then show a resurgence. This is exactly what may be happening now at the end of the first decade of the 2000s, when anecdotal information suggests an increase of first-time users, usually young adolescents, as well as among gay and bisexual men who may have added to their club drug paraphernalia.

What are the Effects of Poppers on the Person?

Poppers are used by inhaling its vapors from a small bottle. Its effects may last from 30 seconds to up to two minutes. There are two main effects to sniffing poppers. One, it dilates or relaxes muscles around blood vessels, which accelerates the heart's blood pumping function, and, two, poppers allow the muscles around the anus and vagina to relax. In the case of the speeding up of the heart, oxygen-rich blood reaches the brain, which produces a highly pleasurable, if brief, sensation. As far as the relaxation of anal and vaginal muscles, the sensation is also pleasurable and is one of the effects that most attracts its users, especially during sexual activity and at the moment of orgasm. Frequent use may cause burns in nasal openings and cause lung irritation, make the person vulnerable to unprotected sexual activity which may lead to infections such as sexually transmitted diseases including HIV (DanceSafe.org, 2007), and potential deleterious effects on the user's immune system.

Who are the Typical Users of Poppers?

As suggested above, anyone may be a user of poppers, but currently in the United States, use tends to concentrate among young adolescents (mostly for the quick rush poppers provide) and gay or bisexual men and women of any age who use poppers for the rush and for sexual enhancement.

Is there a Treatment for Poppers Abuse?

A literature search suggests that there is no treatment for poppers, mostly because very few people become addicted to this drug alone. Its use is done usually in conjunction with other club drugs and alcohol. Hence, any treatment would involve that for other drugs also. In the case of the occasional overdose, medical personnel should be aware of what poppers are and how they affect the body, as described above.

What are the Current Behavioral Research Trends on Poppers?

Poppers have never been the focus of much research in medicine or the social sciences. However this trend may be beginning to change as the drug becomes better known among the public in general. One area of great concern is the interactions that may occur with simultaneous use of poppers and other club drugs, alcohol, and more recently drugs for erectile dysfunction problems, such as Viagra, Levitra, and Cialis.

Case Presentation

"Alex" is a 36-year-old immigrant, who came to the United States at age 23 to pursue an advanced degree. He came out to himself as a gay man at age 25, shortly after a bisexual friend took him to a gay club. Alex enjoyed the experience, and became a regular at the local bars, dance and sex clubs, and the circuit party scene. These outings gave him a sense of freedom, an opportunity to develop a network of friends like himself, and meet sex partners. Eventually, he became involved in some experiences that changed his life style. These experiences included participation in the sex party scene and regular alcohol and drug use. More often that not, the two became intertwined.

When he was about to turn 33, Alex sought therapy with his clinical psychologist. His presenting problems included symptoms of obsessive-compulsive disorder (OCD), difficulties in forming and maintaining romantic relationships, and a sense of "unhappiness" with his life. However, his many intellectual, athletic, and personality strengths made it possible for him to develop a very successful career, to have a small but supportive network of friends, and to have a busy social and sexual life, which was helped by his physical attractiveness and warm and outgoing personality.

After several psychotherapy sessions, Alex confided to his therapist that he was drinking regularly at bars and at home, and using an assortment of club drugs that included Ecstasy and crystal methamphetamine. He stated that he used Ecstasy every weekend, "for the rush it gives me. … It makes me feel hot and attractive, and I can dance all night if I want to." His use of crystal meth was occasional, perhaps twice a month or so, and was done usually in the context of sexual activity, with whomever he was dating at the time, or with anonymous sex partners. The sexual activity occurred in various places, such as at the club itself, at a public venue such as a park, or at a home. Alex insisted that he always was in "control of the situation" and reported that his regular HIV tests were always negative as a result of what he perceived to be consistent condom use.

It is not unusual for this type of scenario to be reported in the context of individual psychotherapy with a private practitioner. The client or patient may come in complaining of depression, anxiety, relationship issues, or, as in this case, with some OCD features. Even though he was asked by the psychologist about drug and alcohol use in the initial evaluation, the client only disclosed his substance use once he felt he could trust this psychotherapist.

As Alex later stated, "I was afraid of being judged negatively by you, and about the legal implications of disclosing this information. I had decided at that point to remain in this country, and didn't want to jeopardize my legal immigration status." There was also some embarrassment on Alex's part, because he did not want to "lose face" as a cultured and well-educated professional who engaged in some behaviors he perceived as "stuff losers do, like those guys who practically live at the bars drinking, smoking, using drugs, and having sex with other losers."

Between the intake evaluation and his disclosure of substance use, treatment consisted of interventions to address Alex's OCD symptoms, which included checking his apartment door multiple times before bed to ensure it was locked, as well as some visible facial tics that embarrassed him in public. All these symptoms, and the underlying anxiety, were addressed through a combination of CBT interventions and anti-anxiety medication prescribed by a psychiatrist. Although the OCD symptoms did not disappear completely, they did subside in frequency and intensity, which Alex found very satisfactory and manageable.

Over the following two years of therapy, his OCD symptoms remained infrequent and short-lived. His romantic relationship issues consisted of difficulties in developing the type of bond he felt he wanted and needed, a combination of physical attraction, intellectual compatibility, mutual emotional support, and common goals. Furthermore, Alex wanted his partner to be interested in his culture of origin, and to be monogamous. He moved from an incipient relationship to another, never satisfied with the man he was with and always searching for his ideal partner. All these issues were explored extensively over a period of two years, using an eclectic combination of CBT techniques, psychodynamic psychotherapy, and some elements of Acceptance Commitment Therapy (ACT); (Hayes, Strosahl, & Wilson, 1999).

Alex made substantial progress and became more flexible regarding his idealized version of the perfect lover, more reasonable in his expectations from the other, and less hard on himself for not having the stable and durable relationship for which he longed. Eventually he met a much younger man, someone who fulfilled most of his criteria. By the time of his termination from therapy, they were living together happily in a monogamous relationship that was sexually, emotionally, and intellectually satisfying to both, as per Alex's report.

Addressing the matter of his substance abuse proved to be trickier. Alex denied his weekend club drug use was a problem, emphasizing his continued physical and emotional well-being, his ability to "control" use, and his need to enjoy club drugs with his new lover. All efforts to educate him further about club drugs in general and crystal meth in particular met with resistance. This situation was compounded by the lack of specific treatment facilities, programs, or even support groups for club drug users in his locality.

However, he was able to explore the roots of such resistance, which turned out to be fear of a resurgence of his OCD symptoms; being a "stick in the mud" in his social network, many of whose members were regular club drug users; and becoming "just another ageing gay guy who was out of the loop with the younger crowd." He was reassured that the CBT techniques he had learned in therapy and implemented in his daily life, along with the anti-anxiety medication he was taking would impede a resurging and increase of his OCD symptoms. He was encouraged to expand his network of friends and acquaintances to include people who were nonusers of club or any other drugs.

Interventions that addressed his fear of becoming older in a community that focuses on youth, beauty, and fitness were helpful, in particular the aspect of his being partnered with a man 14 years his junior, whom he feared would abandon him as he got older and lost some of his good looks. Moreover, Alex began reading and educating himself on the potential disadvantages of club drug use, in particular his two drugs of choice, Ecstasy and crystal meth. The greatest challenge when discussing his substance use was in getting Alex to accept that although he had some control over the extent of his use, this could change quickly at any moment from occasional use to an out-of-control situation that would affect all aspects of his life.

By appealing to his sense of responsibility for self, the importance he gave to fitness and grooming, and the great importance he gave to his career, he began making some lifestyle changes. He reduced by half his alcohol intake, from 15 cocktails or glasses of wine per week; he began socializing more in friends' homes or in his own; and he decreased the frequency of Ecstasy and crystal meth to once every three months or so, when he and his partner would travel to New York City or abroad. Lastly, work was done on getting Alex to find alternative sources of fun and pleasure that did not involve substance use. He increased his workouts at the gym and began spending more time at home with his lover, instead of going out to the bars during the week. At follow-up, some six months after the termination of therapy, he reported being very happy with his life, very much in love with his partner, and less anxious than at the beginning of therapy. He also reported that his drinking and drugging had become minimal, and that he was concentrating on athletic pursuits and on a possible career change.

In many ways, Alex was the ideal client. He was bright and introspective, eager to work on most issues he presented, and responsible with his attendance to all therapy sessions. He was willing to make behavioral changes that led to an improvement in his overall symptomatology and substance use. His gradual improvement reinforced the maintenance of those behaviors. This is not always the case, particularly with clients who do not accept that their use or abuse is a problem; those who refuse to recognize the havoc club drug abuse may be having on their careers, relationships, health, mental stability, and finances; those who after years of use are too fearful of life without their drug of choice; those who only see the presumed advantages of their drugs, such as pleasure, a reduction in shyness, and enhanced sexuality, and those who have to attend therapy sessions because of some legal problems that have gotten them involved with the criminal justice system.

As helping professionals who work with substance abusers know well, Alex's profile and history suggest likely success in treatment. Such is not the case for people who have a greater involvement in club drug use and abuse, as measured by its intensity, duration, and frequency, as well as the specific drugs being used and the unwillingness of users to seek treatment. This situation is further complicated by the relative lack of treatment programs and facilities that would help these users, as well as by the relative lack of information on club drugs that is readily available in the places where users may congregate.

Furthermore, many clinicians, including social workers, counselors, psychiatrists, and psychologists may lack some of the basic knowledge and expertise that are necessary in order to effectively treat club drug users who may come to them for help in private practice situations or in substance abuse programs. Lastly, stigma may also play a role in refusal to seek treatment. Meanwhile, club drug use, particularly crystal meth, continues to expand across the nation and become more hidden, which may affect the efficacy of prevention and treatment efforts.

Other Considerations Regarding Club Drugs

Why are Culture and Context Important when we Try to Understand Club Drug Use?

Music Club drug use is clearly linked to certain types of music, in the context of raves, and circuit and after-hours parties. Lewes & Ross (1995) described the importance some specific types of music in the gay male circuit party scene of Sidney, where *house* and *techno* were the predominant rhythms. Camí & Farré (1996) found that *acid house* was the precursor music for this type of party scene in Europe in the 1980s, and that it evolved over time into *techno music* which then became popular in North America shortly thereafter. This *techno* music consists of a fast-paced repetitive percussion-laden rhythm, usually played loudly and in conjunction with video and laser light shows. In this context, the disc jockey plays a rather important role, as the person who chooses and plays the music that is most likely to be a good fit with the rave party clientele. The purpose of a particular music choice is to enable every patron to have fun, stay in the establishment for long periods of time, consume beverages including alcoholic drinks, and become a regular rave party attendee.

Legislation and Law Enforcement

The Controlled Substance Act (CSA), Title II of the Comprehensive Drug Abuse Prevention and Control Act of 1970 has included club drugs in its schedules (DEA, 2005). Ecstasy is Schedule I as of 1998, Rohypnol is Schedule IV as of 1984, ketamine is Schedule III as of 1999, and GHB is Schedule I as of 2000. The lower the schedule number the more dangerous the drug is considered by the Drug Enforcement Administration (DEA). Hence, Ecstasy and GHB are considered dangerous narcotics (along with heroin and LSD) with potential for abuse. Their manufacture, possession, or distribution may carry serious legal penalties, including heavy fines and incarceration. These legal ramifications may play a considerable role in making club drug use move from bars, clubs, and the circuit party scene to an underground network of private homes and sex parties, which attendees usually learn about through the Internet.

What Club Drug Research may be Needed in the Foreseeable Future?

Despite the availability of club drugs in the United States for decades, and the substantial number of research studies that have been done, much more hard data are still needed to understand the range of implications of club drug use and abuse. Psychologists, psychiatrists, anthropologists, sociologists, public health experts, and epidemiologists have been at the forefront of physiological, behavioral, and psychosocial research that has helped our understanding of club drug use. Their contributions include knowledge about the incidence and prevalence of club drug use, the contexts in which these drugs are obtained and consumed, the street names given to these substances in various locales, the profile of the typical consumer, and the effects these drugs have on the user's emotions, mental and cognitive processes, behavior, interpersonal relationships, as well as to the effects on communities or groups. Likewise, physicians, chemists, pharmacologists, microbiologists, neurophysiologists, neurologists, and other specialists in the health sciences have made substantial contributions to our understanding of the ways club drugs affect the human body, especially the brain.

The need to continue conducting research on club drugs is unquestionable. We need to learn more about the emotional, mental/cognitive, behavioral, and other effects on users and abusers of club drugs, especially by studying users over time and even after regular use has ceased. Prospective or longitudinal studies would be particularly useful to obtain this information. Prevention and treatment is another area of research that merits particular attention. Is a club drug abuse treatment protocol possible, or even wise to consider? It is possible that because of the differences across club drugs, as shown above, specific treatments or best-practices protocols will be the best way to treat abusers of specific club drugs. The complication here would be how best to treat a polydrug abuser who consumes either various club drugs, or club drugs and alcohol, or another illicit drug such as cocaine, heroin, or marijuana.

For more information on material related to club drugs, there is a substantial number of websites, many of which are sponsored by the U.S. government, mostly through the National Institutes of Mental Health. A brief listing of these websites for your perusal appears in Table 20.2.

TABLE 20.2
Club Drug Resources

Ecstasy:

http://www.brown.edu/Student_Services/Health_Services/Health_Education/atod/od_ecstasy.htm

http://teens.drugabuse.gov/stories/story_xtc1.asp

http://www.nida.nih.gov/infofacts/ecstasy.html

http://www.baysidemarin.com/resources/ecstasy.html

Rohypnol and GHB:

http://www.brown.edu/Student_Services/Health_Services/Health_Education/atod/od_rohypnol.htm

http://www.smith.edu/sao/sexualassaultresources/rohypnol.php

http://www.baysidemarin.com/resources/rohypnol_ghb.html

http://www.brown.edu/Student_Services/Health_Services/Health_Education/atod/od_rohypnol.htm

http://www.teen-drug-abuse.org/Rohypnol-and-GHB.htm

http://www.redribbonworks.org/resource_home.asp?parent=2&PageId=51

http://www.drugstats.org/features/dis/rohyandghb.cfm

http://www.dea.gov/concern/flunitrazepam.html

http://ncadi.samhsa.gov/newsroom/abuseInformation/default.aspx?s=rohypnol

Ketamine:

http://olin.msu.edu/factsheet.php?ID=5

http://www.mendezfoundation.org/resources/druginfo/ketamine.htm

http://ncadi.samhsa.gov/newsroom/abuseInformation/default.aspx?s=ketamine

http://www.brown.edu/Student_Services/Health_Services/Health_Education/atod/od_ketamine.htm

Poppers:

http://dancesafe.org

http://www.brookes.ac.uk/health/libra/nitrite.html

Crystal Methamphetamine:

http://www.lifeormeth.com/

http://www.drugfree.org/Portal/DrugIssue/Meth/resources.html

http://www.thebody.com/sfaf/crystal_meth.html

http://www.thebody.com/bp/oct04/crystal_meth.html

http://www.dea.gov/concern/meth.html

http://www.gaycenter.org/Surveys/crystal/

http://www.crystal-meth.us/resources.htm

http://www.whitehousedrugpolicy.gov/drugfact/methamphetamine/index.html

http://chp-pcs.gc.ca/CHP/index_e.jsp/pageid/4005/odp/Top/Health/Youth/Addictions/Drugs/Crystal_Meth

http://www.thecentersd.org/methinfo.php

Additional Resources of Interest:

http://www.whitehousedrugpolicy.gov/drugfact/club/index.html

References

American Association of Medicinal Review Officers. MRO profile of MDMA. Available at http://www.aamro.com/mroalert.html. Accessed January 22, 2007.

Anglin, M. D., Burke, C., Perrochet, B., Stamper, E., & Dawud-Noursi, S. (2000). History of the methamphetamine problem. *Journal of Psychoactive Drugs, 32*, 137–141.

Baggott, M. J. (2002). Preventing problems in ecstasy users: Reduce use to reduce harm. *Journal of Psychoactive Drugs, 34,* 145–162.

Barker, W. D., & Antia, U. (2006). A study of the use of Ephedra in the manufacture of methamphetamine. *Forensic Science International, 166*, 102–109.

Beebe, D. K., & Walley, E. (1995). Smokable methamphetamine ('ice'): An old drug in a different form. *American Family Physician, 51*, 449–453.

Berman, R. M., Cappiello, A., Anand, A., Oren, D. A., Heninger, G. R., Charney, D. S., et al. (2000). Antidepressant effects of ketamine in depressed patients. *Biological Psychiatry, 47*, 351–354.

Bogart, L. M., Kral, A. H., Scott, A., Anderson, R., Flynn, N. Gilbert, M. L., et al. (2005). Sexual risk among injection drug users recruited from syringe exchange programs in California. *Sexually Transmitted Diseases, 32*, 27–34.

Booth, B. M., Leukefeld, C., Falck, R., Wang, J., & Carlson, R. (2006). Correlates of rural methamphetamine and cocaine users: Results from a multistate community study. *Journal of Studies on Alcohol, 67*, 493–501.

Brecht, M. L., Greenwell, L., & Anglin, M. D. (2005). Methamphetamine treatment: Trends and predictors of retention and completion in a large state treatment system (1992–2002). *Journal of Substance Abuse Treatment, 29*, 295–306.

Camí, J., & Farré, M. (1996). Éxtasis, la droga de la ruta del bakalao. *Medicina Clínica, 106*, 711–716.

Center for Substance Abuse Research (CESAR), University of Maryland at College Park. *CESAR Fax report*, December 6, 2004, *13*.

Center for Substance Abuse Research (CESAR), University of Maryland at College Park. *CESAR Fax report*, September 11, 2006, *15*.

Colfax, G., & Guzman, R. (2006). Club drugs and HIV infection: A review. *Clinical Infectious Diseases 42*, 1463–1469.

Covey, H. C. (2007). What is methamphetamine and how and why is it used. In H. C. Covey (Ed.). *The Methamphetamine Crisis* (pp. 3–22). Westport, CT: Praeger Publishers.DanceSafe.org, retrieved on April 2, 2007.

Derlet, R. W., & Heischober, B. (1990). Methamphetamine. Stimulant of the 1990s? *Western Journal of Medicine, 153*, 625–628.

Díaz, R. M., Heckert, A. L., & Sánchez, J. (2005). Reasons for stimulant use among Latino gay men in San Francisco: A comparison between methamphetamine and cocaine users. *Journal of Urban Health, 82*, 71–78.

Drug Enforcement Administration (DEA). (2005). *Drugs of abuse*. Retrieved September 15, 2005, from http://www.usdoj.gov/dea/pubs/abuse/doa-p.pdf.

Green, A. I., & Halkitis, P. N. (2006). Crystal methamphetamine and sexual sociality in an urban gay subculture: An elective affinity. *Cult Health Sex, 8*, 317–333.

Harris, D. S., Boxenbaum, H., Everhart, E. T., Sequeira, G., Mendelson, J. E., & Jones, R. T. (2003). The bioavailability of intranasal and smoked methamphetamine. *Clinical Pharmacology Therapy, 74*, 475–486.

Hayes, S. C., Strosahl, K. D., & Wilson, K. G. (1999). *Acceptance and commitment therapy: An experiential approach to behavior change.* New York: Guilford Press.

Johnston, J., Barratt, M. J., Fry, C. L., Kinner, S., Stoove, M., Degenhardt, L., et al. (2006). A survey of regular ecstasy users' knowledge and practices around determining pill content and purity: Implications for policy and practice. *International Journal of Drug Policy, 17*, 464–472.

Johnston, L. D., O'Malley, P. M., & Bachman, J. G. (2001). *Rise in ecstasy use among American teens begins to slow.* University of Michigan News and Information Services. Available from: www.monitoringthefuture.org.

Khamsi, R. (2006). Ketamine relieves depression within hours. *New Scientist.* Retrieved August 8, 2006 from http://www.newscientist.com/article/dn9696-ketamine-relieves-depression-within-hours.html

Kim, I., Oyler, J. M., Moolchan, E. T., Cone, E. J., & Huestis, M. A. (2004). Urinary pharmacokinetics of methamphetamine and its metabolite, amphetamine following controlled oral administration to humans. *Therapy Drug Monitor, 26,* 664–672.

Lankenau, S. E., & Clatts, M. C. (2005). Patterns of polydrug use among ketamine injectors in New York City. *Substance Use and Misuse, 40,* 1381–1397.

Lewes, L. A., & Ross, M. W. (1995). *A select body: The gay dance party subculture and the HIV/AIDS pandemic.* London: Cassell.

Maglione, M., Chao, B., & Anglin, M. D. (1998). Methamphetamine abuse in California: Correlates of injection use. *AIDS and Behavior, 2,* 257–261.

Mattison, A., M., Ross, M. W., Wolfsan, T., & Franklin, D. (2001). Circuit party attendance, club drug use, and unsafe sex in gay men. *Journal of Substance Abuse, 13,* 119–126.

Maxwell, J. C. (2005). Implications of research for treatment: GHB. Gulf Coast Addiction Technology Transfer Center. U. T. Center for Social Work Research.

Maxwell, J. C. (2005). Implications of research for treatment: Rohypnol. Gulf Coast Addiction Technology Transfer Center. U. T. Center for Social Work Research.

McDaniel, C. H., & Miotto, K. A. (2001). Gamma hydroxybutyrate (GHB) and gamma butyrolactone (GBL) withdrawal: Five case studies. *Journal of Psychoactive Drugs, 33,* 143–149.

McElrath, K. (2005). MDMA and sexual behavior: Ecstasy users' perceptions about sexuality and sexual risk. *Substance Use & Misuse, 40,* 1461–1477.

National Institute on Drug Abuse (NIDA) (2007). Methamphetamine. *Info Facts.* Bethesda, MD: Author. Retrieved May 15, 2007 from http://www.drugabuse.gov/infofacts/methamphetamine.html.

National Institute on Drug Abuse (NIDA). (2008a). *InfoFacts: MDMA (Ecstasy).* NIDA Retrieved August 25, 2008 from http://www.nida.nih.gov/PDF/Infofacts/MDMA08.pdf

National Institute on Drug Abuse NIDA (2008b). NIDA Infofacts: Club Drugs (GHB, Ketamine, and Rohypnol). Retrieved August 25, 2008 from http://www.nida.nih.gov/pdf/infofacts/ClubDrugs08.pdf.

Novoa, R. A., Ompad, D. C., Wu, Y., Vlahov, D., & Galea, S. (2005). Ecstasy use and its association with sexual behaviors among drug users in New York City. *Journal of Community Health, 30,* 331–343.

NSDUH Report. (2005). *Substance use among past year ecstasy users.* Office of Applied Studies, Substance Abuse and Mental Health Services Administration (SAMHSA), April 29, 2005.

Panagopoulos, I., & Ricciardelli, L. A. (2005). Harm reduction and decision making among recreational ecstasy users. *International Journal of Drug Policy, 16,* 54–64.

Parsons, J. T., & Bimbi, D. S. (2006). Intentional unprotected anal intercourse among men who have sex with men: Barebacking, from behavior to identity. *AIDS and Behavior, 11,* 277–287.

Porrata, T. (2006). Ketamine. *GHB Project.* Retrieved on August 23, 2006, from http://www.projectghb.org/ketamine.htm.

Puder, K. S., Kagan, D. V., & Morgan, J. P. (1988). Illicit methamphetamine: Analysis, synthesis, and availability. *American Journal of Drug and Alcohol Abuse, 14,* 463–473.

Rawson, R. A., Anglin, M. D., & Ling, W. (2002). Will the methamphetamine problem go away? *Journal of Addictive Diseases, 21,* 5–19.

Richards, J.R., & Brofeldt, B.T. (2000, Aug.). Patterns of tooth wear associated with methamphetamine use. *Journal of Periodontology, 71,* 1371–1374.

Semple, S. J., Zians, J., Grant, I., & Patterson, T. L. (2006). Sexual compulsivity in a sample of hiv-positive methamphetamine-using gay and bisexual men. *AIDS and Behavior, 10,* 587–598.

Semple, S. J., Patterson, T. L., & Grant, I. (2004). Determinants of condom use stage of change among heterosexually-identified methamphetamine users. *AIDS and Behavior, 8,* 391–400.

Shoptaw, S., Reback, C. J., Peck, J. A., Yang, X., Rotheram-Fuller, E., Larkins, S., et al. (2005). Behavioral treatment approaches for methamphetamine dependence and HIV-related sexual risk behaviors among urban gay and bisexual men. *Drug Alcohol Depend, 78,* 125–134.

Strote, J., Lee, J. E., & Wechsler, H. (2002). Increasing MDMA use among college students: Results of anational survey. *Journal of Adolescent Health, 30,* 64–72.

Substance Abuse and Mental Health Services Administration (SAMSHA), Office of Applied Studies. *Drug abuse warning network report*, 2003.

Substance Abuse and Mental Health Services Administration (SAMHSA). (September 2006). *Results from the 2005 National Survey on Drug Use and Health: National Findings*. Retrieved October 15, 2007, from http://www.oas.samhsa.gov/NSDUH/2k5NSDUH/2k5results.htm.

Tatarsky, A. (2003). Harm reduction psychotherapy: Extending the reach of traditional substance use treatment. *Journal of Substance Abuse Treatment, 25,* 249–256.

Wiener, S. W., Hexdall, A., McStay, C. M., Nelson, L. S., & Hoffman, R. S. (2004). Booty bumping: A novel route of methamphetamine abuse. *Journal of Toxicology: Clinical Toxicology, 42,* 553.

Wohl, A. R., Johnson, D. F., Lu, S., Jordan, W., Beall, G., Currier, J., et al. (2002). HIV risk behaviors among African American men in Los Angeles County who self-identify as heterosexual. *JAIDS Journal of Acquired Immune Deficiency Syndromes, 31,* 354–360.

Wu, L. T., Pilowsky, D. J., Wechsberg, W. M., & Schlenger, W. E. (2004). Injection drug use among stimulant users in a national sample. *The American Journal of Drug and Alcohol Abuse, 30,* 61–83.

Zárate, C. A. Jr., Singh, J. B., Carlson, P. J., Brutsche, N. E., Ameli, R., Luckenbaugh, D. A., et al. (2006). A randomized trial of an N-methyl-D-aspartate antagonist in treatment-resistant major depression. *Archives of General Psychiatry, 63,* 856–864.

Part IV

Special Topics

Dennis E. Mc Chargue
University of Nebraska-Lincoln

Introduction

The majority of the book has built a framework from conceptual to assessment and treatment topics that allows the reader to evaluate the evidence associated with substance use treatment. Part IV attempts to fill in the holes by addressing seemingly disparate but related special topics. Similar to prior chapters, chapters within the Special Topics section approaches each topic within an evidence-based approach.

For example, Chapter 23 addresses the unique population of adolescent substance users. Utilizing Kazdin's (1994) approach to treatment development, Henderson and colleagues illustrate evidence that supports Multidimensional Family Therapy as an efficacious treatment for adolescent substance users. The appeal of Multidimensional Family Therapy is its tailored approach that addresses idiosyncratic aspects of each person. Within the chapter, Henderson and colleagues also compare Multidimensional Family Therapy to other treatment modalities. They progress through the chapter to addressing individual, parental, family, and cultural factors that may influence treatment outcome. The authors also discuss how clinical judgment and adherence are important when assessing effectiveness of such treatments. The chapter then discusses the use of such a treatment for prevention, within a female population and within individuals with comorbid psychopathology. Lastly, dissemination efforts within a variety of populations and agencies are addressed.

In Chapter 24, Roman and Knudsen discuss the special topic of drug testing and workplace issues. The authors begin with a description of the types of drug testing and how prevalent such testing is within the United States. Second, the chapter illustrates the types of agencies that would employ drug testing and segues into state-level policies. Third, the chapter addresses employers' responses and attitudes to drug testing before discussing how drug testing impacts the work environment.

In Chapter 25, al'Absi clearly delineates the effects of stress on substance use initiation, maintenance, and relapse. The chapter conceptualizes stress as a physiological reaction to adverse psychological environmental stimuli. This conceptualization aids in our understanding of the rewarding effects of drugs during stress, as illustrated later in the chapter. The author's conceptualization also allows the reader to clearly understand how individual differences, labeled as moderators, may enhance one's probability of becoming addicted to substances. Specific individual difference factors discussed within the chapter include gender differences, genetic differences, and coping.

Chapter 26 examines the influence of behavioral economics within substance abuse. Simply put, behavioral economics addresses contextual factors that influence substance behavior and consumption. Murphy and colleagues provide one of the most succinct and clear reviews of behavioral economics within this chapter. First, they illustrate the influence of behavioral economics within addiction theory. Second, the authors apply and provide evidence of behavioral economic applicability to assessment and treatment domains. Lastly, the authors discuss behavioral economic factors of drug reinforcement.

Meredith and colleagues then detail the current knowledge of pharmacotherapy with substance use disorders in Chapter 27. The authors start with alcohol and move from one drug classification to another reporting the evidence of efficacious pharmacotherapy for substance use disorders. This chapter is another clear illustration that is easily perused for a current reference of pharmacotherapy.

Although a number of chapters briefly discuss Motivational Interviewing as a treatment for or a component of many substance use treatments, Baer and colleagues give a detailed documentation of the theoretical underpinnings of Motivational Interviewing and treatment efficacy of such a treatment in Chapter 28. They also address how to measure Motivational Interviewing to assess whether the therapist is conducting Motivational Interviewing correctly. Lastly and possibly most important, the authors illustrate the need for training and maintenance of skills through continued training. Despite the intuitive appeal of Motivational Interviewing and its apparent efficacy, extensive training is needed to become proficient in the use of its skills.

Faith has been intimately connected with substance use treatment for decades. Indeed faith-based treatments pervade many treatment agencies. Yet, little has been written about the evidence that supports these efforts beyond Alcohol Anonymous approaches. Chapter 29 may be one of the first well-written works on a variety of faith-based approaches. Johnson discusses the historical precedence of the faith-based movement, derivations of such treatments and the evidence that supports the use of such treatments.

21

Development and Evolution of an Evidence-Based Practice: Multidimensional Family Therapy as Treatment System

Cynthia L. Rowe, Howard A. Liddle,
Gayle A. Dakof, and Craig E. Henderson

*University of Miami Center for Treatment Research
on Adolescent Drug Abuse*

Contents

"Evidence-based practice" can be considered the sign of the times in the substance abuse treatment field as in other areas of psychology. The phrase is so commonly (and perhaps carelessly) used that its full meaning may be obscured to researchers and practitioners alike. Multiple constituents have a stake in the use and promotion of evidence-based practice (e.g., policy makers, community agency directors, community treatment providers, etc.). Policy makers have successfully used best-practice guidelines to encourage the adoption of empirically based treatments (NIDA, 2004; NIMH, 2004). Such policies have had a broad impact on community agency program directors and community treatment providers, as well as treatment researchers. However well-intentioned, pressure from funders to adopt evidence-based practices without sufficient resources to do so places the average community-based provider at a disadvantage in maintaining funding and providing quality services. The merits of evidence-based practice are often hotly debated in relation to the effort and funds needed to implement them. What may get lost in these discussions is that evidence-based practice is not just about the "evidence base" but about developing and using clinical expertise and knowledge of different client groups, activities that have been fundamental in the evolution of certain treatments.

The Institute of Medicine (2001) defined evidence-based practice as "the integration of best research evidence with clinical expertise and client values." The editors of this volume provide a straightforward definition that reflects the IOM (2001) and APA (2005) statements on EBP: "knowledge and use of the most recent evidence to support clinical decision making" (Collins, Leffingwell, Callahan, & Cohen, this volume). Although many controversies exist in terms of the exact nature of evidence-based practice, and establishment of a research base to support and guide implementation of evidence-based practices is just beginning (Miller, Zweben, & Johnson, 2005), there are examples in the adolescent substance abuse field of models demonstrating a true integration of research evidence with clinical expertise in the context of patient characteristics, culture, and preferences (APA, 2005). One such treatment is Multidimensional Family Therapy (MDFT; Liddle, 2002a), which is the focus of this chapter.

We illustrate the ways in which the clinical development and validation of MDFT has been accomplished in the context of a series of randomized clinical trials as well as a set of process studies that have examined specific and change-relevant clinical processes. We also discuss the adaptability and suitability of the model with diverse client groups. The discussion is organized along the three pillars of evidenced-based practice: research evidence, clinical judgment and expertise, and consideration of client characteristics. The chapter concludes with a discussion of a fourth aspect (a potential fourth pillar?) of MDFT's evidence base: the empirically established implementation potential of MDFT in different clinical settings.

MDFT's research foundation includes documented effectiveness on a range of outcomes in controlled efficacy and effectiveness studies. Second, clinical judgment and decision making are discussed in terms of MDFT process studies that link hypothesized clinical mechanisms to client outcomes. Clinical expertise is also substantiated through MDFT adherence studies which show that therapists can be trained to deliver the model with a high degree of fidelity in both clinical research and community-based settings. Third, the model's acceptability to and its effects with diverse clinical groups demonstrate MDFT's flexibility as a treatment system rather than a "one-size-fits-all" approach (a common complaint of practitioners about EBPs). Over the more than 20 years in which MDFT has been studied and refined, we have developed different versions of MDFT specifically designed to match client and family characteristics. We have also established MDFT's potential for successful implementation in different practice settings, and for improving clinical outcomes over standard practice.

A framework that has been influential in shaping MDFT's growth over the past two decades has been Kazdin's (1994) "treatment development" approach (see Table 21.1). This framework, entirely consistent with the IOM (2001) and APA (2005) EBP guidelines, posits that the evolution of an EBP balances sound scientific principles with a cognizance of the need for treatment research to be relevant to multiple constituencies and in different contexts.

Steps 1–4 in Kazdin's framework describe the systematic development of MDFT since the early 1980s, from a thorough understanding and use of basic and applied research on developmental psychopathology and the contexts and processes of normative adolescent

---

TABLE 21.1
Steps in Treatment Development (Kazdin, 1994)

1. Conceptualization of the Dysfunction

   Conceptualization of key areas that relate to the development, onset, and escalation of dysfunction, proposal of key processes that are antecedents to some facet of conduct disorder and the mechanisms by which these processes emerge or operate.

2. Research on Processes Related to Dysfunction

   Research that examines the relations of processes proposed to be critical to the dysfunction (conduct disorder) to test the model.

3. Conceptualization of Treatment

   Conceptualization of the treatment focus, how specific procedures relate to other processes implicated in the dysfunction and to desired treatment outcomes.

4. Specification of Treatment

   Concrete operationalization of the treatment, preferably in manual form, so that the integrity of treatment can be evaluated, the material learned from treatment trials can be codified, and the treatment procedures can be replicated.

5. Tests of Treatment Process

   Studies to identify whether the intervention techniques, methods, and procedures within treatment actually affect those processes that are critical to the model.

6. Tests of Treatment Outcome

   Treatment studies to evaluate the impact of treatment. A wide range of treatment tests (e.g., open [uncontrolled] studies, single-case designs, full-fledged clinical trials) can provide evidence that change is produced. Several types of studies (e.g., dismantling, parametric, and comparative outcome) are relevant.

7. Tests of the Boundary Conditions and Moderators

   Examination of the child, parent, family, and contextual factors with which treatment interacts. The boundary conditions or limits of application are identified through interactions of treatment X diverse attributes within empirical tests.

development (Liddle, Rowe, Dakof, & Lyke, 1998; Liddle et al., 2000) to the specification of the intervention manual and protocols designed to target the specific risk and protective factors linked to adolescent problem behaviors (Liddle, 2002a; Liddle, Rodriguez, Dakof, Kanzki, & Marvel, 2005). The process research described in Step 5 has articulated details about MDFT treatment and clinical decision making that predict variations of therapeutic response (e.g., Diamond & Liddle, 1996; Robbins et al., 2006). A series of outcome studies (Step 6) has established the robust effects of MDFT over standard practice and other highly regarded treatments for adolescent drug abuse (e.g., individual CBT and peer group therapy). Step 7 in Kazdin's framework examines the limits or variations of treatment effectiveness, established through tests of treatment effectiveness with understudied populations and in different clinical contexts. In tests of the boundary conditions of MDFT, we have established its generalizability and ecological validity across variable contexts and addressing diverse client characteristics.

MDFT is an integrative outpatient treatment that has blended family therapy, individual therapy, drug counseling, and multiple-systems-oriented intervention approaches (Liddle, 1999). Interventions target the interconnected domains of adolescent development, and within these contexts, the circumstances and processes known to create and/or continue dysfunction (Bronfenbrenner, 1979; Hawkins, Catalano, & Miller, 1992). MDFT interventions work in four domains: changes in the adolescent (individual developmental functioning, including peer relationships), the parent(s) (individual functioning of the parent as well as parenting), the family environment (family transactional patterns), and extrafamilial systems of influence on the adolescent and family (e.g., working with schools [advocacy work on behalf of the teen, coaching parents to work with school personnel], social service agencies, or the juvenile justice system).

MDFT is a treatment system and not a singular, "one-size-fits-all- approach." It has been adapted and tested in various forms or versions according to target population and contextual characteristics in community-based clinical trials with samples of mainly juvenile justice involved, substance-abusing teens. The approach strives for a consistent and obvious connection among its organizational levels: theory, principles of intervention, interventions strategies and methods, and clinical assessment of family progress. MDFT has been recognized nationally and internationally as among the most effective treatment approaches for adolescent drug abuse and delinquency (Annie E. Casey Foundation, 2002; CSAP/OJJDP, 2000; CSAT, 1998; DHHS, 2002; DrugScope/Drug and Alcohol Findings, 2002; Drug Strategies, 2003; Rigter, NIDA, 1999; Van Gageldonk, & Ketelaars, 2005).

The conceptualization of MDFT as a treatment system is basic to our research program. Implicit in this conceptualization are the notions of treatment adaptation and variability, core features addressed in the consideration of EBP. Akin to specifying and manipulating an independent variable in a classic experimental research design (Campbell & Stanley, 1966), defining a treatment as a treatment system places the approach itself in the forefront of what is manipulated and tested. Through a series of studies, the effects of the treatment adaptation are observed, and, based on data, the treatment is specified further and manipulated to address additional facets of the treatment's boundary conditions. This has been the modus operandi of the MDFT research program over the past two decades. We now turn our attention to specific studies conducted in the MDFT research program.

MDFT Research Evidence

MDFT Versus Peer Group Treatment and Multifamily Educational Groups

MDFT efficacy in reducing adolescent substance abuse and associated behavior problems has been established in five completed controlled trials conducted since the mid-1980s. In the first, Liddle et al. (2001) examined the efficacy of MDFT in comparison to two manualized active treatments, Adolescent Group Therapy (AGT) and Multifamily Educational Intervention (MFEI). The study was conducted at several community clinics in the San Francisco Bay area. Each treatment involved 14–16 office-based sessions provided weekly in the clinic. One hundred and eighty-two marijuana and alcohol-abusing adolescents were randomized to MDFT, AGT, or MFEI and followed for up to a year. Participants were primarily male, and came largely from low-income, single-parent households. Approximately 50% were ethnic minorities. Youth were primarily polydrug users, coupling near-daily use of marijuana and alcohol with weekly use of cocaine, hallucinogens, or amphetamines, and averaged 2.5 years of drug abuse. The results revealed significant decreases in substance use and problem behaviors at termination for all treatments, with youth receiving MDFT showing significantly less substance use than the two comparison treatments. At the one-year follow-up, MDFT youth again decreased their substance use to a greater extent than either treatment. In addition, MDFT showed significantly greater improvements in school performance than the comparison treatments and was also the only treatment in which youth showed improvements in their family functioning as measured by objective behavioral ratings using a videotaped family interaction scale.

MDFT Versus Individual CBT

The second outcome study compared MDFT to an empirically supported, individual-based adolescent treatment, Cognitive Behavior Therapy (CBT; Liddle, 2002b). This study is noteworthy because MDFT was compared to one of the most efficacious and commonly used behavioral treatments for adolescent drug abuse (Kaminer, 1999). Two hundred twenty-four adolescents referred to a community clinic for substance abuse treatment were randomly assigned to one of the two active treatments. This North Philadelphia urban sample was primarily male, African-American, and low income. All youth were substance users, with 78% meeting diagnostic criteria for substance dependence and 17% meeting diagnostic criteria for substance abuse. From intake to discharge, both MDFT and CBT reduced marijuana use and psychological involvement with drugs. However, youth who received MDFT showed more rapid decreases in psychological involvement with drugs through the 12-month follow-up. In addition, youth receiving MDFT continued to improve following treatment discharge, so that at the 6- and 12-month follow-up assessments their psychological involvement with drugs was lower than that of youth receiving CBT. Only MDFT affected hard drug use. Finally, a greater proportion of youth receiving MDFT (64% vs. 44%) reported no or one occasion of drug use at the 12-month follow-up.* In sum, the advantages of MDFT over CBT were its

---

*Of those MDFT youth reporting no or one occasion of drug use (64% of the total MDFT sample), 87% reported being abstinent over the previous 30 days. Of those CBT youth reporting no or one occasion of drug use (44% of the CBT sample), 82% reported being abstinent.

ability to sustain the effects of treatment beyond termination and to effectively affect harder drug use.

MDFT Versus Peer Group Therapy for Young Teens

A third trial tested MDFT as an early intervention for young adolescent alcohol and drug users (ages 11–15) in Miami. Both MDFT and the comparison peer group treatment were delivered by clinicians employed by a local community drug abuse treatment agency. Eighty-three adolescents were randomized to receive MDFT or peer group treatment (Liddle et al., 2004). Intake to discharge findings revealed significant treatment effects favoring MDFT in several major risk domains: (a) individual, (b) family, (c) peer, and (d) school influences. Most important, MDFT participants showed greater decreases in marijuana and alcohol abuse than youth receiving the peer group treatment. Looking further to 12-month follow-up, results indicate that the intake to discharge findings are maintained. MDFT more effectively reduces risks in individual, family, peer, and school domains. Furthermore, youth receiving MDFT were more likely to abstain from drug use, report no problems associated with drug use, and decrease their delinquent behavior more rapidly than youth receiving peer group treatment over 12 months following treatment. The encouraging results of this study indicate that MDFT can be effective with a clinically referred sample of young adolescents.

MDFT in the CYT Study

MDFT was also one of the treatments tested in the multisite Cannabis Youth Treatment (CYT) Study (Dennis et al., 2004). The version of MDFT employed in the CYT study was delivered once a week at outpatient clinics in urban Philadelphia and rural Illinois over a 12–14-week period. Teens who received MDFT in the CYT were primarily male, White non-Hispanic, or African-American, and involved in the juvenile justice system. Consistent with findings from previous trials, MDFT had a positive impact on drug use and other problem behaviors, and it also showed the capacity to sustain gains made in treatment through a 12-month follow-up period (e.g., youth receiving MDFT decreased their substance-related problems over 50% from intake through the 12-month follow-up). The improvements associated with MFDT were similar to those achieved by the other empirically supported active comparison treatments (Motivational Enhancement Therapy/CBT, Adolescent Community Reinforcement Approach) in the CYT study (Dennis et al., 2004).

MDFT as a Prevention Approach for High-Risk Youth

In the fifth completed controlled trial, Multidimensional Family Prevention (MDFP) was tested as a prevention approach with a sample of at-risk, inner-city young adolescents and their families in North Philadelphia (Hogue, Liddle, Becker, & Johnson-Leckrone, 2002). Study participants were early adolescents (mean age 12.5 years), predominantly girls (56%), almost entirely African-American (97%), and mostly low income. Intervention effects were examined for nine targeted outcomes within four domains of functioning: self-competence, family functioning, school involvement, and peer associations. As in the early intervention study described above, these domains are considered to be proximal mediators—that is, indices of risk and protection—of the ultimate behavioral symptoms to be prevented: substance use and antisocial behavior. Youth in MDFP showed greater gains than controls on four of the nine outcomes (one outcome in each of these four domains): increased self-concept, a trend toward increased family cohesion, increased bonding to school, and decreased antisocial behavior by peers. These results offer preliminary evidence for the short-term efficacy of family based prevention counseling for at-risk young adolescents. Although controls experienced decreases in family cohesion and school bonding and an increase in peer delinquency, MDFP subjects reported strengthened family and school bonds and reduced peer delinquency. Overall, these gains were small to moderate in magnitude, and they were evident regardless of the adolescent's sex, age, or initial severity of behavioral symptoms.

In sum, the research evidence supporting MDFT's effects is strong in several respects. First, the studies have shown favorable outcomes for youth in MDFT in comparison to other state-of-the-art, well articulated, and carefully monitored treatments. Second, youths' and families' functioning in a range of domains have been shown to improve during treatment and to maintain gains up to a year following treatment. Third, the studies have recruited clinically referred samples with a range of problems and we have achieved effects within community clinics, demonstrating MDFT's effectiveness in real-world settings as well as its efficacy.

Clinical Judgment and Expertise: MDFT Process and Adherence Research

Clinical judgment and expertise can be established through treatment research focused on processes of change (Kazdin, 2001), as well as adherence research showing that therapists can be trained to deliver the approach with high fidelity to the manual specifications (Waltz, Addis, Koerner, & Jacobson, 1993). MDFT process studies have revealed details about treatment that predict variations of therapeutic response (e.g., Diamond & Liddle, 1996; Robbins, et al., 2006). These studies of the treatment's interior have served to advance manualization and refinement of the approach, as well as substantiating core hypothesized mechanisms of change and helping guide clinical decision making. Our understanding of the mechanisms of change that account for successful outcome in EBPs is far from complete (Kazdin & Nock, 2003), however, progress has been made. In addition, treatment adherence procedures verify that MDFT therapists deliver the interventions with high fidelity to model specifications.

MDFT process research has confirmed the importance of some core hypothesized mechanisms of change in facilitating change during treatment, consistent with the model's theory of change. For instance, interesting results of a recent process study showed that family focused, and not adolescent-focused interventions, predicted posttreatment improvements in drug use, externalizing, and internalizing symptoms within both MDFT and individual CBT (Hogue, Liddle, Dauber, & Samoulis, 2004). Other MDFT process studies, described below, have systematically studied therapist and client contributions to the development of an effective therapeutic alliance (Diamond, Liddle, Hogue, & Dakof, 2000), improvements in parenting (Schmidt, Liddle, & Dakof, 1996), and the resolution of in-session therapeutic impasses (Diamond & Liddle, 1996).

Adolescent Domain: Building Therapeutic Alliances

One of the MDFT therapist's first tasks in treatment is to establish a strong therapeutic relationship with the teen to create a collaborative atmosphere that will facilitate later requests for change. The MDFT theory of change is epigenetic: establishing the alliance with the teen is a fundamental building block that creates the foundation for later therapeutic work. Teen substance abusers are notoriously difficult to engage in therapy, and it can often be a challenge to identify ways that the treatment can be meaningful for them. The critical process of establishing the alliance with teens has thus been an important focus in a series of MDFT process studies.

We first examined the impact of adolescent engagement interventions on improving initially poor therapist–adolescent alliances (Diamond, Liddle, Hogue, & Dakof, 2000). The sample was juvenile justice involved, substance-abusing inner-city teens, most of whom had a dual diagnosis of substance abuse and a mental health disorder. Cases with weak therapist–adolescent alliances in the first treatment session were observed over the course of the first three sessions. Significant gains in working alliance were evident when therapists emphasized the following alliance-building interventions: attending to the adolescent's experience, formulating personally meaningful goals, and presenting one's self as the adolescent's ally. Lack of improvement or deterioration in alliance was associated with the therapist continually socializing the adolescent to the nature of therapy. Moreover, in improved alliance cases therapists increased their use of alliance-building interventions from session two to session three (therapist perseverance), whereas therapists in unimproved cases decreased their use (therapist resignation). These results indicate that although it is an instrumental early stage therapist method, when therapists over-focus on and become stuck in orienting adolescents to therapy, and thus wait too long to discuss how the therapy can be personally meaningful for the teenager, a productive working relationship is not formed.

More recent studies link the development of the therapeutic alliance with teens' and families' overall clinical outcomes. For instance, Shelef, Diamond, Diamond, and Liddle (2005) found that both adolescent–therapist and parent–therapist alliances made important contributions to treatment retention and outcome. Whereas the strength of the parent–therapist alliance predicted treatment retention, once the family engaged in treatment, it was the quality of the adolescent–therapist alliance that predicted decreases in the adolescents' drug-using behavior. In addition, MDFT therapeutic alliances are linked to and predict treatment completion (Robbins et al., 2006).

Parenting Domain: Changing Parenting Practices

The simultaneous development of a strong working alliance with parents sets the stage for change efforts in the parenting realm. When engagement in the program and motivation for change has been facilitated with parents (see Liddle, Rowe, Dakof, & Lyke, 1998 for details about early stage work with parents), the intensive work of targeting ineffective parenting practices and building upon competent parenting strategies can be initiated. Using behavioral ratings of videotaped therapy sessions, Schmidt, Liddle, and Dakof (1996) investigated the nature and extent of change in parenting behaviors, as well as the link between parental subsystem change and reduction in adolescent symptomatology. In a sample of parents whose teenagers were juvenile justice referred and evidenced serious drug and mental health problems, parents showed significant decreases in negative parenting behaviors (e.g., negative affect, verbal aggression) and increases in positive parenting (e.g., monitoring and limit-setting, positive affect, and commitment) over the course of MDFT. These improvements in parenting behaviors were associated with reductions in adolescent drug use and problem behaviors. Four different patterns of parent–adolescent tandem change were identified: 59% of families showed improvement in both parenting practices and adolescent symptomatology, 21% evidenced improved parenting but no change in adolescent problems, 10% showed improved adolescent symptoms in the absence of improved parenting, and 10% showed no improvement in either parenting or adolescent functioning. These results support an elemental tenet of family based treatments: change in a fundamental aspect of the family system (parenting practices) is related to change at the critical level of interest: reduction of adolescent symptoms, including drug abuse.

Family Domain: Resolving Therapeutic Impasses

A third illustration of the potential of process research to empirically support clinical decision making in MDFT addressed one of the core challenges of family based therapy: moving beyond stalemates and promoting healing and real relationship change within families. G. S. Diamond and Liddle (1999) used task analysis, again by studying therapy videotapes, to identify the combination of clinical interventions and family interactions necessary to resolve in-session impasses. These are clinical situations characterized by negative exchanges, emotional disengagement, and poor problem solving between parents and adolescents. The sample in this process study was substance-abusing, juvenile justice-referred teenagers and their families.

Therapist behaviors that contributed to changing these negative interactions included: (a) actively blocking, diverting, or addressing and working with negative emotions; (b) offering, evoking, and amplifying thoughts and feelings that promote constructive discussion; and (c) creating emotional treaties among family members by alternately working in session with parents alone and adolescents alone and then together, a kind of shuttle diplomacy. In cases with successful resolution of the impasse, the therapist transformed the nature and tone of the conversation in the session. The therapist shifted the parent's blaming and hopelessness to attention to their feelings of regret and loss and sometimes sadness about what was occurring with their child. At the same time, the therapist elicited the adolescent's thoughts and feelings about relationship roadblocks with the parent and others. These in-session shifts of attention and emotion made new conversations between parent and adolescent possible. In so doing, the parents developed empathy for the difficult experiences of their teenager and offered support for their teen's coping. These interventions and processes facilitated personal disclosure by the adolescent, decreased defensiveness, and created give and take exchanges.

This study yielded insights about clinical judgment and decision making in several areas. First, we found a theory-based way to reliably define and identify family transactional processes that are known determinants of poor developmental outcomes in children and teenagers. Second, we broke down in behavioral terms the components of the impasse, defining the unfolding sequential contributions of both parent and adolescent. Third, we specified the relation of different therapist actions to the impasse. Fourth, we demonstrated that therapists can change an in-session therapeutic impasse and thus affect one of the predictors of developmental dysfunction related to drug abuse.

MDFT Adherence Evaluation and Monitoring to Support Clinical Judgment and Decision Making

Process-based adherence research has also confirmed that MDFT can be implemented with a high degree of clinical skill and fidelity to the treatment model's prescriptions (Hogue et al., 1998). This line of research also supports clinical decision making by demonstrating that MDFT therapists adhere to interventions consistent with model guidelines and they can be differentiated from therapists delivering other treatment approaches. We compared intervention techniques of MDFT therapists to intervention techniques of cognitive-behavioral therapists in a controlled trial with adolescent substance abusers. Nonparticipant coders observed videotapes of randomly selected sessions from the MDFT and cognitive-behavioral conditions using an adherence evaluation instrument designed to identify therapeutic techniques and facilitative interventions associated with the two treatment models. Coders estimated both the frequency and the thoroughness (i.e., depth, complexity, or persistence) with which techniques were delivered.

Results demonstrated that MDFT therapists reliably utilized the model's core interventions: focusing on and enhancing individual teen and parenting functioning, shaping parenting practices, preparing for and coaching multiparticipant interactions in session, and facilitating change directly with multiple family members (Hogue et al., 1998). Moreover, in keeping with MDFT's commitment to working on family attachment bonds and developmental themes (Liddle & Schwartz, 2002), MDFT therapists focused on establishing a supportive therapeutic environment, encouraging expression and discussion of emotions, engaging clients in crafting a collaborative treatment agenda, and exploring everyday behavior related to normative adolescent development. This study illustrates how fine-grained process-oriented adherence evaluation can contribute to therapist training that shapes clinical decision making. Having a rigorous systematic adherence evaluation system in place enables the level of clinical expertise and quality of clinical decision making to be regularly monitored and adjustments to be made as needed in supervision.

Client Characteristics and Values: The Different "Looks" of MDFT

The previous sections have described the research evidence for MDFT's effects, as well as process and adherence studies supporting the clinical judgment and expertise of MDFT therapists trained along manual guidelines. The next section describes how variations of the MDFT approach have been developed to meet the needs of different client groups (e.g., ethnic minorities, youth with comorbid mental health problems, and girls).

MDFT with Different Cultural Groups

MDFT is noteworthy among treatment approaches for adolescent substance abuse and delinquency because it has been developed and tested with a broad range of cultural and ethnic groups across the United States and more recently in Europe. Almost all of the youth and families with whom we have worked over these years have been from minority groups: primarily African-American and Hispanic. Our engagement and retention rates attest to the acceptability of the treatment with different cultural groups. MDFT clients stay in treatment longer than clients in other outpatient and residential comparison treatments (Dakof, Rowe, Liddle, & Henderson, 2003). Specifically, 96% of clients (a sample that was approximately half African-American and half Hispanic) in intensive outpatient MDFT completed treatment, compared to 78% of youth in group therapy. Recent U.S. national figures indicate that only 27% of youth stay in standard outpatient for 90 days (Hser, Haikang, Chou, Messer, & Anglin, 2001). Although retention rates are a good indicator of the acceptability of MDFT with families of different ethnicities, a major focus of our treatment improvement and development efforts have been directed toward making our approach culturally appropriate and more efficacious for diverse families.

Early treatment development research on MDFT examined key cultural themes important for working effectively with inner-city, African-American youth (Jackson-Gilfort, Liddle, Tejeda, & Dakof, 2001). We investigated whether therapeutic discussion of culturally relevant themes enhanced treatment engagement of African-American male youths residing in urban North Philadelphia. A total of 187 videotaped therapy sessions with African-American male adolescents were coded for in-session discussion of developmentally and culturally related content themes. Exploration of anger and rage, alienation, and the journey from boyhood to manhood (i.e., what it means to become an African-American man) were associated with both increased participation and decreased negativity by adolescents in the very next treatment session. The extent of the adolescent's participation in session was also linked to more open communication and dialogue about the youth's journey from boyhood to manhood in the next therapy session. Interestingly, discussions of racial identity/socialization were found to have no association with adolescent engagement. These results suggest that articulation of particular culturally meaningful themes is directly linked to adolescent investment in the treatment process (Liddle, Jackson-Gilfort, & Marvel, 2006).

Ongoing treatment development work with youth and families in Miami has focused on outlining cultural themes that are most relevant in working effectively with Hispanic and Haitian teens and families. Specifically, MDFT investigators have identified a number of salient content themes and relational patterns, many surrounding the immigration experience and acculturation process, that affect intervention focus and outcome in MDFT. This work has included eliciting the family's immigration story as a fundamental component of treatment engagement, expanding interventions to work within and influence Hispanic and Haitian families' conceptualizations of adolescent development, addressing acculturation differences among family members, and developing culturally syntonic protocols for parents to reconnect with their adolescents.

Our work in exploring cultural themes and making MDFT suitable and maximally effective for other cultural groups continues in Western Europe. We have successfully implemented the model in five countries in Europe (Belgium, France, Germany, the Netherlands, and Switzerland) through a collaborative study financed by the Health Ministries of these nations. A pilot study of MDFT's potential for implementation established the feasibility of training European therapists from a range of backgrounds in MDFT and demonstrated that youth and families from all five countries responded well to the treatment with minimal adaptations of core interventions. The European therapists delivered MDFT at comparable adherence and competence levels to MDFT therapists trained by the model developer in our controlled trials in the United States (Rigter, 2006). Based on the success of the pilot study, the five countries have embarked on a multinational randomized trial comparing MDFT with treatment as usual (TAU) for cannabis-dependent adolescents. Another NIDA-funded study examines the acceptability and effects of MDFT for youth and families treated by addiction workers in Glasgow, Scotland. Responses of the providers and their clients have been positive, and as in the Western European study, few significant adaptations have been needed to implement the model in Scotland. The adaptations tend to have been along the lines of the most salient themes and particular content developed in sessions, as well as systems-level issues, rather than changes to core interventions.

MDFT with Adolescent Girls and their Families

MDFT has also been tested and refined with delinquent and drug-abusing adolescent girls, who face daunting challenges (Dakof, 2000). Their problems are as severe as boys', yet because they tend to internalize their distress to a greater extent than boys (Rowe, Liddle, Greenbaum, & Henderson, 2004), they often do not come to the attention of social service agencies until they are in serious trouble. For instance, an alarmingly large percentage of the girls assessed in Miami-Dade County's Juvenile Detention experienced significant trauma (84%), suffered from mental health and substance abuse disorders (78%), had serious family problems (e.g., 61% with history of family criminality), and were sexually active (79%; Lederman, Dakof, Larrea, & Li, 2004). Moreover, the more girls became involved in the juvenile justice system, the greater the severity of many of their problems. When these girls grow up, they are at high risk for drug addiction, psychiatric problems, HIV infection, poor physical health, domestic violence, losing custody rights of their children, incarceration, and increased mortality if they do not receive the help they need.

Behavioral sciences theory about female adolescent development and the psychology of women, especially Miller's (1987) "self-in-relation" theory, and empirical findings from studies on adolescent female development, combined with our years of clinical experience with adolescent females, have guided the development of a comprehensive intervention specifically for adolescent girls. The approach integrates basic behavioral sciences theory and empirical findings on female adolescent development and the psychology of women with MDFT theory (Dakof, 2000). Given the importance of interpersonal relationships to the well-being of adolescent females, the primary focus of the intervention is relational. Developmental research and clinical findings consistently highlight the importance of healthy and nurturing relationships to adolescent girls, suggesting that in clinical samples, therapists must help heal key relationships to heal the girl. We have developed a gender-specific version of MDFT that aims to repair the relationship between the adolescent girl and her family, instill a positive sense of self in relation to others, and improve her social skills and prosocial opportunities so she is able to increase her affiliations with healthy same-sex and opposite-sex peers.

MDFT for Youth with Comorbid Mental Health Problems

Our work with youth who suffer from serious comorbid mental health problems (see Rowe et al., 2004) facilitated the development of a more intensive and comprehensive version of MDFT to address youths' multiple impairments. The success of comprehensive interventions with their intensity of service delivery, case management components, and home-based service delivery contexts (Henggeler, 1999; Olds et al., 1998) led us to develop a highly intensive version of MDFT incorporating case management and face-to-face therapy sessions primarily delivered in the home and offered more than once per week (Rowe, Liddle, McClintic, & Quille, 2002). We then set out to test whether this intensive family based treatment could achieve comparable outcomes to residential treatment with youth referred for inpatient treatment due to severe substance abuse, previous failure in outpatient programs, family dysfunction, and comorbid mental health disorders. The study also includes a comprehensive benefit-cost analysis of the treatments, and follows youth and their parents each year for four years.

Although this study is ongoing, our preliminary findings are promising (Liddle et al., 2004). Significantly greater proportions of MDFT participants are retained in treatment (87% vs. 68%). In addition, from intake to discharge, despite living at home, MDFT participants decrease their drug use and psychological involvement with drugs at approximately the same rate as residential treatment participants. Furthermore, between intake and discharge, youth receiving MDFT were arrested at approximately the same rate as youth receiving residential treatment (18% vs. 15%), despite the fact that youth in MDFT were "at large" in the community and residential youth were housed securely in their program. Additional preliminary findings show that between treatment discharge and 18-months follow-up, MDFT youth spend fewer days in controlled environments than youth coming from the residential program. Preliminary cost estimates (as measured by the DATCAP) indicate that the cost of delivering intensive MDFT is approximately one-third the cost of delivering the residential treatment ($384 vs. $1,138; Zavala et al., 2005).

Additional support for the benefits of MDFT for youth with severe comorbid conditions comes from additional analyses of the second clinical trial data described above, in which MDFT was tested against a strong individual CBT approach (Liddle, 2002b). Henderson, Dakof, Rowe, Greenbaum, and Liddle (2004) used growth mixture modeling analyses to uncover two distinct subgroups differentiated by their baseline severity in psychological involvement with drugs. The more severe substance-abusing group was also characterized by more baseline family conflict, externalizing symptoms, and comorbid externalizing disorders. Both subgroups showed similar (statistically significant) decreases in their psychological involvement with drugs over time. Treatment comparisons were then conducted within each latent class. For the less severe class, MDFT and CBT were equally effective in reducing substance abuse; however, for the more severe class, MDFT was more effective than CBT. These results suggest that more severely impaired youth benefit significantly from more comprehensive, family based treatments.

Finally, a new study set in the New Orleans area tests an integrative family based approach to treating comorbid substance abuse and trauma among teens and families in the wake of Hurricane Katrina. This randomized trial has a treatment development component in which MDFT developers have systematically incorporated trauma-focused interventions within the model (Rowe & Liddle, 2008). The approach is unique in that few trauma-focused interventions have been truly integrated within an empirically supported substance abuse program. In addition, few empirically based trauma interventions concurrently address the stress and coping of teens and their parents, or leverage the healing potential of the family as a larger unit. Taken as a whole, our systematic work to adapt MDFT for youth with diverse problems has been fruitful, paving the way for new developments. One of our next steps is to devise and test a version of MDFT that can be used in adolescent residential settings, and then, continued upon the youth's discharge back home and to the community.

Pillar 4: MDFT's Potential for Dissemination in Diverse Practice Settings

The transportation of empirically based practices (EBPs) to practice settings is a topic of much conversation in the field of treatment research (IOM, 1998; NIDA, 2004; NIMH, 2004). However, there are multiple factors in clinical settings that may dilute treatment effects, such as insufficient monitoring and compromised adherence to treatment protocols (Henggeler, Melton, Brondino, Scherer, & Hanley, 1997), heterogeneity of the clinical population (Weisz, Doneberg, Han, & Weiss, 1995), and restrictions on treatment delivery (e.g., insufficient time or resources to deliver EBP as specified; Willenbring et al., 2004). Lacking knowledge about how empirically supported treatments work, with whom they are most effective, and how to disseminate them effectively, EBPs ultimately may be ineffective in clinical settings (Kazdin, 2001).

We are increasingly prepared to face these challenges, having launched a series of new studies translating our knowledge about how to execute critical components of the MDFT model into interventions that help systems prepare for and adopt MDFT within their existing structures and realities (Liddle et al., 2002). Our extensive experience in training and supervising family therapists (Liddle, Becker, & Diamond, 1997; Liddle, Breunlin, & Schwartz, 1988;) has been instrumental in our ability to effectively train multidisciplinary clinical teams with a wide range of backgrounds, clinical training, and treatment experiences. Our quest to understand how to most effectively train community clinicians in delivering MDFT continues in our ongoing studies. We are examining how to integrate MDFT into complex and challenging clinical systems (e.g., Juvenile Drug Court and Juvenile Detention) and how to integrate technological aids (i.e., interactive on-line training curriculum, personal digital assistant [PDA]) into core training methods. Our current studies aim to improve outcomes in community-based clinical settings by helping providers learn and integrate MDFT into their day-to-day work.

Transporting Family Therapy into Adolescent Day Treatment

Our first systematic "technology transfer" study tested the effects of MDFT as implemented within the context of an existing intensive, outpatient adolescent day treatment program

(ADTP). Our goals were: (1) to determine if the treatment staff would be able to effectively deliver the MDFT model with fidelity, (2) to examine adolescent outcomes in response to the training, (3) to determine if therapists would continue to be adherent to MDFT following removal of monitoring and supervision by the MDFT team, and (4) to assess the impact of the technology transfer on the organizational climate of the ADTP. A significant aspect of this study was that all ADTP employees (therapists, program director, medical staff, and teachers) were trained in MDFT interventions. Additionally, MDFT was adapted to fit within the existing service delivery characteristics of the ADTP (for details see Liddle et al., 2002). The study utilized an interrupted time series design, divided into study phases: (1) Baseline, in which provider practices, program environment, and client outcomes were assessed but no training was provided; (2) Training/Exposure, in which MDFT developers trained all day treatment staff in MDFT; (3) Implementation, in which MDFT developers provided ongoing supervision and booster training as needed and the impact of training was assessed; and (4) Durability, in which MDFT trainers and research staff withdrew from the ADTP and the sustainability of the training was assessed.

Liddle et al. (2006) reported the impact of training in MDFT on provider practices, program and environmental factors, and client outcomes. First, we investigated whether the intervention effectively changed therapist practices in accordance with MDFT guidelines. Analyses of therapeutic contacts indicated that therapists did indeed hold more treatment sessions with the individual adolescents, their families, and extrafamilial others (e.g., juvenile probation officers and school officials), as prescribed by the MDFT model, following training in MDFT than in the pretraining Baseline phase. Although we expected that the adherence to MDFT parameters would dissipate some in the Durability phase of the study when supervision and monitoring were withdrawn, we found that the number of therapy sessions and extrafamilial contacts either remained stable or increased. All parameters remained significantly above baseline levels. In addition to changing provider practices, content analyses of session notes indicated that therapists were more likely to deal with core MDFT principles in their sessions during the Implementation and Durability phases. As a more powerful test of adherence to MDFT interventions, nonparticipant observers rated actual therapy sessions of day treatment providers during the Baseline, Implementation, and Durability phases using the adherence system described above (Hogue et al., 1998). As hypothesized, day treatment providers utilized more MDFT interventions in the Implementation and Durability Phases than in Baseline.

In addition, the training affected the organizational climate of the ADTP. Clients reported that the ADTP was more orderly in the Implementation phase of the study than in the Baseline phase. Furthermore, clients reported that the staff were clearer about the program rules and expectations and provided a more practical focus to their problems following training.

Perhaps most important, clients showed more improvement in the Implementation and Durability phases than the Baseline phase. Specifically, substance use and comorbid internalizing and externalizing symptoms decreased more rapidly in Implementation and Durability. In addition, youth in the Baseline phase were more likely to be placed in a controlled environment (39%) than youth in the Implementation (8%) and Durability (0%) phases. Finally, client outcomes, specifically substance use and externalizing symptoms, showed greater decreases in Implementation than Baseline. These findings indicate that MDFT can be successfully adapted and transported into an existing community-based drug treatment program, with sustained impact on therapist practice patterns, the organizational climate of the treatment program, and client outcomes. Furthermore, the success of this transportation project supports the dissemination potential of MDFT.

Family-Based Juvenile Drug Court Services

Despite the widespread support and enthusiasm for juvenile drug courts and some promising results, treatments within these systems and the courts themselves tend to lack empirical validation (Belenko & Dembo, 2003). In order to improve the outcomes of court-involved youth, we collaborated with the Miami-Dade County Juvenile Drug Court to adapt MDFT for incorporation into their system. An ongoing randomized trial is comparing the acceptability, efficacy, and benefit-cost of MDFT versus services as usual within the drug court program. As an effectiveness trial, the inclusion and exclusion criteria are set by the court itself and community-based clinicians deliver both treatments. We are interested not only in the comparative effects of MDFT in this setting, but also the mediators and moderators of outcomes (the mechanisms by which both treatments achieve their effects and any variations in clients' response to the treatments). Findings will shed light on key questions, such as whether the effects of drug court are enhanced when empirically supported treatments are implemented, what processes predict the effects of drug courts, and whether drug courts are differentially effective for certain teens or families.

MDFT-DTC: "Detention to Community"

A second current study targeting drug-abusing juvenile offenders tests an integrative, cross-systems family based intervention model that aims to reduce drug abuse, delinquency, and high-risk sexual behavior and other individual and family problems among adolescents detained in juvenile detention and as they return to the community following release. Expanding the boundaries of MDFT, the MDFT-DTC ("Detention to Community") intervention is designed to provide seamless services that bridge the transition between youths' incarceration and their return to the community. This bridge is created by linking the in-detention and outpatient treatment components in ways that reflect the consensus in the literature regarding the need for integrative comprehensive interventions for criminal justice involved, substance-abusing individuals (Altschuler & Armstrong, 1999). The MDFT therapist targets multiple systems influential to a teen's developmental outcomes, including the adolescent's family and school, the judiciary, and social service agencies. This cross-systems intervention includes three principal components: an in-detention family based intervention, an outpatient family based intervention, and an HIV/STD prevention intervention. Each component targets change in the four core areas of MDFT: adolescent, parent, family, and other systems. The MDFT-DTC intervention is currently being tested in a randomized clinical trial in two sites of NIDA's Criminal Justice-Drug Abuse Treatment Studies, a collaborative of drug abuse and criminal justice experts around the country.

Brief-Family Based Therapy for Adolescent Drug Abuse

In addition to our focused efforts to improve services for drug-abusing youth in juvenile justice settings, the success of the initial day treatment study led us to adapt the MDFT treatment approach to be more "community-friendly" for a wide range of substance abuse agencies. Dissemination research documents that existing EBPs rarely conform to the parameters that guide community-based practice (IOM, 1998). Community clinic therapists typically handle large caseloads and have limited opportunity to learn the intricacies of complex manualized treatments (Foster-Fishman, et al., 1997). Furthermore, the resources needed to implement multifaceted treatments are rarely in place in most community-based programs. Thus, even agencies eager to adopt empirically supported treatments may lack the resources to sustain their use. In contrast, brief treatments fit within the contextual realities faced by community practitioners, including delivering effective treatments within timeframes imposed by managed care regulations (Giles & Marafiote, 1998) and needing to treat a large number of clients to more efficiently meet the demands of overtaxed service delivery systems (Bloom, 2000). These factors provided the impetus for our group to develop and test a brief, "community-friendly" version of MDFT that would be less difficult for providers to master and sustain in practice.

This new "brief" version of MDFT represents a marked departure from previous versions, which have typically been anywhere from 12 weeks (CYT version) to 6 months (intensive home-based version) in duration. To enhance its real-world applicability, we refined and then pilot tested an 8-week/8-session version of MDFT in a community setting with agency treatment providers. The new treatment, MDFT-B (Brief), was compared to community TAU (TAU, with a standard length of 4–6 months) and assessments of the new treatment's feasibility and acceptability to the adolescents, parents, and counselors were conducted. Drug use outcomes and changes in prosocial functioning were assessed from adolescent and parent perspectives up to 9 months post-intake. Although results are not yet available, we are hopeful that MDFT-Brief can advance technology transfer efforts by providing community treatment agencies with an EBP that fits within the contextual and structural realities of their day-to-day practice.

Training Community-Based Providers in MDFT

A final ongoing study aimed at increasing the dissemination of MDFT into practice examines the training practices and tools that help community providers implement MDFT with maximal effects. An ongoing pilot study tests the feasibility, acceptability, and effectiveness of a comprehensive, technology-based training program in changing clinician practices and clinical outcomes of providers. The project aims to develop and evaluate a training package that can be used to teach an EBP (MDFT) to a diverse and representative group of community therapists who work with teenagers. We are using methods that integrate new technologies (a Web-based interactive training program and handheld PDA) with existing training methods to facilitate the learning, mastery, and continued high-level use of MDFT following training. The study employs the same interrupted time-series design used successfully in the day treatment study described above (Liddle et al., 2006) to test training effects on providers' practices, organizational factors, and their clients' outcomes. The results will help inform us about more efficient and effective training strategies to help providers adopt EBPs in their agencies.

This final pillar of EBP is the last frontier for clinical researchers and has become the main focus of the MDFT program of research in recent years. Considerable effort has gone into developing and manualizing the model, establishing its efficacy, identifying core mechanisms of action, and adapting the approach for specific populations over the past 20 years. Further refinements and improvements of the model are underway in the projects described to facilitate adoption of the approach in diverse practice settings.

Summary and Conclusions

The field of adolescent substance abuse treatment research has evolved significantly over the past two decades (Liddle & Rowe, 2006). Key among these advances has been the establishment of several empirically based practices for teens with multiple problems. In this chapter, we have shown how MDFT's program of research demonstrates its evidence base consistent with all three pillars of EBPs. We have also provided examples of how MDFT research, along the lines of Kazdin's (1994) concept of testing boundary conditions, supports its dissemination potential in diverse clinical practice settings and systems.

As treatment researchers, we often lament the fact that research findings do not have more impact on national drug policies (Prendergast & Podus, 2000). Yet we need to recognize that part of the problem, as Gregrich[†] (2003) notes, is that a great deal of treatment research does not address the most pressing questions facing policy makers. Such questions include studies identifying the essential elements of treatments, the modalities most suited to specific populations, and studies exploring the costs and economic benefits associated with treatment. Others have also pointed to the critical role that economic evaluations of treatment and its effects have on policy decisions (French, 2001). In the field of substance abuse treatment, the State of Washington has used data from economic evaluations to design funding streams for the state substance abuse treatment system (French, Salomé, & Carney, 2002). Policy makers are influenced by research findings if they are perceived as policy relevant (Backer, 2000). Studies demonstrating the most effective treatment modalities for different populations are needed to make more informed policy decisions (Gregrich, 2003).

MDFT researchers have attempted to address the interests of policy makers in several ways. First, we have designed studies to make MDFT more community-friendly. Recent MDFT studies are each designed to maximize the effectiveness of MDFT in nonresearch settings and have involved adapting the treatment based on a realistic appraisal of the context in which MDFT is being implemented. Second, we have become involved in the systematic study of the process by which community providers can be trained to implement research-based therapy in existing practice. In NIDA-funded studies, training contracts with jurisdictions such as the State of Connecticut (DCF), and international research conducted with European research partners, we are examining and improving the ways we teach and certify MDFT therapists in adolescent outpatient drug treatment programs. Third, we have initiated several studies evaluating the economic impact of MDFT, and preliminary results from these studies have been encouraging, indicating that the costs of MDFT are less than the costs of community treatments of comparable intensity and duration (French et al., 2002; Zavala et al., 2005). Furthermore, in the CYT study, MDFT reduced costs to society (e.g., societal

---

[†] John Gregrich is Senior Policy Analyst, Treatment Office of Demand Reduction Office of National Drug Control Policy.

costs incurred as a result of criminal activity) up to 12 months following treatment intake (French et al., 2003). Benefit-cost analyses comparing MDFT to comparison treatments are ongoing.

Thus, although dramatic strides have been made in developing and testing EBPs for adolescent substance abuse in the past decade, there are many challenges ahead. Given the push to disseminate empirically supported treatments to naturalistic practice settings while maintaining adequate treatment fidelity, it is incumbent on treatment researchers to empirically identify the core elements of their treatments. Further studies are needed to explicate mechanisms of action and evaluate the relative influence on outcome of different components of family based treatment, as well as their costs and economic benefits. Questions remain about the level of adherence to EBPs needed to obtain effects comparable to those in randomized trials. Much more research is needed to facilitate the adoption of EBPs across different service delivery contexts/settings and patient populations. The push for greater treatment dissemination both within the United States and abroad is making further research on the social and cultural appropriateness of treatments even more important (Rigter et al., 2005). Workforce issues such as therapist turnover have been infrequently studied and remain a formidable barrier to the adoption of EBPs. The challenges are considerable, and the opportunities limitless.

References

Altschuler, D. M., &. Armstrong, T. L. (1999). *Reintegrative confinement and intensive aftercare.* Washington, DC: Office of Juvenile Justice and Delinquency Prevention, Office of Justice Programs, U. S. Department of Justice.

American Psychological Association. (2005). *American Psychological Association statement: Policy statement on evidence-based practice in psychology.* Retrieved online at http://www2.apa.org/practice/ebpstatement.pdf.

Annie E. Casey Foundation. (2002). Family affair. *Annie E. Casey Foundation Magazine, 4,* 12–19.

Backer, T. E. (2000). The failure of success: Challenges of disseminating effective substance abuse prevention programs. *Journal of Community Psychology, 28*(3), 363–373.

Belenko, S., & Dembo, R. (2003). Treating adolescent substance abuse problems in the juvenile drug court. *International Journal of Law and Psychiatry, 26,* 87–110.

Bloom, B. (2000). Planned short-term psychotherapies. In C. R. Snyder & R. E. Ingram (Eds.), *Handbook of psychological change: Psychotherapy processes & practices for the 21st century* (pp. 429–454). New York: John Wiley and Sons.

Bronfenbrenner, U. (1979). *The ecology of human development: Experiments by nature and design.* Cambridge, MA: Harvard University Press.

Campbell, D. T., & Stanley, J. C. (1966). *Experimental and quasi-experimental designs for research.* Skokie, IL: Rand McNally.

Center for Substance Abuse Prevention. (2000). *Strengthening America's families: Model family programs for substance abuse and delinquency prevention.* Salt Lake City: University of Utah.

Center for Substance Abuse Treatment. (1998). *Adolescent substance abuse: Assessment and treatment* (CSAT Treatment Improvement Protocol Series). Rockville, MD: SAMSHA.

Dakof, G. A. (2000). Understanding gender differences in adolescent drug abuse: Issues of comorbidity and family functioning. *Journal of Psychoactive Drugs, 32,* 25–32.

Dakof, G. A., Rowe, C. L., Liddle, H. A., & Henderson, C. (2003, March). Engaging and retaining drug abusing youth in home-based Multidimensional Family Therapy. *Beyond the Clinic Walls: Expanding Mental Health, Drug and Alcohol Services Research Outside the Specialty Care System.* Poster presented at the NIMH/NIDA/NIAAA Conference, Washington, DC.

Dennis, M. L., Godley, S. H., Diamond, G. S., Tims, F. M., Babor, T., Donaldson, J., et al. (2004). The Cannabis Youth Treatment (CYT) study: Main findings from two randomized trials. *Journal of Substance Abuse Treatment, 27*, 197–213.

Department of Health and Human Services. (2002). *Best practice initiative: Multidimensional Family Therapy for adolescent substance abuse.* Retrieved on June 15, 2004 from http://phs.os.dhhs.gov/ophs/BestPractice/mdft_miami.htm.

Diamond, G. M., Liddle, H. A., Hogue, A., & Dakof, G. A. (2000). Alliance building interventions with adolescents in family therapy: A process study. *Psychotherapy: Theory, Research, Practice, & Training, 36*, 355–368.

Diamond, G. S., & Liddle, H. A. (1996). Resolving a therapeutic impasse between parents and adolescents in Multidimensional Family Therapy. *Journal of Consulting and Clinical Psychology, 64*, 481–488.

Diamond, G. S., & Liddle, H. A. (1999). Transforming negative parent-adolescent interactions: From impasse to dialogue. *Family Process, 38*, 5–26.

Drug Scope/Drug and Alcohol Findings. (2002). *Linking practice to research/research to practice: What works, what doesn't, what could be done better, 7*, 13.

Drug Strategies. (2003). *Treating teens: A guide to adolescent drug problems.* Washington, DC: Author.

Foster-Fishman, P. G., Perkins, D. G., & Davidson, W. S. (1997). Developing effective evaluation partnerships: Paradigmatic and contextual barriers. *Analise Psychologica, 3*, 389–403.

French, M. T. (2001). The role of health economics in substance abuse research: Recent advances and future opportunities. In M. Galanter (Ed.), *Recent developments in alcoholism, Volume 15: Services research in the era of managed care* (pp. 201–208). New York: Kluwer Academic/Plenum.

French, M. T., Roebuck, M. C., Dennis, M. L., Diamond, G., Godley, S., Tims, F., et al. (2002). The economic cost of outpatient marijuana treatment for adolescents: Findings from a multisite field experiment. *Addiction, 97*, 84–97.

French, M. T., Roebuck, M. C., Dennis, M. L., Godley, S. H., Liddle, H. A., & Tims, F. M. (2003). Outpatient marijuana treatment for adolescents: Economic evaluation of a multisite field experiment. *Evaluation Review, 27*, 421–459.

French, M. T., Salomé, H. J., & Carney, M. (2002). Using the DATCAP and ASI to estimate the costs and benefits of residential addiction treatment in the State of Washington, *Social Science & Medicine, 55*, 2267–2282.

Giles, T., & Marfiote, R. (1998). Managed care and the practitioner: A call for unity. *Clinical Psychology: Science and Practice, 8*, 405–417.

Gregrich, R. J. (2003). A note to researchers: Communicating science to policy makers and practitioners. *Journal of Substance Abuse Treatment, 25*, 233–237.

Hawkins, J. D., Catalano, R. F., & Miller, J. Y. (1992). Risk and protective factors for alcohol and other drug problems in adolescence and early adulthood: Implications for substance abuse prevention. *Psychological Bulletin, 112*, 64–105.

Henggeler, S. W. (1999). Multisystemic therapy: An overview of clinical procedures, outcomes, and policy implications. *Child Psychology and Psychiatry Review, 4*, 2–10.

Henggeler, S. W., Melton, G. B., Brondino, M. J., Scherer, D. B., & Hanley, J. H. (1997). Multisystemic therapy with violent and chronic juvenile offenders and their families: The role of treatment fidelity in successful dissemination. *Journal of Consulting and Clinical Psychology, 65*, 821–833.

Hogue, A., Liddle, H. A., Becker, D., & Johnson-Leckrone, J. (2002) Family-based prevention counseling for high-risk young adolescent: Immediate outcomes. *Journal of Community Psychology, 30*, 1–22.

Hogue, A., Liddle, H. A., Dauber, S., & Samoulis, J. (2004). Linking session focus to treatment outcome in evidence-based treatments for adolescent substance abuse. *Psychotherapy: Theory, Research, Practice, and Training, 33*, 332–345.

Hogue, A., Liddle, H. A., Rowe, C., Turner, R. M., Dakof, G. A., & LaPann, K. (1998). Treatment adherence and differentiation in individual versus family therapy for adolescent substance abuse. *Journal of Counseling Psychology, 45*, 104–114.

Hser, Y. I., Haikang, S., Chou, C. P., Messer, S. C., & Anglin, M. D. (2001). Analytic approaches for assessing long-term treatment effects: Examples of empirical applications and findings. *Evaluation Review, 25,* 233–262.

Institute of Medicine. (1998). *Bridging the gap between practice and research: Forging partnerships with community-based drugs and alcohol treatment.* Washington, DC: National Academy Press.

Institute of Medicine. (2001). *Crossing the quality chasm: A new health system for the 21st century.* Washington, DC: National Academy Press.

Jackson-Gilfort, A., Liddle, H. A., Tejeda, M. J., & Dakof, G. A. (2001). Facilitating engagement of African American male adolescents in family therapy: A cultural theme process study. *Journal of Black Psychology, 27,* 321-340.

Jessor, R. (1993). Successful adolescent development among youth in high risk settings. *American Psychologist, 48,* 117–126.

Kaminer, Y. (1999). Addictive disorders in adolescents. *Psychiatric Clinics of North America, 22*(2), 275–288.

Kazdin, A. E. (1994). Methodology, design, and evaluation in psychotherapy research. In A. E. Bergin & S. L. Garfield (Eds.), *Handbook of psychotherapy and behavior change* (4th ed., pp. 19–71). New York: John Wiley & Sons.

Kazdin, A. E. (2001). Progression of therapy research and clinical application of treatment require better understanding of the change process. *American Psychological Association, 8*(2), 143–151.

Kazdin, A. E., & Nock, M. R. (2003). Delineating mechanisms of change in child and adolescent therapy: Methodological issues and research recommendations. *Journal of Child Psychology and Psychiatry and Allied Disciplines, 44,* 1116–1129.

Lederman, C., Dakof, G. A., Larrea, M., & Li, H. (2004). Characteristics of adolescent females in juvenile detention. *International Journal of Law and Psychiatry, 27,* 321–337.

Liddle, H. A. (1999). Theory development in a family-based therapy for adolescent drug abuse. *Journal of Clinical Child Psychology, 28,* 521–532.

Liddle, H. A. (2002a). *Multidimensional family therapy for adolescent cannabis users, Cannabis Youth Treatment (CYT) Series, Volume 5.* Center for Substance Abuse Treatment (CSAT), Rockville, MD.

Liddle, H. A. (2002b). Advances in family-based therapy for adolescent substance abuse: Findings from the Multidimensional Family Therapy research program. In L. S. Harris (Ed.), *Problems of drug dependence 2001: Proceedings of the 63rd annual scientific meeting* (NIDA Research Monograph No. 182, pp. 113–115). Bethesda, MD: National Institute on Drug Abuse.

Liddle, H. A., Becker, D., & Diamond, G. M. (1997). Family therapy supervision. In C. Watkins (Ed.), *Handbook of psychotherapy supervision* (pp. 400–418). New York: John Wiley & Sons.

Liddle, H. A., Dakof, G. A., Parker, K., Diamond, G. S., Barrett, K., & Tejeda, M. (2001). Multidimensional Family Therapy for adolescent drug abuse: Results of a randomized clinical trial. *American Journal of Drug and Alcohol Abuse, 27,* 651–687.

Liddle, H. A., Dakof, G. A., Rowe, C., Henderson, C., Colon, L., Kanzki, E., et al. (2004). Is an in-home alternative to residential treatment viable? In H. Liddle (Chair), *Family-based treatment for adolescent drug abuse: New findings.* Symposium presented at the Annual Meeting of the American Psychological Association, Honolulu, Hawaii.

Liddle, H. A., Jackson-Gilfort, A., & Marvel, F. A. (2006). An empirically-supported and culturally specific engagement and intervention strategy for African American adolescent males. *Journal of Orthopsychiatry, 76,* 215–225.

Liddle, H. A., Rodriguez, R. A., Dakof, G. A., Kanzki, E., & Marvel, F. A. (2005). Multidimensional Family Therapy: A science-based treatment for adolescent drug abuse. In J. Lebow (Ed.), *Handbook of clinical family therapy* (pp.128–163). New York: John Wiley and Sons.

Liddle, H. A., & Rowe, C. L. (Eds.). (2006). *Adolescent substance abuse: Research and clinical advances.* London: Cambridge University Press.

Liddle, H. A., Rowe, C., Dakof, G., & Lyke, J. (1998). Translating parenting research into clinical interventions for families of adolescents (Special issue). *Clinical Child Psychology and Psychiatry, 3,* 419–443.

Liddle, H. A., Rowe, C., Diamond, G. M., Sessa, F. M., Schmidt, S., & Ettinger, D. (2000). Towards a developmental family therapy: The clinical utility of research on adolescence. *Journal of Marital and Family Therapy, 26,* 485–499.

Liddle, H. A., Rowe, C. L., Gonzalez, A., Henderson, C. E., Dakof, G. A., & Greenbaum, P. E. (2006). Changing provider practices, program environment, and improving outcomes by transporting multidimensional family therapy to an adolescent drug treatment setting. *American Journal on Addictions, 15,* 1–11.

Liddle, H. A., Rowe, C. L., Quille, T., Dakof, G., Mills, D., Sakran, E., et al. (2002). Transporting a research-based adolescent drug treatment into practice. *Journal of Substance Abuse Treatment, 22,* 1–13.

Liddle, H. A., & Schwartz, S. J. (2002). Attachment and family therapy: Clinical utility of adolescent-family attachment research. *Family Process, 41,* 455–476.

Miller, W. R., Zweben, J. E., & Johnson, W. (2005). Evidence-based treatment: Why, what, where, when and how? *Journal of Substance Abuse Treatment, 29,* 267–276.

National Institute of Mental Health. (2004). *State implementation of evidence-based practices II: Bridging science and service.* (Rep. No. RFA-MH-05-004).

National Institute on Drug Abuse. (1999). *Scientifically based approaches to drug addiction treatment. In Principles of Drug Addiction Treatment: A research-based guide.* (Rep. No. NIH publication No. 99-4180). Rockville, MD: National Institute on Drug Abuse.

National Institute on Drug Abuse. (2004). *Enhancing state capacity to foster adoption of science-based practices.* (Rep. No. RFA-DA-05-002).

Olds, D., Henderson, C. R., Cole, R., Eckenrode, J., Kitzman, H., Luckey, D., et al. (1998). Long-term effects of nurse home visitation on childrens criminal and antisocial behavior: 15 year follow up of a randomized controlled trial. *Journal of the American Medical Association, 280,* 1238–1244.

Prendergast, M. L., & Podus, D. (2000). Drug treatment effectiveness: An examination of conceptual and policy issues. *Substance Use and Misuse, 35,* 1629–1657.

Rigter, H. (2006). *INCANT: INternational CAnnabis Need for Treatment: Results of a pilot study of Multidimensional Family Therapy in five European nations. Report to the Steering Committee of the Cannabis Research Action Plan.*

Rigter, H., Van Gageldonk, A., & Ketelaars, T. (2005). *Treatment and other interventions targeting drug use and addiction: State of the art 2004.* Utrecht: National Drug Monitor (of the Netherlands).

Robbins, M. S., Liddle, H. A., Turner, C. W., Dakof, G. A., Alexander, J. F., & Kogan, S. M. (2006). Adolescent and parent therapeutic alliances as predictors of dropout in Multidimensional Family Therapy. *Journal of Family Psychology, 20,* 108–116.

Rowe, C. L., & Liddle, H. A. (2008). When the levee breaks: Adolescents and families in the aftermath of Hurricane Katrina. *Journal of Marital and Family Therapy, 34,* 132–148.

Rowe, C. L., Liddle, H. A., Greenbaum, P. E. & Henderson, C. E. (2004). Impact of psychiatric comorbidity on treatment of adolescent drug abusers. *Journal of Substance Abuse Treatment, 26,* 1–12.

Rowe C. L., Liddle H. A., McClintic K., & Quille, T. (2002). Integrative treatment development: Multidimensional family therapy for adolescent substance abuse. In F. Kaslow & J. Lebow (Eds.), *Comprehensive handbook of psychotherapy, Vol. 4: Integrative/Eclectic Therapies* (pp. 133–161). New York: John Wiley and Sons.

Schmidt, S. E., Liddle, H. A., & Dakof, G. A. (1996). Changes in parental practices and adolescent drug abuse during multi-dimensional family therapy. *Journal of Family Psychology, 10,* 12–27.

Shelef, K., Diamond, G. M., Diamond, G. S., & Liddle, H. A. (2005). Adolescent and parent alliance and treatment outcome in Multidimensional Family Therapy. *Journal of Consulting and Clinical Psychology, 73,* 689–698.

Waltz, J., Addis, M. E., Koerner, K., & Jacobson, N. S. (1993). Testing the integrity of a psychotherapy protocol: Assessment of adherence and competence. *Journal of Consulting and Clinical Psychology, 61,* 620–630.

Weisz, J. R., Doneberg, G. R., Han, S. S., & Weiss, B. (1995). Bridging the gap between laboratory and clinic in child and adolescent psychotherapy. *Journal of Consulting and Clinical Psychology, 63,* 688–701.

Willenbring, M. L., Kivlahan, D., Kenny, M., Grillo, M., Hagedorn, H., & Postier, A. (2004). Beliefs about evidence-based practices in addiction treatment: A survey of Veterans Administration program leaders. *Journal of Substance Abuse Treatment, 26,* 79–85.

Zavala, S. K., French, M. T., Henderson, C. E., Alberga, L., Rowe, C. L., & Liddle, H. A. (2005). Guidelines and challenges for estimating the economic costs and benefits of adolescent substance abuse treatments. *Journal of Substance Abuse Treatment, 29,* 191–205.

22

Drug Testing, the Workplace, and Other Applications

Paul M. Roman

University of Georgia

Hannah K. Knudsen

University of Kentucky

Contents

Testing human beings for evidence of drug use is a fascinating example of a technological innovation that can be productively examined within the framework of the diffusion and adoption of evidence-based practices.

The movement to test potential and active workers for evidence of the use of certain drugs has not only diffused massively throughout the population of American workplaces, but has also been accepted in other prominent venues: the world of sports, widely defined, and, in a related mode, among students desiring to participate in athletic activities.

Although not submitted to randomized clinical trials, evidence from a wide range of long-range posttreatment outcome studies indicates that drug testing can be a useful and even powerful tool in motivating abstinence during the recovery process. The use of drug testing as an adjunct to treatment is not without controversy, inasmuch as it assumes a goal of abstinence in the treatment process, an assumption that many regard as self-defeating, particularly as they proclaim addiction to be a chronic disease characterized by relapses.

The "match" between the needs of treatment follow-up, particularly when the criminal justice system and its requirement of objective measurement is involved, is far clearer than the match with the requirements of the workplace. Although evidence of the sequence of diffusion is not presently available, it appears quite clear that drug testing's controversial application to the workplace diffused into the treatment process, where the fit of application is much clearer.

Careful distinctions need to be drawn about the use of drug testing in the workplace. The widest and best-known application is in pre-employment screening. This event is often dreaded by individuals who may not have used drugs but have been in the company of those who have been using, that is, smoking marijuana. Because there is no legal relationship between job applicants and potential employers, there are no laws or even customs guiding whether potential employers are bound to reveal the results of drug tests. However, it is generally assumed that testing positive for the presence of illegal drug residues in one's urine leads to denial of employment.

As may also be evident, there is considerable discretion on the part of the employer, given that there may be circumstances where an excuse not to hire an individual is needed or where a particular valuable employment prospect is needed, regardless of drug testing results. The absence of a legal framework thus adds to the potency of drug testing as a workplace tool. Although there are no known data on the extent of the practice, there are many reports of settings where job applicants are required to pay the full costs of the drug test "up front," that is, before the testing actually occurs. Further in the chapter we explore several issues about the goals of pre-employment drug testing.

Probably equally well known is the practice of random drug testing in the workplace. A parallel to this practice in everyday American life is the police roadblock used to screen drivers for evidence of driving while intoxicated. The potential for this kind of screening is much greater than its actual use, and in fact its use is precluded on crowded busy highways where the potential impact of the drunken driver may be much greater than on a secondary road.

Random drug testing carries draconian implications through the idea that the employer has the right to demand a urine specimen at any time during work hours. Courts have not upheld this practice for most public employment settings, with the clear exception of those occupations that are in some manner "safety-sensitive." Nonetheless, policies allowing for random drug testing, whether used or not, persist in a numerically large number of workplaces.

The third type of drug testing may be viewed as within the employer–employee relationship, and it stems from long-term rules in most blue-collar workplaces that those coming to work must be "fit for duty" and remain so throughout the work shift. This is typically referred to as "for-cause" testing, and it occurs when the employer has a reasonable basis for suspicion that the employee is unfit for duty. Acting irrationally or displaying hostility are examples of such circumstances. An extremely common basis for challenging an employee's fitness for duty is the occurrence of a workplace accident or the sustaining of a workplace injury. Under such circumstances, the discovery of an employee's impaired condition may free the employer from liability, including the possibility of denying the employee insurance coverage for the costs of medical care.

What Is the Prevalence of Workplace Drug Testing (WDT) Programs?

There are limited nationally representative data on the prevalence of drug testing programs in American workplaces, particularly regarding prior to the 1990s. One of the few studies examining the expansion of drug testing through the 1980s and 1990s reports data from firms in Georgia (Spell & Blum, 2005). They reported that the "take-off" in drug testing occurred in the late 1980s, which may partly reflect President Reagan's declaration in 1986 of the "War on Drugs" and the federal legislation promoting drug-free workplaces that was enacted two years later. These data from Georgia are consistent with other reports linking the expansion of drug testing to the latter 1980s and attributing the adoption of Workplace Drug Testing (WDT) to these political forces (Axel, 1990; Boyes-Watson, 1997; Gerber, Jensen, Schreck, & Babcock, 1990; Macdonald, Wells, & Fry, 1993).

In the 1990s, the National Household Survey on Drug Abuse (now known as the National Survey on Drug Use & Health) included measures of workplace drug testing in surveys conducted in 1994 and 1997; these data were later released as a report (Office of Applied Studies, 1999). Based on reports from full-time workers about their employers, there was some evidence of increasing prevalence of drug testing programs. In 1994, about 35% of full-time workers reported that their employer screened applicants for drug use; this rate of pre-employment screening increased to 39% in 1997. Likewise, random drug testing programs increased from 20% of workplaces in 1994 to 25% in 1997. For-cause testing programs increased to a lesser extent from 28% in 1994 to 30% in 1997.

Data from the National Employee Survey (NES) provide similar evidence about the expansion of workplace drug testing programs and include more recent data. Random-digit dialing was utilized to generate nationally representative samples of full-time employees in 1993, 1997, and 2002. Notably, the NES data indicate continued expansion of the three types of drug testing programs over time. About half of these full-time workers indicated that their employers screened job candidates prior to hiring and tested employees if there was probable cause. Random testing programs continued to be less prevalent than the other two types of testing, but there was still an increase in the percentage of respondents indicating that their employers utilized random testing. See Table 22.1.

The three types of drug testing are also interrelated, such that the adoption of each type of drug testing is positively associated with the likelihood that an organization has adopted the other two types. The data from the 2002 NES also indicate that these associations are

TABLE 22.1
Prevalence of Workplace Drug Testing Programs

	1993 (%)	1997 (%)	2002 (%)
Pre-employment screening	33.5	45.2	49.5
For-cause testing	33.1	41.2	47.6
Random testing	22.4	28.3	31.6

Source. National Employee Survey, University of Georgia.

considerable in magnitude. The correlation between pre-employment screening and for-cause testing was 0.60, the correlation between screening and random testing was 0.48, and the correlation between for-cause and random testing was 0.61.

What Types of Organizations Are More Likely to Have Adopted Workplace Drug Testing?

As workplace drug testing programs have increased over time, some organizational researchers have become interested in understanding what types of employers are more likely to adopt WDT. The literature examining the associations between organizational characteristics and workplace drug testing programs is relatively small, but has drawn on several theoretical traditions. Central among these theoretical perspectives are arguments related to organizational compatibility (Rogers, 1995), strategic choice (Pfeffer & Salancik, 1978), and institutional pressures (DiMaggio & Powell, 1991).

One approach to examining the adoption of WDT has relied heavily on the work of Rogers (1995) and his arguments regarding organizational compatibility. According to Rogers, organizational compatibility, or the "fit" between the characteristics of the innovation itself and the characteristics of the adopting organization, is a critical aspect of the process of innovation adoption. In particular, innovations are more likely to be adopted when they fit with the available resources of the organization, meet a key organizational need, and are consistent with ideas and innovations that have been previously introduced into the organization.

A key variable that has been considered in analyses of workplace drug testing is organizational size. There are several arguments that may explain potential relationships between size and workplace drug testing programs. First, organizational size is often conceptualized as a measure of "slack" resources, meaning that larger organizations are likely to have more resources that they can direct toward innovation adoption (Rogers, 1995; Scott, 2001). Furthermore, larger organizations may have greater employee surveillance needs (Borg, 2000). Specifically, as organizations employ more workers, direct observation and management of employees becomes less feasible (Borg & Arnold, 1997). Instead, larger organizations must turn to more formal mechanisms in order to monitor (and control) employees. Such an argument would be consistent with both Rogers' argument about organizational compatibility as well as the strategic choice perspective, which hypothesizes that innovation adoption decisions reflect attempts by managers to address organizational needs (Pfeffer & Salancik, 1978). Finally, some have argued that larger organizations are more visible within their field, that greater visibility comes with enhanced environmental demands related to legitimacy (Spell & Blum, 2005). This hypothesized relationship between organizational size, as measured by the number of employees, and workplace drug testing programs has been documented in the literature (Knudsen, Roman, & Johnson, 2003). We also examined this association using data from the 2002 National Employee Survey. As seen in Figure 22.1, the presence of the three types of drug testing increases in larger organizations.

In addition to organizational size, some researchers have considered the prevalence of workplace drug testing programs across different industries. The logic underpinning this hypothesized relationship is also drawn from Rogers (1995), particularly his arguments about organizational needs, and is also consistent with the strategic choice perspective (Pfeffer &

FIGURE 22.1
Presence of Workplace Drug Testing by Organizational Size.

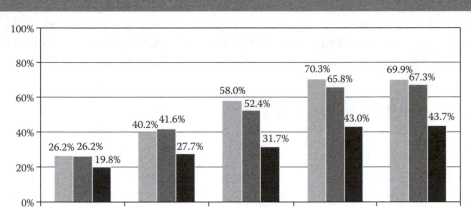

Salancik, 1978). WDT programs have often been constructed as a mechanism to increase employee safety in the workplace, particularly by decreasing accidents. Not all industries are at the same risk of accidents, suggesting there is variability in this particular organizational need. Using the transportation industry as the reference point, Kesselring and Pittman (2002) found that injuries are more prevalent in agriculture, construction, and manufacturing, whereas injuries were lower in wholesale trade, retail trade, services, and finance. Organizations in these "lower injury" industries were significantly less likely to have adopted WDT programs than organizations in the transportation industry, based on data from the NES (Knudsen et al., 2003). The findings for industry were less clear in the "higher injury" industries, which may have been due to the fact that the analyses controlled for the degree of mechanization in the workplace. Mechanization, as measured by the degree to which machines control the pace and performance of work, was positively associated with all three types of WDT; this finding was consistent with Rogers' argument about organizational needs.

In addition to organizational needs, the literature on innovation adoption suggests that such adoption is more likely if the innovation is consistent with organizational norms (Rogers, 1995). For example, organizations may vary in the extent to which they are governed by formalized rules that are enforced. A heavier emphasis on formalized rules suggests an organizational culture that is committed to greater control over its workers. Workplace drug testing programs, which clearly have an element of social control, would likely be consistent with such a rules-based culture. Indeed, data from the NES support such an assertion, with the likelihood of each of the three types of testing increasing in more rule-oriented employment contexts (Knudsen et al., 2003).

A final dimension of organizational compatibility that has relevance in understanding the adoption of workplace drug testing is the notion of previously introduced ideas. Rogers (1995) argues that some innovations may be more likely to be adopted if they are consistent with previously adopted technologies. In the context of WDT programs, employee assistance programs (EAPs), which are mechanisms that link employees with services to address personal needs, have been identified as a predictor of WDT adoption (Hartwell, Steele,

French, & Rodman, 1996). The presence of an EAP within a workplace suggests that the employer has already made a commitment to addressing substance abuse-related issues in its workforce. Furthermore, EAPs provide employers with a method for addressing drug-using employees that are identified through WDT programs. Consistent with the work of Hartwell et al., data from the NES indicate that the presence of an EAP increases the probability of each of the types of workplace drug testing (Knudsen et al., 2003).

State-Level Policies and WDT

Although organizational characteristics are clearly associated with the adoption of workplace drug testing programs, those adoption decisions are embedded within a broader institutional context that includes external pressures that come from state governments. As noted by DiMaggio and Powell (1991), these external pressures on organizations to adopt (or not adopt) a particular innovation may represent "coercive isomorphism." In the context of WDT adoption, there is variability in the supportiveness of state laws with regard to these programs, which may also be associated with the presence of these programs in the workplace. These laws and regulations can be conceptualized as representing a continuum ranging from supportive to restrictive of WDT (Kesselring & Pittman, 2002).

The U.S. Department of Labor maintains a website that tracks the WDT-related laws and policies by state. We examined the summaries of these laws, and four main themes emerged. First, some states offer incentives to organizations that adopt WDT programs, such as reduced workers' compensation premiums. Second, some state laws allow WDT if guidelines related to implementation are followed. The third type of WDT regulations related to offering legal protections to organizations that adopt these programs. At the other end of the continuum, however, some states have placed restrictions on WDT programs, such as specifying the types of situations in which testing is allowable.

Of the four types of laws, the most common category was laws that allowed WDT testing if certain procedures were followed in the implementation WDT (24 states). Ten states offered discounts on worker's compensation premiums, and six states offered legal protections to employers who adopt WDT. Restrictions on WDT were present in eight states.

Drawing on these four types of state laws related to WDT, we examined whether these laws were related to the presence of WDT among respondents to the 2002 NES. Based on the states in which they lived, respondents were coded for whether their state had each of the four types of laws and whether their organization used each of the three kinds of drug testing. We estimated logistic regression models of the three type of WDT on these four laws while controlling for establishment size.

There were mixed results with regard to the association between state laws and the presence of WDT programs. As seen in Table 22.2, state laws that offered discounts in worker's compensation premiums increased the likelihood of each of the three types of drug testing. Laws that provide legal protections to employers were positively associated with the odds of pre-employment screening and for-cause testing. There was a trend for pre-employment screening and random testing being more likely if the state's laws allowed WDT if certain procedures were followed. Laws restricting drug testing were not associated with any of the types

TABLE 22.2
Logistic Regression of Adoption of WDT Programs on State Laws and Establishment Size

	Pre-Employment Screening Odds Ratio	For-Cause Testing Odds Ratio	Random Testing Odds Ratio
State allows WDT if procedures are followed	1.26[†]	1.26	1.30[†]
State offers discount on worker's compensation premiums	1.31*	1.47**	1.68*
State offers legal protections for WDT	1.72*	1.65*	1.30
State places restrictions on WDT	.83	.81	.72
Establishment size			
<25 workers	Reference	Reference	Reference
25–99 workers	1.84***	1.91***	1.50*
100–249 workers	4.16***	3.35***	1.85**
250–499 workers	6.94***	5.48***	3.13***
500+ workers	6.66***	6.24***	3.19***

Source. National Employee Survey, University of Georgia.
[†]$p<.10$, *$p<.05$, **$p<.01$, ***$p<.001$

of WDT, but this may reflect the fact that only a small percentage of respondents (6.2%) live in states with these restrictions. However, an analysis of 69 organizations in the construction industry demonstrated that such restrictions were a barrier to the adoption of WDT programs (Gerber & Yacoubian, 2002).

Thus, there is some evidence of the external environment, particularly in terms of state-level regulations and policies, having some influence on the likelihood that an organization engages in drug testing. State laws that offer employers reductions in their worker's compensation premiums appear to be an incentive that facilitates the adoption of WDT. In this case, WDT may represent a way for organizations to increase their legitimacy because their state government is clearly indicating that testing is a valued mechanism for addressing workplace drug problems (DiMaggio & Powell, 1991). Adoption of WDT may also be perceived as a means of improving the company's image (Gerber & Yacoubian, 2002). Additionally, these laws offer a tangible incentive to organizations that adopt drug testing; as such, WDT may also represent a strategic choice (Pfeffer & Salancik, 1978).

Employer Responses to Positive Tests—Organizational Factors

Although employers may hope that drug testing will deter employees from using drugs, some tests will yield positive results. According to a drug testing laboratory that processed 7.1 million tests in 2003, about 28.2% of for-cause tests were positive (Quest Diagnostics,

2004); the rates for pre-employment screening (4.1%) and random testing (6.6%) were much lower. The question for employers then becomes how to respond to positive results. The likely response for pre-employment screening is to exclude the applicant from employment. In the case of for-cause and random testing, employers have a broader range of options. Roman and Blum (1999) conceptualize these responses as ranging from "externalization" to "internalization." The concept of externalization generally refers to practices in which organizations push certain "costs" to the external environment. In the context of drug-using employees, termination of the employment relationship would represent a form of externalization because it would then become the responsibility of other entities to deal with the drug-using individual. Internalization would include responses that maintain the employment relationship. However, some employers may choose responses that rehabilitate employees by sending them to counseling whereas others elect more punitive responses.

We examined the issue of employers' responses to positive drug tests according to full-time workers participating in the 1997 and 2002 National Employee Surveys. During both time periods, the most common response was that the employee was sent to counseling, which represents a form of internalization that is rehabilitative in nature. However, the percentage of workers reporting this type of response decreased from 55.8% in 1997 to 45.5% in 2002. Consequently, there was evidence of an increase in punitive responses. The percentage of workers reporting that their employers externalize drug-using employees through termination increased from 29.1% in 1997 to 34.2% in 2002. Likewise, a greater percentage of workers indicated that their employer punished (but did not fire) drug-using employees in 2002 (12.1%) relative to 1997 (6.2%). The percentage of respondents indicating that an unspecified "other" response occurred remained stable (8.9% in 1997; 8.2% in 2002).

Just as organizational factors are associated with the likelihood that organizations adopt workplace drug testing, it is also likely that some of the variability in these responses to positive drug tests is explained by organizational characteristics. Using data from the 1997 NES, we examined the odds of punitive responses relative to the rehabilitative response of sending employees to counseling (Knudsen, Roman, & Johnson, 2004). In estimating the odds of termination versus counseling, three organizational characteristics were relevant. First, the presence of unionized employees reduced the odds of termination being the organization's response; this is perhaps not surprising inasmuch as unions often oppose the dismissal of employees who fail drug tests (Seeber & Lehman, 1989). Another protective factor that reduced the likelihood of termination was the presence of an employee assistance program (EAP); again, this finding is intuitive inasmuch as EAPs are charged with helping employees to address personal problems that are negatively influencing their job performance (Roman & Blum, 1985). However, one aspect of organizational culture that increased the odds that employers terminate rather than rehabilitate drug-using employees is the organization's rules orientation. Workplaces in which rules are more formalized and enforced were more likely to terminate drug-using employees; such a response would be consistent with an orientation toward rules enforcement.

These data also offered insight into the organizational characteristics that increased the likelihood of a punitive response (that maintains the employment relationship) relative to the likelihood of a rehabilitative response. In this case, neither unionization nor the organization's rules orientation was significant. However, the presence of an EAP continued to have a protective effect, reducing the likelihood of a punitive response relative to a rehabilitative response. Two other organizational characteristics were significant. Relative to larger organizations, there was a greater risk of a punitive response in small and medium-sized establishments. Also, when compared to public sector organizations, service sector organizations and productive sector organizations (e.g., construction, manufacturing) were at lower risk of a punitive response.

Employee Attitudes toward Workplace Drug Testing

Critiques of employee drug testing programs often invoke arguments related to the invasion of employees' privacy. If such concerns are salient from the perspective of employees, it would be expected that employees would not approve of the three types of drug testing. However, data from the 2002 NES suggest the opposite; in general, the majority of employees approve of all three types of drug testing, particularly when the testing is based on reasonable suspicions of employee drug use (Table 22.3). There is perhaps more ambivalence about random testing programs, but even for this type of drug testing, about 70% of full-time employees report approving of random testing. These high levels of support for workplace drug testing in the NES data are consistent with general opinion polls that suggest about 70–80% of Americans approve of such programs (Fendrich & Kim, 2002).

When compared to earlier NES data, there is mixed evidence about whether employee attitudes toward workplace drug testing have changed over time. Attitudes toward random testing and for-cause testing appear not to have changed between 1993 and 2002. However, in the case of pre-employment testing, there is evidence that employees have become more supportive of such programs over time. For example, about 34.4% of employees strongly approved of pre-employment screening in 1993; by 2002, about 43.3% indicated strongly approving of such testing.

Impact of Workplace Drug Testing

Despite the growing expansion of drug testing in the workplace, the key question about whether such tests are "effective" in the sense of reducing or deterring drug use has not been definitively answered. Analyses of the impacts of WDT programs are few in number and often

TABLE 22.3
Employee Attitudes toward Workplace Drug Testing

Generic Name	Pre-Employment Screening (%)	For-Cause Testing (%)	Random Testing (%)
Strongly approve	43.0	47.6	32.7
Approve	37.5	41.7	38.5
Disapprove	11.4	6.4	14.6
Strongly disapprove	8.1	4.3	14.2

Source. 2002 National Employee Survey, University of Georgia.

suffer from problematic research designs. However, there are some data available that partly address the issue of the impact of WDT on employee drug use and workplace accidents.

Part of the challenge in assessing the impact of workplace drug testing is that examinations of WDT on employee drug use generally rely on self-report data. For example, data from the 1994 National Household Survey on Drug Abuse (NHSDA) suggested that working for an employer with a random testing program was negatively associated with past-month drug use; a similar association was found for working for an organization that screenings potential employees before hiring them (OAS, 1999). When data from the 1997 NHSDA were examined, these associations were not statistically significant. Further complicating the answer were the findings of French, Roebuck, and Alexandre (2004), who reanalyzed the 1997 NHSDA data in conjunction with the 1998 NHSDA data. They considered any drug use in the past year and chronic drug use, as measured by use at least once a week for the past year. In the combined 1997–1998 data, the likelihood of any self-reported drug use in the past year was 24.2% lower when employees worked for organizations with some form of drug testing. In addition, the odds of chronic drug use were 38.6% lower in organizations with at least one type of drug testing.

What remains unclear in these studies that rely on self-report data is the "mechanism of action" by which these lower odds of drug use are produced. For example, it is not clear whether drug-using employees stop or reduce their use once they enter a workplace with a drug testing program. Alternatively, it may be the case that the presence of such programs deters drug users from entering (or staying) with employers that have adopted drug testing. Some evidence from the NHSDA supports the latter explanation. Participants in the NHSDA were asked if they would be less likely to choose an employer based on whether that organization had adopted the three types of drug testing. Comparisons of nondrug users and current drug users suggest that current drug users were much more likely to indicate they would not choose that employer than nondrug users. For example, only 6% of nondrug users reported that they would be less likely to choose an employer that engages in random drug testing compared to 29% of current drug users. Despite this difference, it seems notable that even among current drug users, the majority would not be deterred from choosing to work for an employer that randomly tests for drug use. From this perspective, it would seem that the impact of drug testing on employees' drug use may be limited.

Another method for addressing the impact of drug testing on employee drug use may be to examine trends in the rate of positive drug tests over time. Sources of such data are quite limited, but one SAMHSA-accredited drug testing company has released rates of drug-positive tests over time (Quest Diagnostics, 2004). These data suggest that the rate of positive drug tests has declined considerably since the 1980s, with each year between 1988 and 2003 showing a lower rate of positive tests. For example, the overall positive rate for the combined U.S. workforce was 13.6% in 1988; it had declined to 4.5% in 2003. Of course, it is impossible to draw causal linkages regarding whether this decline is due to drug testing programs per se or simply reflect broader trends of declining illegal drug use among Americans.

The literature on the impact of drug testing on workplace safety is also limited. There are some indications that WDT may reduce accidents. Gerber and Yacoubian (2002) examined injury incident rates in the construction industry and found that companies that implemented workplace drug testing programs were able to achieve reductions in these rates over time.

Conclusions

1. There has been an expansion in WDT over the past decade.
2. Variations in WDT can be explained, in part, by organizational characteristics.
3. There is some evidence that state policies are related to WDT.
4. Organizational characteristics also partly explain differences in how employers respond to positive drug tests.
5. There is some evidence that employers are becoming more punitive in their responses to positive drug tests.
6. There is widespread support among full-time workers for WDT. Self-report data suggest lower drug use among those employed by organizations with WDT. The rate of positive drug tests has decreased since the late 1980s. More research is needed about the "effectiveness" of WDT.

References

Axel, H. (1990). *Corporate experiences with drug testing programs.* New York: Conference Board.

Borg, M. J. (1997). Social monitoring as social control: The case of drug testing in a medical workplace. *Sociological Forum, 12,* 441–460.

Borg, M. J. (2000). Drug testing in organizations: Applying Horwitz's theory of the effectiveness of social control. *Deviant Behavior, 21,* 123–154.

Boyes-Watson, C. (1997). Corporations as drug warriors: The symbolic significance of employee drug testing. *Studies in Law, Politics, and Society, 17,* 185–223.

DiMaggio, P. J., & Powell, W. W. (1991). The iron cage revisited: Institutional isomorphism and collective rationality in organizational fields. In W. W. Powell and P. J. DiMaggio (Eds.), *The new institutionalism in organizational analysis* (pp. 63–82). Chicago: University of Chicago Press.

Fendrich, M., & Kim, J. Y. S. (2002). The experience and acceptability of drug testing: Poll trends. *Journal of Drug Issues, 32,* 81–96.

French, M. T., Roebuck, M. C., & Alexandre, P. K. (2004). To test or not to test: Do employee drug testing programs discourage employee drug use. *Social Science Research, 33,* 45–63.

Gerber, J., Jensen, E. L., Schreck, M., & Babcock, G. M. (1990). Drug testing and social control: Implications for state theory. *Contemporary Crises, 14,* 243–258.

Gerber, J. K., & Yacoubian, G. S., Jr. (2002). An assessment of drug testing within the construction industry. *Journal of Drug Education, 32,* 53–68.

Hartwell, T. D., Steele, P. D., French, M. T., & Rodman, N. F. (1996). Prevalence of drug testing in the workplace. *Monthly Labor Review, 121,* 27–34.

Kesserling, R. G., & Pittman, J. R. (2002). Drug testing laws and employment injuries. *Journal of Labor Research, 23,* 293–301.

Knudsen, H. K., Roman, P. M., & Johnson, J. A. (2003). Organizational compatibility and workplace drug testing: Modeling the adoption of innovative social control practices. *Sociological Forum, 18,* 621–640.

Knudsen, H. K., Roman, P. M., & Johnson, J. A. (2004). The management of workplace deviance: Organizational responses to employee drug use. *Journal of Drug Issues, 34,* 121–144.

Macdonald, S., Wells, S., & Fry, R. (1993). The limitations of drug screening in the workplace. *International Labour Review, 132,* 95–113.

Office of Applied Studies. (1999). *Worker drug use and workplace policies and programs: Results from the 1994 and 1997 NHSDA* (DHHS Pub No. 99-3352). Rockville, MD: SAMHSA.

Office of Applied Studies. (September 27, 2002). *Awareness of workplace substance use policies and programs.* The NHSDA report. Available online at http://www.oas.samhsa.gov/2k2/workpolicies/workpolicies.htm.

Pfeffer, J., & Salancik, G. (1978). *The external control of organizations*. New York: Harper & Row.

Quest Diagnostics. (2004). *Increased use of amphetamines linked to rising workplace drug use, according to Quest Diagnostics' 2003 Drug Testing Index*. Available online at http://www.questdiagnositcs.com/employersolutions/dti_07_2004/dti_index.pdf. Accessed on January 19, 2007.

Rogers, E. M. (1995). *Diffusion of innovations* (4th ed.). New York: Free Press.

Roman, P. M., & Blum, T. C. (1985). The core technology of employee assistance programs. *The ALMACAN, 15*, 8–9, 16–19.

Roman, P. M., & Blum, T. C. (1999). Externalization and internalization as frames for understanding workplace deviance. *Research in the Sociology of Work, 8*, 139–164.

Scott, W. R. (2001). *Institutions and organizations* (2nd ed.). Thousand Oaks, CA: Sage.

Seeber, R. L., & Lehman, M. (1989). The union response to employer-initiated drug testing programs. *Employee Responsibilities and Rights Journal, 25*, 471–503.

Spell, C. S., & Blum, T. C. (2005). Adoption of workplace substance abuse prevention programs: Strategic choice and institutional perspectives. *Academy of Management Journal, 48*, 1152–1142.

23

Mechanisms of Stress Effects on Substance Abuse Initiation, Maintenance, and Relapse: Intervention Implications

Mustafa al'Absi

University of Minnesota Medical School

Contents

Introduction

Stress is linked to all stages of the addiction process, including initiation, maintenance, and relapse. It is widely cited by drug users as the reason they use drugs or abuse alcohol or relapse to cigarette smoking. Although it is clear that addiction is a very complex phenomenon that involves multiple pharmacological, psychosocial, and behavioral processes, there is growing evidence that suggests perceived stress and expectation of relief as important motivators for drug use. This evidence is further solidified by the discovery of multiple neurobiological pathways mediating this link between stress and drug addiction, including the hypothalamic-pituitary-adrenocortical (HPA) axis and the endogenous opioid activity (Adinoff, 2004; Adinoff et al., 2005a; al'Absi, 2006; Goeders, 2007; Mendelson et al., 1988). In this chapter, we present a brief review of the biological and physiological systems involved in regulating the stress response and the psychosocial and situational determinants of this response. We then describe how these systems are involved in mediating the stress effects on drug use initiation, maintenance, and difficulties in recovery.

Definitions

Early in the last century several authors (Cannon, 1928; Selye, 1947) developed the contemporary concept of psychological stress. The focus was on addressing effects of psychological stress on physiological changes in a variety of systems that are similar to those produced by physical or chemical challenges. Selye defined *stress* as a nonspecific response of the body to any demand and described the role of glucocorticoids in mediating potential harmful effects of stress. He discussed the stages of coping the organism encounters when under stress by coining the concept of General Adaptation Syndrome (GAS). The GAS includes the following stages: alarm reaction, resistance, and exhaustion. Later research (Mason, 1975; Ursin & Olff, 1993) has modified the concept of nonspecific reaction to stress by introducing the roles of situational, psychological, and cognitive factors, such as novelty, uncontrollability, unpredictability, and anticipation of negative consequences as discussed later. Cognitive-transactional definitions of stress have also influenced stress research and have focused on the role of cognitive appraisal of the stressful event in determining the impact of a stressor on the individual (Lazarus, 1999). Other definitions specifically focus on the role of individual–environmental transactions in determining the biological responses to stress (e.g., Levine, 2005). These definitions incorporate the role of multiple social and biological determinants of the stress response, including gender, developmental processes, social status, and genetic factors.

Responses to Psychological Stress

Several brain structures are involved in the perception of external and internal events and in regulating the responses to these events. Recent research has focused on two brain structures, the amygdala and the dorsal anterior cingulated cortex (dACC) and found that activation of these structures is associated with threat detection (Hariri, Tessitore, Mattay, Fera, &

Weinberger, 2002b; Ochsner, Bunge, Gross, & Gabrieli, 2002). During a threat situation both the amygdala and dACC serve to mobilize other brain regions, such as the lateral prefrontal cortex (LPFC) and the hypothalamus, and these in turn initiate a series of changes in response to this threat.

Neuroimaging evidence has demonstrated that the amygdala is sensitive to environmental cues signaling danger or novelty (Ochsner et al., 2002) and the degree to which negative stimuli are reported to be unpleasant (Lane et al., 1997). Similarly, the dACC seems to function as a threat detector, evaluating incoming information in terms of congruence of external events with expectation (Carter et al., 2000). Research has also shown that dACC is involved in the response to the threat of social rejection and related social distress experience (Eisenberger, Lieberman, & Williams, 2003).

The activation of these structures sets in motion a cascade of responses via projections to the hypothalamus and LPFC (Carter et al., 2000; Ledoux, 1992) in order to respond to the threat signals. Another region that is also involved in regulating these threat responses is the ventrolateral PFC (VLPFC; Lieberman, Hariri, Jarcho, Eisenberger, & Bookheimer, 2005). Activation of the right VLPFC results in attenuated activation of the amygdala and dACC(Eisenberger et al., 2003; Lieberman et al., 2005; Hariri et al., 2002a). This suggests that LPFC may exert a regulatory influence that modulates activation of the amygdala and dACC in response to external threats.

These central structures are extensively connected to various subcortical and indirectly to peripheral systems involved in orchestrating the peripheral stress response. For example, it is well established that the amygdala has extensive projections to the hypothalamus (Ghashghaei & Barbas, 2002), and that the dACC projects to the paraventricular nucleus of the hypothalamus (Risold, Thompson, & Swanson, 1997). Early experiments measuring peripheral output of these systems have shown that stimulation of the amygdala and the ACC leads to the elevation of blood pressure and cortisol levels in both animals and humans (Frankel, Jenkins, & Wright, 1978; Setekleiv, Skaug, & Kaada, 1961).

These structures directly regulate the two systems that are involved in the stress response, the HPA and the sympatho-adrenomedullary (SAM) system. In addition to their functions in mounting an adaptive response when the organism faces a stressful situation, these two systems also interact closely and influence each other in coordinating this response. In the following sections we briefly describe these two systems.

HPA Axis

The HPA axis performs a central function in organizing the neuroendocrine response to stress and plays a critical role as a mediator of the influence of psychosocial stress on health (McEwen, 1998; Chrousos & Gold, 1992). This axis involves three brain and peripheral structures, the hypothalamus, the pituitary, and the cortical part of the adrenals. The activity of this system is set on by the release of corticotropic-releasing factor (CRF) from neuronal cell bodies of the paraventricular nucleus. Corticotropin-releasing factor travels from the median eminence of the hypothalamus through the portal circulation system and reaches the anterior part of the pituitary gland where it binds CRF receptors, and this leads to the synthesis of proopiomelanocortin. The proopiomelanocortin is a large precursor protein that is cleaved to produce

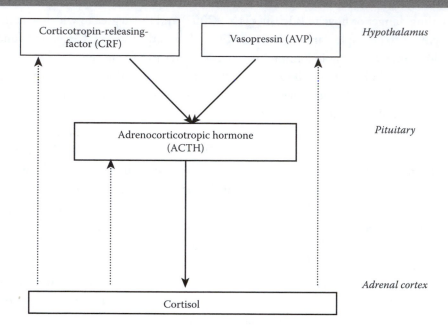

FIGURE 23.1
Structures and Hormones of the Hypothalamic-Pituitary-Adrenocortical Axis. Broken Lines Indicate a Negative Feedback Loop.

both β-endorphin and adrenocorticotropic hormone. In addition to corticotropin-releasing factor, vasopressin is also synthesized and secreted in the paraventricular nucleus. Vasopressin participates in stimulating adrenocorticotropic hormone release. Although vasopressin is a weak secretagogue at adrenocorticotropic hormone-producing cells, when it is combined with CRF it markedly potentiates adrenocorticotropic hormone synthesis and release. Studies have shown that this component of the HPA activity is sensitive to the inhibitory feedback effect of glucocorticoids(Dallman, 1993; Swanson & Simmons, 1989; see Figure 23.1).

Adrenocorticotropic hormone travels through the peripheral circulation to reach the adrenal cortex where it leads to the synthesis and release of corticosteroids, most notably in human cortisol. Corticosteroids, including cortisol, are derived from a common precursor, cholesterol, formed from circulating lipoprotein. The formation of cortisol takes place in the Zona fasciculata (ZF), the intermediate zone of the adrenal cortex. At ZF a cascade of hydroxylation of progesterone to 17-alpha-hydroxyprogestrone to 11-hydroxycortisol and then to cortisol occurs. About 95% of cortisol is bound to corticosteroid-binding globulin (CBG). The remaining free cortisol enters cells to affect their metabolic activity. The liver is the main site for cortisol metabolism, and free cortisol (40–100 ug/day) is excreted in urine.

Cortisol Functions and Corticosteroid Receptors. There are several critical functions performed by the hormone cortisol that are important for normal functioning. These include facilitating the coping process during exposure to acute stress and regulating the manner by which the body reacts to long-term or excessive exposure to stress physiological response

(McEwen, 1997b; Munck, Guyre, & Holbrook, 1984). Cortisol also influences various central nervous system processes that are involved in perceiving and appraising challenging events and in developing appropriate responses to these events (Sapolsky, Romero, & Munck, 2000).

The manner by which cortisol influences brain and other organ functions is determined by the type of receptor being targeted. There are two types of corticosteroid receptors. Type I mineralcorticoid receptor, found primarily in the limbic system, has a high affinity for cortisol, and is progressively occupied over the range of 0–3 ug/dl of cortisol. When occupied, it serves as the major receptor regulator of normal activity of the HPA axis. Type II glucocorticoid receptor (GR), which is more wide spread than Type I, has a lower affinity for cortisol, and becomes occupied when there are higher levels of circulating cortisol. During diurnal peak or after stress this receptor may be up to 60% occupied (Dallman, 1993). The distribution of these two types of receptors allows for a wide range of peripheral and central nervous system functions.

Once released into the circulation, cortisol also exerts numerous peripheral effects, including metabolic, immune, and cardiovascular effects. One of its main functions in the periphery is to make energy stores available for use throughout the body, by increasing protein catabolism and gluconeogenesis, and by decreasing glucose uptake by cells resulting in increased plasma concentrations of amino acids and glucose (Vander, Sherman, & Luciano, 1994). Additionally, cortisol serves to enhance the actions of the sympathetic nervous system by stimulating phenylethanolamine-N-methyltransferase (PNMT), resulting in increased epinephrine synthesis and by inhibiting the catabolic actions of catechol-o-methyltransferase (COMT) on catecholamines (Wilson & Foster, 1992).

Recent research has demonstrated significant influence of cortisol on a wide range of central nervous system functions (Sapolsky, 2000a, 2000b; Lupien et al., 1997). For example, experimental evidence has demonstrated the impact of both cortisol and CRF on neuronal functions and morphology, indicating that excessive exposure to these hormones produce long-term neuronal alterations (Gould, Woolley, & McEwen, 1991; McEwen & Sapolsky, 1995; Sapolsky, 1996). These changes may increase risk for emotional and behavioral problems during adulthood (Heim, Ehlert, Hanker, & Hellhammer, 1998; Heim, Ehlert, & Hellhammer, 2000). The consequences are likely to result from numerous neurochemical changes. Cortisol influences action of the biogenic amines and it influences gene expression of beta-adrenoreceptors and therefore regulates effects of catecholamines that interact with these receptors (Hadcock & Malbon, 1988).

Cortisol plays an important function in regulating its own secretion through its effects on the pituitary, hippocampus, medial region of the frontal cortex, and central amygdala (Diorio, Viau, & Meaney, 1993; Makino, Gold, & Schulkin, 1994a, 1994b). Through these actions, cortisol influences CRF expression (Swanson et al., 1989), as well as the expression of vasopressin (Fink, Robinson, & Tannahill, 1988). It also decreases secretion of adrenocorticotropic hormone from the pituitary (Drouin et al., 1993).

Cortisol elevations in response to stress are important to restore heightened immune activation induced by stress. This is consistent with the hypothesis that stress-related glucocorticoids activity helps curtail the activity of endogenous cytokines and other stress-reactive immune functions (Munck et al., 1984; McEwen, 1997a, 1998). This "braking" mechanism prevents the occurrence of harmful effects that may be produced by an unchecked immune response. Although the cortisol response to acute stress has a survival value, persistently elevated cortisol may lead to various metabolic and cardiovascular effects (Brindley & Rolland, 1989; Rosmond, Dallman, & Bjorntorp, 1998; Rosmond & Bjorntorp, 1998b), and these changes may mediate the stress effects on risk for cardiovascular disease, diabetes, and stroke (Brindley et al., 1989; Rosmond et al., 1998b; Rosmond & Bjorntorp, 1998a).

Sympathetic System

The sympathetic nervous system, in concert with the parasympathetic nervous system, plays an essential role in the body's adjustments to normal demands, and it is critical for the integration and expression of the fight–flight response during times of stress. This system increases heart rate, blood pressure, shifts blood flow to skeletal muscles, increases blood glucose, and leads to the dilation of the pupils and the increase in respiration. This pattern of activation facilitates the organism's ability to face the challenging situation or escape from it.

The sympathetic nervous system controls the activity of smooth muscles or cardiac muscles by secreting norepinephrine (NE) at specialized synaptic junctions. NE enhances the rate and force of contraction of the innervated smooth muscles. Thus, the sympathetic nervous system generally increases activation and function of the organs it innervates. One important element of this system is the sympathetic innervations of the medulla of the adrenal glands. The adrenal medulla receives sympathetic preganglionic fibers directly from the spinal cord. These fibers secrete acetylcholine causing the adrenal medulla to release epinephrine and NE into the circulation where epinephrine acts as an endocrine messenger. Norepinephrine is secreted at the same time as epinephrine, but its effect on tissues via circulation is limited (Steptoe, 1987; Goldstein & Kopin, 1990).

Role of the Locus Coeruleus.   The locus coeruleus, located in the brainstem, contains 90% of the NE-synthesizing cell bodies in the central nervous system. It projects down in the spinal cord and upward to several subcortical and cortical systems (Aston-Jones, Ennis, Pieribone, Nickell, & Shipley, 1986). When this system is activated it causes the release of NE from noradrenergic neurons in various brain loci. This NE release facilitates a heightened state of attention and vigilance and may contribute to increased anxiety (Dinan, 1996; Chrousos et al., 1992; Redmond & Huang, 1979). These processes are enhanced during stress.

In addition to the activation of the HPA and NE-sympathetic system, research has also demonstrated that stress is associated with changes in proinflammatory cytokine activity (Kiecolt-Glaser, McGuire, Robles, & Glaser, 2002; Maier & Watkins, 1998). These immune-related changes are also dynamically related to NE-sympathetic and HPA axis activity. For example, experiments have shown that under conditions of stress there is an increase in proinflammatory cytokine activity, as measured by variables such as interleukin-6 and tumor necrosis factor, and that this increase is linked to the negative emotional consequences of these conditions (Maier et al., 1998). As indicated above, some of these stress-related changes are protective in the short term. However, when this activation state continues in a chronic fashion, then adverse consequences may ensue resulting in enhanced risk for various behavioral and physiological disorders, including problems such as depression and cardiovascular diseases (e.g., Kiecolt-Glaser et al., 2002).

Central Integration of the Stress Response

Over the last two decades, research has demonstrated directly that stress effects of the HPA and NE-sympathetic system are centrally regulated through complex interactive pathways (Holsboer & Barden, 1996). One such important interaction involves CRF and locus coeruleus-NE systems. These two systems form a basic arousal unit that mediates behavioral responses to stressful events, and their interaction contributes to a coordinated response to stress. This interaction is demonstrated by the findings that CRF secreting neurons project from the paraventricular nucleus to the brain stem (Saper, Swanson, & Cowan, 1979). Catecholaminergic neurons project from the locus cerelus to the paraventricular nucleus (Cunningham, Bohn, & Sawchenko, 1990; Chrousos et al., 1992), and locus coeruleus neurons firing rate is increased by the application of corticotropin-releasing factor (Valentino & Foote, 1988; Valentino & Van Bockstaele, 2001;).

The close neuronal interaction between the locus coeruleus and the paraventricular nucleus is also augmented by separate projections from the paraventricular nucleus and locus coeruleus to other brain structures involved in coordinating an emotional response to stress (Makino et al., 1994b). For example, locus coeruleus projects to other areas in the brain from which it may have an indirect contribution to the increased NE action in the paraventricular nucleus, which in turn activates the HPA. CRF on the other hand may facilitate sensory and attention processes during stress through increased catcholamine input to CRF cells (Dallman, 1993). Epinephrine and NE have a stimulatory effect on adrenocorticotropic hormone (Tilders, Berkenbosch, Vermes, Linton, & Smelik, 1985); an effect that is exerted through catecholamine effects on CRF (Cunningham et al., 1990; Szafarczyk et al., 1988). Blockage of CRF release can prevent this effect (Tilders et al., 1985). Stress-induced catecholamine changes, therefore, contribute to the release of corticotropin-releasing factor and adrenocorticotropic hormone (Rivier & Vale, 1983).

Additional neuroechmical systems are also involved in regulating the stress response. For example, the central serotonergic system has an excitatory effect on the HPA axis and may contribute to stress-related HPA activity (Tuomisto & Mannisto, 1985). Experiments have shown that tryptophan hydroxylase and monoamine oxidase are present in the pituitary (Chaouloff, 1993). Studies using lesions in certain nuclei of the brain found that lesions of central serotonergic nerves lead to a disruption of the adrenocorticotropic hormone and corticosterone circadian variations (Weiner & Ganong, 1978). On the other hand, experiments using electrical stimulation show that stimulation of the raphe nucleus increases serotonin metabolism in the paraventricular nucleus. These results indicate the presence of a direct effect of serotonin activity on CRF-producing neurons (Petersen, Hartman, & Barraclough, 1989). Serotonin has an excitatory effect on other stress-related systems, including the adrenomedullary activity (Chaouloff, 1993; Di Sciullo et al., 1990). HPA hormones, on the other hand, exert control on the serotonin system (Ruggiero, Underwood, Rice, Mann, & Arango, 1999), including activating tryptophan hydroxylase activity during stress (Singh, Corley, Krieg, Phan, & Boadle-Biber, 1994; Boadle-Biber, Singh, Corley, Phan, & Dilts, 1993).

In sum, the HPA and the locus coeruleus–brain stem mechanisms interact dynamically, and both systems have a complex interaction with various brain regions that have functional significance in facilitating the central nervous system actions in a stressful situation. One primary outcome of this interaction is the activation of the adrenal cortex to produce cortisol during states of stress and in response to multiple drugs of abuse.

Modulators of the Stress Response

The influence of stress on the HPA activation is influenced by multiple situational and individual difference factors. Lazarus (1999) views the effect of stress as a product of the individual–environment interaction. The individual's perception of the stressful situation and the availability of ways to cope with this situation determine the effect of this stress (Lazarus, 1999). Under this formulation, stressful situations are appraised and judged as to whether they are threatening or challenging. Persons engage in primary appraisals that include potential threat, perceived control, situation ambiguity, and personal beliefs. Secondary appraisals include the evaluation of one's resources and abilities in dealing with the stressor and the likely effectiveness of such coping efforts. A situation may be perceived as threatening if the individual does not have control and appraises his or her resources as less efficacious in dealing with that situation.

In addition to the individuals' appraisal and beliefs about their ability to cope, the psychological characteristics of stressful situations themselves influence the extent to which the response will involve the activation of the HPA axis. Distressing situations, for example, those characterized by the anticipation of aversive outcome, are associated with an increase in cortisol release (Lundberg & Frankenhaeuser, 1980; Lovallo, Pincomb, Brackett, & Wilson, 1990). We have shown greater increases in cortisol response to behavioral tasks that are characterized by novelty, uncertainty, and negative affect (al'Absi, Lovallo, McKey, & Pincomb, 1994; al'Absi & Lovallo, 1993).

Animal experiments have demonstrated that control of a stressor influences intensity of the HPA response (Davis, Gass, & Bassett, 1981; Ursin et al., 1993). Control of a stressor seems to facilitate behavioral efforts to cope and therefore reduce HPA response (Overmier & Murison, 2005). Similarly, environmental novelty seems to increase HPA activation (Hennessy, Mendoza, Mason, & Moberg, 1995), an effect that seems to be ameliorated by social support (Levine & Coe, 1993). Another dimension that modulates the influence of acute stress is the emotional tone of the stressful situation and whether it is perceived as challenging or distressing (Frankenhaeuser, 1980; Lundberg et al., 1980; Lundberg, 1984). For example, research has shown that the HPA response is activated in situations where the participants perceive the situation as being uncontrollable and report distress (Henry, 1992, 1993). On the other hand, situations perceived as challenging and requiring effort, but seeming surmountable, activate the sympathetic-adrenal-medullary system. There is evidence to suggest that neurophysiologically, these different patterns of responses and associated psychological profiles rely on a specific neural circuit that involves multiple brain structures, including the paraventricular nucleus, the medial prefrontal cortex, the hippocampus, and the bed nucleus of the stria terminalis (Diorio et al., 1993; Herman & Cullinan, 1997).

Human laboratory studies have introduced various manipulations to test the effects of these constructs in the laboratory. One recent review of the literature (Dickerson & Kemeny, 2004) indicated that HPA responses to stress can be reliably induced by using challenges that were characterized by uncontrollability and social evaluation threat. One good example of these challenges is the Trier Social Stress task (Kirschbaum, Pirke, & Hellhammer, 1993). A similar challenge was developed earlier and was found to be useful in laboratory stress studies that assess neuroendocrine function (al'Absi, Bongard, Buchanan, Pincomb, & Licinio, 1997). The task includes a combination of public speaking stress and math stressor and uses a prolonged and repeated exposure to both types of tasks. Both tasks produced substantial cardiovascular, adrenocorticotropic hormone, and cortisol responses; public speaking produced greater changes. When comparing the two types of tasks, we found that the public speaking challenge was more advantageous with repeated presentations of this challenge producing a stable pattern of cardiac activation, whereas repetitions of the mental arithmetic initially produced large cardiac responses that changed to a more vascular pattern across task periods. Furthermore, we found that both tasks increased negative affect, but correlations among the endocrine, cardiovascular, and negative affects were significant only during the public speaking stressor (al'Absi et al., 1997). These observations were replicated in several subsequent studies conducted in other laboratories indicating the usefulness of the public speaking task as a socially relevant experimental protocol for studying reactivity in the laboratory setting and eliciting a relatively high, stable, and homogeneous stress response.

Summary

Both central and peripheral factors play a role in coordinating the behavioral and physiological activation that guides the organism's response to stress. There is clear evidence that the manner and the intensity by which individuals respond to stress can be modulated by several situational and depositional factors. These include how novel the stressor is, how much control the individual has on that stressor, what is the level of uncertainty about the source and potential outcome of that stressor, and what are the types of emotion stirred by this stressor. This distinction is important when speculating about the potential harmful effects of stress. For example, cortisol responses to acute stress are related to reported distress and perceived aversiveness suggesting that HPA activity is specifically related to expenditure of mental effort and emotional salience. Acute stressful challenges in daily life that are prolonged and characterized by negative emotional tone may generate sustained physiological activation that may predispose a person to increased risk of disease. This activation may also mediate stress effects on the propensity to use drugs as we discuss in the following sections of this chapter.

Stress and Addiction

Drug Effects of the Stress Response Systems

The stimulating effects of acute use of drugs of abuse on the HPA, sympathetic, and endogenous opioid system have been documented in many animal and human experiments (see Figure 23.2), and these findings indicate that drug effects are analogous to those produced by stress,

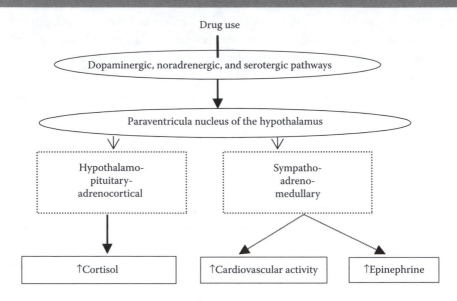

FIGURE 23.2
Effects of Substance Use on Stress-Related Psychobiological Systems.

demonstrating the involvement of these systems in regulating multiple neurochemical and behavioral effects of the drug (Borowsky & Kuhn, 1991; Kirschbaum, Wust, & Strasburger, 1992; Mendelson et al., 1988; Rivier & Vale, 1987b, 1987a; Sarnyai, Mello, Mendelson, Eros-Sarnyai, & Mercer, 1996; Wilkins et al., 1982). Effects of many of the drugs of abuse are centrally mediated through hypothalamic and extra-hypothalamic structures and through multiple neubiological pathways, including dopaminergic, noradrenergic, and serotonergic meurotransmission (Mendelson, Mello, Teoh, Ellingboe, & Cochin, 1989; Mendelson, Teoh, Mello, Ellingboe, & Rhoades, 1992; Sarnyai et al., 1996; Cheeta, Irvine, Kenny, & File, 2001; Fu, Matta, Brower, & Sharp, 2001; George, Verrico, Picciotto, & Roth, 2000; Salokangas et al., 2000; Rose & Corrigall, 1997; Pontieri, Tanda, Orzi, & Di Chiara, 1996).

Stress Response Interactions with Drug Reward Pathway

The hypothalamic-pituitary-adrenocortical system closely interacts with multiple reward pathways, including the endogenous opioid system and the dopaminergic system. Experimental evidence has shown that stress increases dopamine synaptic transmission, and this effect is prevented by administering GR antagonist (Saal, Dong, Bonci, & Malenka, 2003). These stress-related increases in dopamine synaptic transmission seem to be related to CRF reactivity, because administering CRF leads to the potentiation of N-methyl-D-aspartate receptor-mediated increase in dopamine transmission (Ungless et al., 2003; Marinelli, 2007). Suppression of glucocrticoids using adrenalectomy reduces dopamine concentration in the nucleus accumbens (Barrot et al., 2000). This effect seems to be due to suppression of corticosterone, inasmuch as administering this hormone reversed the effect of adenalectomy. The relevance of stress in this interaction is further reinforced by the observations that effects of glcuocorticoids on dopamine seem to be mediated by the GRs rather than mineralcorticoid receptors, because administration of mineralcorticoid receptor antagonist does not influence dopamine, whereas GR antagonists decreased dopamine levels (Marinelli, Aouizerate, Barrot, Le Moal, & Piazza, 1998). Another line of evidence linking the HPA and dopaminergic activity in mediating drug reward has emerged from experiments using administration of glucocorticoids. These experiments have shown that using in vivo microdialysis techniques where administration of corticosterone increases dopamine level in the nucleus accumbens (Mittleman, Jones, & Robbins, 1991; Mittleman, Blaha, & Phillips, 1992; Marinelli, 2007).

Effects of HPA on dopaminergic transmission are likely mediated by multiple mechanisms. There is evidence indicating that (1) HPA stress response may modify dopamine neuron activity and release and that HPA response facilitates glutamate-induced activity (Marinelli, 2007; Overton, Tong, Brain, & Clark, 1996) which in turn may stimulate dopamine release; (2) HPA stress response may modify dopamine synthesis, because glucocorticoids facilitate the action of tyrosin hydroxylase (the rate-limiting enzyme of dopamine synthesis; Ortiz et al., 1995); (3) HPA stress response may modify metabolism and clearance of DA, because glucocorticoids decrease the activity of dopamine-metabolizing enzymes, such as monoamine oxidase (Veals et al., 1977); and (4) HPA hormones may act at the level of dopamine transporter sites and therefore influence dopamine transmission, because glucocorticoid suppression reduces the number of dopamine binding sites in the nucleus accumbens, and administration reverses this effect (Sarnyai, McKittrick, McEwen, & Kreek, 1998). Consistent with this, studies using chronic stress showed increase in dopamine transporters functions (Copeland, Neff, & Hadjiconstantinou, 2005).

Role of Stress in Initiation of Substance Abuse

There is growing evidence from both animal and human research that suggests effects of various stressful conditions on risk for addiction. Animal experiments have shown that manipulations involving social separation or isolation increase self-administration of different drugs of abuse (e.g., Alexander, Beyerstein, Hadaway, & Coambs, 1981; Alexander, Coambs, & Hadaway, 1978; Schenk, Lacelle, Gorman, & Amit, 1987). Rhesus monkeys reared by their peers during the first six months of their life consumed more alcohol than monkeys reared by their mothers (Higley, Hasert, Suomi, & Linnolia, 1998; Higley et al., 1993). Similar findings were obtained in adult monkeys where social separation led to increases in alcohol consumption comparable to those seen in the peer-reared monkeys suggesting that exposure to stress, whether during childhood or later in life increases drug self-administration.

Human studies have shown similar results. Adverse childhood experiences, such as emotional, physical, and sexual abuse, are associated with increased risk for addiction and with initiation of substance abuse at an early age (Dembo, Dertke, Borders, Washburn, & Schmeidler, 1988; Harrison, Fulkerson, & Beebe, 1997; Widom, Weiler, & Cottler, 1999). Exposure to physical or sexual abuse increases likelihood to continue drug use (e.g., Harrison et al., 1997), and high levels of social and environmental stress predict a rapid progression in tobacco, marijuana, and alcohol use (Wills, 1986; Wills, Sandy, & Yaeger, 2002). Studies have also demonstrated increased frequency of history of trauma among drug-dependent individuals, especially women, than nondrug users (Cottler, Compton, III, Mager, Spitznagel, & Janca, 1992; Najavits et al., 1998). In addition, individuals suffering from posttraumatic stress disorder (PTSD) are at increased risk for substance abuse. There is additional evidence indicating a clear relationship between PTSD and increased substance use. Rates of substance abuse among individuals with PTSD have been reported to be as high as 60–80%, and rates of PTSD among substance abusers have also been reported between 40–60% (Brady & Sinha, 2005; Donovan, Padin-Rivera, & Kowaliw, 2001). Patients with PTSD report a higher lifetime use of nicotine, alcohol, cocaine, and heroin than those who do not suffer from the disorder (Keane & Kaloupek, 1997; Zaslav, 1994). In addition to traumatic stress, other types of stress have also been linked with drugs, including being in unhappy marriages and dissatisfaction with employment (Breslau & Davis, 1992; Breslau, Davis, & Schultz, 2003; Gianoulakis, 1998; Kessler, Sonnega, Bromet, Hughes, & Nelson, 1995). Exposure to traumatic stress seems to particularly increase risk for comorbid PTSD and substance abuse in women than in men (Newton-Taylor, DeWit, & Gliksman, 1998).

Mediators of Stress Effects on Substance Use

Factors that mediate effects of early stress on vulnerability for substance abuse are likely to include biological, social, and behavioral processes reflecting the long-term consequences of childhood stress. These effects may also resemble those produced by chronic stress. There is evidence indicating that chronic stress and exposure to hardship in early life contribute to significant alterations in the stress response neurobiological systems. For example, research has shown that animals who were reared under various stressful conditions exhibited significant alterations in the HPA stress response throughout development and adult life (Plotsky & Meaney, 1993). Increased levels of CRF in the cerebrospinal fluid were found in chronically stressed infant monkeys, reflecting enhanced output of the corticotrophin-releasing factor-HPA system similar to that found in mood disorders (Arborelius, Owens, Plotsky, & Nemeroff, 1999; Coplan et al., 1996).

Extensive basic research also suggests the possibility that stress-related effects on dopaminergic activity may be one mechanism through which stress increases the risk for drug addiction. Animals with higher reactivity to mild stress exhibit enhanced dopaminergic activity relative to animals with lower reactivity (Marinelli, 2007). Increased reactivity was defined in terms of greater or longer corticosterone or greater or longer locomotor response to a stressful situation (Kabbaj, Devine, Savage, & Akil, 2000; Marinelli, 2007). There is also a close interaction between the HPA activity and mesolimbic dopamine (DA) in the context of drug-seeking behaviors (Piazza & Le Moal, 1998). Mesolimbic dopamine is activated by many drugs of abuse (Epping-Jordan, Watkins, Koob, & Markou, 1998; Salamone, 1994; Wise, 1996), and is directly involved in the reinforcing and mood regulating effects of drug use. This system is stimulated by aversive conditions (Salamone, 1994) and may facilitate coping with these conditions (Salamone, 1994). Experiments have shown that stress-induced increases in dopamine synaptic transmission are blocked by GR antagonist (Saal et al., 2003). A relevant line of research shows that administration of corticosterone produces an increase in dopamine in the nucleus accumbens (Imperato, Puglisi-Allegra, Casolini, & Angelucci, 1991; Mittleman et al., 1992).

In humans there is evidence to suggest that stress-related vulnerability may be due to a dysregulated or blunted stress response by the HPA axis. This is supported by results showing that nonalcoholics with a family history of alcoholism exhibit blunted responses to stress (Dai, Thavundayil, & Gianoulakis, 2005). Research has also shown lower levels of plasma β-endorphin in individuals with positive family history for alcoholism than in those without a positive family history (Gianoulakis et al., 2005). Furthermore, alcohol consumption was associated with increased plasma β-endorphin levels in the high-risk but not in the low-risk group (Gianoulakis, 1996), and consumption of alcohol was associated with smaller attenuation of plasma β-endorphin responses to stress in individuals with positive family history for alcoholism (Dai, Thavundayil, & Gianoulakis, 2002). A similar pattern of reactivity was also found in individuals at high risk for addictive problems, including boys with persistent antisocial behaviors (Snoek, Van Goozen, Matthys, Buitelaar, & van Engeland, 2004) and women with increased trait anxiety (Chong et al., 2006).

It has been suggested that alterations in HPA functions in those at risk for drug abuse are linked to reduced central opioid tone (Wand & Schumann, 1998). Experiments assessing HPA response to opioid receptor blockade have found that compared to individuals with negative family history for alcoholism, individuals with a positive family history require lower concentrations of naloxone to remove the opioid inhibitory control of the CRF neurons (Wand et al., 1998). They also exhibit higher adrenocorticotropic hormone and cortisol responses to administration of similar doses of naloxone and naltrexone (Wand et al., 2002) (Hernandez-Avila, Oncken, Van Kirk, Wand, & Kranzler, 2002). We should note, however that blunted HPA stress response has also been documented in abstinent alcoholics (Adinoff, Junghanns, Kiefer, & Krishnan-Sarin, 2005; Adinoff et al., 2005b) and smokers (al'Absi, Wittmers, Erickson, Hatsukami, & Crouse, 2003). This attenuated HPA activity may represent a risk factor associated with vulnerability to drug dependence.

In summary, exposure to stressful events early in life or to chronic stress may increase vulnerability to addiction. Mechanisms of this risk may include altered HPA and endogenous opioid stress response. Stress-related effects on dopaminergic activity may also be a mechanism, although results have not been systematically confirmed in humans. For example, although animal experiments suggest that stress-related hyper-responsiveness predicts risk for drug self-administration, human studies suggest that it is the hypoactivation of the stress response systems that seem to relate to risk for drug addiction.

Stress and Maintenance of Drug Abuse

Accumulating evidence supports the role of stress in maintaining drug use, and this seems to be particularly the case when there are expectations that drug use will alleviate withdrawal-related symptoms (Kassel et al., 2007). Abstinence from drug use is usually associated with several aversive affective states, including anxiety, depression, restlessness, irritability, physical symptoms, and detriments in cognitive performance (American Psychiatric Association, 1994; Hughes, 1992; Pritchard, Robinson, & Guy, 1992; Snyder, Davis, & Henningfield, 1989; Stitzer & Gross, 1988). The intensity of these withdrawal symptoms is influenced by multiple factors including: (1) the length of time since the last drug use and level of drug dependence, (2) situational demands (e.g., acute stressors, demanding challenges, or drug-related cues;

al'Absi, Amunrud, & Wittmers, 2002; Koval & Pederson, 1999), (3) the person's disposition and skills (e.g., coping resources, history of psychopathology, etc.; Gilbert, 1995; Jamner, Girdler, Shapiro, & Jarvik, 1998; Jamner, Shapiro, & Jarvik, 1999).

The detrimental effects of abstinence on mood may contribute to the experience of a high level of stress, and therefore, enhance craving (Brown, Lejuez, Kahler, & Strong, 2002; Drobes & Tiffany, 1997; Heishman, 1999). This heightened perceived stress may result from internal and external cues conditioned to withdrawal symptoms (such as craving), and exposure to these cues after cessation may elicit withdrawal symptoms (Carey, Kalra, Carey, Halperin, & Richards, 1993; Perkins & Grobe, 1992). The reduction of these negative affective states by drug use reinforces this behavior, increasing the likelihood in the future of experiencing craving for drugs in the presence of stress-related cues and negative affective states. These conditions may also play a significant role in relapse. Both correlational and laboratory-based studies have demonstrated the role of stress-related cues as triggers for relapse (Fox et al., 2005; McFall, Mackay, & Donovan, 1992; McKay, Rutherford, Alterman, Cacciola, & Kaplan, 1995). Animal experiments have noted a role for exposure to aversive experiences in reinstatement and relapse (Kreek & Koob, 1998).

Because abstinence from drug use increases perceived stress (File, Dinnis, Heard, & Irvine, 2002; Parrott, 1999), it is possible that those who experience heightened negative affect after initial abstinence are at high risk for early relapse (Burgess et al., 2002; Kenford et al., 2002; al'Absi, Hatsukami, Davis, & Wittmers, 2004). To that end, we have used laboratory-based procedures to identify predictors of smoking relapse (al'Absi, Hatsukami, & Davis, 2005). In one study we found that smokers who relapsed within four weeks of a quit attempt showed attenuated hormonal and cardiovascular responses to stress, exaggerated withdrawal symptoms, and mood deterioration after quitting. When analyzing the data using regression analyses we found that attenuated responses to stress predicted a shorter time to relapse (al'Absi et al., 2005). Other studies using recall and imaginary experiences have also been useful. Studies using guided imagery involving recall of personal stressful experiences were found to increase craving for cocaine and alcohol in abstinent cocaine dependent participants (Fox et al., 2005; Sinha, Catapano, & O'Malley, 1999), and these reports predicted the incidence of relapse following treatment (Fox et al., 2005).

There are several neurobiological and behavioral mechanisms that have been proposed as possible mechanisms that mediate effects of stress on relapse. For example, experiments using pharmacological, neurochemical, and behavioral methods have demonstrated the role of CRF in stress-induced relapse (Erb, 2007). Other mechanisms include dopamine and glutamatergic systems activity within the nucleus accumbens and the prefrontal cortex and may involve projections to multiple other brain structures that are involved in emotion regulation and affective response to stress (McFarland, Davidge, Lapish, & Kalivas, 2004). These pathways may represent the substrate through which the stress response interfaces with addiction relapse.

In summary, evidence to date suggests that stress and negative affect play a significant role in maintaining drug use and can precipitate relapse. Because drug use reduces effects of stress and negative affective states, a negative reinforcement contingency takes place increasing the effects of future exposure to stress-related cues on craving and drug use. There seems to be multiple biological and neurochemical pathways that mediate these associations including those related to the CRF and dopamine systems, and approaches to this problem will have to account for these multiple causes and mechanisms of drug use and relapse.

Potential Moderators of the Influence of Stress on Substance Abuse

Sex Differences

Accumulating evidence from both human and animal studies suggests that gender moderates effects of stress on drug administration. For example, animal experiments show that early life stress has greater effects on cocaine self-administration in female rats than in controls (Kosten & Kehoe, 2007). Drugs, such as cocaine, produce greater behavioral and hormonal responses in female than in male rats, and these effects seem to be independent of ovarian hormones (Bowman et al., 1999; Kuhn & Francis, 1997). Neonatal isolation facilitates acquisition and maintenance of food intake in female but not in male rats (Kosten & Ambrosio, 2002; Kosten, Miserendino, & kehoe, 2000; Kosten, Sanchez, Zhang, & Kehoe, 2004). Effects of stress on drug administration may also be mediated by different neurophysiological changes in males and females. For example, experiments found that N-methyl-D-aspartate receptor binding in dorsal striatum was up-regulated in isolated males but down-regulated in isolated females (Sircar, Mallinson, Goldbloom, & Kehoe, 2001). Similar sex differences were found showing that neonatal isolation was associated with increased corticosterone levels in female but not in male pups (Knuth & Etgen, 2005).

Clinical and epidemiological studies also indicate that stress has different effects in men and women. Stress is more frequently reported by women than men with addiction problems, and it is more frequently cited as a reason for drug use, maintenance, and relapse in women than in men (e.g., Najavits et al., 1998). Earlier studies have reported that women who experienced childhood sexual abuse exhibited a fourfold increase in risk for lifetime prevalence of both alcoholism and other drug abuse relative to women who did not experience such abuse (Wilsnack, Vogeltanz, Klassen, & Harris, 1997; Winfield, George, Swartz, & Blazer, 1990). Women are also more likely to have symptoms of posttraumatic stress disorder and comorbid substance abuse problems than men (Newton-Taylor et al., 1998).

There are indications that environmental context plays a greater role in determining perception of drug effects in women than in men (Perkins, 1999). For example, sensory cues related to smoking seem to have greater effects in women than in men in triggering craving (Perkins, 1999). Women who smoke are more likely to use smoking to cope with negative affect than men (Dicken, 1978; File, Fluck, & Leahy, 2001). They report more urges to smoke (Abrams et al., 1987) and more distress after exposure to acutely stressful situations and to smoking-specific stimuli than male smokers (Abrams et al., 1987; Swan, Ward, Jack, & Javitz, 1993), and they are less likely to maintain long-term smoking abstinence than men (Bowen, McTiernan, Powers, & Feng, 2000; D'Angelo, Reid, Brown, & Pipe, 2001; Ward, Klesges, Zbikowski, Bliss, & Garvey, 1997; Wetter et al., 1999).

Stress-related effects on addiction may work through different mechanisms in men and women and this may contribute to these differences in patterns and severity of addiction

(Grunberg, Winders, & Wewers, 1991; Staley et al., 2001). For example, in one study that used responses to stress as potential predictors of relapse, we found different patterns of relapse predictors in men and women. Attenuated cortisol and adrenocorticotropic hormone responses to stress were better predictors of early relapse in men. Intensity of withdrawal symptoms after exposure to acute stress predicted time to relapse in women (al'Absi, 2006).

In summary, there is ample evidence of the existence of sex differences in the patterns of addiction vulnerability, motivators for drug use, and risk factors for relapse. Clinical and epidemiological studies suggest that stress may be a more potent risk factor for drug initiation, maintenance, and relapse in women than in men. There are no specific mechanisms that have been identified to account for these sex differences, but multiple systems are likely to be involved, including systems that generate and integrate the stress response and reinforcement regulation. Observed sex differences should be taken into consideration when assessing and treating stress-related disorders and substance abuse.

Genetic Factors

There is preliminary evidence to suggest direct involvement of genetic factors in increasing vulnerability and moderating effects of stress on drug abuse and relapse. Research to identify polymorphisms associated with the opioid system functions has demonstrated that the functional polymorphism Asn40Asp (+118A/G) in the mu-opioid receptor gene (OPRM1) is closely involved in regulating the functions of the HPA system. This polymporphism is associated with a threefold increase in mu-endorphin binding affinity and potency. Thus, it is likely that this polymorphism is also associated with increased inhibition of the corticotropin-releasing factor neurons (Bond et al., 1998).

Recent studies have also shown that relative to Asn40 allele, OPRM1 Asp40 variant was associated with lower cortisol responses to psychological stressors in healthy men (Chong, Uhart, & Wand, 2007). Consistent with these results, OPRM1 Asp40 was associated with enhanced HPA activation, as evidenced by larger cortisol responses to opioid receptor blockade (Hernandez-Avila et al., 2002; Wand et al., 2002). Research in rhesus monkeys provides consistent information demonstrating that a similar polymorphism was associated with reduced ACTH-stimulated plasma cortisol levels (Miller et al., 2004), although the association of this polymorphism with drug dependence has not been established (Arias, Feinn, & Kranzler, 2006).

The extent to which these polymorphisms may help in developing new intervention strategies is the focus of ongoing research. Previous work has shown that opioid receptor antagonists may be useful in the treatment of alcoholism (O'Malley, Krishnan-Sarin, Farren, Sinha, & Kreek, 2002). Opioid-related polymorphisms may enhance the matching of this treatment with the appropriate candidate. Recent research, for example, has shown that alcoholics with one or two copies of the Asp40 allele who were treated with naltrexone had significantly lower relapse rates and moderated their drinking for a longer period of time compared with Asn40 homozygotes alcoholics (Oslin et al., 2003).

Coping Resources

Individuals with adequate coping and social support resources are able to overcome stress and minimize its effects on addiction vulnerability than those with minimal coping resources.

It is therefore possible that by teaching individuals who have addiction problems coping skills and cognitive behavioral strategies to address stress they may be able to sustain their recovery (Carroll et al., 1994). Although this is intuitive, it is surprising that interventions to address stress in the context of addictive problems remain relatively less developed. It is well recognized that exposure to ongoing or childhood stress when combined with addictive problems presents complicated challenges to researchers and clinicians, and this in turns requires sophisticated approaches to address this comorbidity.

Reviews of research on comorbidity indicate that individuals with substance use problems and who suffer from psychological problems may face significant hurdles in their efforts to overcome their addictions (Donahue & Kushner, 2007; Roberts, Moore, & Beckham, 2007). The reasons may include their history of using substances to cope with negative affective states. The negative reinforcement of this drug-using behavior increases chances of using the drug to cope with stress or negative affect in the future, including those caused by temporary abstinence (Ahmed & Koob, 2005; Childress et al., 1994), with the result being a vicious cycle of substance use to regulate affect. This cycle occurs during active drug use as well as in precipitating relapse. In this context, it is important to recognize and account for the role of expectancy in the interaction between stress and addiction, inasmuch as expectancy may be one mechanism through which the link between substance use and stress or negative affect is reinforced (Kassel et al., 2007).

Discussion and Future Directions

Efforts that address specific risk factors for addiction and relapse are sorely needed, and existing treatment strategies to address substance abuse remain crude and largely ineffective. New treatments should integrate multiple biobehavioral approaches and focus on helping patients at multiple levels, including gaining insight into the role of stress and negative affect in their addictions. One particular strategy to help individuals inflicted with addiction problems is to help them develop and use effective coping skills to deal with ongoing or daily stressors, and this approach should take into consideration the role played by expectations that drug use may help in reducing negative affect. Related to this coping-focused strategy, it is important to integrate other approaches, such as developing an abstinence-focused social support network and promoting self-efficacy about the ability to cope with stress. In addition to these psychosocial interventions it is important to take advantage of available pharmacological treatments.

The fact that stress effect on drug use is mediated by multiple neurobiological and social factors makes a hybrid approach to treatment most sensible in reducing stress-triggered drug use and relapse. There is still a need to learn about how these multimodal treatments can be integrated and who may benefit more from this type of stress-focused approach. For example, it is conceivable that patients with stress-related problems, such as those who have been exposed to trauma, would benefit from stress-coping focused treatment. A proactive approach to care for this high-risk group may be needed in order to prevent escalation of their problems. One approach for this will be to screen for these problems early and tailor management of addiction liability in conjunction with approaches to address stress-related complications.

There are also new lines of research that seek to discover direct interventions addressing the stress-related neurobiological pathways. Evidence demonstrates the role of corticotropin-releasing factor as an extra-hypothalamic neuromodulator directly involved in integrating different facets of the stress response, including autonomic, hormonal, and immune responses (Koob & Heinrichs, 1999) and interacting with several key structures, such as the amygdale, ventral tegmental area, cortex, and hippocampus, that are involved in addictive processes (Dunn, Swiergiel, & Palamarchouk, 2004; Ungless et al., 2003; Wang et al., 2005). These interactions have stimulated efforts to explore pharmacological agents that interact with this system. There is now evidence from animal studies showing that systemic injections of CRF receptor antagonists or alpha-2 adrenoceptor agonists prevent stress-induced reinstatement. There is also evidence demonstrating effectiveness of CRF receptor antagonists in treating ongoing addiction and reducing risk for relapse in response to stress and drug-related cues (Goeders, 2007). Research is still needed to identify potential therapeutic effects of CRF-probing agents. It is also important to understand how the corticotropin-releasing system interacts with the endogenous opioid and dopaminergic systems in the context of stress and addiction. Translational extension of this work to human laboratory studies is critical in guiding future discoveries for treatment of stress-related problems and addiction.

Conclusions

The recent decade has witnessed significant growth in research on the neurobiological circuitry linking stress to substance use. This progress has been complemented by progress on research investigating effects of early life stress on the stress response regulation, and effects of early stressful experiences on motivated behavior and addiction vulnerability. Research related to the role of genetics in addiction and stress neurobiology has also advanced noticeably over the recent decade. Additional progress has been achieved in improving tools to assess addiction and stress. Notwithstanding these advances, there remains much to be achieved, especially to translate the wealth of basic information into treatment research, including the focus on identifying HPA-related pharmacological interventions in humans. Furthermore, strategies such as learning means to reduce and cope with stress should be integrated into addiction treatments as tools to manage triggers that may promote drug use and relapse. In addition, combining existing pharmacotherapies targeting stress response systems and cognitive behavioral stress management techniques may prove effective in managing stress-related triggers of drug use and abuse.

References

Abrams, D. B., Monti, P. M., Pinto, R. P., Elder, J. P., Brown, R. A., & Jacobus, S. I. (1987). Psychosocial stress and coping in smokers who relapse or quit. *Health Psychology, 6,* 289–303.

Adinoff, B. (2004). Neurobiologic processes in drug reward and addiction. *Harvard Review of Psychiatry, 12,* 305–320.

Adinoff, B., Junghanns, K., Kiefer, F., & Krishnan-Sarin, S. (2005). Suppression of the HPA axis stress-response: Implications for relapse. *Alcoholism: Clinical and Experimental Research, 29,* 1351–1355.

Adinoff, B., Krebaum, S. R., Chandler, P. A., Ye, W., Brown, M. B., & Williams, M. J. (2005a). Dissection of hypothalamic-pituitary-adrenal axis pathology in 1-month-abstinent alcohol-dependent men, part 1: Adrenocortical and pituitary glucocorticoid responsiveness. *Alcoholism: Clinical and Experimental Research, 29,* 517–527.

Adinoff, B., Krebaum, S. R., Chandler, P. A., Ye, W., Brown, M. B., & Williams, M. J. (2005b). Dissection of hypothalamic-pituitary-adrenal axis pathology in 1-month-abstinent alcohol-dependent men, part 2: Response to ovine corticotropin-releasing factor and naloxone. *Alcoholism: Clinical and Experimental Research, 29,* 528–537.

Ahmed, S. H., & Koob, G. F. (2005). Transition to drug addiction: A negative reinforcement model based on an allostatic decrease in reward function. *Psychopharmacology (Berl), 180,* 473–490.

al'Absi, M. (2006). Hypothalamic-pituitary-adrenocortical responses to psychological stress and risk for smoking relapse. *International Journal of Psychophysiology, 59,* 218–227.

al'Absi, M., Amunrud, T., & Wittmers, L. E. (2002). Psychophysiological effects of abstinence and behavioral challenges in habitual smokers. *Pharmacology Biochemistry & Behavior, 72,* 707–716.

al'Absi, M., Bongard, S., Buchanan, T., Pincomb, G. A., & Licinio, J. (1997). Cardiovascular and neuroendocrine adjustment to public speaking and mental arithmetic stressors. *Psychophysiology, 34,* 266–275.

al'Absi, M., Hatsukami, D., & Davis, G. L. (2005). Attenuated adrenocorticotropic responses to psychological stress are associated with early smoking relapse. *Psychopharmacology (Berl), 181,* 107–117.

al'Absi, M., Hatsukami, D., Davis, G. L., & Wittmers, L. E. (2004). Prospective examination of effects of smoking abstinence on cortisol and withdrawal symptoms as predictors of early smoking relapse. *Drug and Alcohol Dependence, 73,* 267–278.

al'Absi, M., & Lovallo, W. R. (1993). Cortisol concentrations in serum of borderline hypertensive men exposed to a novel experimental setting. *Psychoneuroendocrinology, 18,* 355–363.

al'Absi, M., Lovallo, W. R., McKey, B., & Pincomb, G. (1994). Borderline hypertensives produce exaggerated adrenocortical responses to mental stress. *Psychosomatic Medicine, 56,* 245–250.

al'Absi, M., Wittmers, L. E., Erickson, J., Hatsukami, D. K., & Crouse, B. (2003). Attenuated adrenocortical and blood pressure responses to psychological stress in ad libitum and abstinent smokers. *Pharmacology Biochemistry and Behavior, 74,* 401–410.

Alexander, B. K., Beyerstein, B. L., Hadaway, P. F., & Coambs, R. B. (1981). Effect of early and later colony housing on oral ingestion of morphine in rats. *Pharmacology Biochemistry and Behavior, 15,* 571–576.

Alexander, B. K., Coambs, R. B., & Hadaway, P. F. (1978). The effect of housing and gender on morphine self-administration in rats. *Psychopharmacology (Berl), 58,* 175–179.

American Psychiatric Association (1994). *Diagnostic and Statistical Manual of Mental Disorders* (4th ed.). Washington, DC: Author.

Arborelius, L., Owens, M. J., Plotsky, P. M., & Nemeroff, C. B. (1999). The role of corticotropin-releasing factor in depression and anxiety disorders. *Journal of Endocrinology, 160,* 1–12.

Arias, A., Feinn, R., & Kranzler, H. R. (2006). Association of an Asn40Asp (A118G) polymorphism in the mu-opioid receptor gene with substance dependence: A meta-analysis. *Drug and Alcohol Dependence, 83,* 262–268.

Aston-Jones, G., Ennis, M., Pieribone, V. A., Nickell, W. T., & Shipley, M. T. (1986). The brain nucleus locus coeruleus: Restricted afferent control of a broad efferent network. *Science, 234,* 734–737.

Barrot, M., Marinelli, M., Abrous, D. N., Rouge-Pont, F., Le Moal, M., & Piazza, P. V. (2000). The dopaminergic hyper-responsiveness of the shell of the nucleus accumbens is hormone-dependent. *European Journal of Neuroscience, 12,* 973–979.

Boadle-Biber, M. C., Singh, V. B., Corley, K. C., Phan, T. H., & Dilts, R. P. (1993). Evidence that corticotropin-releasing factor within the extended amygdala mediates the activation of tryptophan hydroxylase produced by sound stress in the rat. *Brain Research, 628,* 105–114.

Bond, C., LaForge, K. S., Tian, M., Melia, D., Zhang, S., Borg, L., et al. (1998). Single-nucleotide polymorphism in the human mu opioid receptor gene alters beta-endorphin binding and activity: Possible implications for opiate addiction. *Proceedings of the National Academy of Sciences (US), 95,* 9608–9613.

Borowsky, B., & Kuhn, C. M. (1991). Chronic cocaine administration sensitizes behavioral but not neuroendocrine responses. *Brain Research, 543,* 301–306.

Bowen, D. J., McTiernan, A., Powers, D., & Feng, Z. (2000). Recruiting women into a smoking cessation program: Who might quit? *Women Health, 31,* 41–58.

Bowman, B. P., Vaughan, S. R., Walker, Q. D., Davis, S. L., Little, P. J., Scheffler, N. M., et al. (1999). Effects of sex and gonadectomy on cocaine metabolism in the rat. *Journal of Pharmacology and Experiemental Therapeutics, 290,* 1316–1323.

Brady, K. T., & Sinha, R. (2005). Co-occurring mental and substance use disorders: The neurobiological effects of chronic stress. *American Journal of Psychiatry, 162,* 1483–1493.

Breslau, N., & Davis, G. C. (1992). Posttraumatic stress disorder in an urban population of young adults: Risk factors for chronicity. *American Journal of Psychiatry, 149,* 671–675.

Breslau, N., Davis, G. C., & Schultz, L. R. (2003). Posttraumatic stress disorder and the incidence of nicotine, alcohol, and other drug disorders in persons who have experienced trauma. *Archives of General Psychiatry, 60,* 289–294.

Brindley, D., & Rolland, Y. (1989). Possible connections between stress, diabetes, obesity, hypertension, and adrenal lipoprotein metabolism that may result in artherosclerosis. *Clinical Science, 49,* 282–291.

Brown, R. A., Lejuez, C. W., Kahler, C. W., & Strong, D. R. (2002). Distress tolerance and duration of past smoking cessation attempts. *Journal of Abnormal Pschology, 111,* 180–185.

Burgess, E. S., Brown, R. A., Kahler, C. W., Niaura, R., Abrams, D. B., Goldstein, M. G., et al. (2002). Patterns of change in depressive symptoms during smoking cessation: Who's at risk for relapse? *Journal of Consulting and Clinical Psychology, 70,* 356–361.

Cannon, W. B. (1928). The mechanisms of emotional disturbance of body function. *New England Journal of Medicine, 198,* 877–884.

Carey, M. P., Kalra, D. L., Carey, K. B., Halperin, S., & Richards, C. S. (1993). Stress and unaided smoking cessation: A prospective investigation. *Journal of Consulting and Clinical Psychology, 61,* 831–838.

Carroll, K. M., Rounsaville, B. J., Gordon, L. T., Nich, C., Jatlow, P., Bisighini, R. M., et al. (1994). Psychotherapy and pharmacotherapy for ambulatory cocaine abusers. *Archives of General Psychology, 51,* 177–187.

Carter, C. S., Macdonald, A. M., Botvinick, M., Ross, L. L., Stenger, V. A., Noll, D., et al. (2000). Parsing executive processes: Strategic vs. evaluative functions of the anterior cingulate cortex. *Proceedings of the National Academy of Sciences (US), 97,* 1944–1948.

Chaouloff, F. (1993). Physiopharmacological interactions between stress hormones and central serotonergic systems. *Brain Research Brain Research Reviews, 18,* 1–32.

Cheeta, S., Irvine, E. E., Kenny, P. J., & File, S. E. (2001). The dorsal raphe nucleus is a crucial structure mediating nicotine's anxiolytic effects and the development of tolerance and withdrawal responses. *Psychopharmacology (Berl), 155,* 78–85.

Childress, A. R., Ehrman, R., McLellan, A. T., MacRae, J., Natale, M., & O'Brien, C. P. (1994). Can induced moods trigger drug-related responses in opiate abuse patients? *Journal of Substance Abuse Treatment, 11,* 17–23.

Chong, R. Y., Oswald, L., Yang, X., Uhart, M., Lin, P. I., & Wand, G. S. (2006). The micro-opioid receptor polymorphism A118G predicts cortisol responses to naloxone and stress. *Neuropsychopharmacology, 31,* 204–211.

Chong, R. Y., Uhart, M., & Wand, G. S. (2007). Endogenous opiates, addiction, and stress response. In M.al'Absi (Ed.), *Stress and Addiction: Biological and Psychological Mechanisms* (pp. 85–104). London: Academic Press/Elsevier.

Chrousos, G. P., & Gold, P. W. (1992). The concepts of stress and stress system disorders. Overview of physical and behavioral homeostasis. *Journal of the American Medical Association, 267,* 1244–1252.

Copeland, B. J., Neff, N. H., & Hadjiconstantinou, M. (2005). Enhanced dopamine uptake in the striatum following repeated restraint stress. *Synapse, 57,* 167–174.

Coplan, J. D., Andrews, M. W., Rosenblum, L. A., Owens, M. J., Friedman, S., Gorman, J. M., & Nemeroff, C. B. (1996). Persistent elevations of cerebrospinal fluid concentrations of corticotropin-releasing factor in adult nonhuman primates exposed to early-life stressors: Implications for the pathophysiology of mood and anxiety disorders. *Proceedings of the National Academy of Science (US), 93,* 1619–1623.

Cottler, L. B., Compton, W. M., III, Mager, D., Spitznagel, E. L., & Janca, A. (1992). Posttraumatic stress disorder among substance users from the general population. *American Journal of Psychiatry, 149,* 664–670.

Cunningham, E. T. J., Bohn, M. C., & Sawchenko, P. E. (1990). Organization of adrenergic inputs to the paraventricular and supraoptic nuclei of the hypothalamus in the rat. *Journal of Comparative Neurology, 292,* 651–667.

D'Angelo, M. E., Reid, R. D., Brown, K. S., & Pipe, A. L. (2001). Gender differences in predictors for long-term smoking cessation following physician advice and nicotine replacement therapy. *Canadian Journal of Public Health, 92,* 418–422.

Dai, X., Thavundayil, J., & Gianoulakis, C. (2002). Differences in the responses of the pituitary beta-endorphin and cardiovascular system to ethanol and stress as a function of family history. *Alcoholism: Clinical and Experimental Research, 26,* 1171–1180.

Dai, X., Thavundayil, J., & Gianoulakis, C. (2005). Differences in the peripheral levels of beta-endorphin in response to alcohol and stress as a function of alcohol dependence and family history of alcoholism. *Alcoholism: Clinical and Experimental Research, 29,* 1965–1975.

Dallman, M. (1993). Stress update: Adaptation of the hypothalamic-pituitary-adrenal axis to chronic stress. *Trends in Endocrinology and Metabolism, 4,* 62–69.

Davis, H., Gass, G., & Bassett, J. (1981). Serum cortisol response to incremental work in experienced and naive subjects. *Psychosomatic Medicine, 43,* 127–132.

Dembo, R., Dertke, M., Borders, S., Washburn, M., & Schmeidler, J. (1988). The relationship between physical and sexual abuse and tobacco, alcohol, and illicit drug use among youths in a juvenile detention center. *International Journal of Addiction, 23,* 351–378.

Di Sciullo, A., Bluet-Pajot, M. T., Mounier, F., Oliver, C., Schmidt, B., & Kordon, C. (1990). Changes in anterior pituitary hormone levels after serotonin 1A receptor stimulation. *Endocrinology, 127,* 567–572.

Dicken, C. (1978). Sex roles, smoking, and smoking cessation. *Journal of Health and Social Behavior, 19,* 324–334.

Dickerson, S. S., & Kemeny, M. E. (2004). Acute stressors and cortisol responses: A theoretical integration and synthesis of laboratory research. *Psychological Bulletin, 130,* 355–391.

Dinan, T. G. (1996). Serotonin and the regulation of hypothalamic-pituitary-adrenal axis function. *Life Sciences, 58,* 1683–1694.

Diorio, D., Viau, V., & Meaney, M. (1993). The role of the medial prefrontal cortex (cingulate gyrus) in the regulation of hypothalamic-pituitary-adrenal responses to stress. *Journal of Neuroscience, 13,* 3839–3847.

Donahue, C. B., & Kushner, M. G. (2007). Stress, anxiety, and addiction: Intervention strategies. In M.al'Absi (Ed.), *Stress and addiction: Biological and psychological mechanisms* (pp. 301–314). London: Academic Press/Elsevier.

Donovan, B., Padin-Rivera, E., & Kowaliw, S. (2001). "Transcend": Initial outcomes from a post-traumatic stress disorder/substance abuse treatment program. *Journal of Traumatic Stress., 14,* 757–772.

Drobes, D. J., & Tiffany, S. T. (1997). Induction of smoking urge through imaginal and in vivo procedures: Physiological and self-report manifestations. *Journal of Abnormal Psychology, 106,* 15–25.

Drouin, J., Sun, Y. L., Chamberland, M., Gauthier, Y., De Lean, A., Nemer, M., et al. (1993). Novel glucocorticoid receptor complex with DNA element of the hormone- repressed POMC gene. *European Molecular Biology Organization, 12,* 145–156.

Dunn, A. J., Swiergiel, A. H., & Palamarchouk, V. (2004). Brain circuits involved in corticotropin-releasing factor-norepinephrine interactions during stress. *Annals of the New York Academy of Sciences, 1018,* 25–34.

Eisenberger, N. I., Lieberman, M. D., & Williams, K. D. (2003). Does rejection hurt? An FMRI study of social exclusion. *Science, 302,* 290–292.

Epping-Jordan, M. P., Watkins, S. S., Koob, G. F., & Markou, A. (1998). Dramatic decreases in brain reward function during nicotine withdrawal. *Nature, 393,* 76–79.

Erb, S. (2007). Neurobiology of stress and risk for relapse. In M.al'Absi (Ed.), *Stress and addiction: Biological and psychological mechanisms* (pp. 147–169). London: Academic Press/Elsevier.

File, S. E., Dinnis, A. K., Heard, J. E., & Irvine, E. E. (2002). Mood differences between male and female light smokers and nonsmokers. *Pharmacology Biochemistry and Behavior 72*, 681–689.

File, S. E., Fluck, E., & Leahy, A. (2001). Nicotine has calming effects on stress-induced mood changes in females, but enhances aggressive mood in males. *International Journal of Neuropsychopharmacology, 4*, 371–376.

Fink, G., Robinson, I. C., & Tannahill, L. A. (1988). Effects of adrenalectomy and glucocorticoids on the peptides CRF-41, AVP and oxytocin in rat hypophysial portal blood [published erratum appears in *J Physiol (Lond)* 1988 Nov;405:785]. *Journal of Physiology (London), 401*, 329–345.

Fox, H. C., Talih, M., Malison, R., Anderson, G. M., Kreek, M. J., & Sinha, R. (2005). Frequency of recent cocaine and alcohol use affects drug craving and associated responses to stress and drug-related cues. *Psychoneuroendocrinology, 30*, 880–891.

Frankel, R. J., Jenkins, J. S., & Wright, J. J. (1978). Pituitary-adrenal response to stimulation of the limbic system and lateral hypothalamus in the rhesus monkey (Macacca mulatta). *Acta Endocrinologica (Copenh), 88*, 209–216.

Frankenhaeuser, M. (1980). Psychobiological aspects of life stress. In S. Levine & H. Ursin (Eds.), *Coping and health* (pp. 203–223). Plenum.

Fu, Y., Matta, S. G., Brower, V. G., & Sharp, B. M. (2001). Norepinephrine secretion in the hypothalamic paraventricular nucleus of rats during unlimited access to self-administered nicotine: An in vivo microdialysis study. *Journal of Neuroscience, 21*, 8979–8989.

George, T. P., Verrico, C. D., Picciotto, M. R., & Roth, R. H. (2000). Nicotinic modulation of mesoprefrontal dopamine neurons: Pharmacologic and neuroanatomic characterization. *Journal of Pharmacology and Experimental Therapeutics, 295*, 58–66.

Ghashghaei, H. T., & Barbas, H. (2002). Pathways for emotion: Interactions of prefrontal and anterior temporal pathways in the amygdala of the rhesus monkey. *Neuroscience, 115*, 1261–1279.

Gianoulakis, C. (1996). Implications of endogenous opioids and dopamine in alcoholism: Human and basic science studies. *Alcohol and Alcoholism - Supplement, 1*, 33–42.

Gianoulakis, C. (1998). Alcohol-seeking behavior: The roles of the hypothalamic-pituitary-adrenal axis and the endogenous opioid system. *Alcohol Health and Research World, 22*, 202–210.

Gilbert, D. G. (1995). *Smoking: Individual differences, psychopathology, and emotion.* Washington, DC: Taylor & Francis.

Goeders, N. E. (2007). The hypothalamic-pituitary-adrenocortical axis and addiction. In M.al'Absi (Ed.), *Stress and addiction: Biological and psychological mechanisms* (pp. 21–40). London: Academic Press/Elsevier.

Goldstein, D. & Kopin, I. (1990). The autonomic nervous system and catecholamines in normal blood pressure control and in hypertension. In J. Laragh & B. Brenner (Eds.), *Hypertension: Pathophysiology, diagnosis, and management* (pp. 711–747). New York: Raven Press.

Gould, E., Woolley, C., & McEwen, B. (1991). The hippocampal formation: Morphological changes induced by thyroid, gonadal, and adrenal hormones. *Psychoneuroendocrinology, 16*, 67–84.

Grunberg, N. E., Winders, S. E., & Wewers, M. E. (1991). Gender differences in tobacco use. *Health Psychology, 10*, 143–153.

Hadcock, J. R., & Malbon, C. C. (1988). Regulation of beta-adrenergic receptors by "permissive" hormones: Glucocorticoids increase steady-state levels of receptor mRNA. *Proceedings of the National Academy of Sciences (U S), 85*, 8415–8419.

Hariri, A. R., Mattay, V. S., Tessitore, A., Kolachana, B., Fera, F., Goldman, D., et al.. (2002a). Serotonin transporter genetic variation and the response of the human amygdala. *Science, 297*, 400–403.

Hariri, A. R., Tessitore, A., Mattay, V. S., Fera, F., & Weinberger, D. R. (2002b). The amygdala response to emotional stimuli: A comparison of faces and scenes. *Neuroimage, 17*, 317–323.

Harrison, P. A., Fulkerson, J. A., & Beebe, T. J. (1997). Multiple substance use among adolescent physical and sexual abuse victims. *Child Abuse and Neglect, 21*, 529–539.

Heim, C., Ehlert, U., Hanker, J. P., & Hellhammer, D. H. (1998). Abuse-related posttraumatic stress disorder and alterations of the hypothalamic-pituitary-adrenal axis in women with chronic pelvic pain. *Psychosomatic Medicine, 60*, 309–318.

Heim, C., Ehlert, U., & Hellhammer, D. H. (2000). The potential role of hypocortisolism in the pathophysiology of stress-related bodily disorders. *Psychoneuroendocrinology, 25*, 1–35.

Heishman, S. J. (1999). Behavioral and cognitive effects of smoking: Relationship to nicotine addiction. *Nicotine and Tobacco Research, 1* (Suppl 2) S143–S147.

Hennessy, M. B., Mendoza, S. P., Mason, W. A., & Moberg, G. P. (1995). Endocrine sensitivity to novelty in squirrel monkeys and titi monkeys: Species differences in characteristic modes of responding to the environment. *Physiology and Behavior, 57,* 331–338.

Henry, J. P. (1992). Biological basis of the stress response. *Integrative Physiological Behavioral Science, 27,* 66–83.

Henry, J. P. (1993). Psychological and physiological responses to stress: The right hemisphere and the hypothalamo-pituitary-adrenal axis, an inquiry into problems of human bonding. *Integrative Physiological & Behavioral Science, 28,* 369–387.

Herman, J. P., & Cullinan, W. E. (1997). Neurocircuitry of stress: Central control of the hypothalamo-pituitary-adrenocortical axis. *Trends in Neurosciences, 20,* 78–84.

Hernandez-Avila, C. A., Oncken, C., Van Kirk, J., Wand, G., & Kranzler, H. R. (2002). Adrenocorticotropin and cortisol responses to a naloxone challenge and risk of alcoholism. *Biological Psychiatry, 51,* 652–658.

Higley, J., Hasert, M., Suomi, S., & Linnolia, M. (1998). The serotonin reuptake inhibitor sertraline reduces excessive alcohol consumption in nonhuman primates: Effect of stress. *Neuropsychopharmacology, 18,* 431–443.

Higley, J. D., Thompson, W. W., Champoux, M., Goldman, D., Hasert, M. F., Kraemer, G. W., et al. (1993). Paternal and maternal genetic and environmental contributions to cerebrospinal fluid monoamine metabolites in rhesus monkeys (Macaca mulatta). *Archives of General Psychiatry, 50,* 615–623.

Holsboer, F., & Barden, N. (1996). Antidepressants and hypothalamic-pituitary-adrenocortical regulation. *Endocrine Reviews, 17,* 187–205.

Hughes, J. R. (1992). Tobacco withdrawal in self-quitters. *Journal of Consulting and Clinical Psychology, 60,* 689–697.

Imperato, A., Puglisi-Allegra, S., Casolini, P., & Angelucci, L. (1991). Changes in brain dopamine and acetylcholine release during and following stress are independent of the pituitary-adrenocortical axis. *Brain Research, 538,* 111–117.

Jamner, L. D., Girdler, S. S., Shapiro, D., & Jarvik, M. E. (1998). Pain inhibition, nictotine, and gender. *Experimental and Clinical Psychopharmacology, 6,* 96–106.

Jamner, L. D., Shapiro, D., & Jarvik, M. E. (1999). Nicotine reduces the frequency of anger reports in smokers and nonsmokers with high but not low hostility: An ambulatory study. *Experimental and Clinical Psychopharmacology, 7,* 454–463.

Kabbaj, M., Devine, D. P., Savage, V. R., & Akil, H. (2000). Neurobiological correlates of individual differences in novelty-seeking behavior in the rat: Differential expression of stress-related molecules. *Journal of Neuroscience, 20,* 6983–6988.

Kassel, J. D., Veilleux, J. C., Wardle, M. C., Yates, M. C., Greenstein, J. E., Evatt, D. P., et al. (2007). Negative affect and addiction. In M.al'Absi (Ed.), *Stress and addiction: Biological and psychological mechanisms* (pp. 171–190). London: Academic Press/Elsevier.

Keane, T. M., & Kaloupek, D. G. (1997). Comorbid psychiatric disorders in PTSD. Implications for research. *Annals of the New York Academy of Sciences, 821,* 24–34.

Kenford, S. L., Smith, S. S., Wetter, D. W., Jorenby, D. E., Fiore, M. C., & Baker, T. B. (2002). Predicting relapse back to smoking: Contrasting affective and physical models of dependence. *Journal of Consulting and Clinical Psychology, 70,* 216–227.

Kessler, R. C., Sonnega, A., Bromet, E., Hughes, M., & Nelson, C. B. (1995). Posttraumatic stress disorder in the National Comorbidity Survey. *Archives of General Psychiatry, 52,* 1048–1060.

Kiecolt-Glaser, J. K., McGuire, L., Robles, T. F., & Glaser, R. (2002). Psychoneuroimmunology: Psychological influences on immune function and health. *Journal of Consulting and Clinical Psychology, 70,* 537–547.

Kirschbaum, C., Pirke, K., & Hellhammer, D. H. (1993). The 'Trier Social Stress Test'—A tool for investigating psychobiological stress responses in a laboratory setting. *Neuropsychobiology, 28,* 76–81.

Kirschbaum, C., Wust, S., & Strasburger, C. J. (1992). Normal cigarette smoking increases free cortisol in habitual smokers. *Life Sciences, 50,* 435–442.

Knuth, E. D., & Etgen, A. M. (2005). Corticosterone secretion induced by chronic isolation in neonatal rats is sexually dimorphic and accompanied by elevated ACTH. *Hormones and Behavior, 47,* 65–75.

Koob, G. F., & Heinrichs, S. C. (1999). A role for corticotropin releasing factor and urocortin in behavioral responses to stressors. *Brain Research, 848,* 141–152.

Kosten, T. A., & Ambrosio, E. (2002). HPA axis function and drug addictive behaviors: Insights from studies with Lewis and Fischer 344 inbred rats. *Psychoneuroendocrinology, 27,* 35–69.

Kosten, T. A., & Kehoe, P. (2007). Early life stress and vulnerability to addiction. In M.al'Absi (Ed.), *Stress and addiction: Biological and psychological mechanisms* (pp. 105–126). London: Academic Press/Elsevier.

Kosten, T. A., Miserendino, M. J., & Kehoe, P. (2000). Enhanced acquisition of cocaine self-administration in adult rats with neonatal isolation stress experience. *Brain Research, 875,* 44–50.

Kosten, T. A., Sanchez, H., Zhang, X. Y., & Kehoe, P. (2004). Neonatal isolation enhances acquisition of cocaine self-administration and food responding in female rats. *Behavioural Brain Research, 151,* 137–149.

Koval, J. J., & Pederson, L. L. (1999). Stress-coping and other psychosocial risk factors: A model for smoking in grade 6 students. *Addictive Behaviors, 24,* 207–218.

Kreek, M. J., & Koob, G. F. (1998). Drug dependence: Stress and dysregulation of brain reward pathways. *Drug and Alcohol Dependence, 51,* 23–47.

Kuhn, C., & Francis, R. (1997). Gender difference in cocaine-induced HPA axis activation. *Neuropsychopharmacology, 16,* 399–407.

Lane, R. D., Reiman, E. M., Bradley, M. M., Lang, P. J., Ahern, G. L., Davidson, R. J., et al. (1997). Neuroanatomical correlates of pleasant and unpleasant emotion. *Neuropsychologia, 35,* 1437–1444.

Lazarus, R. (1999). *Stress and emotion: A new synthesis.* New York: Springer.

Ledoux, J. E. (1992). Emotion and the amygdala. In John P. Aggleton (Ed.), *The amygdala: Neurobiological aspects of emotion, memory, and mental dysfunction* (pp. 339–351). New York: Wiley-Liss.

Levine, S. (2005). Developmental determinants of sensitivity and resistance to stress. *Psychoneuroendocrinology, 30,* 939–946.

Lieberman, M. D., Hariri, A., Jarcho, J. M., Eisenberger, N. I., & Bookheimer, S. Y. (2005). An fMRI investigation of race-related amygdala activity in African-American and Caucasian-American individuals. *Nature Neuroscience, 8,* 720–722.

Lovallo, W. R., Pincomb, G. A., Brackett, D. J., & Wilson, M. F. (1990). Heart rate reactivity as a predictor of neuroendocrine responses to aversive and appetitive challenges. *Psychosomatic Medicine, 52,* 17–26.

Lundberg, U. (1984). Human psychobiology in Scandinavia: II. Psychoneuroendocrinology- human stress and coping processes. *Scandinavian Journal of Psychology, 25,* 214–226.

Lundberg, U., & Frankenhaeuser, M. (1980). Pituitary-adrenal and sympathetic-adrenal correlates of distress and effort. *Journal of Psychosomatic Research, 24,* 125–130.

Lupien, S. J., Gaudreau, S., Tchiteya, B. M., Maheu, F., Sharma, S., Nair, N. P., et al. (1997). Stress-induced declarative memory impairment in healthy elderly subjects: Relationship to cortisol reactivity. *Journal of Clinical Endocrinology and Metabolism, 82,* 2070–2075.

Maier, S. F. & Watkins, L. R. (1998). Cytokines for psychologists: Implications of bidirectional immune-to-brain communication for understanding behavior, mood, and cognition. *Psychological Review, 105,* 83–107.

Makino, S., Gold, P. W., & Schulkin, J. (1994a). Corticosterone effects on corticotropin-releasing hormone mRNA in the central nucleus of the amygdala and the parvocellular region of the paraventricular nucleus of the hypothalamus. *Brain Research, 640,* 105–112.

Makino, S., Gold, P. W., & Schulkin, J. (1994b). Effects of corticosterone on CRH mRNA and content in the bed nucleus of the stria terminalis; comparison with the effects in the central nucleus of the amygdala and the paraventricular nucleus of the hypothalamus. *Brain Research, 657,* 141–149.

Marinelli, M. (2007). Dopaminergic reward pathways and effects of stress. In M.al'Absi (Ed.), *Stress and addiction: Biological and psychological mechanisms* (pp. 41–83). London: Academic Press/Elsevier.

Marinelli, M., Aouizerate, B., Barrot, M., Le Moal, M., & Piazza, P. (1998). Dopamine-dependent responses to morphine depend on glucocortoid receptors. *Neurobiology, 95,* 7742–7747.

Mason, J. W. (1975). A historical view of the stress field. *Journal of Human Stress, 1,* 22–36.

McEwen, B. S. (1997b). The brain is an important target of adrenal steroid actions. A comparison of synthetic and natural steroids. *Annals of the New York Academy of Sciences, 823,* 201–213.

McEwen, B. S. (1997a). The brain is an important target of adrenal steroid actions. A comparison of synthetic and natural steroids. *Annals of the New York Academy of Sciences, 823,* 201–213.

McEwen, B. S. (1998). Protective and damaging effects of stress mediators. *New England Journal of Medicine, 338,* 171–179.

McEwen, B. S., & Sapolsky, R. M. (1995). Stress and cognitive function. *Current Opinion in Neurobiology, 5,* 205–216.

McFall, M. E., Mackay, P. W., & Donovan, D. M. (1992). Combat-related posttraumatic stress disorder and severity of substance abuse in Vietnam veterans. *Journal of Studies on Alcohol, 53,* 357–363.

McFarland, K., Davidge, S. B., Lapish, C. C., & Kalivas, P. W. (2004). Limbic and motor circuitry underlying footshock-induced reinstatement of cocaine-seeking behavior. *Journal of Neuroscience, 24,* 1551–1560.

McKay, J. R., Rutherford, M. J., Alterman, A. I., Cacciola, J. S., & Kaplan, M. R. (1995). An examination of the cocaine relapse process. *Drug and Alcohol Dependence, 38,* 35–43.

Mendelson, J. H., Mello, N. K., Teoh, S. K., Ellingboe, J., & Cochin, J. (1989). Cocaine effects on pulsatile secretion of anterior pituitary, gonadal, and adrenal hormones. *Journal of Clinical Endocrinology and Metabolism, 69,* 1256–1260.

Mendelson, J. H., Teoh, S. K., Lange, U., Mello, N. K., Weiss, R., Skupny, A., et al. (1988). Anterior pituitary, adrenal, and gonadal hormones during cocaine withdrawal. *American Journal of Psychiatry, 145,* 1094–1098.

Mendelson, J. H., Teoh, S. K., Mello, N. K., Ellingboe, J., & Rhoades, E. (1992). Acute effects of cocaine on plasma adrenocorticotropic hormone, luteinizing hormone and prolactin levels in cocaine-dependent men. *Journal of Pharmacology and Experimental Therapeutics, 263,* 505–509.

Miller, G. M., Bendor, J., Tiefenbacher, S., Yang, H., Novak, M. A., & Madras, B. K. (2004). A mu-opioid receptor single nucleotide polymorphism in rhesus monkey: Association with stress response and aggression. *Molecular Psychiatry, 9,* 99–108.

Mittleman, G., Blaha, C. D., & Phillips, A. G. (1992). Pituitary-adrenal and dopaminergic modulation of schedule-induced polydipsia: Behavioral and neurochemical evidence. *Behavioral Neuroscience, 106,* 408–420.

Mittleman, G., Jones, G. H., & Robbins, T. W. (1991). Sensitization of amphetamine-stereotypy reduces plasma corticosterone: Implications for stereotypy as a coping response. *Behavioral and Neural Biology, 56,* 170–182.

Munck, A., Guyre, P. M., & Holbrook, N. J. (1984). Physiological functions of glucocorticoids in stress and their relation to pharmacological actions. *Endocrinology Review, 5,* 25–44.

Najavits, L. M., Gastfriend, D. R., Barber, J. P., Reif, S., Muenz, L. R., Blaine, J., et al. (1998). Cocaine dependence with and without PTSD among subjects in the National Institute on Drug Abuse Collaborative Cocaine Treatment Study. *American Journal of Psychiatry, 155,* 214–219.

Newton-Taylor, B., DeWit, D., & Gliksman, L. (1998). Prevalence and factors associated with physical and sexual assault of female university students in Ontario. *Health Care Women International, 19,* 155–164.

Ochsner, K. N., Bunge, S. A., Gross, J. J., & Gabrieli, J. D. (2002). Rethinking feelings: An FMRI study of the cognitive regulation of emotion. *Journal of Cognitive Neuroscience, 14,* 1215–1229.

O'Malley, S. S., Krishnan-Sarin, S., Farren, C., Sinha, R., & Kreek, J. (2002). Naltrexone decreases craving and alcohol self-administration in alcohol-dependent subjects and activates the hypothalamo-pituitary-adrenocortical axis. *Psychopharmacology (Berl), 160,* 19–29.

Oslin, D. W., Berrettini, W., Kranzler, H. R., Pettinati, H., Gelernter, J., Volpicelli, J. R., et al. (2003). A functional polymorphism of the mu-opioid receptor gene is associated with naltrexone response in alcohol-dependent patients. *Neuropsychopharmacology, 28,* 1546–1552.

Overmier, J. B., & Murison, R. (2005). Trauma and resulting sensitization effects are modulated by psychological factors. *Psychoneuroendocrinology, 30,* 965–973.

Overton, P. G., Tong, Z. Y., Brain, P. F., & Clark, D. (1996). Preferential occupation of mineralocorticoid receptors by corticosterone enhances glutamate-induced burst firing in rat midbrain dopaminergic neurons. *Brain Research, 737,* 146–154.

Parrott, A. (1999). Does cigarette smoking cause stress? *American Psychologist, 54,* 817–820.

Perkins, K. A. (1999). Nicotine discrimination in men and women [In Process Citation]. *Pharmacology Biochemistry and Behavior, 64,* 295–299.

Perkins, K. A., & Grobe, J. E. (1992). Increased desire to smoke during acute stress. *British Journal of Addiction, 87,* 1037–1040.

Petersen, S. L., Hartman, R. D., & Barraclough, C. A. (1989). An analysis of serotonin secretion in hypothalamic regions based on 5- hydroxytryptophan accumulation or push-pull perfusion. Effects of mesencephalic raphe or locus coeruleus stimulation and correlated changes in plasma luteinizing hormone. *Brain Research, 495,* 9–19.

Piazza, P. V., & Le Moal, M. (1998). The role of stress in drug self-administration. *Trends in Pharmacological Sciences, 19,* 67–74.

Plotsky, P. M., & Meaney, M. J. (1993). Early, postnatal experience alters hypothalamic corticotropin-releasing factor (CRF) mRNA, median eminence CRF content and stress-induced release in adult rats. *Molecular Brain Research, 18,* 195–200.

Pontieri, F. E., Tanda, G., Orzi, F., & Di Chiara, G. (1996). Effects of nicotine on the nucleus accumbens and similarity to those of addictive drugs. *Nature, 382,* 255–257.

Pritchard, W. S., Robinson, J. H., & Guy, T. D. (1992). Enhancement of continuous performance task reaction time by smoking in non-deprived smokers. *Psychopharmacology (Berl), 108,* 437–442.

Redmond, D. E. J., & Huang, Y. H. (1979). Current concepts. II. New evidence for a locus coeruleus-norepinephrine connection with anxiety. *Life Sciences, 25,* 2149–2162.

Risold, P. Y., Thompson, R. H., & Swanson, L. W. (1997). The structural organization of connections between hypothalamus and cerebral cortex. *Brain Research Brain Research Reviews, 24,* 197–254.

Rivier, C., & Vale, W. (1983). Modulation of stress-induced ACTH release by corticotropin-releasing factor, catecholamines and vasopressin. *Nature, 305,* 325–327.

Rivier, C., & Vale, W. (1987a). Cocaine stimulates adrenocorticotropin (ACTH) secretion through a corticotropin-releasing factor (CRF)-mediated mechanism. *Brain Research, 422,* 403–406.

Rivier, C., & Vale, W. (1987b). Diminished responsiveness of the hypothalamic-pituitary-adrenal axis of the rat during exposure to prolonged stress: A pituitary-mediated mechanism. *Endocrinology, 121,* 1320–1328.

Roberts, M. E., Moore, S. D., & Beckham, J. C. (2007). Posttraumatic stress disorder and substance use disorders. In M.al'Absi (Ed.), *Stress and addiction: Biological and psychological mechanisms* (pp. 315–332). London: Academic Press/Elsevier.

Rose, J. E., & Corrigall, W. A. (1997). Nicotine self-administration in animals and humans: similarities and differences. *Psychopharmacology (Berl), 130,* 28–40.

Rosmond, R., & Bjorntorp, P. (1998a). Blood pressure in relation to obesity, insulin and the hypothalamic-pituitary-adrenal axis in Swedish men. *Journal of Hypertension, 16,* 1721–1726.

Rosmond, R., & Bjorntorp, P. (1998b). Endocrine and metabolic aberrations in men with abdominal obesity in relation to anxio-depressive infirmity. *Metabolism, 47,* 1187–1193.

Rosmond, R., Dallman, M. F., & Bjorntorp, P. (1998). Stress-related cortisol secretion in men: Relationships with abdominal obesity and endocrine, metabolic and hemodynamic abnormalities. *Journal of Clinical Endocrinology and Metabolism, 83,* 1853–1859.

Ruggiero, D. A., Underwood, M. D., Rice, P. M., Mann, J. J., & Arango, V. (1999). Corticotropic-releasing hormone and serotonin interact in the human brainstem: Behavioral implications. *Neuroscience, 91,* 1343–1354.

Saal, D., Dong, Y., Bonci, A., & Malenka, R. C. (2003). Drugs of abuse and stress trigger a common synaptic adaptation in dopamine neurons. *Neuron, 37,* 577–582.

Salamone, J. D. (1994). The involvement of nucleus accumbens dopamine in appetitive and aversive motivation. *Behavioural Brain Research, 61,* 117–133.

Salokangas, R. K., Vilkman, H., Ilonen, T., Taiminen, T., Bergman, J., Haaparanta, M., et al. (2000). High levels of dopamine activity in the basal ganglia of cigarette smokers. *American Journal of Psychiatry, 157,* 632–634.

Saper, C. B., Swanson, L. W., & Cowan, W. M. (1979). An autoradiographic study of the efferent connections of the lateral hypothalamic area in the rat. *Journal of Comparative Neurology, 183,* 689–706.

Sapolsky, R. M. (1996). Why stress is bad for your brain. *Science, 273,* 749–750.

Sapolsky, R. M. (2000a). Glucocorticoids and hippocampal atrophy in neuropsychiatric disorders. *Archives of General Psychiatry, 57,* 925–935.

Sapolsky, R. M. (2000b). The possibility of neurotoxicity in the hippocampus in major depression: a primer on neuron death. *Biological Psychiatry, 48,* 755–765.

Sapolsky, R. M., Romero, L. M., & Munck, A. U. (2000). How do glucocorticoids influence stress responses? Integrating permissive, suppressive, stimulatory, and preparative actions. *Endocrinology Reviews., 21,* 55–89.

Sarnyai, Z., McKittrick, C. R., McEwen, B. S., & Kreek, M. J. (1998). Selective regulation of dopamine transporter binding in the shell of the nucleus accumbens by adrenalectomy and corticosterone-replacement. *Synapse, 30,* 334–337.

Sarnyai, Z., Mello, N. K., Mendelson, J. H., Eros-Sarnyai, M., & Mercer, G. (1996). Effects of cocaine on pulsatile activity of hypothalamic-pituitary-adrenal axis in male rhesus monkeys: Neuroendocrine and behavioral correlates. *Journal of Pharmacology and Experimental Therapeutics, 277,* 225–234.

Schenk, S., Lacelle, G., Gorman, K., & Amit, Z. (1987). Cocaine self-administration in rats influenced by environmental conditions: Implications for the etiology of drug abuse. *Neuroscience Letters, 81,* 227–231.

Selye, H. (1947). *The general adaptation syndrome and diseases of adaptation.* Montreal: Montreal University.

Setekleiv, J., Skaug, O. E., & Kaada, B. R. (1961). Increase of plasma 17-hydroxycorticosteroids by cerebral cortical and amygdaloid stimulation in the cat. *Journal of Endocrinology, 22,* 119–127.

Singh, V. B., Corley, K. C., Krieg, R. J., Phan, T. H., & Boadle-Biber, M. C. (1994). Sound stress activation of tryptophan hydroxylase blocked by hypophysectomy and intracranial RU 38486. *European Journal of Pharmacology, 256,* 177–184.

Sinha, R., Catapano, D., & O'Malley, S. (1999). Stress-induced craving and stress response in cocaine dependent individuals. *Psychopharmacology (Berl), 142,* 343–351.

Sircar, R., Mallinson, K., Goldbloom, L. M., & Kehoe, P. (2001). Postnatal stress selectively upregulates striatal N-methyl-D-aspartate receptors in male rats. *Brain Research, 904,* 145–148.

Snoek, H., Van Goozen, S. H., Matthys, W., Buitelaar, J. K., & van Engeland, H. (2004). Stress responsivity in children with externalizing behavior disorders. *Developmental Psychopathology, 16,* 389–406.

Snyder, F. R., Davis, F. C., & Henningfield, J. E. (1989). The tobacco withdrawal syndrome: performance decrements assessed on a computerized test battery. *Drug and Alcohol Dependence, 23,* 259–266.

Staley, J. K., Krishnan-Sarin, S., Zoghbi, S., Tamagnan, G., Fujita, M., Seibyl, J. P., et al. (2001). Sex differences in [123I]beta-CIT SPECT measures of dopamine and serotonin transporter availability in healthy smokers and nonsmokers. *Synapse, 41,* 275–284.

Steptoe, A. (1987). The assessment of sympathetic nervous function in human stress research. *Journal of Psychosomatic Research, 31,* 141–152.

Stitzer, M. L., & Gross, J. (1988). Smoking relapse: The role of pharmacological and behavioral factors. *Progress in Clinical Biological Research, 261,* 163–184.

Swan, G. E., Ward, M. M., Jack, L. M., & Javitz, H. S. (1993). Cardiovascular reactivity as a predictor of relapse in male and female smokers. *Health Psychology, 12,* 451–458.

Swanson, L. W., & Simmons, D. M. (1989). Differential steroid hormone and neural influences on peptide mRNA levels in CRH cells of the paraventricular nucleus: A hybridization histochemical study in the rat. *Journal of Comparative Neurology, 285,* 413–435.

Szafarczyk, A., Guillaume, V., Conte-Devolx, B., Alonso, G., Malaval, F., Pares-Herbute, N., et al. (1988). Central catecholaminergic system stimulates secretion of CRH at different sites. *American Journal of Physiology, 255,* E463–E468.

Tilders, F. J., Berkenbosch, F., Vermes, I., Linton, E. A., & Smelik, P. G. (1985). Role of epinephrine and vasopressin in the control of the pituitary-adrenal response to stress. *Federation Proceedings, 44,* 155–160.

Tuomisto, J., & Mannisto, P. (1985). Neurotransmitter regulation of anterior pituitary hormones. *Pharmacological Reviews, 37,* 249–332.

Ungless, M. A., Singh, V., Crowder, T. L., Yaka, R., Ron, D., & Bonci, A. (2003). Corticotropin-releasing factor requires CRF binding protein to potentiate NMDA receptors via CRF receptor 2 in dopamine neurons. *Neuron, 39,* 401–407.

Ursin, H., & Olff, M. (1993). Psychobiology of coping and defence strategies. *Neuropsychobiology, 28,* 66–71.

Valentino, R. J., & Foote, S. L. (1988). Corticotropin-releasing hormone increases tonic but not sensory-evoked activity of noradrenergic locus coeruleus neurons in unanesthetized rats. *Journal of Neuroscience, 8,* 1016–1025.

Valentino, R. J., & Van Bockstaele, E. (2001). Opposing regulation of the locus coeruleus by corticotropin-releasing factor and opioids. Potential for reciprocal interactions between stress and opioid sensitivity. *Psychopharmacology (Berl), 158,* 331–342.

Vander, A. J., Sherman, J. H., & Luciano, D. S. (1994). *Human physiology* (6th ed.). New York: McGraw-Hill.

Wand, G. S., McCaul, M., Yang, X., Reynolds, J., Gotjen, D., Lee, S., et al. (2002). The mu-opioid receptor gene polymorphism (A118G) alters HPA axis activation induced by opioid receptor blockade. *Neuropsychopharmacology, 26,* 106–114.

Wand, G. S., & Schumann, H. (1998). Relationship between plasma adrenocorticotropin, hypothalamic opioid tone, and plasma leptin. *Journal of Clinical Endocrinology and Metabolism, 83,* 2138–2142.

Wang, B., Shaham, Y., Zitzman, D., Azari, S., Wise, R. A., & You, Z. B. (2005). Cocaine experience establishes control of midbrain glutamate and dopamine by corticotropin-releasing factor: A role in stress-induced relapse to drug seeking. *Journal of Neuroscience., 25,* 5389–5396.

Ward, K. D., Klesges, R. C., Zbikowski, S. M., Bliss, R. E., & Garvey, A. J. (1997). Gender differences in the outcome of an unaided smoking cessation attempt. *Addictive Behaviors, 22,* 521–533.

Weiner, R. I., & Ganong, W. F. (1978). Role of brain monoamines and histamine in regulation of anterior pituitary secretion. *Physiological Reviews, 58,* 905–976.

Wetter, D. W., Kenford, S. L., Smith, S. S., Fiore, M. C., Jorenby, D. E., & Baker, T. B. (1999). Gender differences in smoking cessation [In Process Citation]. *Journal of Consulting and Clinical Psychology, 67,* 555–562.

Widom, C. S., Weiler, B. L., & Cottler, L. B. (1999). Childhood victimization and drug abuse: A comparison of prospective and retrospective findings. *Journal of Consulting and Clinical Psychology, 67,* 867–880.

Wilkins, J. N., Carlson, H. E., Van Vunakis, H., Hill, M. A., Gritz, E., & Jarvik, M. E. (1982). Nicotine from cigarette smoking increases circulating levels of cortisol, growth hormone, and prolactin in male chronic smokers. *Psychopharmacology, 78,* 305–308.

Wills, T. A. (1986). Stress and coping in early adolescence: Relationships to substance use in urban school samples. *Health Psychology, 5,* 503–529.

Wills, T. A., Sandy, J. M., & Yaeger, A. M. (2002). Stress and smoking in adolescence: A test of directional hypotheses. *Health Psychology, 21,* 122–130.

Wilsnack, S. C., Vogeltanz, N. D., Klassen, A. D., & Harris, T. R. (1997). Childhood sexual abuse and women's substance abuse: National survey findings. *Journal of Studies on Alcohol, 58,* 264–271.

Wilson, J. D., & Foster, D. W. (1992). *Williams textbook of endocrinology* (8th ed.). Pheladelphia: Saunders.

Winfield, I., George, L. K., Swartz, M., & Blazer, D. G. (1990). Sexual assault and psychiatric disorders among a community sample of women. *American Journal of Psychiatry, 147,* 335–341.

Wise, R. A. (1996). Neurobiology of addiction. *Currrnt Opinion in Neurobiology, 6,* 243–251.

Zaslav, M. R. (1994). Psychology of comorbid posttraumatic stress disorder and substance abuse: Lessons from combat veterans. *Journal of Psychoactive Drugs, 26,* 393–400.

24

Behavioral Economics of Substance Abuse

James G. Murphy
University of Memphis

Christopher J. Corriea
Auburn University

Rudy E. Vuchinich
University of Alabama

Contents

Behavioral Economic Theories of Addiction

Most modern theories of addiction view drug self-administration as an operant that is maintained by the reinforcing properties of drugs (Schuster & Thompson, 1969). Widely abused drugs such as morphine, cocaine, and ethanol reliably reinforce the behavior that leads to their administration (Schuster & Thompson, 1969). A key task of any theory of drug use, however, is to predict the conditions in which drugs will be highly preferred or valued reinforcers. Behavioral economic theory uses the term *reinforcing value*, which in laboratory settings is quantified by the amount of behavior (e.g., lever presses, time) allocated to gain access to the reinforcer, and to describe the relative level of preference for a reinforcer such as alcohol or drugs. According to behavioral economics, the reinforcing value of a given drug is a dynamic and contextually determined function of the reinforcing effects of the drug and the availability of alternative reinforcers, rather than a fixed property of the drug or a characteristic of the individual (Bickel, Madden, & Petry, 1998; Bickel, Marsch, & Carroll, 2000; Heyman, 2003; MacKillop et al., 2008; Murphy et al., 2005; Vuchinich & Heather, 2003). Thus, compared to most other theories of addiction (Leonard & Blane, 1999), a distinguishing feature of behavioral economic theory is the focus on contextual determinants of drug use. Relative to theories that focus largely on stable individual differences in personality, cognitions, or biology as explanations for addiction, a strength of behavioral economics theories is their ability to account for the substantial fluctuations in drug use within an individual over time that have been repeatedly demonstrated in clinical and epidemiological research (Del Boca, Darkes, Greenbaum, & Goldman, 2004; Moos, Finney, & Cronkite, 1990; Tucker, 1999). The following sections describe several key features of behavioral economic theories of addiction.

Drug Use is Influenced by the Availability and Price of Drugs and Alternative Reinforcers

Behavioral economic theory predicts that the primary contextual influences on drug use are both constraints on access to drugs and the availability and value of alternative substance-free sources of reinforcement (Vuchinich & Tucker, 1988). Although several authors have developed formal behavioral economic theories of addiction (Becker & Murphy, 1988; Herrnstein & Prelec, 1992; Rachlin, 1997), and there are substantive differences among the theories (Vuchinich & Heather, 2003), all view the decision to use drugs as a cost-benefit analysis that is based on the relative availability and value of drugs versus alternative activities. Stated most simply, behavioral economic theory predicts that drug use is most likely when there are minimal constraints on drug use and substantial constraints on access to valued nondrug reinforcers. This postulate is supported by data indicating that: (1) rates of substance use, in both laboratory and naturalistic settings, are highly sensitive to alterations in the response cost or price associated with drug use (Hursh & Winger, 1995; Murphy & MacKillop, 2006), (2) high rates of substance use are most likely in contexts devoid of substance-free sources of reinforcement, and (3) that substance use will generally decrease if access to alternative reinforcers is increased (Cohen, Britt, & Collins, 1999; Correia et al., 2005; Higgins, Heil, & Plebani-Lussier, 2004). Regarding postulates (2) and (3), we should point out that although several studies have identified alternative reinforcers that substitute for drug use (an inverse relation between levels of drug use and levels of the drug-free activity), drugs and alternative reinforcers can also be independents (no relation between levels of drug use and levels of the drug-free activity) or complements (positive relation between levels of drug use and levels of the drug-free activity; Petry & Bickel, 1998). For example, whereas employment and religious activity are generally substitutes for drug and alcohol use (Anthony, Warner, & Kessler, 1994; Miller, 1998), spending drug-free time with substance users may have a complementary relationship to substance use (Martin & Hoffman, 1993).

It is important to point out that behavioral economics is a *molar theory*, which means that its goal is to account for patterns of behavioral allocation toward drugs and alternatives over time, rather than discrete instances of drug use (Rachlin, 1997; Vuchinich & Heather, 2003; Vuchinich & Tucker, 1996). Drug use is assumed to vary predictably in relation to the relative availability of drugs and alternatives, but no predictions are made about whether an individual will use drugs in a given instance. In contrast, biological, social learning, and cognitive theories of addiction focus on proximal explanations for specific instances of drug use (e.g., craving, expectancies, peer pressure). In Aristotelian terms, behavioral economics focuses on final rather than efficient causes (Rachlin, 1997).

Relative Value of Drugs Versus Alternative Changes as a Function of Engagement in these Activities

A key assumption of behavioral economic theories of addiction is that the cost-benefit ratio of drug consumption versus engagement in other activities changes as a function of the amount of engagement in these respective activities. The nature of the change in the cost-benefit ratio as a function of consumption (or participation), however, is markedly different for drugs versus many potential substitute activities (Rachlin, 1997, 2000). Drugs are viewed as price-habituated activities, which means that there is a negative relation between the amount of consumption over time and the benefit derived from a given consumption episode. This is consistent with the observation that tolerance reduces the rewarding effects of a given drug dose in experienced drug users. In contrast, many substance-free activities are price-sensitized, which means that there is a positive relation between participation and the benefits derived from the activity. Interpersonal relationships, exercise/sports, and hobbies such as chess and playing piano are examples of activities that will generally result in increased benefits over time, as intimacy (in the case of relationships) and skill generally increases with repeated engagement in these activities. If these activities are neglected, conversely, their cost-benefit ratio will decrease (e.g., playing tennis when out of practice, attempting to access social support after a period of social isolation, attending calculus class after missing the previous three classes).

Behavioral economic theories suggest that the central dynamic of addiction is the relative distribution of behavior over time to constructive price-sensitized activities versus drug use (Heyman, 2003; Rachlin, 1997; Vuchinich & Tucker, 1996). Because drug use is price-habituated it is in theory a self-limiting activity. Whereas moderate substance use (e.g., a glass of wine with dinner, or several drinks during a weekly happy hour) results in reliable benefits (euphoria, relaxation, social facilitation), regular heavy drug use diminishes the value of any single unit of use, perhaps due to acute or extended tolerance. Indeed, the fact that the number of moderate drinkers and drug users far exceeds the number of heavy users is consistent with this self-limiting prediction (Kandel & Yamaguchi, 2002). However, there are several conditions that could result in increased drug use, including (1) an event that results in a reduction in substance-free substitutes (e.g., losing a job or relationship, moving to a new environment, retirement, an injury or illness), (2) reduced price of drug use (e.g., moving into a fraternity house or a neighborhood where alcohol/drugs are readily available, or turning 21 and being able to purchase alcohol legally), or (3) social contingencies that reinforce drug use (e.g., beginning a relationship with a heavy drinker, or a job that includes weekly happy hours). Because drug use and many substance-free activities are mutually substitutable, an increase in drug use will result in decreased engagement in substance-free activities (Green & Fisher, 2000; Petry & Bickel, 1998; Rachlin, 1997, 2000). This decrease will in turn reduce the value of the price-sensitized substance-free activities, resulting in greater behavioral allocation toward substance use.

Although the value of any occasion of substance use will continue to decrease as use escalates, the concurrent reduction in the value of price-sensitized substance-free substitutes will often make drug use the option with the greatest immediate benefit. This progression toward greater drug use is exacerbated by the fact that drug use often has a direct negative impact on other activities (e.g., hangover-related impairment, alcohol-related arguments, social stigma, legal fines/sanctions) in addition to the price-sensitized effect associated with diminished engagement in substance-free activities (Heyman, 2003; Rachlin, 1997, 2000). It is also possible, however, for contextual events, such as in increase in the price of drugs or a decrease in the price of substance-free activities, to increase the cost-benefit ratio of substance-free activities, leading to reduced drug use (Vuchinich & Tucker, 1996). Later in this chapter we discuss several treatment approaches that attempt to achieve these shifts in the price of drugs and alternatives (Murphy et al., 2007).

Temporal Influences on Choice between Drugs and Alternatives

The choice dynamic described above is critically dependent on the temporal context of the decisions. Drug choices will often maximize utility (i.e., happiness, satisfaction) if the timeframe for maximization is short (Heyman, 2003; Heyman & Dunn, 2002). Using drugs on one particular day might maximize utility for that day compared to going to work, for example. If the temporal context is extended (e.g., one month or year), however, behavioral allocation toward constructive, price-sensitized activities would maximize utility. Herrnstein and Prelec (1992) point out that addiction entails a series of "distributed choices" (e.g., drinking vs. abstaining on a given night) rather than a discrete choice (to be an alcoholic vs. an abstainer), and that the frame of reference used to estimate the relative value of a series of choices concerning drug use will determine the amount of drug use over time (Heyman, 2003; Heyman & Dunn, 2002; Tucker, Vuchinich, & Rippins, 2006).

Although behavioral economic theories of addiction focus primarily on contextual influences on drug use, individual differences in the extent to which decisions are made on the basis of relatively short-term versus long-term outcomes are understood as an important contributor to addiction (Bickel & Marsh, 2001; Green & Myerson, 2004; Heyman, 2003). For example, although the value of all rewards decreases as their receipt is delayed (i.e., delay discounting), there are substantial individual differences in the degree of discounting of delayed rewards, and behavioral economic theory suggests that this discounting phenomenon may be a core feature of substance abuse (Bickel & Marsch, 2001). That is, consistently using drugs instead of engaging in activities with greater long-term benefit (e.g., work, relationships, school) may be due to sharp devaluing of these delayed rewards relative to the immediate benefits of drug use. Research with humans and animals suggests that relative preference for smaller sooner rewards increases sharply as the receipt of the smaller reward is imminent (Ainslie & Monterosso, 2003; reviewed by Green & Myerson, 2004; Reynolds, 2006). This choice pattern is well described by a hyperbolic discount function and is remarkably consistent with the choice dynamics associated with substance abuse, including switching preference from larger delayed rewards (e.g., academic or vocational pursuits, physical health) to substance use when drugs are immediately available.

Studies have found that college student alcohol abusers (Vuchinich & Simpson, 1998), adult heroin users (Madden et al., 1997; Petry et al., 1998), problem gamblers (Petry, 2001), cocaine users (Heil et al., 2006), and smokers (Bickel et al., 1999) discount delayed monetary rewards more steeply than controls (Bickel & Marsch, 2001). Although delay discounting rates are fairly stable over time (Ohmura, Takahashi, & Kitamura, 2006; Simpson and Vuchinich, 2000a) and are viewed by some as a stable personality variable (Dom, D'haene, & Hulstijn, 2006), the state versus trait nature of discounting remains unresolved (Bickel & Yi, 2006; Field, Santarcangelo, & Sumnall, 2006; Reynolds, 2006), and, as discussed later in this chapter, researchers have begun to identify techniques to extend individual's time horizon (Logue, 2000).

Behavioral Economic Variables that are Relevant to the Assessment and Treatment of Addictive Behaviors

It is important to point out that there have not been comprehensive evaluations of the ability of behavioral economic models of addiction to predict the development, progression, and remission of addictive behavior (Vuchinich & Heather, 2003). Therefore, although the theory's central assumptions are consistent with well-supported principles of economics, behavioral pharmacology, and operant psychology, future research is needed to establish the validity of the overall account of addiction, and in particular the dynamic explanation for how addiction develops and changes (Herrnstein & Prelec, 1992; Rachlin, 1997). However, several of the key elements of behavioral economic theories of addiction have been supported by both laboratory and naturalistic studies and hold promise as a means of improving applied efforts to predict and reduce substance use (Murphy et al., 2005; Tucker et al., 2002, 2006; Vuchinich and Tucker, 1996). The following sections discuss four behavioral economic variables that have demonstrated consistent relations to substance use. After first presenting a brief review of the data supporting the relevance of each variable to substance use, we discuss the implications of each variable for the assessment and treatment of substance abuse. Because several previous reviews have clearly outlined the influence of these variables in laboratory settings (Carroll, 1996; Higgins et al., 2004), we focus primarily on recent applied studies and on the clinical implications of each behavioral economic variable.

Drug Price

As predicted by the law of demand, consumption of most commodities, including alcohol and other psychoactive drugs, is inversely related to price or response requirement (reviewed by DeGrandpre & Bickel, 1996). However, there are cross-commodity (Hursh & Winger, 1995; Jacobs & Bickel, 1999) as well as individual (MacKillop & Murphy, 2007; Murphy & MacKillop, 2006) differences in the relative price-sensitivity or elasticity of consumption. Demand for a reinforcer is unit-elastic when increases in price lead to proportional decreases in consumption (resulting in no change in overall expenditures on that reinforcer) and elastic when increases in price lead to greater-than proportional decreases in consumption (resulting in a reduction in overall expenditures on that reinforcer). Demand for nonessential and/ or luxury items, such as restaurant meals, is generally elastic. Alternatively, demand for a reinforcer is inelastic when increases in price lead to less-than-proportional decreases in consumption, resulting in an increase in overall expenditures on that reinforcer (e.g., demand for home heating oil during a cold winter). It is worth noting that the elasticity of a good may be partially moderated by the income of a consumer. In behavioral terms, income is defined as the total amount money, time, energy, or other resources that can be allocated to various reinforcers. The behavior of consumers with a relatively high income may be less sensitive to price increases than those with relatively low income. Thus, individuals with large amounts of free time (e.g., college students, unemployed adults) are more likely to "spend" large amounts of time procuring and using drugs (Anthony, Warner, & Kessler, 1994; Bickel & DeGrandpre, 1995; Wechsler et al., 1995).

In considering the effects of price on consumption, it is important to note that the behavioral economic definition of price goes beyond the simple monetary cost. Chaloupka and Pacula (2000) provided a comprehensive review of a variety of factors that can influence decisions about smoking, including the monetary costs of purchasing cigarettes, restrictions on where and when people can smoke, the fines and other legal consequences of smoking at unauthorized locations, and awareness of the short- and long-term health risks associated with smoking. More generally, the full price of any good, service, or reinforcer consists of the basic components: (1) monetary cost, (2) time and effort costs, (3) potential legal cost, and (4) potential health cost. Increases in any of these costs can lead to decreases in substance use, and, conversely, lowering the cost can lead to increases (DeGrandpre & Bickel, 1996).

Several laboratory studies have modeled the relationship between price and alcohol consumption. Murphy and MacKillop (2006) used a simulated alcohol purchase task to assess levels of alcohol consumption across a range of prices in a sample of social drinkers. The average number of standard drinks consumed was approximately seven when the price was $0.25 or less per drink, remained at or above five drinks at prices up to $1.50 per drink, and then became more elastic and showed a steady linear decrease as prices increased. Not surprisingly, participants with a history of engaging in heavy episodic drinking were willing to spend more to consume alcohol, demonstrating that individual difference factors such as history of use and dependence can play a role in the demand elasticity of alcohol. A much earlier laboratory study demonstrated that alcohol consumption increases under price manipulations meant to simulate "happy hour" conditions (i.e., much cheaper drinks available during discrete periods of time; Babor, Mendelson, Greenberg, & Kuehnle, 1978). Several other studies have demonstrated that increasing the effort required to obtain a drug (also referred to as response requirement) leads to decreased consumption (Bigelow, Griffiths, & Liebson 1976; Liebson et al., 1971; Van Etten, Higgins, & Bickel, 1995).

An abundance of population-based research also supports the notion that an increase in the monetary price of alcohol leads to decreases in consumption, making demand for alcohol fairly elastic (see Osterberg, 2001, or Chaloupka, Grossman, & Saffer, 2002, for comprehensive reviews). However, recent studies suggest that the relationship between price and consumption is quite complex. An analysis of Swedish alcohol price and sales data collected between 1984 and 1994 (Gruenewald, Ponicki, Holder, & Romelsjo, 2006) confirmed that increases in price led to decreases in consumption for spirits, wine, and beer, but also revealed that increases in price led some consumers to switch to lower-quality (and lower-priced) products so that they could maintain their level of consumption. The authors noted that many nations enact price-based policies as part of their prevention efforts, and that a more complete understanding of how both consumers and manufacturers respond to various forms of price manipulation is needed to optimize their effectiveness in decreasing total consumption.

Clinical Implications

Research on the relationship between price and consumption has been successfully translated into a number of effective intervention strategies. One of the clearest examples is the development of contingency management (CM) procedure to reduce the use of a variety of psychoactive substances. CM has been described as the "systematic application of behavioral consequences for drug use and abstinence" (Higgins, 1999, p. 5). CM procedures have been used effectively to reduce the use of a number of substances, including cigarettes (Correia & Benson, 2006), alcohol (Petry, Martin, Cooney, & Kranzler, 2000), cocaine (Higgins et al., 1993), marijuana (Sigmon et al., 2000), and opiates (Silverman et al., 1996). The conceptual framework for the treatment, which is based on basic operant and behavioral economic research, calls for changes in the user's environment such that (a) drug use and abstinence are readily detected, (b) drug abstinence is readily reinforced, (c) drug use results in a loss of reinforcement, and (d) the density of reinforcement derived from nondrug sources is increased to compete with the reinforcing effects of drug use (Higgins et al., 1991). Thus, one of the active mechanisms of CM is the increased costs (loss of reinforcement) associated with the detection of drug use.

Brief motivational interventions have emerged as an effective strategy for reducing problematic alcohol use among a variety of populations (Hettema, Steele, & Miller, 2006). These interventions tend to target individuals with mild to moderate substance-related problems who may not seek traditional forms of substance abuse treatment such as hospitalization or 12-Step support groups (Zweben & Fleming, 1999). We have previously written on the areas of theoretical and practical overlap between behavioral economics and brief interventions (Henslee, Irons, & Correia, 2007; Murphy et al., 2005). One of the primary goals of brief motivational interventions is to increase the client's motivation to change her substance-related behavior by fostering awareness regarding the costs and consequences of substance use (additional goals include strengthening an individual's beliefs about his ability and commitment to change, and utilizing specific techniques that will facilitate change; Zweben & Fleming, 1999). Although brief interventions do not necessarily increase the actual costs of substance use, they do attempt to make those costs more explicit.

In many brief interventions, including Motivational Enhancement Therapy (DiClemente, 2003) and the Brief Alcohol Screening and Intervention for College Students program (Dimeff, Baer, Kivlahan, & Marlatt, 1999), information about the costs of alcohol is provided to clients in the form of personalized feedback forms. The feedback form typically includes normative information about how a client's beliefs about alcohol use, and her drinking practices, compared to actual drinking behavior in the general population or on campus. Personalized feedback often includes a review of information about estimated blood alcohol content on a typical or heavy night of alcohol use, which can highlight potential legal and health costs. A review of relevant risk factors for the development of longer-term drinking problems, and of the frequency and severity of previously experienced alcohol-related consequences, is also a component of many feedback forms. Finally, some brief interventions incorporate a decisional balance exercise designed to highlight both the positive and negative effects of substance use. All of these strategies encourage clients to consider the total costs of substance use, relative to the overall benefits, and are designed to motivate self-regulation and more informed decision making (DiClemente, 2003).

There are a number of rather simple ways that clients and therapists can work to increase the costs of substance use. Stimulus control, which entails avoiding stimuli that elicit a problem behavior, can be achieved by removing triggers from the environment (Prochaska & Norcross, 2007). From a behavioral economic perspective, removing all cigarettes and ashtrays from the home not only removes powerful triggers but also increases the effort costs associated with obtaining new cigarettes. Various forms of monitoring can also be used to increase the costs of substance use, and the increasing availability of low-cost point-of-contact drug testing kits make their use much more feasible in both clinical and nonclinical settings. Having to submit to occasional drug testing for employers, parole officers, spouses, or parents can increase the legal costs of substance use and provide an opportunity to arrange positive contingencies for abstinence and explicit costs for substance use. Parental monitoring can also foster a greater awareness of the tangible costs of substance use among children and adolescents. An evaluation of a communitywide adolescent alcohol prevention program revealed that a adolescent's awareness of the specific costs of alcohol use (e.g., my family has rules against young people drinking alcohol, my parents have told me what would happen if I were caught drinking alcohol) were predictive of successful outcomes, whereas discussion about more general and potentially distal effects of alcohol (my parents talk with me about problems alcohol can cause young people) did not contribute to outcomes (Komro, Perry, Williams, Farbakhsh,

& Veblen-Mortenson, 2001). Indeed, research on basic decision making suggests that immediate consequences are more likely to influence behavior than more distal consequences such as potential declines in health (Bickel and Marsch, 2000).

Drug-Free Reinforcement

Several laboratory paradigms have been used to demonstrate a relationship between the reinforcing effects of drugs and the presence of substance-free alternative reinforcers. The dependent variable is typically a measure of drug use preference, such as the amount of the drug consumed, the amount of effort devoted to obtaining a drug, or the number of times drug use is chosen over an alternative reinforcer (Bickel et al., 1995; Campbell & Carroll, 2000; Higgins et al., 2004). Independent variables involve manipulations of the availability, magnitude, and delay associated with an alternative reinforcer. The relationship has been studied across a wide range of drugs, including cigarettes (Roll, Reilly, & Johanson, 2000), alcohol (Little & Correia, 2006; Vuchinich & Tucker, 1983), cocaine (Hart, Haney, Foltin, & Fischman, 2000; Higgins, Roll, & Bickel, 1996), and heroin (Comer et al., 1998). Across these laboratory studies, participants generally showed a greater preference for drug use when the value of the alternative reinforcer was small, the alternative reinforcer was delayed, or when the price of the alternative reinforcer was increased. In summarizing the literature on drug use and alternative reinforcers, Vuchinich and Tucker (1988) concluded that drug use may emerge as a highly preferred activity when constraints on psychoactive substances are minimal and alternative reinforcers are either sparse or constraints on their access make them difficult to acquire (see Higgins, Heil, & Lussier, 2004, for a more recent review).

A growing literature has also documented the relationship between drug use and alternative reinforcers in the natural environment. Several of these studies have used measures of behavioral allocation, such as the Pleasant Events Schedule (PES; MacPhillamy & Lewinsohn, 1976) to measure engagement in a range of potentially reinforcing activities. Van Etten, Higgins, Budney, and Badger (1998) used the PES to compare the density of naturally occurring positive substance-free reinforcement experienced by cocaine abusers to the density experienced by a matched control group. Cocaine abusers reported a lower frequency of engagement in nonsocial, introverted, passive outdoor, and mood-related activities relative to the control group. Similar findings were reported in a study of college student binge drinkers (Correia, Carey, Simons, & Borsari, 2003). Relative to the comparison group of lighter-drinking undergraduates, students who engaged in frequent binge drinking derived less reinforcement from a variety of substance-free activities. Other recent studies applying a behavioral framework to college student drinking in the natural environment have demonstrated that the frequency, quantity, and negative consequences of alcohol use are predicted by the amount of reinforcement derived from drug-free activities (e.g., school work, relationships, employment; Correia, Carey, & Borsari, 2002; Correia, Simons, Carey, & Borsari, 1998); that substance-free reinforcement is associated with increased motivation to change alcohol use (Murphy, Barnett, Goldstein, & Colby, 2007); that increases in substance-free activities such as exercise can lead to decreases in substance use (Correia, Benson, & Carey, 2005); and that reduced drinking following a brief motivational intervention is associated with an increase in substance-free reinforcement (Murphy et al., 2005). One study found that, among college students, the inverse relationship between substance-free reinforcement and substance use held only for women, perhaps because college men are especially reliant on drinking as a means of social facilitation (Murphy, Barnett, & Colby, 2006; Murphy et al., 2007).

Clinical Implications

With regard to the assessment of addictive behaviors, Murphy and Vuchinich (2002) suggest that a primary implication of behavioral economics is to assess activities and domains outside of substance use, inasmuch as access to and utilization of potentially reinforcing alternative activities are predictive of alcohol consumption and therefore an important treatment target. Several reinforcement surveys, such as the revised PES (Pleasant Events Schedule; MacPhillamy & Lewinsohn, 1982; see also Correia, Carey, & Borsari, 2002) or the revised Adolescent Reinforcement Survey Schedule (ARSS; Murphy et al., 2005) have been used to identify rewarding substance-free reinforcers. These surveys measure the frequency and subjective pleasure of potentially reinforcing events and activities. The data could be used to help clients identify activities that are highly pleasurable but engaged in infrequently, and behavioral activation strategies could then be used to increase engagement in these targeted behaviors (Lejuez, Hopko, & Hopko, 2001). Alternatively, people with very few or no highly pleasurable activities could benefit from social skills training and treatment programs that expose them to novel sources of reinforcement, such as activity-oriented groups (i.e., ceramics, hiking). This type of information, if presented early in treatment, may help motivate clients who are reluctant to give up the reinforcement derived from drug use by making them more aware of underutilized substance-free sources of reinforcement.

The basic research reviewed above has spawned several treatment approaches that explicitly target substance-free reinforcement. An early application, termed the Community Reinforcement Approach (CRA), was implemented to treat alcoholics admitted to a public hospital for inpatient treatment (Hunt & Azrin, 1973). The CRA continues to be used to treat clients who abuse alcohol (Smith, Meyers, & Delaney, 1998), marijuana (Diamond et al., 2002), cocaine (NIDA manual), opiates (Bickel, Amass, Higgins, Badger, & Esh, 1997), and cigarettes (Roozen et al., 2006). According to Smith and Meyers (1995), "CRA acknowledges the powerful role of environmental contingencies in encouraging or discouraging drinking, and attempts to rearrange these contingencies such that sober behavior is more rewarding than drinking behavior (p. 251)." In the original Hunt and Azrin (1973) study, CRA participants were provided with counseling designed to improve employment prospects, marital and family relationships, and nondrinking social and recreational interactions. Some CRA participants with limited financial resources were provided with radios or televisions, subscriptions to local newspapers, telephones, and fees to obtain a driver's license. These goods and services were provided to help clients access alternative sources of reinforcement by providing entertainment, or facilitating communication with employers and social partners. More recent approaches have been expanded to include a stronger family therapy component (e.g., Meyers, Miller, Hill, & Tonigan, 1998), or abstinent contingent incentives or vouchers (e.g., Higgins et al., 2003). A recent meta-analysis concluded that CRA is more effective than usual care, and that the addition of incentives for abstinence leads to improved outcomes (Roozen et al., 2003).

We have already discussed the use of CM to provide an immediate tangible cost for substance use (i.e., the loss of a voucher incentive). In addition to this direct contingency on drug use, CM approaches attempt to increase alternatives by ensuring that the vouchers are exchanged for goods or services that support constructive substance-free activities (e.g., tuition for vocational training, sporting equipment, movie tickets; Higgins, 1993; Higgins et al., 2004). A study with opioid-dependent patients demonstrated that CM can also be effective when vouchers are used to directly reinforce engagement in substance-free activities that are consistent with treatment goals (Iguchi et al., 1997). Participants were randomly assigned to one of three treatment conditions: urinalysis-based reinforcement (UA), treatment-plan-based reinforcement condition (TP), and standard care (STD). Participants in the UA and TP conditions could earn vouchers, described as treatment assistance coupons, redeemable for expenses linked to a treatment plan (i.e., clothing for job interview). Participants in the UA condition earned vouchers for opioid-negative urine specimens. Vouchers were awarded to the TP participants for meeting objectively defined and clearly verifiable treatment plan tasks. For example, vouchers could be earned for obtaining paperwork regarding job training courses.

In each case, treatment plan tasks were individually tailored for each client, and vouchers were used to shape behavior toward long-range treatment goals. Standard care consisted of counseling sessions and a system of privilege levels for take-home medication eligibility. Results indicated that participants in the TP conditions demonstrated significant improvement in abstinence rates over the course of the study. Despite the fact that only the UA participants were directly reinforced for abstaining, the TP condition participants were more than twice as likely to produce negative urine specimens, highlighting the importance of reinforcing drug-free alternatives. Note that gains were maintained six weeks after the discontinuation of the treatment program. These results support the notion that clients who are brought into contact with drug-free reinforcers occurring naturally in their environment are most likely to maintain behavioral changes after removal of the experimental contingencies. However, because a more recent study (Petry et al., 2006) reported that reinforcing goal-related activities was not as efficacious in decreasing drug use as directly reinforcing abstinence, additional research is needed to determine the most effective strategies for simultaneously decreasing drug use and increasing engagement in drug-free activities.

The Therapeutic Workplace, developed by Kenneth Silverman and colleagues (Silverman, Svikis, Robles, Stitzer, & Bigelow, 2001; Silverman et al., 2002) is another example of a CM treatment approach that directly targets engagement in drug-free activities. In one series of studies, drug-abusing pregnant and postpartum women are able to earn a livable wage by working and/or acquiring job skills related to data entry. Each day, when a participant reports to the workplace, she is required to provide a urine sample, and if the sample is drug-free, she is allowed to work that day. After completing a three-hour work shift, she receives a payment voucher. A recent 3-year outcome study demonstrated the effectiveness of the Therapeutic Workplace with pregnant and postpartum women (Silverman et al., 2002), and research with homeless alcoholics is underway (Wong et al., 2005).

Several treatment approaches that were not developed within the behavioral economic framework nevertheless highlight the various ways in which substance-free reinforcers can be developed and used to reduce drug use. For example, several treatment approaches focus on the development of substance-free coping and social skills (Carroll, 1996; Marlatt & Gordon, 1985; Monti, Rohsenow, Colby, & Abrams, 1995). These approaches are designed to address basic skill deficits that prevent clients from adequately coping with emotions and deriving satisfaction from a social-interpersonal situations at work, with friends, and with significant others. By building better interpersonal skill and improving skills for dealing with stressful life events, the treatment aims to increase positive and decrease negative social interactions. One specific example of a well-articulated and evaluated skills-based approach is the Coping Skills Training (CST) program developed by Peter Monti and colleagues (Monti, Rohsenow, Colby, & Abrams, 1995). CST modules include delivering positive and negative feedback, listening skills, conversation skills, developing a sober support network, and assertiveness training. Behavioral activation therapy (e.g., Lejuez, Hopko, & Hopko, 2001) also promotes the development of skills to promote engagement in substance-free reinforcers. Although originally intended to treat depression, behavioral activation has recently been applied to substance use disorders (Daughters et al., 2008). From a behavioral economic perspective the CST and behavioral activation serve to decrease the reinforcing value of drug use by increasing the reinforcing value of substance-free social interactions and activities. Both treatments have been effectively used to reduce alcohol and cocaine use in range of patient populations (e.g., Daughters et al., 2007; Monti, Kadden, Rohsenow, Cooney, & Abrams, 2002; Rohsenow et al., 2004).

O'Farrell and Fals-Stewart (2000) developed a behavioral couples therapy for drug and alcohol abuse. The treatment assumes that drug-abusing patients are less likely to relapse when they are involved in happy and cohesive relationships, and one of the explicit goals is to help every member of the family experience reinforcement in an environment that supports abstinence. Daily sobriety contracts and ingestion of Antabuse® (when indicated) are acknowledged and verbally reinforced by the spouse. Other assignments, such as "Catch Your Partner Doing Something Nice" and "Shared Rewarding Activities" are designed to involve the couple in rewarding drug-free activities and increase the rate of reinforcement derived from behaviors aimed at improving the couple's day-to-day interactions. Behavioral couples therapy has been effective with both male and female drug-abuses (Fals-Stewart, O'Farrell, & Birchler, 2004), and a brief version has also shown promise as an effective intervention (Fals-Stewart, Klostermann, Yates, O'Farrell, & Birchler, 2005).

Relative Reinforcement Value

Behavioral economic theory views addiction as an acquired state in which the relative reinforcement from substance use remains high compared to other available reinforcers, despite the negative physical and psychosocial consequences of continued use (Ainslie & Monterusso, 2003; Bickel et al., 2000; Herrnstein & Prelec, 1992; Rachlin, 1997, 2000; Vuchinich & Tucker, 1988, 1996). In laboratory settings, the relative reinforcing value (RRV) of drugs is generally measured by the levels of operant responding for a drug, the quantity of the drug and drug-free reinforcer earned or consumed during the session, or the proportional response rate toward drugs (Bickel et al. 2000; Hursh & Winger, 1995; MacKillop & Murphy, 2007). Herrnstein's (1970) matching law ($\log B_1/B_2 = a \log r_1/r_2 + \log c$), for example, states that the proportional resource allocation directed toward available activities (B_1/B_2) equals the proportion of reinforcement obtained from the activities (r_1/r_2). The a and c parameters reflect sensitivity to reinforcement frequency and bias for one or the other alternative, respectively.

The matching law has accurately predicted choice in numerous laboratory studies involving a variety of species and reinforcers (Mazur, 1991), including studies examining drug administration (Anderson & Woolverton, 2000). RRV measures that plot the sensitivity of drug consumption and drug-reinforced responding to increases in price (demand curves) have also been used to predict the abuse liability of drugs (Hursh & Winger, 1995). Despite a strong empirical and theoretical foundation there has been relatively little translation of the existing experimental measures of RRV into clinical contexts. The lack of translational research is regrettably common in behavioral science (Onken & Bootzin, 1998; National Advisory Mental Health Council Behavioral Science Workgroup, 2000) and is unfortunate in this case because these measures might provide unique information on strength of preference for drugs that cannot be gleaned from existing measures (Murphy et al., 2007; Murphy & Mackillop, 2006; Tucker et al., 2006).

There are several measures of RRV that can be administered to human participants in clinical settings, and some recent studies provide initial support for the validity of these novel measures of substance abuse problem severity. Tucker and colleagues (2002, 2006) developed a measure of RRV based on proportional discretionary monetary expenditures to alcohol. Their discretionary expenditure measure, which is modeled after laboratory paradigms that consider response output and consumption as distinct facets of RRV (Bickel et al., 2000), is based on the premise that alcohol is a more valued reinforcer for an individual who allocates 45% of her expenditures to alcohol consumption than it would be for an individual who allocates only 10% of her expenditures to alcohol consumption, even if these individuals had similar alcohol consumption levels. In two studies of natural recovery from alcohol dependence, Tucker et al. (2002, 2006) assessed the proportion of discretionary income allocated to alcohol in alcohol dependent individuals prior to a quit attempt. The results indicated that relative resource allocation to alcohol predicted drinking outcomes whereas traditional measures of consumption and dependence did not. Participants who relapsed within the two-year follow-up period allocated a greater proportion of their money to alcohol in the year prior to the attempted resolution, even though their levels of alcohol consumption and problems during this period were similar to resolved participants. Thus, consistent with behavioral economic predictions, RRV measures based on resource allocation appear to have utility in predicting clinically relevant changes in drinking.

Another way to measure reinforcement is to assess the frequency of specific, rewarding activities. Reinforcement surveys such as the Pleasant Events Schedule (PES; MacPhillamy & Lewinsohn, 1982) and the ARSS (Adolescent Reinforcement Survey Schedule; Holmes et al., 1991) measure the frequency of participation in, and subjective enjoyment derived from, various activities (e.g., eating good meals, meeting someone new, gardening, etc.). The cross product of the frequency and enjoyment ratings provides an approximation of obtained reinforcement (e.g., the sum of recent time spent in enjoyable activities; Correia & Carey, 1999; Murphy et al., 2005). Participants make two sets of frequency and enjoyment ratings for each item: one for drug-free activities and one for activities that take place while using drugs or alcohol (Correia et al., 1998). The substance-related reinforcement score is a measure of drug-related enhancement of other activities (e.g., socializing while high) rather than a direct index of the reinforcing effects of drug use (e.g., sedation, euphoria). The substance-free cross-product score provides an index of substance-free reinforcement. The primary score derived from the modified reinforcement surveys is the ratio of substance-related reinforcement to total reinforcement; an index of the RRV of substance use. Correia and colleagues derived this index from Herrnstein's (1970) matching law: Substance-Related Reinforcement/(Substance-Free Reinforcement + Substance-Related Reinforcement). Cross-sectional studies with college drinkers (Correia, Simons, Carey, & Borsari, 1998) and psychiatric patients (Correia & Carey, 1999) demonstrated that the ratio measure predicted unique variance in drinking quantity beyond the effect of substance-related reinforcement alone.

Another study examined whether this reinforcement survey measure of RRV was related (prospectively) to drinking outcomes among heavy-drinking college students who completed a brief alcohol intervention (Murphy et al., 2005). Only women showed a significant reduction in drinking at the six-month follow-up, and RRV accounted for unique variance in their drinking outcomes. Women who derived a smaller proportion of their total reinforcement from substance use at baseline reported lower levels of follow-up drinking, even after controlling for their baseline drinking level. Thus, individuals who have a number of enjoyable alternatives to drinking may have an easier time reducing their consumption following an intervention (see also Tucker et al., 2006). Men and women who reduced their drinking by at least five drinks per week showed increased proportional reinforcement from substance-free activities at follow-up, which suggests that successful drinking reductions are associated with more global changes in lifestyle and activity participation (Tucker, 1999; Vuchinich & Tucker, 1996).

Another analysis from this treatment trial examined a reinforcement measure derived from a hypothetical alcohol purchase task wherein participants report the number of drinks they would purchase across 14 different prices (0–$13.00; MacKillop & Murphy, 2007). Reported consumption and expenditures are plotted as a function of price (demand curves), which are in turn used to generate several indices of RRV (Hursh & Winger, 1995; Jacobs & Bickel, 1999), such as maximum level of alcohol consumption at low cost (intensity of demand), maximum level of alcohol expenditure (O_{max}), and several measures that reflect the degree to which consumption decreases with increasing price (breakpoint, P_{max}, and elasticity of demand; Bickel et al., 2000). As hypothesized, a number of the facets of reinforcement predicted weekly alcohol consumption and heavy drinking at the six-month postintervention follow-up assessment. Participants who at baseline reported greater maximum expenditure (i.e., O_{max}) for alcohol and lower price sensitivity (i.e., breakpoint, P_{max}, and elasticity) reported greater follow-up weekly drinking (MacKillop & Murphy, 2007). Little and Correia (2006) provided further evidence for the construct validity and potential utility of self-report reinforcement measures that utilize hypothetical alcohol purchases. Hypothetical alcohol purchases on the Multiple Choice Procedure (Griffiths, Rush, & Puhala, 1996) were significantly correlated with measures of alcohol consumption and problems and with a laboratory paradigm that included real choices between alcohol and monetary amounts. Another recent study found that RRV measures derived from hypothetical cigarette demand curves demonstrated significant associations with smoking and nicotine dependence (MacKillop et al., 2008). Thus, RRV measures that are based on simulated drug purchases appear to be valid and to show meaningful relations to real world patterns of substance use and problems.

Clinical Implications

Behavioral economic indices of RRV are consistent with well-established laboratory paradigms for determining reinforcer value (Anderson & Woolverton, 2000; Bickel et al., 2000) and provide unique information about the value or strength of preference for substance use that is not typically included in clinical or applied research contexts. Existing substance abuse measures provide important information on consumption levels and the immediate risks and harmful effects of drinking/drug use, but they do not describe the relative prominence of substance use in an individual's overall lifestyle or the amount of resources allocated to substance use, which may be more predictive of the course of substance use over time (Murphy et al., 2007; Tucker et al., 2006). Proportional reinforcement from substance use relative to substance-free activities operationalizes an important feature of substance misuse: devoting considerable time/resources to substance use and neglecting other important activities. This concept is included in the *DSM–IV* dependence criteria, but is not explicitly measured in traditional substance use assessment batteries (Tucker, Vuchinich, & Murphy, 2002). RRV may be an especially useful means of discriminating between individuals with similar substance use patterns, but different levels of risk (and need for treatment) based on their overall pattern of behavioral allocation/reinforcement (Murphy et al., 2005). For an individual who engages in a number of reinforcing activities other than substance use, an addictive behavior pattern may change relatively easily in response to a brief intervention or life event (Miller & Rollnick, 2002; Tucker, 1999), a change that would be facilitated by a reallocation of behavior toward already established reinforcing activities (e.g., educational pursuits, a rewarding relationship or hobby). If substance use accounts for a large proportion of total reinforcement, conversely, and there are few valued alternatives, more intensive interventions such as CM or CRA might be necessary to increase drug-free sources of reinforcement (e.g., Higgins et al., 2004; Higgins & Silverman, 1999).

In addition to assessing substance abuse problem severity, RRV measures might also be used as motivational feedback that demonstrates the client's reliance on substance use relative to other activities. For clients with harm reduction goals, RRV might be measured repeatedly as an index of progress toward reducing the relative reliance on drug-related reinforcement. Given that RRV has only recently been translated into naturalistic measures, however, more research is needed to establish its clinical utility and to develop practical assessment tools (Murphy & Vuchinich, 2002). In the meantime, clinicians interested in measuring RRV could adopt one of the approaches described above. The PES and ARSS, for example, have been validated with several populations and can be easily modified to generate separate substance-related and substance-free subscores. Similar information could also be derived from activity logs or time allocation diaries, both of which are commonly used as part of behavioral approaches to treating addiction (Vuchinich et al., 1988; Murphy & Vuchinich, 2002).

Delay Discounting

Impulsivity is included in the *DSM–IV* criteria for a number of disorders and has been implicated as a symptom or correlate of a wide range of problematic behaviors, including antisocial and borderline personality disorders; bipolar disorder, depression, and suicide; ADHD and conduct disorder; substance abuse; gambling and excessive spending; binge eating and failure to exercise; and aggressive, delinquent, and criminal behaviors (Bickel & Marsch, 2001; Evenden, 1999; Moeller et al., 2001). Behavioral economic researchers measure impulsivity with an operant model that quantifies individuals' relative preference between larger delayed and smaller sooner rewards (Green & Myerson, 2004; Reynolds et al., 2006). Although the value of all rewards decreases as their receipt is delayed (i.e., delay discounting), there are substantial individual differences in the degree that delayed rewards are discounted, and this discounting phenomenon may be a core feature of substance abuse (Bickel & Marsch, 2001; Vuchinich & Simpson, 1998). That is, consistently using drugs instead of engaging in activities with greater long-term benefit (e.g., work, relationships, school) may be due to sharp devaluing of these delayed rewards relative to the immediate benefits of drug use.

Research with humans and animals suggests that relative preference for smaller sooner rewards increases sharply as the receipt of the smaller reward is imminent (Ainslie & Monterosso, 2003; reviewed by Green & Myerson, 2004). This choice pattern is well described by a hyperbolic discount function and is remarkably consistent with the choice dynamics associated with substance abuse, including switching preference from larger delayed rewards (e.g., academic or vocational pursuits, physical health) to substance use when drugs are immediately available (Ainslie & Monterosso, 2003). Studies have found that substance abusers discount delayed monetary rewards more steeply than controls (Bickel & Marsch, 2001), that delay discounting predicts the acquisition of drug administration in rats (Perry et al., 2005), and that delay discounting may increase in response to acute intoxication (Reynolds et al., 2006, but see also de Wit et al., 2002) and withdrawal (Field et al., 2006; Giordano et al., 2002). Thus, delay discounting may be a central mechanism by which individuals make seemingly irrational decisions to use drugs despite the myriad physical, social, and legal risks (Bickel & Marsch, 2001).

Clinical Implications

A primary clinical implication of the delay discounting literature is that substance abusers are less sensitive to the delayed rewards that might substitute for drug use (e.g., employment, relationships, physical health) and the delayed costs of substance use (e.g., physical, occupation, psychological, and social impairment, legal repercussions). Whenever feasible, interventions should try to increase the immediacy of the reinforcers associated with abstinence and the aversive consequences associated with drug use. Indeed, efficacious interventions such as CRA, CM, and Antabuse® do just that (Higgins et al., 2004). Although in many clinical contexts it may not be feasible for the clinician to directly manipulate the immediacy of these outcomes associated with substance use and abstinence, less intensive approaches, such as behavioral couples therapy (Fals-Stewart, Klostermann, Yates, O'Farrell, & Birchler, 2005), may be able to achieve a similar restructuring of contingencies.

Short of reducing the delay to alternatives or establishing immediate consequences for drug use, interventions might attempt to counteract sharp discounting by increasing the salience of delayed outcomes. Indeed, several authors have pointed out that many of the important larger delayed rewards that would compete with substance abuse are diffuse and abstract outcomes that occur over extended periods of time (e.g., health, relationship satisfaction, career success;

Correia, 2004; Simpson & Vuchinich, 2000b; Vuchinich & Tucker, 1996). Logue (2000) suggested a technique wherein people are taught to analyze a choice situation in terms of all of the possible costs and benefits associated with each possible outcome, including what opportunities may be lost through making a particular choice (i.e., opportunity cost). Similarly, the decisional balance exercise, often used in cognitive-behavioral and motivational interventions, may help clients to consider the full range of negative and positive consequences of their behaviors (Miller & Rollnick, 2002). The exercise follows from the notion that a behavior will change when the perceived costs of the behavior begin to outweigh the perceived benefits. Personalized feedback about the health risks, financial costs, and negative consequences associated with an addictive behavior pattern might also help to increase the salience of the delayed outcomes associated with substance abuse and is often combined with the aforementioned motivational enhancement exercises (Marlatt et al., 1998; Miller & Rollnick, 2002; Murphy et al., 2001). Indeed, personalized feedback appears to be one of the key ingredients of successful brief interventions for substance abuse (Lewis and Neighbors, 2006). The goals of feedback-based interventions are consistent with basic behavioral economic research suggesting that self-control choices are more likely when behavior is seen as part of a cohesive pattern, rather than a discrete choice (Heyman & Dunn, 2002; Rachlin, 1995; Simpson & Vuchinich, 2000b). For example, after learning that you have high cholesterol the decision to eat a bacon cheeseburger versus a turkey sandwich becomes part of a general pattern of behavior related to the goal of reducing cholesterol rather than a discrete decision related to preference.

Basic research on delay discounting has identified another potential strategy for reducing substance abusers' tendency to devalue delayed outcomes. As described earlier, humans and animals make choices between larger delayed and smaller immediate rewards in a manner that is well described by a hyperbolic decay function (Green & Myerson, 2004). Larger more delayed rewards may be preferred over smaller sooner rewards when both are delayed, but when receipt of the smaller sooner reward is imminent, preference switches and the smaller reward is selected over the larger delayed reward. Consider, for example, an individual who decides that physical fitness is more important than sleeping late, and thus makes the decision the night before to exercise in the morning, only to switch preference to sleep the next morning when the opportunity to sleep is immediately available. However, if given the opportunity, humans and animals will often elect to "precommit" to the self-control choice (larger reward), by, for example, pressing a lever that eliminates the later opportunity to select the smaller immediate reward (Monterosso & Ainslie, 1999; Siegal & Rachlin, 1995). This laboratory observation is consistent with common behavioral strategies that attempt to circumvent delay discounting by removing the possibility of making an impulsive choice. The would-be exerciser described above, for example, might set his alarm clock for 6:00AM and arrange to meet with a running partner at 6:30AM as a means of "precommitting" and reducing the possibility of switching preference to the smaller reward (sleep). Other common precommitment strategies relevant to addiction include avoiding places where alcohol and drugs are available, throwing out cigarettes in preparation for a quit attempt, and taking Antabuse® or agonists that block the reinforcing effects of drugs (e.g., Buprenorphine, Naltrexone; Swift, 2003). Clinicians should encourage such commitment strategies, especially among clients who are motivated to abstain, but have a history of impulsive relapse episodes.

Conclusions

We have attempted to provide an introduction to behavioral economic approaches to studying addiction, and in particular to highlight the implications for the assessment and treatment of addictive behaviors. Interestingly, the reader may find the ideas presented herein to be a juxtaposition of the old and the new; although behavioral economics incorporates familiar concepts such as the law of demand and reinforcement that are supported by decades of empirical and theoretical work within mircoeconomics and operant psychology, the synthesis of these disciplines and application to a complex behavioral problem such as addiction is new, and has generated a flurry of empirical activity over the past 5 to 10 years. Although there is little doubt that variables such as price, alternatives, and reward delay influence decisions about drug use and other clinically relevant behaviors, an important goal for future research is to continue the process of translating these theoretical and laboratory concepts so that they can contribute to efforts to understand and treat addiction.

References

Ainslie, G., & Monterosso, J. (2003). Hyperbolic discounting as a factor in addiction: A critical analysis. In R. E. Vuchinich, & B. N. Heather (Eds.), *Choice, behavioral economics, and addiction.* (pp. 35–61) Oxford: Elsevier.

Anderson, K. G., & Woolverton, W. L. (2000). Concurrent variable-interval drug self-administration and the generalized matching law: A drug-class comparison. *Behavioral Pharmacology, 11,* 413–420.

Anthony, J. C., Warner, L. A., & Kessler, R. C. (1994). Comparative epidemiology of dependence on tobacco, alcohol, controlled substances, and inhalants: Basic findings from the national comorbidity survey. *Experimental and clinical psychopharmacology, 2,* 244–268.

Becker, G. S., & Murphy, K. M. (1988). A theory of rational addiction. *Journal of Political Economy, 96,* 675–700.

Bickel, W. K., Amass, L., Higgins, S. T., Badger, G. J., & Esch, R. A. (1997). Effects of adding behavioral treatment to opioid detoxification with buprenorphine. *Journal of Consulting and Clinical Psychology, 65,* 803–810.

Bickel, W. K., & DeGrandpre, R. J. (1995). Price and alternatives: Suggestions for drug policy from psychology. *The International Journal of drug policy, 6* (2) 93–105.

Bickel, W. K., DeGrandpre, R. J., & Higgins, S. T. (1995). The behavioral economics of concurrent drug reinforcers: A review and reanalysis of drug self-administration research. *Psychopharmacology, 118,* 250–259.

Bickel, W. K., Madden, G. J., & Petry, N. M. (1998). The price of change: The behavioral economics of drug consumption. *Behavior Therapy, 29,* 545–565.

Bickel, W. K., & Marsch, L. A. (2000). The tyranny of small decisions: Origins, outcomes, and proposed solutions. In W. K. Bickel & R. E. Vuchinich (Eds.), *Reframing health behavior change with behavioral economics* (pp. 341–392). Mahwah, NJ: Lawrence Erlbaum.

Bickel, W. K., & Marsch, L. (2001). Toward a behavioral economic understanding of drug dependence: Delay discounting processes. *Addiction, 96,* 73–86.

Bickel. W. K, Marsch, L. A., & Carroll, M. E. (2000). Deconstructing relative reinforcing efficacy and situating the measures of pharmacological reinforcement with behavioral economics: A theoretical proposal. *Psychopharmacology, 153,* 44–56.

Bickel, W. K., Odum, A. L., & Madden, G. J. (1999). Impulsivity and cigarette smoking: Delay discounting in current, never, and ex-smokers. *Psychopharmacology, 146,* 447–454.

Bickel, W. K., & Yi, R. (2006). What came first? Comment on Dom et al. (2006). *Addiction, 101,* 291–292.

Bigelow, G. E., Griffiths, R. R., & Liebson, I. A. (1976). Effects of response requirement upon human sedative self-administration and drug-seeking behavior. *Pharmacology Biochemistry & Behavior, 5,* 681–685.

Borsari, B. E., & Carey, K. B. (1999). Understanding fraternity drinking: Five recurring themes in the literature, 1980–1998. *Journal of American College Health, 48,* 30–37.

Budney, A. J., & Higgins, S. T. (1998). *A community reinforcement approach plus vouchers approach: Treating cocaine addiction, NIDA Therapy Manuals for Drug Addiction.* NIH publication no. 98-4309, Washington DC.

Campbell, U.C., & Carroll, K.E. (2000). Acquisition of drug self-administration: Environmental and pharmacological interventions. *Experimental and Clinical Psychology, 8,* 312–325.

Carroll, M. E. (1996). Reducing drug abuse by enriching the environment with alternative non- drug reinforcers. In J. Kagel & L. Green (Eds.), *Advances in behavioral economics* (Vol. 3, pp. 37–68). Norwood, NJ: Ablex.

Carroll, M. E. (1999). Income alters the relative reinforcing effects of drug and nondrug reinforcers. In F. J. Chaloupka, M. Grossman, W. K. Bickel, & H. Safer (Eds.), *The economic analysis of substance use and abuse: An integration of econometric and behavioral economic research* (pp. 311–326). Chicago: University of Chicago Press.

Chaloupka, F. J., Grossman, M., & Saffer, H. (2002). The effects of price on alcohol consumption and alcohol-related problems. *Alcohol Research and Health, 26,* 22–34.

Chaloupka, F. J., & Pacula, R. L. (2000). Economics and antihealth behavior: The economic analysis of substance use and abuse. In W. K. Bickel & R. E. Vuchinich (Eds.), *Reframing health behavior change with behavioral economics* (pp. 89–114). Mahwah, NJ: Lawrence Erlbaum.

Cohen, L. M., Britt, D. M., & Collins, F. L. (1999). Chewing gum affects smoking topography. *Experimental and Clinical Psychopharmacology, 7,* 444–447.

Comer, S. D., Collins, E. D., Wilson, S. T., Donovan, M., Foltin, R. W., & Fischman, M. W. (1998). Effects of an alternative reinforcer on intravenous heroin self-administration by humans. *European Journal of Pharmacology, 345,* 13–26.

Correia, C. J. (2004). Behavioral economics: Basic concepts and clinical applications. In W. M. Cox & E. Klinger (Eds.), *Handbook of motivational counseling.* West Sussex, England: Wiley.

Correia, C. J., & Benson, T. A. (2006). The use of contingency management to reduce cigarette smoking among college students. *Experimental and Clinical Psychopharmacology, 14,* 171–179.

Correia, C. J., Benson, T., & Carey, K. B. (2005). Decreased substance use following increases in alternative behaviors: A preliminary investigation. *Addictive Behaviors, 30,* 19–27.

Correia, C. J., & Carey, K. B. (1999). Applying behavioral theories of choice to substance use in a sample of psychiatric outpatients. *Psychology of Addictive Behaviors, 134,* 207–212.

Correia, C. J., Carey, K. B., & Borsari, B. (2002). Measuring substance-free and substance-related reinforcement in the natural environment. *Psychology of Addictive Behaviors, 16,* 28–34.

Correia, C. J., Carey, K. B., Simons, J., & Borsari, B. E. (2003). Relationships between binge drinking and substance-free reinforcement in a sample of college students: A preliminary investigation. *Addictive Behaviors, 28,* 361–368.

Correia, C. J., Simons, J., Carey, K. B., & Borsari, B. E. (1998). Predicting drug abuse: Application of behavioral theories of choice. *Addictive Behaviors, 23,* 705–709.

Cox, W. M., & Klinger, E. (2004). *Handbook of motivational counseling: Concepts, approaches, and assessment.* West Sussex, England: Wiley.

Daughters, S. B., Braun, A. R., Sargeant, M. N., Reynolds, E. R., Hopko, D., Blanco, C., et al. (2008). Effectiveness of a brief behavioral treatment for inner-city illicit drug users with elevated depressive symptoms: The Life Enhancement Treatment for Substance Use (LETS ACT!). *The Journal of Clinical Psychiatry, 69,* 122–129.

DeGrandpre, R. J., & Bickel, W. K. (1996). Drug dependence as consumer demand. In L. Green & J. Kagel (Eds.), *Advances in behavioral economics* (Vol. 3, pp. 1–36). Norwood, NJ: Ablex.

Del Boca, F. K., Darkes, J., Greenbaum, P. E., & Goldman, M. S. (2004). Up close and personal: Temporal variability in the drinking of individual college students during their first year. *Journal of Consulting and Clinical Psychology, 72,* 155–164.

Diamond, G., Godley, S. H., Liddle, H. A., Sampl, S., Webb, C., Tims, F. M., et al. (2002). Five outpatient treatment models for adolescent marijuana use: A description of the Cannabis Youth Treatment Interventions. *Addiction, 97,* 70–83.

DiClemente, C. C. (2003) *Addiction and change*. New York: Guilford.

Dimeff, L. A., Baer, J. S., Kivlahan, D. R., & Marlatt, G. A. (1999). *Brief alcohol screening and interventions for college students: A harm reduction approach*. New York: Guilford Press.

Dom, G., D'haene, P., & Hulstijn, W. (2006). Impulsivity in abstinent early- and late-onset alcoholics: Differences in self-report measures and a discounting task. *Addiction, 101,* 50–59.

Dowdall, G. W., & Wechsler, H. (2002). Studying college alcohol use: Widening the lens, sharpening the focus. *Journal of Studies on Alcohol,* (Suppl. 14), 14–22.

Evenden, J. L. (1999). Varieties of impulsivity. *Psychopharmacology, 146,* 348–361.

Fals-Stewart, W., Klostermann, K., Yates, B. T., O'Farrell, T. J., & Birchler, G. R. (2005). Brief relationship therapy for alcoholism: A randomized clinical trial examining clinical efficacy and cost-effectiveness. *Psychology of Addictive Behavior, 19,* 363–371.

Fals-Stewart, W., O'Farrell, T. J., & Birchler, G. R. (2004). Behavioral couples therapy for substance abuse: Rationale, methods, and findings. *Science and Practice Perspectives, 2,* 30–41.

Field, M., Santarcangelo, M., & Sumnall, H. (2006). Delay discounting and the behavioural economics of cigarette purchases in smokers: The effects of nicotine deprivation. *Psychopharmacology, 186,* 255–263.

Green, L., & Fisher, E. B. (2000). Economic substitutability: Some implications for health behavior. In W. K. Bickel & R. E. Vuchinich (Eds.) *Reframing health behavior change with behavioral economics* (pp. 115–144). Mahwah, NJ: Erlbaum.

Green, L., & Myerson. J. (2004). A discounting framework for choice with delayed and probabilistic rewards. *Psychological Bulletin, 130,* 769–792.

Griffiths, R. R., Bigelow, G. E., & Liebson, I. (1978). Relationship in social factors to ethanol: Self-administration in alcoholics. In P. E. Nathan, G. A. Marlatt, & T. Loberg (Eds.), *Alcoholism: New directions in behavioral research and treatment* (pp. 351–380). New York: Plenum Press.

Griffiths, R. R., Rush, C. R., & Puhala, K. A. (1996). Validation of the Multiple-Choice Procedure for investigating drug reinforcement in humans. *Experimental and Clinical Psychopharmacology, 4,* 97–106.

Gruenewald, P. J., Ponicki, W. R., Holder, H. D., & Romelsjo, A. (2006). Alcohol prices, beverage quality, and the demand for alcohol: Quality substitutions and price elasticities. *Alcoholism: Clinical and Experimental Research, 30,* 96–105.

Hart, C. L., Haney, M., Foltin, R. W., & Fischman, M. W. (2000). Alternative reinforcers differentially modify cocaine self-administration by humans. *Behavioral Pharmacology, 11,* 87–91.

Heil, S. H., Johnson, M. W., & Higgins, S. T. (2006). Delay discounting in currently using and currently abstinent cocaine-dependent outpatients and non-drug-using matched controls. *Addictive Behaviors, 31,* 1290–1294.

Henslee, A. M., Irons, J. G., & Correia, C. J. (2007). Alcohol use among undergraduate students: From brief interventions to behavioral economics. In P. M. Miller and D. Kavanagh (Eds.), *Translation of addiction science into practice: Update and future directions* (pp. 417–438). United Kingdom: Elsevier.

Herrnstein, R. J. (1970). On the law of effect. *Journal of the Experimental Analysis of Behavior, 13,* 243–266.

Herrnstein, R. J., & Prelec, D. (1992). A theory of addiction. In J. Elster & G. Loewenstein (Eds.), *Choice over time* (pp. 331–360). New York: Guilford Press.

Hettema, J. E., Steele, J. M., & Miller, W. R. (2005). Motivational interviewing. *Annual Review of Clinical Psychology, 1,* 91–111.

Heyman, G. M. (2003). Consumption dependent changes in reward value: A framework for understanding addiction. In R. E. Vuchinich & B. N. Heather, *Choice, behavioral economics, and addiction* (pp. 95–121). Oxford: Elsevier.

Heyman, G. M., & Dunn, B. (2002). Decision biases and persistent illicit drug use: An experimental study of distributed choice and addiction. *Drug and Alcohol Dependence, 67,* 193–203.

Higgins, S. T., Budney, A. J., Bickel, W. K., Hughes, J. R., Foerg, B. A., & Badger, G. (1993). Achieving cocaine abstinence with a behavioral approach. *American Journal of Psychiatry, 150,* 763–769.

Higgins, S. T., Delaney, D. D., Budney, A. J., Bickel, W. K., Hughes, J. R., Foerg, F., et al., (1991). A behavioral approach to achieving initial cocaine abstinence. *American Journal of Psychiatry, 148,* 1218–1124.

Higgins, S. T., Heil, S. H., & Plebani-Lussier, J. (2004). Clinical implications of reinforcement as a determinant of substance use disorders. *Annual Review of Psychology, 55,* 431–461.

Higgins S. T., Roll J. M., & Bickel W. K. (1996). Alcohol pretreatment increases preference for cocaine over monetary reinforcement. *Psychopharmacology, 123,* 1–8.

Higgins, S. T., Sigmon, S. C., Wong, C. J., Heil, S. H., Badger, G. J., Donham, R. et al. (2003). *Archives of General Psychiatry, 60,* 1043–1052.

Higgins, S. T., & Silverman, K. (Eds.). (1999). *Motivating behavior change among illicit-drug abusers.* Washington DC: American Psychological Association.

Holmes, G. R., Sakano, Y., Cautela, J., & Holmes, G. L. (1991). Comparison of factor-analyzed adolescent reinforcement survey schedule (ARSS) responses from Japanese and American adolescents. *Journal of Clinical Psychology, 47,* 749–755.

Hunt, G. M., & Azrin, N. H. (1973). A community reinforcement approach to alcoholism. *Behavior Research and Therapy, 11,* 91–104.

Hursh, S. R., & Winger, G. (1995). Normalized demand for drugs and other reinforcers. *Journal of the Experimental Analysis of Behavior, 64,* 373–384.

Iguchi, M. Y., Belding, M. A., Morral, A. R., Lamb, R. J., & Husband, S. D. (1997). Reinforcing operants other than abstinence in drug abuse treatment: An effective alternative for reducing drug use. *Journal of Consulting and Clinical Psychology, 65,* 421–428.

Jacobs, E. A., & Bickel, W. K. (1999). Modeling drug consumption in the clinic via simulation procedures: Demand for heroin and cigarettes in opioid-dependent outpatients. *Experimental and Clinical Psychopharmacology, 7,* 412–426.

Kandel, D. B., & Yamaguchi, K. (2002). Stages of drug involvement in the U.S. population. In D. B. Kandel (Ed.), *Stages and pathways of drug involvement: Examining the gateway hypothesis.* New York: Cambridge University Press.

Komro, K. A., Perry, C. L., Williams, C. L., Stigler, M. H., Farbakhsh, K., & Veblen-Mortenson, S. (2001). *Health Education Research, 16,* 59–70.

Kuo, M., Wechsler, H., Greenberg, P., & Lee, H. (2003). The marketing of alcohol to college students. *American Journal of Preventative Medicine, 25,* 204–211.

Lejuez, C. W., Hopko, D. R., & Hopko, S. D. (2001). A brief behavioral activation treatment for depression. *Behavior Modification, 25,* 255–286.

Leonard, K. E., & Blaine, H. T. (Eds.). (1999). *Psychological theories of drinking and alcoholism.* New York: Guilford Press.

Liebson, I. A., Cohen, M., Faillace, L. A., & Ward, R. F. (1971). The token economy as a research method in alcoholics. *Psychiatric Quarterly, 45,* 574–581.

Little, C., & Correia, C. J. (2006). use of a multiple-choice procedure with college student drinkers. *Psychology of Addictive Behaviors, 20,* 445–452.

Logue, A. W. (2000). Self control and health behavior. In W. K. Bickel and R. E. Vuchinich (Eds.), *Reframing health behavior change with behavioral economics* (pp.167–192). Mahwah, NJ: Lawrence Erlbaum.

MacKillop, J., & Murphy, J. G. (2007). A behavioral economic measure of demand for alcohol predicts brief intervention outcomes. *Drug and Alcohol Dependence, 89,* 227–233.

MacKillop, J., Murphy, J. G., Ray, L., Eisenberg, D. T. A., Lisman, S. A., Lum, J. K., et al. (2008). Further validation of a cigarette purchase task for assessing the relative reinforcing efficacy of nicotine in smokers. *Experimental and Clinical Psychopharmacology, 16,* 57–65.

MacPhillamy, D. J., & Lewinsohn, P. M. (1982). The Pleasant Events Schedule: Studies on reliability, validity, and scale intercorrelation. *Journal of Consulting and Clinical Psychology, 50,* 363–380.

Madden, G. J., Petry, N. M., Badger, G. J., & Bickel, W. K. (1997) Impulsive and self-control choices in opioid-dependent patients and non-drug-using control participants: Drug and monetary rewards. *Experimental and Clinical Psychopharmacology, 5,* 256–263.

Marlatt, G. A., Baer, J. S., Kivlahan, D. R., Dimeff, L. A., Larimer, M. E., Quigley, L. A., et al. (1998). Screening and brief intervention for high-risk college student drinkers: Results from a two-year follow-up assessment. *Journal of Consulting and Clinical Psychology, 66,* 604–615.

Marlatt, G. A., & Gordon, J. R. (Eds.). (1985). *Relapse prevention: Maintenance strategies in the treatment of addictive behaviors.* New York: Guilford.

Marlatt, G. A., & Kilmer, J. R. (1998). Consumer choice: Implications of behavioral economics for drug use and treatment. *Behavior Therapy, 29,* 567–576.

Martin, C. M., & Hoffman, M. A. (1993). Alcohol expectancies, living environment, peer influence, and gender: A model of college student drinking. *Journal of College Student Development, 34,* 206–211.

Mazur, J. E. (1991). Choice. In I. H. Iverson, & K. A. Lattal (Eds.), *Experimental analysis of behavior* (pp. 219–250). New York: Elsevier.

Meyers, R. J., Miller, W. R., Hill, D. E., & Tonigan, J. S. (1998). Community reinforcement and family training (CRAFT): Engaging unmotivated drug users in treatment. *Journal of Substance Abuse, 10,* 291–308.

Miller, W. R. (1998). Researching the spiritual dimensions of alcohol and other drug problems. *Addiction, 93,* 979–990.

Miller, W. R., & Rollnick, S. (2002). *Motivational interviewing: Preparing people for change* (2nd ed.). New York: Guilford Press.

Moeller F. G., Barratt E. S., Dougherty D. M., Schmitz J. M., & Swann A. C. (2001). Psychiatric aspects of impulsivity. *American Journal of Psychiatry, 158,* 1783–1793.

Monterosso, J., & Ainslie, G. (1999). Beyond discounting: Possible experimental models of impulse control. *Psychopharmacology, 146,* 339–347.

Monti, P. M., Rohsenow, D. J., Colby, S. M., & Abrams, D. B. (1995). Coping and social skills training. In R. K. Hester & W. R. Miller (Eds.), *Handbook of alcoholism treatment strategies* (2nd ed., pp. 221–241). Boston: Allyn & Bacon.

Moos, R. H., Finney, J. W., & Cronkite, R. C. (1990). *Alcoholism treatment: Context, process, and outcome.* New York: Oxford University Press.

Murphy, J. G., Barnett, N. P., & Colby, S. M. (2006). Alcohol-related and alcohol-free activity participation and enjoyment among college students: A behavioral theories of choice analysis. *Experimental and Clinical Psychopharmacology, 14,* 339–349.

Murphy, J. G., Barnett, N. P., Goldstein, A. L., & Colby, S. M. (2007a). Gender moderates the relationship between substance-free activity enjoyment and substance use. *Psychology of Addictive Behaviors, 21,* 261–265.

Murphy, J. G., Correia, C. J., & Barnett, N. P. (2007b). Behavioral economic approaches to reduce college student drinking. *Addictive Behaviors, 32,* 2573–2585.

Murphy, J. G., Correia, C. J., Colby, S. M., & Vuchinich, R. E. (2005). Using behavioral theories of choice to predict drinking outcomes following a brief intervention. *Experimental and Clinical Psychopharmacology, 13,* 93–101.

Murphy, J. G., Duchnick, J. J., Vuchinich, R. E, Davison, J. W., Karg, R., Olson, A. M., et al. (2001). Relative efficacy of a brief motivational intervention for college student drinkers. *Psychology of Addictive Behaviors, 15,* 373–379.

Murphy, J. G., & MacKillop, J. (2006). Relative reinforcing efficacy of alcohol among college student drinkers. *Experimental and Clinical Psychopharmacology, 14,* 219–227.

Murphy, J. G., & Vuchinich, R. E. (2002). Implications of behavioral theories of choice for substance abuse assessment. *The Addictions Newsletter, 9,* 2–6.

National Advisory Mental Health Council Behavioral Science Workgroup. (2000). *Translating behavioral science into action.* Bethesda, MD: National Institute of Mental Health (NIMH).

O'Farrell, T. J., & Fals-Stewart, W. (2000). Behavioral couples therapy for alcoholism and drug abuse. *Journal of Substance Abuse Treatment, 18,* 51–54.

Ohmura, Y., Takahashi, T., & Kitamura, N. (2006). Three-month stability of delay and probability discounting measures. *Experimental and Clinical Psychopharmacology, 14,* 318–328.

O'Malley, P. M., & Johnston, L. D. (2002). Epidemiology of alcohol and other drug use among American college students. *Journal of Studies on Alcohol, 63,* 23–40.

Onken, L. S., & Bootzin, R. R. (1998). Behavioral therapy development and psychological science: If a tree falls in the wood and nobody hears it. *Behavior Therapy, 29,* 539–544.

Osterberg, E. (2001). Effects of price and taxation. In N. Heather, T. J. Peters, & T. Stockwell (Eds.), *International handbook of alcohol dependence and problems* (pp. 685–698). New York: Wiley.

Pearce, D. W. (Ed.). (1992). *The MIT dictionary of modern economics* (3rd ed.). Cambridge, MA: MIT Press.

Perry, J. L., Larson, E. B., & German, J. P. (2005). Impulsivity (delay discounting) as a predictor of acquisition of IV cocaine self-administration in female rats. *Psychopharmacology, 178,* 193–201.

Petry, N. M. (2001). Pathological gamblers, with and without substance use disorders, discount delayed rewards at high rates. *Journal of Abnormal Psychology, 110,* 482–487.

Petry, N. M., Alessi, S. M., Carroll, K. M., Hanson, T., MacKinnon, S., Rounsaville, B., et al. (2006). Contingency management treatments: Reinforcing abstinence versus adherence with goal-related activities. *Journal of Consulting and Clinical Psychology, 74,* 592–601.

Petry, N. M., & Bickel, W. K. (1998). Polydrug abuse in heroin addicts: A behavioral economic analysis. *Addiction, 93,* 321–335.

Petry, N. M., Bickel, W. K., & Arnett, M. (1998). Shortened time horizons and insensitivity to future consequences in heroin addicts. *Addiction, 93,* 729–738.

Petry, N. M., Martin, B., Cooney, J. L., & Kranzler, H. R. (2000) Give them prizes and they will come: Contingency management for treatment of alcohol dependence. *Journal of Consulting and Clinical Psychology, 68,* 250–257.

Prochaska, J. O., & Norcross, J. C. (2007). *Systems of psychotherapy: A transtheoretical analysis.* Pacific Grove, CA: Brooks/Cole.

Rachlin, H. (1995). Self control: Beyond commitment. *Behavioral and Brain Sciences, 18,* 109–159.

Rachlin, H. (1997). Four teleological theories of addiction. *Psychonomic Bulletin and Review, 4,* 462–473.

Rachlin, H. (2000). The lonely addict. In W. K. Bickel & R. E. Vuchinich (Eds.), *Reframing health behavior change with behavioral economics.* Englewood Cliffs, NJ: Prentice Hall.

Redish, A. D. (2004). Addiction as a computational process gone awry. *Science, 306,* 1944–1947.

Reynolds, B. (2006). A review of delay-discounting research with humans: Relations to drug use and gambling. *Behavioural Pharmacology, 17,* 651–667.

Reynolds, B., & Schiffbauer, R. (2004). Measuring changes in human delay discounting: An experiential discounting task. *Behavioral Processes, 67,* 343–356.

Roll, J. M., Reilly, M. P., & Johanson, C. E. (2000). The influence of exchange delays on cigarette versus money choice: A laboratory analog of voucher-based reinforcement therapy. *Experimental and Clinical Psychopharmacology, 8,* 366–370.

Roozen, H. G., Van Beers, S. E. C., Weevers, H. J. A., Breteler, M. H. M., Willemsen, M. C., Postmus, P. E., et al. (2006). Effects on smoking cessation: Naltrexone combined with a cognitive behavioral treatment based on the community reinforcement approach. *Substance Use and Misuse, 41,* 45–60.

Roozen, H. G., Boulogne, J. J., van Tulder, M. W., Brink, W. V. D., DeJong, C. A. J., & Kerkhof, A. J. F. M. (2004). *Drug and Alcohol Dependence, 74,* 1–13.

Schuster, C. R., & Thompson, T. (1969). Self-administration of and behavioral dependence on drugs. *Annual Review of Pharmacology, 9,* 483–502.

Siegel, E., & Rachlin, H. (1995). Soft commitment: Self-control achieved by response persistence. *Journal of the Experimental Analysis of Behavior, 64,* 117–128.

Sigmon, S. C., Steingard, S., Badger, G. J., Anthony, S. L., & Higgins, S. T. (2000). Contingent reinforcement of marijuana abstinence among individuals with serious mental illness: A feasibility study. *Experimental and Clinical Psychopharmacology, 8,* 509–517.

Silverman, K., Svikis, D., Robles, E., Stitzer, M. L., & Bigelow, G. E. (2001). A reinforcement-based therapeutic workplace for the treatment of drug abuse: Six-month abstinence outcomes. *Experimental and Clinical Psychopharmacology, 9,* 14–23.

Silverman, K., Svikis, D., Wong, C. J., Hampton, J., Stitzer, M. L., & Bigelow, G. E. (2002). A reinforcement-based therapeutic workplace for the treatment of drug abuse: Three-year abstinence outcomes. *Experimental and Clinical Psychopharmacology, 10,* 228–240.

Silverman, K., Wong, C. J., Higgins, S. T., Brooner, R. K., Montoya, I. D., Contoreggi, C., et al. (1996). Increasing opiate abstinence through voucher-based reinforcement therapy. *Drug and Alcohol Dependence, 41,* 157–165.

Simpson. C. A., & Vuchinich, R. E. (2000a). Reliability of a measure of temporal discounting. *The Psychological Record, 50,* 3–16.

Simpson, C. A., & Vuchinich, R. E. (2000b). Temporal changes in the value of objects of choice: Discounting, behavior patterns, and health behavior. In W. K. Bickel & R. E. Vuchinich (Eds.), *Reframing Health Behavior Change with Behavioral Economics* (pp. 193–215). Mahwah: Lawrence Erlbaum Associates Publishers.

Smith, J. E., & Meyers, R. J. (1995). *The community reinforcement approach.* In R. K. Hester & W. R. Miller (Eds.), *Handbook of alcoholism treatment strategies* (2nd ed., pp. 251–266). Boston: Allyn & Bacon.

Smith, J. E., Meyers, R. J., & Delaney, H. D. (1998). The community reinforcement approach with homeless alcohol-dependent individuals. *Journal of Consulting and Clinical Psychology, 66,* 541–548.

Spring, B., Pagoto, S., & Kaufmann, P. G. (2005). Invitation to a dialogue between researchers and clinicians about evidence-based behavioral medicine. *Annals of Behavioral Medicine, 30,* 125–137.

Swift, R. M. (2003). Medications. In R. K. Hester & W. R. Miller (Eds.), *Handbook of alcoholism treatment approaches* (3rd ed., pp. 259–281). Boston: Allyn and Bacon.

Tucker, J. (1999). Changing addictive behavior: Historical and contemporary perspectives. In J. Tucker et al. (Eds.), *Changing addictive behaviors: Bridging clinical and public health strategies* (pp. 3–44). New York: Guilford Press.

Tucker, J. A., Vuchinich, R. E., Black, B. C., & Rippens, P. D. (2006). Significance of a behavioral economic index of reward value in predicting drinking problem resolution. *Journal of Consulting and Clinical Psychology, 74,* 317–326.

Tucker, J. A., Vuchinich, R. E., & Murphy, J. G. (2002). Assessment, treatment planning, and outcome evaluation for substance use disorders. In M. H. Anthony & D. H. Barlow (Eds.), *Handbook of assessment and treatment planning* (pp. 415–452). New York: Guilford Press.

Tucker, J. A., Vuchinich, R. E., & Rippins, P. D. (2002). Predicting natural resolution of alcohol- related problems: A prospective behavioral economic analysis. *Experimental and Clinical Psychopharmacology, 10,* 248–257.

Van Etten, M. L., Higgins, S. T., & Bickel, W. K. (1995). Effects of response cost and unit dose on alcohol self-administration in moderate drinkers. *Behavioural Pharmacology, 6,* 754–758.

Van Etten, M. L., Higgins, S. T., Budney, A. J., & Badger, G. J. (1998). Comparison of the frequency and enjoyability of pleasant events in cocaine abusers vs. non-abusers using a standardized behavioral inventory. *Addiction, 93,* 1669–1680.

Vuchinich, R. E., Tucker, J. A., & Harllee, L. M. (1988). Behavioral assessment (of alcohol dependence). In W. R. Miller & N. Heather (Eds.), *Treating addictive behavior: Processes of chance* (2nd ed., pp. 93–104). New York: Plenum.

Vuchinich, R. E., & Heather, B. N. (2003). *Choice, behavioral economics, and addiction.* Oxford, England: Elsevier.

Vuchinich, R. E., & Simpson, C. A. (1998). Hyperbolic temporal discounting in social drinkers and problem drinkers. *Experimental and Clinical Pharmacology, 6,* 292–305.

Vuchinich, R. E., & Tucker, J. A. (1983). Behavioral theories of choice as a framework for studying drinking behavior. *Journal of Abnormal Psychology, 92,* 408–416.

Vuchinich, R. E., & Tucker, J. A. (1988). Contributions from behavioral theories of choice to an analysis of alcohol abuse. *Journal of Abnormal Psychology, 92,* 408–416.

Vuchinich, R. E., & Tucker, J. A. (1996a). Alcoholic relapse, life events, and behavioral theories of choice: A prospective analysis. *Experimental and Clinical Psychopharmacology, 4,* 19–28.

Vuchinich, R. E., & Tucker, J. A. (1996b). The molar context of alcohol abuse. In J. Kagel, & L. Green (Eds.), *Advances in behavioral economics* (Vol. 3, pp. 133–162). Norwood, NJ: Ablex.

Vuchinich, R. E., Tucker, J. A., & Harllee, L. M. (1988). Behavioral assessment (of alcohol dependence). In W. R. Miller, & N. Heather (Eds.), *Treating addictive behavior: Processes of chance* (2nd ed., pp. 93–104). New York: Plenum.

Wechsler, H., Dowdall, G. W., Devenport, A., & Castillo, S. (1995). Correlates of college student binge drinking. *American Journal of Public Health, 85,* 921–926.

Weitzman, E. R., Folkman, A., Lemieux Folkman, K., & Wechsler, H. (2003). The relationship of alcohol outlet density to heavy and frequent drinking and drinking-related problems among college students at eight universities. *Health and Place, 9,* 1–6.

Zweben, A., & Fleming, M. F. (1999). Brief interventions for alcohol and drug problems. In J. A. Tucker, D. M. Donovan, & G. A. Marlatt (Eds.), *Changing addictive behavior: Bridging clinical and public health strategies.* New York: Guilford Press.

25

Pharmacological Approaches to the Treatment of Substance Use Disorders

Ryan M. Caldeiro, Charles W. Meredith,
Andrew J. Saxon, and Donald A. Calsyn

University of Washington

Contents

Introduction

This chapter reviews pharmacological treatments for substance use disorders. The focus primarily rests upon pharmacotherapy for alcohol dependence, opioid dependence, and nicotine dependence, disorders for which we have medications specifically approved by the Food and Drug Administration (FDA) for treatment of those disorders.

The section on alcohol dependence covers medically supervised withdrawal from alcohol as well as four medications approved for ongoing treatment. A brief mention is made of medically supervised withdrawal from sedative-hypnotics inasmuch as the protocols are similar to those for alcohol withdrawal.

Similarly the section on opioid dependence addresses medically supervised withdrawal, maintenance treatment, and antagonist therapy with some discussion of the regulations involved in opioid agonist treatment.

The section on nicotine dependence describes nicotine replacement strategies, antidepressant medications, and a newly approved nicotinic receptor partial, agonist, varenicline. Although all of the approved medications have demonstrated efficacy, none of them is ideal and active research efforts are ongoing to identify new agents. Medications under investigation which do not have FDA approval for alcohol, opioid, or nicotine dependence, but may show promise, are mentioned only in passing. In contrast, because no FDA-approved treatments yet exist for cocaine and methamphetamine (MA) dependence, discussion of pharmacotherapies for these disorders can only convey information about potential agents on the horizon.

Co-occurring psychiatric disorders are frequently encountered in patients with substance use disorders so the pharmacological management of these co-occurring disorders is also alluded to.

An important premise of the chapter, although not discussed at length, is the view that medications for these substance use disorders should generally be prescribed in the context of ongoing behavioral interventions for the disorders, and that most patients will have better outcomes when both behavioral and pharmacotherapeutic interventions are applied in concert. Behavioral interventions could range from referral to self-help groups to a variety of brief intervention techniques to a full course of psychotherapy using cognitive-behavioral, motivational, psychodynamic, or 12-step facilitation approaches.

At present the majority of patients with substance use disorders do not receive efficacious pharmacological treatments. It is hoped that this chapter encourages increased use of these agents to improve treatment outcomes.

Alcohol Intoxication and Withdrawal

Ethyl alcohol is a central nervous system (CNS) depressant that activates ligand-gated receptors of the inhibitory neurotransmitters GABA (Allan & Harris, 1986; Martz, Deitrich, & Harris, 1983; Suzdak, Schwartz, Skolnick, & Paul, 1986; Ticku, Lowrimore, & Lehoullier, 1986) and glycine (Findlay et al., 2002; Quinlan, Ferguson, Jester, Firestone, & Homanics, 2002; Williams, Ferko, Barbieri, & DiGregorio, 1995), leading to increased flux of negatively charged chloride ions. The physiological and behavioral effects of the CNS depressant ethyl alcohol vary, dependent upon an individual's level of tolerance as well as on the concentration of alcohol in the individual's bloodstream. Between concentrations of 0.020 and 0.080, patients tend to experience mild euphoria, a sense of activation, and some loss of physical coordination. Loss of coordination becomes more profound from 0.020 to 0.200, with ataxia and dysarthria. Patients' level of consciousness becomes progressively affected with further increases, as they experience a clouded sensorium and significant nausea and vomiting between 0.200–0.300, marked sedation above 0.300, and risk of coma above 0.400 (CSAT, 2006).

Unless they have developed significant liver damage from their chronic alcoholism, chronic drinkers usually experience marked tolerance. Thus they may very well be able to tolerate alcohol concentrations of above 0.300 or 0.400 and remain not only conscious, but relatively lucid and organized. However as their alcohol concentration drops with decreased or terminated alcohol consumption, they are at marked risk for withdrawal (Johnson & Ait-Daoud, 2005). The CNS experiences a state of increased excitation as the inhibitory GABA system is no longer stimulated by alcohol, leaving the excitatory glutamatergic unopposed (Davis & Wu, 2000). Patients tend to experience insomnia, profound anxiety, nausea and vomiting, tremulousness, diaphoresis, and papillary dilation. In addition, they also frequently experience hyperthermia, tachycardia, and hypertension. Untreated alcohol withdrawal can be complicated by altered mental status, proceeding to delirium tremens in which patients are disoriented, extremely agitated, and experience severe visual and tactile hallucinations as well as significant autonomic hyperactivity. During this stage, patients have died from cardiovascular collapse (Erwin, Williams, & Speir, 1998; Foy, Kay, & Taylor 1997). Untreated patients are also at risk for experiencing generalized seizures after 24–48 hours, and the risk of future seizures in the setting of withdrawal is thought to increase with each past withdrawal-related seizure (Chang & Kosten. 2005). Up to 30% of patients with history of withdrawal-related seizures may go on to experience delirium tremens.

Thiamine for Wernicke's Encephalopathy

Although there do not exist significant pharmacological treatments for acute alcohol intoxication, prolonged intoxication in the setting of poor nutrition can predispose alcohol-dependent individuals to the development of Wernicke's encephalopathy, an acute delirium characterized by the triad of ataxia, opthalmoplegia, and confusion. This is due to depletion of thiamine, vitamin B-1, a biologically active cofactor for three metabolic enzymes involved in the Krebs cycle, glycolysis, and the pentose–monophosphate shunt (Victor, Adams, & Collins 1989). Inactivation of these enzymes leads to demyleination and other neurological damage, resulting in the symptoms of the encephalopathy. Untreated, this reversible syndrome can proceed to the permanent amnestic damage of Korsakoff's psychosis, a form of alcohol-induced dementia. The syndrome is treated with thiamine repletion, traditionally three to five daily oral doses of 100 mg, or up to 6–12 months in the case of Korsakoff's psychosis (Johnson & Ait-Daoud, 2005). Severely ill (i.e., comatose) patients may require 500 mg parenterally, up to twice daily. Treatment with dextrose or glucose prior to thiamine repletion accelerates the neurological damage of Wernicke's encephalopathy, by providing more substrate for the affected biochemical pathways, and effectively depleting any of the remaining limited thiamine stores (Koguchi, Nakatsuji, Abe, & Sakoda, 2004).

Benzodiazepines

There are numerous medication options to treat alcohol withdrawal, although the mainstay of treatment is the use of benzodiazepines (Lejoyeux, Solomon, & Ades, 1998; Mayo-Smith, 1997). Furthermore, this class of medication can be administered via a predetermined schedule, or via a protocol for symptom-triggered therapy. Although one can dose benzodiazepines based on parameters such as vital signs and subjective reports of anxiety, the Clinical Institute Withdrawal Assessment of Alcohol Scale-Revised (CIWA-Ar; Sullivan, Sykora, Schneiderman, Naranjo, & Sellers, 1989) has become the symptom-triggered withdrawal assessment instrument of choice (see Figure 25.1). Application of symptom-triggered therapy with an instrument such as the CIWA-A or CIWA-Ar withdrawal scale has been shown to lead to less administration of total dose of benzodiazepine and shorter treatment courses than have other withdrawal scales or protocols utilizing scheduled doses (Daeppen et al., 2002; Mayo-Smith, 1997; Reoux & Miller, 2000; Saitz et al., 1994). The CIWA-Ar regimen has been shown to be effective with short, intermediate, or long-acting benzodiazepines. Patients with known risk of withdrawal seizures can be safely treated with the CIWA-Ar protocol, but also need to be treated with scheduled doses of a long-acting benzodiazepines for seizure prophylaxis (Weinhouse & Manaker, 2007). Commonly accepted protocols include 50 mg chlodiazepoxide or up to 20 mg diazepam every 6 hours for 4–12 doses (Kosten & O'Connor, 2003).

The disadvantage of a standardized and rigorous symptom-triggered approach such as the CIWA-Ar is that it cannot be performed in centers where the nursing staff has not been trained to administer it. Nor can it be administered in the outpatient setting, necessitating a protocol of scheduled dosing. A commonly used strategy with scheduled dosing is to establish an acute loading dose in the first 24 hours, and then gradually taper over the following 3–4 days. Medications should be held for side effects such as sedation or ataxia. Despite these cautions, the drawback of scheduled dosing regimens is that they cannot control for under-medication or overmedication near as well as a standardized symptom-triggered approach such as the CIWA-Ar. Thus these strategies have higher rates of breakthrough seizures or

FIGURE 25.1
Clinical Institute Withdrawal Assessment of Alcohol Scale (CIWA-Ar).

Patient:_____Date:_____ Time: _____ (24 hour clock, midnight = 00:00)

Pulse or heart rate, taken for one minute:_____ Blood pressure:_____

NAUSEA AND VOMITING—Ask "Do you feel sick to your stomach? Have you vomited?" Observation.
0 no nausea and no vomiting
1 mild nausea with no vomiting
2
3
4 intermittent nausea with dry heaves
5
6
7 constant nausea, frequent dry heaves and vomiting

TACTILE DISTURBANCES—Ask "Have you any itching, pins and needles sensations, any burning, any numbness or do you feel bugs crawling on or nnder your skin" Observation.
0 none
1 very mild itching, pins and needles burning or numbness
2 mild itchmg, pins and needles, burning or numbness
3 moderate itching, pins and needles, burning or numbness
4 moderately severe hallucinations
5 severe hallucinations
6 extremely severe hallucinations
7 continuous hallucinations

TREMOR—Arms extended and fingers spread apart. observation.
0 no tremor
1 not visible, but can be felt fingertip to fingertip
2
3
4 moderate, with patient's arms extended
5
6
7 severe, even with arms not extended

AUDITORY DISTURBANCES—Ask "Are you more aware of sounds around you? Are they harsh? Do they frighten you? Are you hearing anything that is disturbing to you? Are you hearing things you know are not there?" Observation.
0 not present
1 very mild harshness or ability to frighten
2 mild harshness or ability to frighten
3 moderate harshness or ability to frighten
4 moderately severe hallucinations
5 severe hallucinations
6 extremely severe hallucinations
7 continuous hallucinations

PAROXYSMAL SWEATS—observation.
0 no sweat visible
1 barely perceptible sweating, palms moist
2
3
4 beads of sweat obvious on forehead
5
6
7 drenching sweats

VISUAL DISTURBANCES—Ask "Does the light appear to be too bright? Is its color different? Does it hurt your eyes? Are you seeing anything that is disturbing to you? Are you seeing things you know are not there?" Observation.
0 not present
1 very mild sensitivity
2 mild sensitivity
3 moderate sensitivity
4 moderately severe hallucinations
5 severe hallucinations
6 extremely severe hallucinations
7 continuous hallucinations

ANXIETY—Ask "Do you feel nervous?" Observation.
0 no anxiety, at ease
1 mild anxious
2
3
4 moderately anxious, or guarded, so anxiety is inferred
5
6
7 equivalent to acute panic states as seen in severe delirium or acute schizophrenic reacitons

HEADACHE, FULLNESS IN HEAD—Ask "Does your head feel different? Does it feel there is a band around your head?" Do not rate for dizziness or lightheadedness. Otherwise, rate severity.
0 not present
1 very mild
2 mild
3 moderate
4 moderately severe
5 severe
6 very severe
7 extremely severe

FIGURE 25.1
(Continued)

AGITATION—Observation.
0 normal activity
1 somewhat more than normal activity
2
3
4 moderately fidgety and restless
5
6
7 paces back and forth during most of the interview, or constantly thrashes about

ORIENTATION AND CLOUDING OF SENSORIUM—Ask "What day is this? Where are you? Who am I?"
0 oriented and can do serial additions
1 cannot do serial additions or is uncertain about date
2 disoriented for date by no more than 2 calendar days
3 disoriented for date by more than 2 calendar days
4 disoriented for place/or person

Total **CIWA-AR** Score _____
Rater's Initials _____
Maximum Possible Score 67

The **CIWA-AR** is not copyrighted and may be reproduced freely. This assessment for monitoring withdrawal symptoms requires approximately 5 minutes to administer. The maximum score is 67 (see instrument). Patients scoring less than 10 do not usually need additional medication for withdrawal.

Source. Sullivan, J.T.; Sykora, K.; Schneiderman, J.; Naranjo, C.A.; Sellers, E.M. Assessment of alcohol withdrawal: The revised clinical Institute Withdrawal Assessment for Alcohol scale (**CIWA-Ar**). *British Journal of Addiction* 84: 1353–1357, 1989.

TABLE 25.1
Sample Benzodizaepine Fixed-Dosing Strategies

Medication	Day 1	Day 2	Day 3	Day 4
Chlordiazepoxide	100 mg QID	75 mg QID	50 mg QID	25 mg QID
Diazepam	10 mg QID	5 mg QID	5 mg TID	5 mg BID
Lorazepam*	2 mg QID	2 mg TID	2 mg BID	1 mg BID

*Medications with short half-lives, such as lorazepam, likely will need to be dosed via regimens longer than 4 days.

benzodiazepine toxicity than does the CIWA-Ar. Common examples of such strategies are listed in Table 25.1.

Benzodiazepines have significant side effects, and can be dangerous, particularly in the setting of alcohol intoxication. Side effects are dose-dependent and include sedation, ataxia, confusion, and even delirium. Death is possible secondary to respiratory depression. These risks are heightened in elderly patients, or patients with hepatic impairment, making it difficult to adequately metabolize these medications. Although they have been prescribed safely for withdrawal in a home setting via a scheduled regimen, the risk of overdose (especially if the patient actively drinks during the dosing regimen) is not to be ignored. Patients need to be advised to avoid alcohol, as well as driving, operating heavy machinery, or other dangerous activities that require full attention and physical coordination. Alternative treatment options for acute withdrawal include inpatient treatment with benzodiazepines for withdrawal, or inpatient or outpatient treatment with other classes of medications such as anticonvulsants (Kosten & O'Connor, 2003).

Although no benzodiazepine has been clearly shown to be superior to its brethren in the treatment of acute alcohol withdrawal, the advantages of chlordiazepoxide and diazepam are that they both have long half-lives. Consequently, they require less frequent daily dosing, lead to steadier serum levels, and can be more comfortably self-tapered than shorter-lasting medications (Saitz & O'Malley, 1997). Both have satisfactory oral absorption, although diazepam has a quicker onset of action. However, older patients or patients with hepatic compromise may have difficulty metabolizing these medications as both have active metabolites and undergo multiple metabolic steps in their hepatic metabolism. Thus they can accumulate quickly to toxic levels in vulnerable patients, particularly when dosed very aggressively in the first 24 hours, putting these patients at risk for falls secondary to ataxia, benzodiazepine-induced delirium, or respiratory compromise.

Such patients may do better with oxazepam or lorazepam, shorter-lasting benzodiazepines commonly used for treatment of acute alcohol withdrawal that need to be dosed 3–4 times per day due to their short half-lives (Weinhouse & Manaker, 2007; see Table 25.2). Lorazepam has an intermediate half-life of 8–15 hours and oxazepam has a shorter half-life of 6–8 hours. Thus they are less likely to accumulate to toxic levels, but may precipitate breakthrough symptoms in between doses, or even a slightly increased risk of seizure late in the detoxification process (CSAT, 2006). Of note, both medications are glucoronidated by the liver and then renally excreted, making them better tolerated in patients with impaired hepatic metabolism.

Phenobarbital

Due to their improved safety profile, benzodiazepines have replaced the use of barbiturates, which are now reserved for special cases and typically only used in very well medically supervised situations (Kosten & O'Connor, 2003). Although this class of medication was the treatment of choice prior to the advent of benzodiazepines, they have high overdose potential, particularly in alcohol intoxication (Hobbs, Rall, & Verdoorn, 1996). They also tend to be plagued by the development of rapid tolerance, making them difficult to prescribe. The long-lasting phenobarbital is the most commonly used barbiturate today, is metabolized/excreted both hepatically and renally, and needs to be dosed carefully in the elderly, patients with hepatic impairment, and patients with decreased renal clearance. Its use is not recommended in pregnancy, as it has been linked to an increased risk of fetal abnormalities such as facial

---

TABLE 25.2
Benzodiazepine Medications Commonly Involved in Treatment of Withdrawal from Alcohol or Sedative/Hypnotics

Generic Name	Brand Name	Half-Life* (Half-Life of Active Metabolite) (hrs)
Chlordiazepoxide	Librium	5–30 (35–200)
Clonazepam	Klonopin	18–50
Diazepam	Valium	20–100 (35–200)
Lorazepam	Ativan	10–20
Oxazepam	Serax	5–15

*Shorter acting compounds have more abuse potential. Longer-acting compounds may be substituted for shorter ones and tapered in benzodiazepine withdrawal. Half-life from http://www.benzo.org.uk/bzequiv.htm.

abnormalities, decreased cognitive development, decreased head circumference, hip dysplasia, and digital deformities in the hands (Aase, 1974; Kaneko et al., 1992; Seip, 1976; Zellweger, 1974). Common side effects include constipation, nausea and vomiting, sedation or insomnia, and dizziness. It can also precipitate delirium, behavioral disinhibition or agitation, and dose-dependent toxicity leads to somnolence and ataxia. Finally, phenobarbital has been associated with increased risk of the rare but potentially fatal development of Stevens–Johnson syndrome, severe thrombocytopenia, fulminant hepatitis, and aplastic anemia (AMA Department of Drugs, 1992; Kahn, Faguet, Agee, & Middleton, 1984; Sneddon, 1967).

Valproic Acid and Carbamazepine

Given the safety concerns of using benzodiazepines in unsupervised outpatient settings, the anticonvulsants have been shown to be of value, particularly when inpatient treatment is not an option. Valproic acid and carbamazepine are the best studied, and have been shown to prevent the development of seizures and to be as effective as benzodiazepines in mild to moderate alcohol withdrawal (Bjorkqvist, Isohanni, Makela, & Malinen, 1976; Malcolm, Ballenger, Sturgis, & Anton, 1989; Malcolm, Myrick, Brady, & Ballenger, 2001; Reoux, Saxon, Malte, Baer, & Sloan, 2001, see Table 25.3).

Although both can be dangerous in intentional overdose, they have a larger safety margin and much less abuse potential than do unsupervised benzodiazepines. Because they are hepatically metabolized, they may need to be administered at lower doses in patients with compromised hepatic function. Furthermore, carbamazepine is a well-known inducing agent of hepatic metabolic enzymes, and can lead to decreased serum levels of a patient's concurrent medications. Common side effects include nausea and vomiting, sedation, and weight gain (Schachter, 2007). Acute toxicity from elevated serum levels may manifest as ataxia, oversedation, nystagmus, confusion, and dizziness. Rare but fatal side effects include the development of aplastic anemia or fulminant hepatitis (Porter, 1987). Carbamazepine has also been linked to the development of Stevens–Johnson syndrome, particularly in the first 8 weeks of treatment (Rzany, Saxon, Malte, Baer, & Sloan, 1999). Both prior to initiation of therapy and periodically throughout the course of therapy, complete LFT panel and CBC need to be drawn and reviewed. Serum levels of the medication should be obtained throughout the course of therapy as well. A typical dosing strategy by patient's weight would be to titrate towards 10–20 mg/kg, with target serum levels of 4–12 mcg/ml. Of note, carbamazepine is available in extended release formulations that require less frequent dosing and is better tolerated (Ficker et al., 2005).

Common side effects of valproic acid include sedation, diarrhea, weight gain, and nausea and vomiting, although the latter is less common with depakote, the more expensive enteric coated formulation. Acute toxicity from elevated serum levels can lead to nystagmus, ataxia, oversedation, tremor, headache, and confusion. Rare but potentially lethal problems include the development of severe pancreatitis, fulminant hepatitis, or significant thrombocytopenia and thus increased bleeding times.(Dreifuss et al., 1987; Schachter, 2007) Like carbamazepine (Jones, Lacro, Johnson, & Adams, 1989; Rosa, 1991), valproic acid (Abbott, 2006) is contraindicated in pregnancy due to increased risk of neural tube defects, comes in an extended-release formulation with once a day dosing and requires review of CBC, LFTs, and serum levels throughout therapy, as well as review of both CBC and LFTs prior to starting the medication. Target serum levels are 50–100 mcg/ml, although most practitioners will aim for 80–120 mcg/ml and estimate the target dose based on a patient's weight, aiming for 15–20 mg valproic acid/KG weight. Typical dosing duration for acute alcohol withdrawal ranges from 5–14 days.

Gabapentin

Less well-studied than valproic acid or carbamazepine, the advantage of the anticonvulsant gabapentin is that it is excreted renally unchanged, and thus easily dosed in patients with hepatic impairment from chronic alcohol dependence. Supported mainly by case reports (Bonnet et al., 1999; Chatterjee & Ringold, 1999) and open-label trials (Bozikas, Petrikis, Gamvrula, Savvidou, & Karavatos, 2002; Mariani, Rosenthal, Tross, Singh, & Anand, 2006; Voris, Smith, Rao, Thorne, & Flowers, 2003) either in monotherapy or as an add-on to other pharmacotherapy, gabapentin is thought to be less effective in severe withdrawal than valproic acid or carbamazepine. In fact, a large double-blind study found no efficacy for gabapentin as an add-on therapy to clomethiazole, a common agent used in Germany (Bonnet et al. 1999). Gabapentin needs to be administered in reduced doses in patients with renal impairment, and a creatinine should be drawn and reviewed prior to initiation of therapy. Common side effects may include peripheral edema, myalgia, or behavioral activation. Signs of dose-dependent toxicity include nystagmus, tremor, somnolence, and ataxia. Gabapentin has also been associated with the rare but dangerous possibility of developing Stevens–Johnson syndrome, which resolved following discontinuation of the medication (Gonzalez-Sicilia, Cano, Serrano, & Hernandez, 1998). There are no known contraindications to use of this agent in pregnancy, although this has not been well-studied. Gabapentin should be considered still under investigation for acute alcohol withdrawal.

Sedative-Hypnotic Intoxication

Flumazenil

Intoxication and withdrawal syndromes of the sedative-hypnotics share some similarities with those of alcohol. Benzodiazepines are commonly prescribed in medical practice and have significant anxiolytic effects, due to their binding to the GABA-A receptor (Sieghart, 1995; Smith & Olsen, 1995). Subsequently, severe benzodiazepine intoxication can mimic that of alcohol, characterized by dsyarthria, ataxia, loss of physical coordination, altered sensorium, and loss of consciousness. Benzodiazepine overdose can be fatal secondary to respiratory suppression. However, acute life-threatening benzodiazepine toxicity can be treated with 0.2 mg intravenous flumazenil over 30 seconds. If necessary, another 0.3 mg can be repeated after 1 minute, followed by additional 0.5 mg doses at minute intervals to a total of 5 mg. Because it is a short-acting competitive inhibitor that binds to the benzodiazepine binding site of the GABA-A receptor, flumazenil has no effect in overdose of alcohol or other non-benzodiazepines (CSAT, 2006). It has rapid-onset within minutes, and its activity peaks at 10 minutes. It is shorter-lasting than most benzodiazepines and thus patients need close monitoring with repeat dosing if life-threatening sedation returns as flumazenil is metabolized. In the chronic benzodiazepine user, flumazenil treatment can precipitate severe benzodiazepine withdrawal. Similar to that seen with alcohol, this syndrome is commonly associated with tremor, significant anxiety, and profound sympathetic outflow manifesting as hyperpyrexia, tachycardia, and hypertension. The risk of delirium and seizures is extremely significant as well.

Sedative-Hypnotic Dependence

Given the risks of severe complications with benzodiazepine withdrawal, it is recommended to slowly taper benzodiazepines in the chronic user, rather than abrupt discontinuation (CSAT, 2006). Benzodiazepines can be tapered over weeks to months, but patients on short-acting medications may not tolerate such a taper without intermittent withdrawal symptoms. An alternative strategy is to first covert such patients to equivalent doses of longer-lasting benzo-diazepines, such as clonazepam or chlordiazepoxide (Kosten & O'Connor, 2003). This can be potentially risky in outpatients who may not be reliable, or at risk for abuse or diversion of the prescribed benzodiazepine.

Anti-Convulsants and Phenobarbital

Another strategy providers can use is to substitute the benzodiazepine with the anti-convulsants carbamazepine (Garcia-Borreguero, Bronisch, Apelt, Yassouridis, & Emrich, 1991; Neppe & Sindorf, 1991; Ries, Cullison, Horn, & Ward, 1991; Ries, Roy-Byrne, Ward, Neppe, & Cullison,1989; Roy-Byrne, Sullivan, Cowley, & Ries, 1993; Schweizer, Rickels, Case, & Greenblatt, 1991) or valproic acid (Apelt & Emrich, 1990; Roy-Byrne, Ward, & Donnelly, 1989) for both alleviation of withdrawal symptoms as well as seizure prophylaxis. Finally, another commonly accepted strategy is to substitute the benzodiazepine with the long-acting barbitu-rate phenobarbital. Phenobarbital has a large differential between fatal doses and doses at which

TABLE 25.3
Non-Benzodiazepine Medications Involved in Treatment of Intoxication/Withdrawal of Alcohol or Sedative/Hypnotics

Generic Name	Brand Name	Indications for Use*
Carbamazepine	Tegretol Carbatrol Equetro	Withdrawal from alcohol and sedative/hypnotics (off-label)
Flumazenil	Romazicon	Benzodiazepine intoxication/overdose
Gabapentin	Neurontin	Acute alcohol withdrawal (off-label)
Phenobarbitol	Donnatal (oral)	Withdrawal from alcohol and sedative/hypnotics (off-label)
Valproic acid	Depakene	Withdrawal from alcohol and sedative/hypnotics (off-label)
Divalproex	Depakote Depakote ER	

*Only indications discussed in this chapter are listed here.

easily observable toxicity appears, and because it does not produce much disinhibition, it seems to have less abuse potential than benzodiazepines (Wesson, Smith, Ling, & Seymour, 2005). Less popular with the advent of anti-convulsants for benzodiazepine withdrawal, Phenobarbital seems to have fallen out of favor due to a 1–5% frequency of developing rash, and difficulties with approximating the dose conversion (Wesson et al., 2005). Best administered in an inpatient setting, phenobarbitol is dosed in 30 mg equivalents. The starting dose is continued for 2 days, and then the medication is tapered by 30 mg per day. Starting doses above 500 mg are to be avoided and should the starting dose result in signs of toxicity such as dysarthria, nystagmus, ataxia, or confusion, it is reasonable to reduce the starting dose by 50%. For benzodiazepine withdrawal, 30 mg of phenobarbitol approximates to 1 mg of clonazepam or alprazolam (Wesson et al., 2005).

Alcohol Dependence

There are four FDA-approved medications for the treatment of chronic alcohol dependence (see Table 25.7). Disulfiram was approved in 1951 and has long been available in generic form. The μ-opioid antagonist naltrexone received FDA approval for daily oral use in 1994 and then again as a long-acting intramuscular medication in 2006. Finally, after many years of use in Europe, acamprosate was approved by the FDA for the treatment of alcohol dependence in 2004.

Disulfiram

The interaction between disulfiram and alcohol was originally noted by Danish physicians who were testing it as an antibiotic against flatworm infection. These investigators ingested disulfiram themselves to determine its side effects. They noted no side effects but later that evening developed a range of unpleasant effects after drinking alcohol and then recognized that disulfiram had potential in treating alcohol problems. By inhibiting aldehyde dehydrogenase, a key enzyme in the major metabolic pathway for ethanol, disulfiram causes accumulation of acetaldehyde after alcohol ingestion. The buildup of acetaldehyde usually causes, an "alcohol–disulfiram reaction." That typically ensues within minutes of alcohol ingestion. Different individuals exhibit varying degrees of the reaction (see Table 25.4) which may last for several hours. Severe reactions are exceedingly rare. The reaction may continue for several hours in some patients and may rarely require supportive treatment such as oxygen and intravenous antihistamines or antiemetics.

The usual starting dose of disulfiram is 250 mg/day. Genetic variability may determine sensitivity to the medication, and patients with high levels of aldehyde dehydrogenase may be less sensitive to the effects of disulfiram and require higher doses of medication, up to 500 mg/day (Hall-Flavin, Black, Mrazek, & Sanchez-Samper, 2002). Some patients may not tolerate 250 mg/day and should have the dose reduced to 125 mg/day.

Disulfiram is associated with a number of mild side effects such headache, metallic aftertaste, erectile dysfunction, mild fatigue or sedation, and rash. Such side effects frequently dissipate sponataneously or with a dosage decrease. Much more serious adverse events such as optic neuritis, peripheral neuropathy, hepatic injury, or psychotic symptoms or delirium, although rare, necessitate immediate disulfiram discontinuation. Disulfiram-induced hepatic injury can occur

| TABLE 25.4 |
| Characteristics of the Alcohol–Disulfiram Reaction |

Physiological Effects of the Alcohol–Disulfiram Reaction

Moderate	Severe
Dermatological	
–Diaphoresis	
–Warmth and flushing	
Cardiovascular	
–Angina/palpitations	–Cardiovascular collapse
–Hypotension	–Dysrythmia
–Tachycardia	–Acute myocardial infarction
	–Acute congestive heart failure
Respiratory	
–Tachypnea	–Respiratory depression
–Dyspnea	
Gastrointestinal	
–Nausea/vomiting	
HEENT	
–Headache	
–Thirst	
–Blurred vision	
–Acetaldehyde breath odor	
Central Nervous System	
–Vertigo	–Seizures
–Anxiety	–Prolonged loss of consciousness
–Confusion	
–Syncope	

idiosyncratically at an estimated rate of 1/25,000 (Wright, Vafier & Lake, 1988) to 1/30,000 (Chick, 1999) patient treatment years. Disulfiram-induced hepatic injury can rapidly proceed to total liver failure. It most usually occurs within the first 6 months of treatment. Symptoms include extreme fatigue, malaise, anorexia, fever, jaundice, scleral icterus, nausea, vomiting, and billirubinuria. Baseline liver function tests should be obtained prior to initiation of disulfiram treatment and then at 1–2 month intervals during the first 6 months of treatment. With the decreased risk of disulfiram-induced hepatic injury after the first 6 months of treatment, LFT monitoring can subsequently be done every 3–6 months if treatment continues. Many patients who might be considred for disulfiram therapy present with moderately elevated transaminases related to alcohol use (particularly in the context of hepatitis C). These modest transaminase elevations do not represent a total contraindication to disulfiram therapy. Very rapid rises in bilirubin and transaminases occur in disulfiram-induced hepatic injury and indicate the need to stop disulfiram at once. If the medication is discontinued promptly, the signs and symptoms of liver injury typically fully resolve. If the medication is not stopped, total hepatic failure and death can supervene unless a liver transplant is performed.

Patients with pre-existing cirrhosis or other serious liver disease generally are not good candidates for disulfiram. Other contraindications include pregnancy or lactation, history of prior hypersensitivity to disulfiram or significant coronary artery disease. The latter group could experience myocardial ischemia during a severe alcohol–disulfiram reaction.

Disulfiram has greater benefit with monitoring of medication administration. Although the largest study to date demonstrated that disulfiram dosed at 250 mg per day over one year did not lead to increased abstinence rates or longer time to first drink compared to placebo, it did lead to significantly fewer drinking days over the study year (Fuller et al., 1986).

Naltrexone

The μ-opioid antagonist, naltrexone, originally developed to treat opioid dependence (see below) was subsequently approved to treat alcohol dependence in 1994 and is available in generic form. An involvement of the endogenous opioid systems in the reinforcing effects of alcohol seems likely based on the fact that opioid antagonists block the alcohol-induced release of dopamine into the nulceus accumbens (Benjamin, Grant, & Pohorecky, 1993). The ability of alcohol to promote the release of endogenous opioids (De Waele & Gianoulakis, 1994; Olive, Koenig, Nannini, & Hodge, 2001) or to affect opioid receptor binding (Tabakoff & Hoffman, 1983) may account for dopamine release engendered by alcohol and for the blockade of this event by opioid antagonists. Naltrexone, an orally effective μ-opioid antagonist (O'Malley & Froehlich, 2003) with an active metabolite (6-β naltrexol; McCaul et al., 2000b) with some δ-opioid antagonist properties at higher brain concentrations (Lesscher et al., 2003) decreases alcohol consumption in animals (Stromberg et al., 2002; Volpicelli, Davis, & Olgin 1986). Naltrexone also changes the subjective experience of alcohol consumption in humans rendering it less reinforcing and more sedating (King, Volpicelli, Frazer, & O'Brien, 1997; McCaul et al. 2000a; Swift,Whelihan, Kuznetsov, Buongiorno, & Hsuing, 1994).

These laboratory findings accord well with naltrexone's clearly demonstrated efficacy in the treatment of alcohol dependence in numerous (but not all) clinical trials (Kranzler & Van Kirk, 2001; O'Brien, 2001; Srisurapanont & Jarusuraisin, 2002). In addition to delaying and preventing relapse and reducing the percentage of drinking days, naltrexone has demonstrated the capacity to reduce γ-glutamyl transpeptidase (GGT) levels (Balldin et al., 2003; Gastpar et al., 2002; O'Malley & Froehlich,2003; Volpicelli, Alterman, Hayashida, & O'Brien, 1992; Volpicelli et al., 1997), an objective biomarker of both alcohol consumption and hepatic health status (Allen, Sillamaukee, & Anton ,1999).

Naltrexone is rapidly and almost fully absorbed after oral administration, achieves its peak effect after 1 hour, has a half-life of approximately 4 hours (metabolite half-life = 12 hours). The usual dose is 50 mg per day which is sufficient to occupy the majority of μ-opioid receptors (Lee et al., 1988). Many clinicians begin naltrexone at 25 mg per day for a few days to minimize side effects and then titrate up to 50 mg per day. Although data are sparse some clinicians will also increase naltrexone to 100 mg per day if a suboptimal response occurs at 50 mg per day, and the 100 mg/d dose demonstrated modest efficacy in the COMBINE Study (Anton et al., 2006). It is sometime recommended although certainly not essential that patients have been abstinent at least 3 days prior to initiation and all signs of alcohol withdrawal have resolved. Naltrexone will precipitate withdrawal in patients with physiological dependence on opioids and should not be started until such patients have been opioid free for 5–10 days. If concerns about opioid dependence remain, a naloxone challenge test can be performed prior to the administration of naltrexone.

TABLE 25.5
Naltrexone's Side Effect Profile

Common Side Effect Profile of Naltrexone

–Nausea and vomiting	–Fatigue
–Headache	–Sedation
–Dizziness	–Anxiety

Less Common Side Effects from Naltrexone

–GI cramps, constipation, diarrhea	–Diaphoresis and lacrimation
–Insomnia	–Delayed ejaculation/anorgasmia
–Anorexia, increased thirst	–Dysphoria
–Joint or muscle pain	–Rash

Common side effects of naltrexone are typically mild, tend to resolve within the first week of treatment, and are detailed in Table 25.5. Naltrexone does have a blackbox label warning for acute hepatitis, although most of these events occurred at doses of 300 mg per day in clinical trials for obesity, and there is little evidence of hepatotoxicity at currently recommended doses for alcohol dependence. Nevertheless, given the black box warning it is judicious to obtain liver function tests prior to initiation and then at months 1, 3, 6, and 12 during therapy. The medication should be immediately discontinued should the patient develop signs of acute hepatitis such as scelral icterus, jaundice, light-colored urine, suspected billirubinruria, or significant abdominal pain and malaise. It can be safely administered in patients with active liver disease with more frequent laboratory monitoring of their liver function tests, but probably should be avoided in patients with transaminase levels five times above the normal level. Pregnant patients should be carefully counseled regarding the risks/benefits of naltrexone before starting treatment and women of child-bearing age should be counseled to use effective birth control methods during treatment, as naltrexone has been assigned FDA category C in pregnancy.

Because naltrexone blocks μ-opioid receptors, opioid medications will be much less effective in the situation in which an injury or serious medical condition calls for acute pain control. Ideally patients on naltrexone should carry a medicalert card or bracelet to notify emergency medical personnel of the fact that they take this medication in case they need opioid analgesia and cannot communicate about their medication usage. If given in adequate doses (usually higher than would otherwise be required) opioids can generally overcome the blockade, but close monitoring of the patient in an inpatient setting to observe for and manage respiratory depression is advised. Naltrexone should be stopped 3 days before any elective surgery or dental procedures that will require opioid analgesia, and the patient should discontinue of opioids for 3–7 days prior to resuming naltrexone.

Long-Acting Injectable Naltrexone

Although oral naltrexone generally appears efficacious compared to placebo in reducing relapse to heavy drinking (Anton et al., 2006; Bouza, Angeles, Munoz, & Amate, 2004; Mann, 2004), it has not performed well in several studies (Kranzler, Modesto-Lowe, & Van Kirk, 2000; Krystal, Cramer, Krol, Kirk, & Rosenheck, 2001). However, when patients found to be nonadherent for oral naltrexone are factored out in several other studies, naltrexone demonstrates efficacy for treatment of alcohol dependence compared to placebo (Chick et al., 2000; Volpicelli et al., 1997). Consequently, long-acting intramuscular naltrexone, FDA approved in 2006, may alleviate this problem and has been shown to be effective compared to placebo in reducing heavy drinking (Garbutt et al., 2005). Additional advantages of long-acting intramuscular naltrexone include much lower rates of first-pass hepatic metabolism, exposing the liver to significantly lower peak dosages than daily oral dosing, and potentially less risk of dose-dependent hepatotoxicity. The reduced first-pass metabolism of intramuscular naltrexone leads to lower levels of the active metabolite 6β-hydroxynaltrexol, which has been correlated with side effects such as nausea. Lower levels of this metabolite may lead to better toleralability of naltrexone's intramuscular form. Long-acting injectable naltrexone is indicated for patients who have achieved some period of abstinence which could be as brief as several hours. The dosage is one 360 mg gluteal injection every 4 weeks. Patients can be started directly on the injection without a trial on oral medication.

Acamprosate

Acamprosate, which has seen widespread use in Europe for many years, received FDA approval for the treatment of alcohol dependence in 2004. Acamprosate has been extensively studied and in clinical use in Europe for nearly 20 years. Acamprosate is believed to modulate both the major excitatory system in the brain, the glutamate system as well as the major inhibitory system, the GABA system. Alcohol interacts with these systems as well, but when alcohol is stopped after chronic exposure, glutamatergic hyperactivity and GABA hypoactivity contribute substantially to the alcohol withdrawal syndrome. Acamprosate theoretically acts to counteract these imbalances and so may attenuate symptoms associated with subsyndromal, prolonged alcohol withdrawal such as insomnia, anxiety, and restlessness which could provoke alcohol cravings and relapse (Thomsen Healthcare Inc. 2006; Litten, Fertig, Mattson, & Egli, 2005; Myrick & Anton, 2004). Acamprosate also may diminish reinforcement derived from alcohol ingestion (Myrick & Anton, 2004) and the amount of alcohol consumed by patients in treatment who do experience relapse (Chick, Lehert, & Landron 2003). Numerous controlled studies of acamprosate demonstrated higher total abstinence rates and longer time to relapse for acamprosate compared to placebo. For reasons that remain incompletely understood, acamparosate failed to show efficacy in two large clinical trials conducted in the United States (Anton et al., 2006; Mason, Goodman, Chabac, & Lehert, 2006). It has been proposed that subjects in the U.S. studies may not have experienced sufficient prolonged subsyndromal withdrawal to benefit from acamprosate (Kiefer & Mann, 2006).

Acamprosate has very limited oral bioavailability. It acheives steady-state after five days and is not metabolized by the liver but excreted unchanged in the urine. The usual dose is 666 mg (two 333 mg tablets) three times daily. The labeling indicates that acamprosate should be started after a modicum of abstinence has been achieved, but there are no safety issues if acamprosate is taken concomitantly with alcohol and abstinence is not essential. In fact, acamprosate should be continued if a patient relapses to alcohol use.

It is recommended that a serum creatinine level to evaluate kidney function be obtained prior to initiation of therapy because the dose should be lowered in patients with impaired kidney

TABLE 25.6
Acamprosate's Side Effect Profile

Side Effect Profile of Acamprosate

–Diarrhea, flatulence, cramps, or nausea	–Changes in libido
–Insomnia	–Headache
–Pruritus	–Muscle weakness
–Dizziness	–Anxiety

function. Acamprosate is FDA category C, so women of child-bearing age must use an effective method of birth control when on acamprosate. All patients should be monitored for suicidal thoughts because such thoughts occurred more frequently among acamprosate-treated patients than among placebo-treated patients in clinical trials. Most side effects of acamprosate are relatively mild, resolve within the first two weeks of treatment, and are detailed in Table 25.6.

The medication's manufacturer recommends that acamprosate treatment be continued for 12 months, and follow-up studies show increased abstinence rates that persist 1 year after cessation of treatment (Sass, Soyka, Mann, & Zieglgansberger, 1996). Advantages of acamprosate include its lack of drug–drug interactions and the fact that it is not contraindicated in patients with serious liver disease.

Additional Agents

Several GABAergic agents currently show promise under active investigation for the treatment of alcohol dependence (see Table 25.8). Although preclinical studies suggest that the GABA$_B$ agonist baclofen has potential evidence in decreasing alcohol use (Colombo et al., 2004, 2002; Maccioni et al., 2005), baclofen dosed at 10 mg TID over 30 days led to statistically significant reductions on both alcohol craving and consumption (Addolorato et al., 2002). The anticonvulsant topiramate promotes GABAergic activity and antagonizes glutamatergic AMPA/kainite receptors. In a 12 week studies in escalating doses from 25 mg to 300 mg/day, topiramate led to statistically significant reductions in alcohol use, alcohol craving, and reduced harmful drinking consequences (Johnson, Ait-Daoud, Akhtar, & Ma, 2004; Johnson et al., 2003). Both agents are discussed in more depth in this chapter under cocaine dependence.

Management of Opioid Intoxication and Withdrawal

Opioid dependence is a serious problem effecting millions of people worldwide. It is estimated that in 2005, there were 227,000 Americans with heroin dependence or abuse and 1.5 million Americans who used prescription pain relievers for nonmedical reasons (Studies, 2006). There were also 108,000 Americans who used heroin for the first time in 2005. The cost of opioid abuse and dependence is high, with the productivity loss, criminal activities, and medical expenses associated with heroin addiction each exceeding a billion dollars in the United States (Mark, Woody, Juday, & Kleber, 2001). Patients with opioid dependence are often dependent on other substances of abuse, and have comorbid psychiatric problems as well as medical and social problems related to opioid abuse.

TABLE 25.7
FDA-Approved Medications for Treatment of Alcohol Dependence

Generic Name	Brand Name	Indications for Use
Acamprosate	Campral	**Alcohol dependence**
Disulfiram	Antabuse	**Alcohol dependence**
Naltrexone (intramuscular)	Vivitrol (IM)	**Alcohol dependence**
		Opioid dependence (off-label)
Naltrexone (oral)	Revia (oral)	**Alcohol dependence**
	Depade	**Opioid dependence**

TABLE 25.8
Medications Under Investigation for "Off-Label Use" in Treatment of Alcohol Dependence

Generic Name	Brand Name	Indications for Use*
Baclofen	Lioresal	Alcohol dependence (off-label)
		Cocaine dependence (off-label)
Topiramate	Topamax	Alcohol dependence (off-label)
		Cocaine dependence (off-label)

*Only indications discussed in this chapter are listed here. Medications being investigated for "off-label" use are not recommended for this clinical use unless a patient has failed each of the FDA approved agents, or such agents are contraindicated.

Opioid-dependent patients may present for treatment openly seeking treatment for their substance abuse or they may present for medical or psychiatric treatment without disclosing their substance abuse. Diagnosis can be made by taking a history, it may be verified by documentation from previous health care providers of dependence on opioids, urine toxicology detecting the presence of opioid drugs, observation on the skin of intravenous injection sites, and observation of the characteristic signs of withdrawal. *The Diagnostic and Statistical Manual of Mental Disorders–IV (DSM–IV)* defines opioid dependence as a maladaptive pattern of opioid use over a 12-month period, leading to clinically significant impairment or distress, as manifested by three or more of the following: tolerance for opioids, withdrawal syndrome from opioids, opioids being taken in a larger amounts or over longer periods than intended, persistent desire or unsuccessful efforts to cut down or control use of opioids, a great deal of time spent in activities necessary to obtain, use or recover from the use of opioids, important social, occupational, or recreational activities given up or reduced because of opioid use and opioid use continuing in spite of knowledge of persistent or recurrent physical or psychological problems caused by their use (American Psychiatric Association, 2000).

Pharmacological treatments for opioid dependence are targeted at preventing overdose, ameliorating toxicity and withdrawal, and maintenance therapies to prevent illicit opioid use or preventing relapse to opioid use after stopping opioid use (see Table 25.9).

Management of Opioid Intoxication and Overdose

Opioid use and overdose are a significant cause of mortality. Nonfatal and fatal overdose are relatively common among those with opioid dependence, especially heroin addicts. A prospective cohort study of heroin addicts in Los Angeles followed for 33 years found that among this group of patients, there was an average 18.3 years of life lost prior to age 65, of which, 22% was accounted for by death due to overdose (Smyth, Hoffman, Fan, & Hser, 2007) In addition, overdose deaths are increasing worldwide, with a growing role of prescription narcotics in many countries (Drummer, 2005).

Opioids are CNS depressants that produce a characteristic pattern of signs and symptoms during intoxication. Opioid intoxication is characterized by bradycardia, hypotension, hypothermia, sedation, pupillary constriction, slurring of speech, motor retardation, head nodding, euphoria, analgesia, and a sense of calmness. At toxic levels, opioids cause respiratory depression and obtundation.

Naloxone   Naloxone, a complete opioid antagonist with a short half-life, has been the standard agent used in treating opioid toxicity since the 1960s. Treatment with naloxone is commonly done by emergency responders or in the emergency department setting. Use of naloxone in the emergency setting is typically triggered by decreased arousal and respiratory depression or decreased oxygen saturation. Naloxone can be administered intravenously, intramuscularly, or subcutaneously. Intravenous administration should be dosed as a bolus dose of 0.1 mg per minute until the patient has improvement in respiratory rate above 10 per minute, oxygen saturation, and level of consciousness. Intramuscular and subcutaneous dosing should be made as a single bolus of 0.4 mg and 0.8 mg, respectively. Patients should be observed for at least two hours for signs of recurring toxicity, which may require repeated dosing if the patient overdosed on a long-acting opioid (Clarke, Dargan, & Jones, 2005). A particularly worrisome complication of opioid overdose is pulmonary edema.

The effectiveness of naloxone in preventing overdose death has led some governments to allow prescription of naloxone to heroin users for use by friends or family members in the event of overdose and even sale over the counter in Turin, Italy. A pilot project in Chicago, Illinois where more than 3,500 patients were educated and given naloxone kits for emergency use resulted in over 300 reported overdose reversals as well as declining overdose deaths in the county for 3 consecutive years of the study (Maxwell, Bigg, Stanczykiewicz, & Carlberg-Racich, 2006).

Management of Opioid Withdrawal

Many opioid dependent patients seeking treatment for medical, psychiatric, or substance abuse problems, will desire or need medically supervised withdrawal to ease them through the withdrawal period, if they are not receiving or scheduled to receive substitution therapy. Medically supervised withdrawal or detoxification can be done on an inpatient or outpatient basis. For routine medically supervised withdrawal the agents of choice are methadone, buprenorphine, or clonidine.

The opioid withdrawal syndrome is a group of unpleasant signs and symptoms that often contributes to continued use of opioids or relapse in individuals trying to abstain from opioid use. The withdrawal syndrome is characterized by tachycardia, hypertension, hyperthermia, hyperreflexia, diaphoresis, piloerection, dilation of the pupils, lacrimation, yawning, rhinorrhea, muscle aches, "bone" pain, muscle spasm, abdominal cramping, nausea, vomiting, diarrhea, and anxiety. The goal of medically supervised withdrawal is to alleviate these symptoms as opioids are eliminated from the patient's system allowing the patient to transition to abstinence-based psychosocial treatment and/or treatment with an opioid antagonist.

Methadone   Withdrawal from opioids has most commonly been managed with methadone, a long acting, μ-opioid agonist (CSAT, 2006). The use of methadone is highly regulated and can only be used by physicians in certified opioid treatment programs or during hospitalization for another condition. Care should be made in obtaining a history of the patient's opioid use, considering purity of local supplies to determine a starting dose of methadone. Clinicians should not underdose methadone, but care should also be made not to start at too high of a dose as this can lead to overdose. For many patients, a starting dose of 10 mg can be used initially, with withdrawal symptoms being reassessed in 1–2 hours. Individuals with very high levels of dependence may require initial doses of 30–40 mg, which should be sufficient to treat even severe withdrawal. Once a stable dose is established, that alleviates withdrawal symptoms without producing sedation or signs of intoxication, methadone can be tapered over a 3–10 day period by decreasing the daily dose by 5 mg or 10 mg increments. In spite of methadone being considered the gold standard medication for management of withdrawal, a recent systematic review comparing methadone to other pharmacological treatments for withdrawal found no difference between methadone and these other agents either pooled or on an individual head-to-head basis (Amato et al. 2005b). Methadone was, however, superior to placebo.

Buprenorphine   A medication, which has recently been added to the prescribing armamentarium is buprenorphine, a partial μ-opioid agonist with high affinity for the μ-opioid receptor. Unlike methadone, buprenorphine is not restricted to use in opioid treatment programs, however, physicians do need to get additional training that satisfies the requirements of the Drug Addiction Treatment Act (DATA) of 2000 and then apply to the Drug Enforcement Agency (DEA) for a special DEA number in order to prescribe buprenorphine. Because of its high affinity for the μ-opioid receptor and partial agonist effect, buprenorphine can precipitate withdrawal in patients who have recently used opioids or who have high levels of opioids in their system, such as individuals who are on high dose methadone maintenance. There are a number of different protocols that are used for detoxification with buprenorphine. Clinical guidelines developed by the Center for Substance Abuse Treatment recommend stabilizing patients over 2 days on 12 mg to 16 mg of buprenorphine and once patients have ceased use of illicit opioids, this may be gradually tapered with dose reductions in 2 mg increments every 2 to 3 days or slower (CSAT, 2004). Management of withdrawal may be done more quickly, in a safe and comfortable manner over 5 days with doses of 8 mg per day on the first three days, 4 mg on day 4, and 2 mg on day 5 (Oreskovich et al., 2005). A recent systematic review of opioid detoxification using buprenorphine versus clonidine, methadone and other agents examined 18 studies with over 1,300 patients found that buprenorphine is superior to clonidine in treating withdrawal symptoms and in allowing patients to complete withdrawal treatment

(Gowing, Ali, & White, 2006). The reviewers found that buprenorphine was not more effective than methadone although withdrawal symptoms may be alleviated more quickly with buprenorphine.

Clonidine   Prior to the introduction of buprenorphine, clonidine, an α2-adrenergic agonist, was the primary alternative to methadone for management of opioid withdrawal. Clonidine is an antihypertensive medication, which has been used off-label for this purpose since the late 1970s. Clonidine has several advantages to methadone and buprenorphine as an agent to manage opioid withdrawal. Clonidine does not have the regulatory restrictions that methadone and buprenorphine have, making it easier to use and more widely available. It does not act at the opioid receptor so it does not produce euphoria and is not reinforcing. It also allows for detoxification without use of opioids. It has limitations, however, and is fairly ineffective at treating muscle aches, drug craving, and insomnia in the withdrawal setting. Clonidine is also contraindicated in patients with low systolic or diastolic blood pressures. Blood pressure should be checked prior to administering the first dose of clonidine and should generally not be given if the blood pressure parameters are less than 90 systolic or 60 diastolic. The concern about inducing hypotension makes this agent best used for inpatient detoxification and blood pressure as well as withdrawal symptoms should be assessed as often as the medication is being administered. Typically a 0.1 mg test dose is given and withdrawal symptoms assessed afterward. A dose of 0.1 mg to 0.2 mg can be given every 4 to 6 hours for withdrawal symptoms over the first 24 hours. The total dose given over the first 24 hours can then be divided to be given as a standing dose every 4 to 6 hours. This dose is then tapered over the course of 3–5 days (CSAT, 2006). A recent systematic review compared studies of clonidine and another α2-adrenergic agonist, lofexidine, with methadone. There was no difference between α2-adrenergic agonists and methadone in terms of completing detoxification, but patients receiving methadone remained in treatment longer. Additionally, clonidine has more adverse reactions, such as hypotension, dry mouth, dizziness and fatigue, compared to methadone (Gowing, Farrell, Ali, & White, 2004).

Rapid Anesthesia-Assisted Detoxification   In spite of these options, many opioid-dependent patients fear any withdrawal symptoms and wish to complete the detoxification quicker than the typical 5–10 days of most protocols. This helped give rise to anesthesia-assisted rapid detoxification, where patients are sedated by an anesthesiologist while an opioid antagonist, typically naloxone or naltrexone, is administered to attempt to hasten the withdrawal period. A recent randomized trial compared anesthesia-assisted rapid detoxification with buprenorphine and clonidine detoxification followed by induction onto naltrexone maintenance and outpatient treatment in 106 opioid dependent patients (Collins, Kleber, Whittington, & Heitler, 2005). There was no difference in the groups in terms of withdrawal severity or completion of detoxification, however, anesthesia-assisted detoxification and buprenorphine were comparable to each other and superior to clonidine in terms of induction onto naltrexone and retention in treatment at 12 weeks. The anesthesia-assisted rapid detoxification, however, was associated with three life-threatening adverse events. Given the risks associated, great expense, and lack of superiority to other available treatments, use of anesthesia-assisted rapid detoxification is not advisable.

TABLE 25.9

Medications Involved in Treatment of Opioid Intoxication, Withdrawal, and Dependence

Generic Name	Brand Name	Indications for Use*
Buprenorphine	Subutex	Opioid dependence Opioid withrawal (off-label)
Buprenorphine/naloxone	Suboxone	Opioid dependence Opioid withdrawal (off-label)
Clonidine	Catapres Duraclon	Opioid withdrawal
Levomethadyl acetate hydrochloride (LAAM)	Orlaam	Opioid dependence (discontinued in U.S. 9/2003)
Methadone	Dolophine	Opioid dependence
	Methadone	Opioid withdrawal (use only approved in federally licensed facilities)
Naloxone	Narcan	Opioid overdose
Naltrexone (intramuscular)	Vivitrol (IM)	Alcohol dependence Opioid dependence (off-label)
Naltrexone (oral)	Revia (oral)	Alcohol dependence
	Depade	Opioid dependence

*Only indications discussed in this chapter are listed here.

TABLE 25.10

Medications Involved in Treatment of Nicotine Dependence

Generic Name	Brand Name	Indications for Use*
Bupropion	Zyban Wellbutrin	Smoking cessation
Nicotine	Nicoderm CQ (patch) Nicotrol (inhaler/patch) Nicorette (gum) Habitrol (patch/gum) Nicotrol NS (nasal) Commit (lozenge) Endit (inhaler)	Smoking cessation
Nortriptyline	Aventyl Pamelor	Smoking cessation (off-label)
Varenicline	Chantix	Smoking cessation

*Only indications discussed in this chapter are listed here.

Overview   Methadone, buprenorphine, and clonidine each have their advantages and disadvantages in management of opioid withdrawal. Due to the typically small size and heterogeneity of studies, it is difficult to draw strong conclusions about these agents. A recent overview of comparative reviews found that compared to other opioid agonists, methadone relieved withdrawal symptoms best and led to higher rates of completion of detoxification (Amato et al. 2004a). Methadone was also superior to clonidine in retaining patients in treatment and had lower rates of relapse. Buprenorphine was also superior to clonidine in relieving withdrawal symptoms.

In spite of the ability of all of the above treatments to relieve symptoms of opioid withdrawal, detoxification remains a fairly ineffective treatment approach, with patients frequently dropping out of treatment, either during the detoxification or afterward, to resume using opioids. This is due in part to the relative lack of effectiveness of treatment approaches other than opioid agonist therapies. The most typically used nonopioid agonist treatment is naltrexone and this frequently cannot be started immediately after completion of detoxification with clonidine or other agents and suffers from poor compliance in the outpatient setting. Adding to pharmacological treatment for management of opioid withdrawal with psychosocial interventions is one possible way to enhance treatment outcomes. A systematic review of studies adding psychosocial treatments to detoxification with either methadone or buprenorphine examined 8 studies with over 400 subjects (Amato et al. 2004b). This review found that adding any of the psychosocial interventions (contingency management, community reinforcement, structured counseling or family therapy) improved completion of detoxification, compliance, and follow-up results.

Opioid Agonist Therapy

Opioid substitution therapy is by far the most widely used, researched, and effective treatment for opioid dependence. For many years, methadone was the sole agent available for substitution therapy in highly regulated specialty clinics until the FDA approved the use of levo-α-acetyl methadol (LAAM) in 1993 and then in 2002, when buprenorphine was approved for office-based substitution therapy.

Methadone   Methadone is an orally active, μ-opioid agonist with an average half-life greater than 24 hours, which allows for once daily dosing without serious withdrawal discomfort during that interval.

The Substance Abuse and Mental Health Services Administration (SAMHSA) and the DEA provide regulatory oversight of opioid agonist treatment. The legal mandate for this oversight comes from the Controlled Substance Act (1970, Public Law [PL] 91-513), the Narcotic Addict Treatment Act (1974, PL 93-281), and the Drug Addiction Treatment Act 2000 (DATA 2000, PL 106-310, div. B). From 1972 to 2000 the FDA had provided oversight of the treatment services. Regulations strictly govern the use of agonist therapies, but allow for some latitude in program goals, policies, and philosophies. Under the regulations, patients need to have a documented 1 year or greater history of dependence to opioids. They must get a physical exam, serologic testing for syphilis, and tuberculin skin testing on entry. Patients initiating treatment must also show signs of observable withdrawal at the time of evaluation to prevent exposure of nondependent patients to iatrogenic dependence. Programs must provide monthly counseling and patients must have urine toxicology at least 8 times the first year and quarterly thereafter, though this is commonly done more frequently. Programs must be open to dispense methadone at least 6 days per week. After being stable in treatment for 3 months, patients may be allowed to have take-home doses and reduce clinic days with certain limits (CSAT 2005).

Regulations limit the initial dose of methadone to 30 mg and doses on the first day in excess of 40 mg require medical justification. Typically, patients demonstrating opioid withdrawal symptoms are given an initial dose of 20 mg to 30 mg of methadone and reassessed for withdrawal symptoms in 2 to 4 hours. If withdrawal symptoms persist additional doses of 5 mg to 10 mg of methadone are given and monitoring continues at regular intervals. Doses can then be titrated fairly rapidly over the first few weeks to eliminate withdrawal symptoms. Ultimate maintenance doses need to be individualized to avoid opioid intoxication and withdrawal (CSAT, 2005). Although effective dose ranges vary widely and overlap with ineffective doses, individual factors such as presence of psychiatric comorbidity and treatment delivery factors should be considered in dosing patients with methadone (Trafton, Minkel & Humphreys, 2006). Doses ranging between 60 mg and 100 mg per day are more effective than lower doses at retaining patient in treatment and decreasing heroin use (Faggiano, Vigna-Taglianti, Versino, & Lemma, 2003). Higher methadone doses also reduce cocaine use during treatment, which can be a significant problem (Peles, Kreek, Kellogg, & Adelson, 2006).

Opioid-dependent patients rapidly develop tolerance to the opioid effects of methadone, showing little or no signs of intoxication or psychomotor impairment from the medication. As with other opioid medications, however, methadone has typical side effects of constipation and decreased libido. There is no evidence to suggest that chronic methadone administration permanently impairs any organ system although problems with the endocrine system, such as weight gain and low testosterone, are seen in some patients. There have been some reports of torsade de pointes in patients on very high doses of methadone in maintenance treatment programs and receiving methadone for chronic pain treatment (Krantz et al., 2002). The average dose of methadone in this case series, 397 mg per day, is far higher than recommended daily doses of methadone for maintenance therapy.

In maintenance therapy, retention is the primary goal. Retention rates for treatment of opioid dependence with behavioral therapies alone are exceedingly poor. Findings from the Drug Abuse Reporting Program (Simpson & Sells, 1982; Simpson et al., 1990), the Treatment Outcome Prospective Study (Hubbard, Mardsen, & Rachal, 1989), and the Drug Abuse Treatment Outcome Study (DATOS; Simpson et al. 1997) suggest a minimum of one year in methadone maintenance treatment is needed to obtain substantial clinical improvement. All 29 DATOS programs providing methadone maintenance recommended a two year minimum treatment stay. However, only 50% of all clients remained in those programs more than 365 days with the median length of stay ranging from 117 to 583 days (Simpson et al., 1997). A series of recent systematic reviews of currently available maintenance therapies found methadone maintenance to have retention rates of 52–81% in studies lasting between 3 months and 2 years (Amato et al. 2005a).

The objective of maintenance treatment is to reduce illicit opioid use and the many negative consequences associated with this activity. Continued opioid use, determined by urine toxicology or self-report has consistently been shown to be decreased by treatment with methadone. A Cochrane review of methadone versus no opioid replacement treatment found morphine positive urines over the course of treatment in 47% of methadone subjects versus 77% in controls and self-report of heroin use in only 27% of methadone subjects versus 87% of controls (Mattick, Breen, Kimber, & Davoli, 2003).

A major rationale for maintenance therapies such as methadone is to reduce the burden of other significant health problems on these individuals and society at large. Recent reviews have found that methadone maintenance does in fact reduce injection drug use, sharing of needles and other equipment, patients reporting multiple sex partners or exchanging sex for drugs or money, as well as lower prevalence and incidence of HIV/AIDS (Gowing et al., 2006; Sullivan et al., 2005). In spite of this effectiveness, methadone has interactions with many anti-retroviral medications leading to withdrawal symptoms, anti-retroviral toxicity, or elevated levels of methadone if not carefully monitored (McCance-Katz, 2005).

Although methadone is an effective medication, patients in methadone maintenance treatment often have complex medical and psychosocial problems that affect their retention in treatment and overall health. A consensus panel of experts have recommended that all treatment programs have several specific components to address these common problems in this population (CSAT, 2005). Patients should have a comprehensive psychosocial evaluation with goals to specifically identify any co-occurring disorders or neuropsychological problems and family problems. In addition to an initial medical examination, there should be an annual medical examination with laboratory studies. Testing for HIV and hepatitis C virus, with education, counseling, and referral for care should be included in this. Periodic drug testing should be conducted. Counseling services should be targeted at stopping substance abuse as well as managing craving. Referral for additional services identified in the comprehensive evaluation should be made as well.

Drug testing, in addition to being required of treatment programs, is useful in monitoring treatment compliance and effectiveness. Urine toxicology is the most commonly used form of testing because it is inexpensive and easy to obtain, although other forms of testing may be used including serum and oral fluid drug testing. Standard testing should detect methadone and its metabolites, other opioids, cocaine, benzodiazepines, and other drugs depending on local use patterns (e.g., MA, phencyclidine). The consensus panel recommends that testing frequency and randomness be sufficient to be useful in guiding therapy considerations, though they advise against basing clinical decisions solely on testing results (CSAT, 2005). Testing frequency should be higher at the beginning of treatment and increased for individuals who have repeated positive results for illicit drug use to ensure prompt therapeutic response to relapses. Methadone maintenance alone is effective in retaining a large percentage of patients in treatment and significantly reducing illicit drug use and medical consequences of this use, but in many cases it does not eliminate this activity. Psychosocial treatments are a very important component of treatment of patients maintained on methadone just as it is for patients in treatment for substance use disorders other than opioid dependence. A recent Cochrane review of 12 studies involving 981 subjects found any additional psychosocial treatments reduce heroin use during methadone maintenance (Amato et al. 2004b). The interventions in these studies ranged from biofeedback, cognitive-behavioral therapy, contingency management, psychoanalytic-oriented treatment, structured counseling, and a form of short-term interpersonal therapy. Although these added treatments did not significantly increase treatment retention, there was a trend in that direction.

Most treatment programs offer some take-home doses and give these contingent on progress in treatment. Federal regulations permit one take-home dose per week during the first

90 days of treatment, up to two take-home doses per week the second 90 days of treatment, up to 3 take-home doses per week the third 90 days of treatment, and up to 6 take-home doses per week the fourth 90 days of treatment. After the first year of continuous treatment, programs can give up to a 2 weeks supply of take-home doses at a time and after 2 years of continuous treatment, one month's supply of take-home medication can be given at a time. Federal regulation requires that increases in take-home doses must be made by the medical director of the treatment program after considering absence of recent drug or alcohol use, regular program attendance, absence of behavioral problems, recent criminal activity, stability of home environment and social relationships, acceptable length of comprehensive treatment, assurance of safe storage of take-home doses, and determination that benefits of decreased program attendance outweigh the risk of diversion (CSAT, 2005).

LAAM   Due to concerns over diversion of methadone take-home doses and ineffectiveness of methadone in some patients, LAAM was developed and approved for use in opioid treatment programs by the FDA in 1993. Like methadone, LAAM is a long-acting synthetic μ-opioid agonist. LAAM, however, has a 46 hour half-life and is metabolized by the liver to two active metabolites, nor-LAAM and dinor-LAAM, which have average half-lives of 62 and 175 hours. Due to this difference in duration of action, LAAM can be administered in the clinic 3 times per week without the need for take-home doses. Otherwise, LAAM administration must follow the same federal regulations as methadone. Patients may be started on LAAM directly or converted from substitution with methadone. Initial doses for those starting on LAAM cannot exceed 40 mg every other day. In converting patients from methadone to LAAM, the LAAM dose should be calculated by multiplying the daily methadone dose by 1.2 or 1.3 and administering this every other day. Due to the very long half-lives of LAAM and its metabolites, steady-state doses are not achieved for several weeks and can lead to instability in patients, especially during the 72 hour period of the week where they do not get a dose of medication.

A recent Cochrane review of the effectiveness of LAAM looked at 15 studies with over 1000 subjects, comparing LAAM with methadone (Clark et al., 2002). This meta-analysis found LAAM to be more effective than methadone at reducing heroin use, but that patients who begin treatment with LAAM were more likely to stop, although it is not clear if this is due to pharmacological effect or some other reason. Postmarketing analysis of LAAM found an association with prolongation of the QT interval and fatal torsade de pointes, which has led to the FDA placing a black box warning on this medication and subsequently to the voluntary discontinuation of its production by the manufacturer.

Buprenorphine   An increase in heroin use and especially in diseases spread by injection drug use led in part to an Institute of Medicine report which recommended expansion of access to methadone and exploration of other agonist treatments (Rettig & Yarmolinsky, 1995). Another alternative was developing in Europe, where the synthetic partial μ-opioid agonist buprenorphine was being used successfully in office-based maintenance therapy for opioid dependence.

The pharmacological characteristics of buprenorphine make it a very attractive medication for office-based substitution therapy. Its partial agonist action means that it has a ceiling effect for CNS and respiratory depressive effects meaning it is far safer in overdose than methadone and other full μ-opioid agonists. This partial agonist property also makes it easier to withdraw from this medication than methadone, which can be very poorly tolerated by patients. One disadvantage of the partial agonist effect is that patients dependent on very high doses of opioids or who are trying to transition from high-dose methadone maintenance to buprenorphine are likely to experience some withdrawal when they transition. Buprenorphine has a long half-life, allowing for once daily or even thrice weekly dosing. Buprenorphine is poorly absorbed by the oral route, so for maintenance therapy purposes, it is administered sublingually.

Buprenorphine may be administered by opioid treatment programs, regulated in the same fashion as methadone, but it may also be administered in the office setting, which was made possible by the DATA of 2000. DATA allows for office-based opioid maintenance therapy for opioid dependence using Schedule III, IV, or V medications approved for this use by the FDA. In 2002, the FDA approved buprenorphine for this purpose and it is the only medication at this time which has this indication. In order to prescribe buprenorphine, physicians must obtain a waiver from the DEA, which requires specialty training in addictions or completion of approximately 8 hours of training in management of opioid dependence provided by an approved association, and physicians must be able to refer patients to appropriate counseling and ancillary services. The waiver allows physicians to prescribe buprenorphine to up to 100 patients at a given time.

Buprenorphine is available for sublingual administration as a single agent or as a combination buprenorphine–naloxone preparation with a ratio of 4 mg buprenorphine to 1 mg of naloxone. The advantage of the combination buprenorphine–naloxone preparation is the prevention of abuse. Buprenorphine is absorbed sublingually, whereas naloxone is not available sublingually and so has no effect on patients when administered as intended. If the combination medication is dissolved in an attempt to inject buprenorphine, however, naloxone, which has a higher affinity for the μ receptor, will exert its antagonist properties resulting in withdrawal instead of euphoria. The single agent should be reserved for use only in situations where there is no concern for potential abuse, such as in an inpatient setting or in individuals who are at greater risk to potential withdrawal symptoms if exposed to naloxone, such as pregnant women or those transitioning from methadone. Those transitioning from methadone must be on 30 mg per day or less and should be transitioned to the buprenorphine–naloxone combination after several days of starting treatment with buprenorphine. Due to the partial agonist properties of buprenorphine, patients need to be clearly educated that they should not take this medication soon after taking other opioid drugs because this may precipitate withdrawal. Induction of buprenorphine should begin 12–24 hours after last use of a short-acting opioid drug or 24–48 hours after last use of a long-acting opioid drug and patients should be showing signs of withdrawal at the time of initiation of therapy.

On the first day of induction, the maximum dose should not exceed 8–12 mg. Patients transitioning from methadone should be monitored for withdrawal signs every 1 to 2 hours initially. If patients still have withdrawal symptoms after receiving the maximum dose, they should be treated symptomatically with adjunctive agents for specific withdrawal symptoms. Over the course of the next 2–6 days, patients should be assessed for signs and symptoms of withdrawal with increases in buprenorphine given for persistent symptoms up to a total of 16 mg on the second day and a maximum of 32 mg per day by the end of the first week. Withdrawal symptoms beyond this time typically indicate persisting illicit opioid abuse. Following induction, patients will stabilize on a dose over the following 1–2 months and the dose should be adjusted to the lowest effective dose to prevent withdrawal symptoms, prevent craving of opioids, and suppress illicit opioid abuse. Once this dose is established, patients can be maintained on this medication indefinitely or may choose to gradually taper off (CSAT, 2004).

Numerous studies have found buprenorphine to be effective retaining patients in treatment and reducing illicit opioid abuse. A systematic review of studies, which compared 13 studies involving 2,544 subjects in trials of buprenorphine versus either placebo or methadone, found buprenorphine to be effective as a maintenance therapy for opioid dependence when compared to placebo (Mattick et al., 2002). Compared with methadone, however, especially at higher doses of methadone, buprenorphine is not as effective at maintaining patients in treatment or reducing heroin use. In contrast to methadone, however, buprenorphine has little relative interaction with anti-retroviral medications, making HIV-infected patients a special population who may benefit specifically from buprenorphine treatment.

Opioid Antagonist Therapy

In spite of the notable efficacy of agonist therapies, many opioid-dependent patients either do not wish to be on maintenance therapy with an opioid agonist, or are unable to receive maintenance treatment.

Naltrexone   Naltrexone was developed as an alternative medication treatment for opioid dependence and approved by the FDA in 1984. For many of those individuals who successfully withdraw from illicit opioids or from maintenance therapy, the opioid antagonist naltrexone is an ideal medication to aid in continuing abstinence from continued opioid use.

Naltrexone is a long-acting μ-opioid antagonist with a higher affinity for the μ-opioid receptor than heroin. Naltrexone is almost completely absorbed in the gastrointestinal tract, with peak plasma concentrations within one hour of administration. This rapid absorption and receptor affinity, leads to complete blockade of analgesic and euphoric effects of exogenous opioids when the medication is used at sufficient doses. A 50 mg dose of naltrexone blocks the effects of 25 mg of intravenous heroin for 24 hours (Tucker & Ritter, 2000).

Due to its pharmacological profile, patients who have even low levels of opioids will be subject to withdrawal symptoms if the medication is initiated too soon after cessation of opioids. This is an important property of this medication and requires thorough patient education. Patients should be abstinent from short-acting opioids for at least 5 days and long-acting opioids at least 10 days prior to starting treatment with naltrexone to avoid this possibility. When there are still questions about whether a patient has been fully detoxified from opioids prior to starting naltrexone, a challenge dose of 0.8 mg of the short-acting opioid antagonist naloxone may be administered parenterally to observe whether withdrawal will be precipitated. Dosing is straightforward, with most patients being able to tolerate starting at the full dose of 50 mg per day. For those more likely to have side effects (shorter prior abstinence, women, and adolescents) the dose may be started at 25 mg or 12.5 mg daily. Due to its long half-life, naltrexone can be given on a flexible schedule to enhance compliance, with 100 mg given every other day or 150 mg given every third day.

The FDA has issued a black box warning for naltrexone due to concerns over potential hepatotoxicity. Naltrexone is metabolized almost exclusively by the liver. Due to these safety concerns with naltrexone, it is contraindicated in patients with acute hepatitis and liver failure due to its potential hepatotoxic effects, which have been seen at very high doses of 300 mg per day. A recent study looking at high doses of 150 mg per day in very impulsive individuals treated for almost a year, saw no change in serum transaminase levels in these relatively healthy individuals who did not use acetaminophen or NSAIDs (Kim, Grant, Yoon, Williams, & Remmel, 2006). In order to ensure patient safety when using naltrexone, serum transaminases, gamma glutathione transferase, and serum bilirubin levels should be checked prior to initiating treatment and periodically thereafter (e.g., at 1, 3, and 6 months and then yearly) in all patients taking naltrexone. More frequent monitoring of liver functioning should be employed if the patient has high baseline levels, if they have a history of hepatic disease, are taking other potentially hepatotoxic drugs, or if the patient is on doses of naltrexone higher than 50 mg daily. Another concern for patients taking naltrexone is when they will need medical treatment with narcotic pain medications. Patients will need to discontinue naltrexone at least 3 days prior to undergoing operative procedures. After long-term use of naltrexone, opioid receptor upregulation leads to a marked risk of fatal overdose following discontinuation and relapse to opioids (Digiusto, Shakeshaft, Ritter, O'Brien, & Mattick, 2004). Patients should be clearly warned of this possibility before starting treatment.

Naltrexone is generally very well tolerated in individuals who have been fully detoxified from opioids. Most common side effects include nausea, vomiting, diarrhea, headache, decreased mental acuity, fatigue, rashes, depression, and dysphoria, although these have rarely been cited as reasons to discontinue in clinical trials (Tucker & Ritter, 2000). The concern for potential depression as a side effect and susceptibility to overdose of those discontinuing treatment has led some investigators to explore this link further. Although the risk of overdose is high after stopping treatment, most studies have found depressive symptoms to actually improve over the course of treatment (Dean et al., 2006; Miotto et al., 1997; Ngo et al., 2007). Rates of depression are high in opioid dependent patients and depressive symptoms should be monitored in patients receiving naltrexone.

As noted earlier, methadone maintenance is the most effective treatment for opioid dependence. This has not stopped many with opioid dependence from opting for opioid antagonist treatment instead. A recent Cochrane review of 10 studies with 696 total patients found naltrexone or naltrexone plus psychosocial intervention were more effective than placebo or placebo plus psychosocial intervention in reducing heroin use, without a significant effect on retention in treatment. In addition, a small subsample of studies demonstrated that naltrexone plus psychosocial intervention were superior to placebo plus psychosocial intervention at reducing criminal recidivism.(Minozzi et al., 2006) Another recent meta-analysis examining 15 studies involving 1,071 opioid-dependent patients found that naltrexone was only significantly better than placebo at reducing heroin use in a high-retention subgroup where contingency management was used (Johansson, Berglund, & Lindgren 2006). Because ineffectiveness of naltrexone is due in large part to patients discontinuing the medication, it is often useful to have administration observed either in the clinic or by reliable family or friends.

To overcome this limitation of its problems with retention in treatment and nonadherence, very long-acting forms of the medication such as naltrexone implants and depot naltrexone have been developed. Naltrexone implants, which are available in Europe and Australia, can deliver levels of naltrexone sufficient to block heroin effects for over 6 months (Hulse et al., 2004). Early pilot studies of naltrexone implants have shown them to eliminate or greatly reduce the use of opioids while plasma levels of naltrexone were adequate to block opioid effects (Foster, Brewer, & Steele, 2003; Waal et al., 2006), as well as eliminating opioid overdoses during this time period (Hulse et al., 2005). In the United States, a long-acting, injectable form of naltrexone complexed to polylactide glycolide microspheres, Vivitrol, has been approved by the FDA for treatment of alcohol dependence. Vivitrol is designed to provide sustained release naltrexone over 28 days (Harrison, Plosker, & Keam, 2006). In opioid-dependent patients, a different formulation of depot intramuscular naltrexone was shown to reduce the reinforcing and subjective effects of intravenous heroin at up to 25 mg for 4–5 weeks (Sullivan, Vosburg, & Comer, 2006). Currently there is insufficient experience with long-acting forms of naltrexone to say with confidence how they perform compared to better-established treatments, but there is potential for them to offer a good alternative to opioid agonist therapies.

Treatments for Smoking Cessation

Nicotine is one of the most widely abused substances worldwide. In the United States, 20.9% of adults (45.1 million people) are current smokers (Mariolis et al., 2006). Smoking is damaging to nearly every organ in the body and is the number one preventable cause of disease, contributing to over 440,000 deaths in the United States per year, more than any other substance of abuse (DHHS, 2004).

In spite of the well-known and publicized health concerns associated with tobacco use, it is very difficult for most smokers to quit smoking tobacco. Tobacco smoking has a number of positive effects, which become conditioned with mood and environmental factors leading to dependence on nicotine. Nicotine can improve reaction time and attention, reduce anxiety, temporarily relieve hunger, and produce a pleasurable sensation. Nicotine withdrawal is marked by the opposite of many of these effects, with anxiety, confusion, irritability, difficulty concentrating, restlessness, constipation, dizziness, headache, sweating, and craving for nicotine being common.

Smoking tobacco causes extremely rapid absorption of nicotine across the alveolar surface, with nicotine reaching the brain in 7–19 seconds. Smoking cigarettes allows the smoker a great deal of control over their exposure to nicotine as frequency and intensity of inhalation effect the amount of nicotine absorbed, with a typical 1 pack per day smoker absorbing 20–40 mg of nicotine per day. Nicotine is primarily metabolized by the liver, with a half-life of 1–4 hours, but after habitual smoking, nicotine accumulates for 6–8 hours. Nicotine is a direct agonist of presynaptic acetylcholine receptors, which influences acetylcholine, norepinephrine, dopamine and serotonin neurotransmission (Thompson & Hunter, 1998).

The goals of interventions for cessation of tobacco use are to prevent the many associated illnesses, improve overall health, and to reduce health care costs. For these purposes, a number of treatments have been developed including several forms of nicotine replacement, use of antidepressant medications, and nicotine receptor partial antagonists (see Table 25.10).

Nicotine Replacement

Nicotine replacement was the first pharmacological approach for the treatment of nicotine dependence, with the approval of nicotine polacrilex gum in 1984. Subsequently, several different forms of nicotine replacement have been developed, including transdermal patches, nasal spray, inhalers, and lozenges, which are intended to be used to prevent withdrawal symptoms and allow smokers to gradually wean themselves from nicotine use with tapering doses of replacement medications. Nicotine gum, patches, and lozenges are available over the counter, whereas nicotine nasal spray and inhalers are available by prescription only. For all of these forms of treatment, patients should stop smoking when they begin using the replacement therapy. Use of nicotine replacement should be avoided within one month of myocardial infarction, serious arrhythmia, or unstable angina unless the benefits of replacement therapy outweigh the risks.

Nicotine Gum   To be used effectively, nicotine gum must be chewed until a tingling sensation is felt in the gums and then the piece of gum is parked on the gums of the patient to allow nicotine to be absorbed across the buccal mucosa for approximately 30 minutes. Because nicotine is a tertiary amine, ingestion of fluids, such as soft drinks and coffee can interfere with the absorption of nicotine. Heavy smokers should decrease their smoking to one pack per day prior to attempting to quit with nicotine gum. Patients should use no more than 30 pieces of 2 mg gum or 20 pieces of 4 mg gum per day. Patients are able to control their own dosing of nicotine and gradually taper themselves off as they employ behavioral techniques to prevent relapse on cigarettes. Nicotine gum should be used for at least 3 months.

Side effects of using of nicotine gum include oral soreness, sore throat, gastrointestinal side effects (nausea, indigestion, flatulence, and diarrhea), and blisters in the mouth. Use of nicotine gum for long periods is associated with insulin resistance and hyperinsulinemia (Okuyemi, Nollen, & Ahluwalia, 2006; Thompson & Hunter, 1998).

Nicotine Transdermal Patch   Nicotine patches were first approved for use by the FDA in 1991 and allow for once-daily dosing of nicotine replacement. There are several different over-the-counter formulations of nicotine patches including 24-hour patches and 16-hour patches, which are intended to be removed in the evening and allow for a nicotine-free period. Dosing varies by formulation of the patch, but typically, smokers who smoke more than 10 cigarettes per day should use one 21 mg patch per 24 hours for 6–8 weeks, then use one 14 mg patch per 24 hours for 2–4 weeks, then use one 7 mg patch per 24 hours for another 2–4 weeks before stopping altogether.

Smokers who smoke more than a pack per day are likely to have some withdrawal symptoms when starting with the patch. The nicotine patch has many of the same side effects as nicotine gum; however, patch users also commonly have local skin reactions at the site of the patch (itching, erythema, and burning). In addition, some patch users, especially those using 24-hour patches, experience insomnia and vivid strange dreams (Okuyemi, Nollen, & Ahluwalia, 2006; Thompson & Hunter, 1998).

Nicotine Nasal Spray   The nicotine nasal spray allows for very good dose flexibility, but also is the most addictive nicotine replacement therapy available. A dose of nicotine nasal spray contains 1 mg of nicotine and consists of one spray to each nostril. Patients quitting tobacco use should use one to two doses per hour for 3–6 months. Patients may taper the dose gradually by one half per week until completely discontinued. The nicotine nasal spray is associated with watery eyes, nasal irritation, sneezing, runny nose, cough and sore throat, which typically resolves after a week of use (Okuyemi, Nollen, & Ahluwalia 2006).

Nicotine Inhaler   The nicotine inhaler mimics the hand-to-mouth action of smoking, but nicotine is absorbed in the mouth instead of the lungs. The inhaler dose is a cartridge, which delivers 4 mg of nicotine in addition to menthol. Patients should use 6–16 cartridges per day for 3 months and then taper use over the subsequent 6–12 months. Use of the nicotine inhaler can cause mild throat irritation and cough (Okuyemi, Nollen, & Ahluwalia 2006).

Nicotine Lozenge   The nicotine lozenge comes in the same doses as nicotine gum, but delivers more nicotine per dose than does the gum. Patients who smoke within 30 minutes of awakening should use the 4 mg dose. Patients should use one lozenge every 1–2 hours over the first 6 weeks, and then decrease frequency of use to every 2–4 hours over the next 3 weeks and finally decreasing to one lozenge every 4–8 hours over the next 3 weeks before stopping use. Patients using the lozenge must also avoid concurrent beverage use that may change oral pH as with nicotine gum. Users of the lozenge can have mouth soreness and upset stomach (Okuyemi, Nollen, & Ahluwalia 2006).

Effectiveness of Nicotine Replacement   Nicotine replacement, regardless of which form, is an effective aid to achieve abstinence from tobacco products. A recent Cochrane review of 123 studies of nicotine replacement therapies found that all forms of nicotine replacement were significantly better than placebo at achieving abstinence. The odds ratio of achieving abstinence ranged from 1.66 for nicotine gum to 2.35 for nicotine nasal spray. The 12-month abstinence rates for nicotine gum, transdermal patch, nicotine nasal spray, nicotine inhaler and nicotine lozenge were 17.4%, 13.7%, 24%, 17%, and 17%, respectively (Silagy et al., 2004). Although there are sex differences in rates of smoking, a meta-analysis examining this question in studies of the transdermal patch did not find a difference in effectiveness of the patch between sexes (Munafo, Bradburn, Bowes, L., & David, 2004). Investigators have tried to determine which characteristics of smokers would predict a better outcome from among the different forms of nicotine replacement therapies. Two different studies suggest that low or moderately dependent smokers were more likely to benefit from the transdermal patch (Lerman et al., 2004; Yudkin et al., 1996) whereas highly dependent smokers were more likely to benefit from nicotine nasal spray (Lerman et al., 2004).

Nortriptyline

One of the first agents to be used successfully for smoking cessation was the tricyclic antidepressant medication nortriptyline, although it is not FDA approved for this condition. Nortriptyline is an antidepressant, which stimulates serotonergic, noradrenergic, and dopaminergic systems in the brain. It is believed that the properties that make this medication efficacious for smoking cessation are related to its noradrenergic and/or its dopaminergic activity, although it is much more noradrenergic than dopaminergic.

Studies using nortriptyline and subsequent guidelines for its use in smoking cessation recommend starting the medication at 25 mg daily 10 to 28 days prior to the patient's quit date. Over the 10 days to several weeks after starting the medication, it should be titrated as tolerated to a final dose of 75 mg to 100 mg per day. Recommendations are for use of nortriptyline for 12 weeks to 6 months. Blood levels can be checked to ensure compliance and patient safety. Patients should taper off of the medication when discontinuing because of the potential for a discontinuation syndrome when it is abruptly stopped.

At doses recommended for treatment of smoking cessation, nortriptyline is typically as well tolerated as other treatments. Typical side effects include dry mouth, light-headedness, and constipation. Nortriptyline can also be quite sedating, so it is often administered at bedtime. Sedation is even more of a concern if the medication is taken in combination with alcohol or other sedating drugs. Additionally, nortriptyline can be fatal in overdose.

Although the number of studies and total number of subjects studied with nortriptyline is smaller than other forms of treatment, reviews of available studies indicate that nortiptyline is as effective as nicotine replacement or bupropion for smoking cessation (Hughes, Stead, & Lancaster 2005).

Bupropion

Until very recently, the only other clearly recognized pharmacological agent shown to be helpful for tobacco dependence was bupropion, which was approved by the FDA for smoking cessation in 1997. Bupropion is a novel antidepressant, which acts on noradrenergic and dopaminergic systems in the brain.

Using bupropion for smoking cessation is fairly straightforward. Typically the sustained-release formulation is used and started at a dose of 150 mg per day for 3 days and then increased to 150 mg twice a day. Unlike nicotine replacement, patients typically attempt to stop using nicotine a week after starting bupropion.

Bupropion is generally well tolerated; the most common side effects are insomnia and dry mouth, and other less common side effects include nausea, anxiety, and headache. There is also a dose-dependent increased risk for seizures, so patients with a history of seizures, head trauma, anorexia or bulimia, or increased risk for seizures should not use buproprion.

A recent Cochrane review of all antidepressant trials for smoking cessation examined 31 studies with over 10,000 patients of bupropion versus placebo and found similar success to nicotine replacement therapy, with a pooled odds ratio of abstinence of 1.94. There were a limited number of studies of combined therapy with nicotine replacement, which did not indicate a significant benefit to combination therapy (Hughes, Stead, & Lancaster 2007).

Varenicline

In 2006, a new class of medication for smoking cessation became available when the FDA approved varenicline, an $\alpha4\beta2$ nicotinic receptor partial agonist, following completion of phase III trials (Gonzales et al., 2006; Jorenby et al., 2006; Tonstad et al., 2006). Basic science research suggested a role of this particular receptor in the reinforcing properties of nicotine and varenicline was developed from a plant alkaloid.

Varenicline is titrated up over the course of a week, starting at 0.5 mg per day for the first three days, then 0.5 mg twice per day for the next 4 days and then increased to the final dose of 1 mg twice per day. Studies to date have looked at both 12 weeks of treatment with varenicline and at extended treatment with varenicline. Varenicline is fairly well tolerated. The most common side effects are nausea, headaches, insomnia, abnormal dreams, and flatulence.

The evidence at this time is limited to a few well-designed, pharmaceutical company sponsored trials. A Cochrane review of these current studies finds that varenicline improves the odds of smoking cessation three times that of placebo, it is more successful than bupropion in limited studies, and its effectiveness in extended treatment is not yet clear (Cahill, Stead, & Lancaster 2007).

Combination Therapy

Even with use of a pharmacologic agent, relapse rates are high for tobacco smokers. Attempts to improve on the effectiveness by combining pharmacotherapies have been studied in a limited number of studies. Combining nicotine replacement with bupropion does not appear to increase rates of smoking cessation, but combining pharmacotherapy with a number of behavior interventions does improve outcomes (Ingersoll & Cohen 2005). Combining forms of nicotine replacement therapy by adding an ad lib form of nicotine such as nicotine gum, lozenge, nasal spray or inhaler to treatment with the nicotine patch to help patients manage nicotine cravings is more effective than monotherapy (Silagy, Lancaster, Stead, Mant, & Fowler, 2004).

Stimulant Dependence

Cocaine Dependence and Withdrawal

To date, no medication has been FDA approved for cocaine dependence, but a small handful of agents have shown meaningful promise in decreasing cocaine use (see Table 25.11). Several GABA medications have been shown in 10–16 week double-blind, placebo-controlled trials to have gradual efficacy decreasing the frequency of cocaine-positive urines. Dosed at 20 mg three times daily for 16 weeks, the GABA$_B$ agonist baclofen lead to significantly fewer cocaine-positive urine toxicology screens (UDAS) than did placebo, with no difference in side effects (Shoptaw et al., 2003). FDA approved for spasticity, abrupt withdrawal of intrathecal baclofen can put patients at risk for rebound spasticity, fever, mental status changes, and rhabdomyolosis (Medtronic 2002a, 2002b), and abrupt withdrawal of oral baclofen after prolonged treatment may lead to increased risk of seizure (Barker & Grant, 1982). Common side effects include diarrhea, nausea, vomiting, dizziness, sedation, headache, and decreased muscle tone (IVAX, 2001). The majority of baclofen's clearance is via renal excretion (Wuis, Dirks, Termond, Vree, & Van der Kleijn, 1989), although 15% of its clearance occurs through hepatic metabolism. Thus dosing will need to be adjusted to a patient's creatinine clearance.

The anticonvulsant tiagabine increases GABA levels by inhibiting an enzyme involved in its metabolism. Dosed at 24 mg/day, it led to a decrease in cocaine-positive UDAS over the course of 10 weeks in opioid-dependent individuals treated in a methadone program (Gonzalez et al., 2007, 2003). Topiramate promotes GABAergic activity and atagonzies glutamatergic AMPA/kainite receptors. In a 14-week study it was tolerated as well as placebo at a target dose of 200 mg/day and led to significantly higher abstinence rates than did placebo in cocaine-dependent individuals. However, it had to be slowly titrated over 8 weeks, by 25 mg/week (Kampman et al., 2004). Furthermore, a month supply of these anticonvulsants is estimated to cost over $470, compared to about $30/month for baclofen. Both anticonvulsants have also been associated with high rates of both dizziness and asthenia, and at least one case of Stevens–Johnson syndrome (Abbott, 1997; Ortho-McNeil Pharmaceutical, 2004), and topiramate has also been associated with high rates of cognitive slowing and somnolence (Ortho-McNeil Pharmaceutical, 2004). In a recent open label trial, the anticonvulsant vigabatrin showed remarkable promise in decreasing cocaine and MA use (Brodie, Figueroa, Laska, & Dewey, 2005), but this compound is not available in the United States due to a high incidence of associated visual field defects (Brodie, Figueroa & Dewey 2003).

FDA-approved for use in narcolepsy, the wake-promoting agent modafinil blocks reuptake of both dopamine and norepinephrine and enhances glutamatergic activity (Ferraro et al., 1998, 1999), which has been theorized to play a role in cocaine dependence and vulnerability to relapse in preclinical models (Baker et al., 2003; Kalivas et al., 2003). It has been shown to lead to decreased cocaine use and an increased likelihood of 3 continuous weeks of abstinence compared to placebo in an 8-week study in which it was dosed at 400 mg/day (Dackis et al. 2005). Although no one discontinued the study due to side effects, nausea, upper respiratory symptoms, anxiety, dry mouth, and urinary tract infection were the most commonly reported side effects and occurred at twice the frequency than those reported in the placebo group.

Most medications that manipulate catecholamine neurotransmitter systems have shown little success at best in decreasing cocaine use. Neither desipramine (Carroll et al., 1994; McDowell et al., 2005), fluoxetine (Grabowski et al., 1995; Schmitz et al., 2001), nor any other antidepressants (Lima et al. 2003) have shown any sustained efficacy in reducing cocaine use, while the antipsychotics risperidone (Grabowski et al., 2004) and olanzapine (Kampman et al., 2003) have also failed to show any effect or in fact worsened cocaine dependence (Grabowski et al., 2000). d-Amphetamine (Grabowski et al., 2001; Grabowski et al., 2004), but not methylphenidate (Grabowski et al. 1997; Schubiner et al., 2002) has been shown to lead to some decrease in cocaine use, although the utility of this controlled substance is limited by its own abuse potential and subsequent need for frequent, if not daily, monitoring to insure appropriate administration. Trials of the dopaminergic agonist bromocriptine, combined with the dopaminergic/noradrenergic antidepressant bupropion (Montoya et al., 2002) and mazindol (Stine et al., 1995) failed to show any decrease in cocaine use.

The most promising agent at this time for the treatment of cocaine dependence appears to be the dopamine-β-hydroxylase inhibitor, disulfiram, whose side effect and pharmacokinetic

TABLE 25.11
Select Medications Discussed in Treatment of Cocaine Dependence/Withdrawal

Generic Name	Brand Name	FDA Indications
Amantadine	Symmetrel	Influenza A
		Parkinsonism
		Extra-pyramidal disease
Baclofen	Lioresal	Spasticity
Disulfiram	Antabuse	Alcohol dependence
Modafinil	Provigil	Narcolepsy
		Obstructive sleep apnea
		Shift work sleep disorder
Propranolol	Inderal	Hypertension
		Post-myocardial infarction
		Dysrythmia
		Migraine prophylaxis
		Essential tremor
		Angina pectoris, chronic
Tiagabine	Gabitril	Partial seizures
Topiramate	Topamax	Partial seizures
		Generalized seizures
		Lennox-Gestaut syndrome
		Migraine prophylaxis

*No medication is FDA approved for treatment of cocaine dependence or withdrawal. Thus FDA approved uses are listed for medications discussed as having off-label potential for use in cocaine dependence.

TABLE 25.12
Select Medications Discussed in Treatment of Methamphetamine Dependence/Withdrawal

Generic Name	Brand Name	FDA Indications
Desipramine	Norpramin	Depression
Fluoxetine	Prozac	Depression
	Sarafem	Obsessive compulsive disorder
		Panic disorder
		Bullimia nervosa
		Premenstrual dysporic disorder
Imipramine	Tofranil	Depression
		Nocturnal enuresis
Methylphenidate	Ritalin	Narcolepsy
	Concerta	Attention-deficit hyperactivity disorder
	Metadate	
Mirtazapine	Remeron	Depression
Vigabatrin	—	Anticonvulsant not available in U.S. due to safety concerns

*No medication is FDA approved for treatment of mehtamphetamine dependence or withdrawal. Thus FDA approved uses are listed for select medications discussed as either having off-label potential or recently having been investigated for use in methamphetamine dependence.

profile was discussed at length in the section on treatments for alcohol dependence. Disulfiram inhibits the conversion of dopamine to norepinephrine, raising dopamine levels (Karamanakos et al., 2001). It has consistently been associated with decreased cocaine use, dosed at 250 mg/day (Carroll et al., 2004, 1998; George et al., 2000; Petrakis et al., 2000), and costs roughly $15/month. Given its aversive interaction with alcohol, some patients can be reluctant to start this medication, which can be a barrier to use.

Although there are no medications that have shown clear efficacy in the management of cocaine withdrawal or intoxication, initial data suggested that the doapminergic agonist amantadine (Kampman et al., 2000) and the β-adrenergic antagonist propranolol (Kampman et al., 2001) may help to decrease future cocaine use in patients with severe acute cocaine withdrawal. Unfortunately follow-up studies showed no effect of amantadine after ten weeks (Kampman et al., 2006) or four months (Shoptaw et al., 2002), although there appeared to be some benefit of propranolol after 10 weeks in patients who reported strict adherence to the study medication (Kampman et al., 2006).

MA Dependence and Withdrawal

Rigorous data on pharmacological treatments is much more sparse for MA dependence than for cocaine dependence, and as in cocaine dependence, there are currently no medications approved for this condition (Srisurapanont, Kittiratanapaiboon, & Jarusuraisin, 2001, see Table 25.12). Although imipramine 150 mg per day has been shown to keep both MA and cocaine abusers in treatment longer than controls dosed with 10 mg per day, it led to no measurable reduction in MA use or craving (Galloway et al., 1996, 1994). The addition of desipramine to the standardized Matrix behavioral treatment program for MA dependence led to no significant differences compared to a Matrix treatment plus placebo group or to Matrix treatment alone (Shoptaw et al., 1994). Fluoxetine decreases MA self-administration in animal studies, and an unpublished double blind placebo-controlled study in MA-dependent adults demonstrated decreased subjective cravings for MA in the treatment group (Srisurapanont et al., 2001). However, fluoxetine did not decrease subjective reports of MA use or positive urine toxicology screens (Batki et al., 1999). Sertraline was shown to lead to worse outcomes than placebo in a recent 12-week study (Shoptaw et al., 2006). As discussed above, the anticonvulsant vigabatrin led to lower MA (and cocaine) use then otherwise expected in a 9-week open-label trial (Brodie et al., 2005), but the medication is not available in the United States because it has been linked to a high incidence of visual field problems (Brodie, Figueroa, & Dewey, 2003). MA-dependent patients treated for 20 weeks with 15 mg daily of aripiprazole had significantly more MA-positive UDAS than patients treated with placebo, whereas patients treated with 54 mg daily of slow release methylphenidate had significantly fewer MA-positive urines than patients in the placebo group (Tiihonen et al., 2007). Although medications for acute MA detoxification have been even less-studied than have agents for longterm treatment of dependence, a small 2-week study of mirtazapine indicated it reduced anxiety symptoms, compared to placebo, in acute withdrawal (Kongsakon, Papadopoulos, & Saguansiritham, 2005).

Addressing Co-Occuring Psychiatric Disorders in Substance Abuse Treatment

Patients with substance use disorders have high rates of co-occurring Axis I psychiatric disorders (Brooner et al., 1997; Kessler et al., 1996; Regier et al., 1990). In practice it is important, although often difficult, to establish whether co-occurring disorders are primary or are substance induced (Hasin et al., 2002; Nunes et al., 2006; Schuckit, 2006). If co-occurring disorders are substance-induced, the generally held belief is that they will remit spontaneously with some period of abstinence and that pharmacological treatment is not necessary. Primary disorders will typically require both pharmacological and psychotherapeutic treatment.

Evidence that a co-occurring psychiatric disorder is primary can be gleaned from the history that it had its onset prior to the onset of the substance use disorder or that it occurred during a prior episode of abstinence and remission from the substance use disorder. A family history of the co-occurring disorder provides adjunctive help in making this determination. Lack of such historical evidence does not prove that the disorder is not primary, but it would encourage an attempt to observe the patient over a 4- through 6-week period of abstinence to see if psychiatric symptomatology resolves without specific treatment. Not infrequently the psychiatric symptomatology appears to interfere with attempts to achieve abstinence. In that circumstance it makes sense to initiate pharmacological treatment with the hope of ameliorating the psychiatric symptoms and then attaining abstinence, although no research data specifically support this approach.

Precisely the same pharmacologic treatments are used for co-occurring psychiatric disorders as would be used for psychiatric disorders without co-occurring substance use (Green, 2006; Nunes & Levin, 2006; Vornik & Brown, 2006). Evidence to date suggests that active treatment of co-occurring psychiatric disorders in the context of substance use treatment improves the outcome of the psychiatric disorder and may at times benefit the course of the substance use disorder (Carpenter, Brooks, Vosburg, & Nunes, 2004; Cornelius et al., 1997; McDowell et al., 2005; McGrath et al., 1996; Nunes et al., 1998).

Conclusions

Abuse and dependence of tobacco, alcohol, and illicit drugs pose a major health problem to many patients in addition to constituting significant social and legal problems for society at large. The scope and complexity of these disorders necessitates a broad approach encompassing, prevention, treatment, and public policy. This chapter has focused on one component, pharmacological treatments, of addressing this group of disorders, where treatment of these disorders should include behavioral treatments as well as addressing any co-occurring disorders that are commonly present in these populations.

We have reviewed pharmacological treatments that are effective in treating tobacco dependence, acute intoxication, withdrawal, and dependence on alcohol, opioids, and sedative-hypnotics, as well as withdrawal from and dependence on cocaine and MA. Although this represents a number of effective treatments, all of the medications discussed in this chapter have limitations and research on new treatments is being conducted by many investigators throughout the world. Effective strategies for treating tobacco dependence include various forms of nicotine replacement that can be used as a monotherapy or in combined therapy with each other, select antidepressants such as bupropion and nortriptyline and the new nicotine receptor partial agonist varenicline. Treatment of alcohol abuse and dependence ranges from using benzodiazepines, barbiturates, and anticonvulsants to treat acute withdrawal to using the aversive agent disulfiram, the opioid antagonist naltrexone to reduce craving, and the GABA and glutamate modulator acamprosate. Management of opioid intoxication is best done with the short-acting opioid antagonist naloxone, whereas acute withdrawal is most safely treated with a short course of the opioid agonist methadone, partial opioid agonist buprenorphine, or the α2-adrenergic agonist clonidine. The most effective and best studied treatment for opioid dependence is methadone maintenance, but access is limited to treatment in regulated opioid treatment programs. Buprenorphine is similarly effective, however, it is available for use in office-based practices by providers who have obtained special authorization. Antagonist therapy with naltrexone is less effective than agonist therapies for opioid dependence, but new delivery methods may enhance its effectiveness. Benzodiazepine toxicity is treated with the competitive inhibitor flumazenil, and an approach to management of withdrawal from these drugs is by gradual taper with a benzodiazepine, use of the anticonvulsants carbamazepine or valproic acid or the barbiturate phenobarbitol. Cocaine and MA abuse and dependence are widespread but, to date, these are the drugs for which we have the least evidence for effective pharmacological treatments. For cocaine dependence, there is limited evidence to support the use of the antispasmodic baclofen, the anticonvulsants tiagabine and topiramate, the dopamine and norepinephrine reuptake inhibitor modafinil, and the dopamine-β-hydroxylase inhibitor disulfiram. There is currently no evidence for safe and effective pharmacological treatments for MA dependence.

The complex and varied set of behaviors that constitute addiction in humans are the result of alterations at the cellular level in several brain structures causing long-term changes in responsiveness of the circuits that connect these regions. The sum of these changes is that certain stimuli attain elevated importance because of their association with drugs of abuse such that their subsequent presence is sufficient to trigger directed "drug-seeking" behaviors. The currently available pharmacotherapies discussed in this chapter have been developed in ways ranging from serendipitous discovery to calculated design to affect some step in the process of addiction to a specific substance of abuse. As the neurobiological basis of addictive disorders becomes better understood, common patterns between the various drugs of abuse are developing such that there appears to be a final common pathway to development of addiction consisting of glutamatergic circuits involving the prefrontal cortex, nucleus accumbens core and the ventral pallidum (Kalivas & Volkow, 2005).

Effective medications target different steps on this pathway, but the theory is supported by the fact that several medications discussed in this chapter can serve to treat different substances of dependence. For example, naltrexone has some efficacy in both opioid and alcohol dependence, and disulfiram, baclofen, and topiramate may have efficacy in both alcohol and cocaine dependence. It is hoped that as knowledge grows, new therapies may be developed that will target this common pathway producing more effective treatments that are effective for addictions to all drugs of abuse.

References

Aase, J.M. (1974). Letter: Anticonvulsant drugs and congenital abnormalities. *American Journal of Disease Children, 127*–758.

Abbott (2006). *Product information: DEPAKOTE(R) ER extended-release tablet, divalproex sodium extended-release tablet.* North Chicago, IL: Abbott Laboratories.

Abbott (1997). *Product information: Gabitril(R), tiagabine.* North Chicago, IL: Abbott Laboratories.

Addolorato, G., Caputo, F., Capristo, E., Domenicali, M., Bernardi, M., Janiri, L., et al. (2002). Baclofen efficacy in reducing alcohol craving and intake: A preliminary double-blind randomized controlled study. *Alcohol and Alcoholism, 37*, 504–508.

Allan, A. M., & Harris, R. A. (1986). Gamma-aminobutyric acid and alcohol actions: Neurochemical studies of long sleep and short sleep mice. *Life Sciences, 39*, 2005–2015.

Allen, J. P., Sillamaukee, P., & Anton, R. (1999). Contribution of carbohydrate deficient transferrin to gamma glutamyl transpeptidase in evaluating progress of patients in treatment for alcoholism. *Alcoholism: Clinical & Experimental Research, 23*,115–120.

AMA Department of Drugs. (1992). *AMA evaluations subscription.* Chicago, IL.: American Medical Association.

Amato, L., Davoli, M., C, A. P., Ferri, M., Faggiano, F., & Mattick, R. P. (2005a). An overview of systematic reviews of the effectiveness of opiate maintenance therapies: Available evidence to inform clinical practice and research. *Journal of Substance Abuse Treatment, 28*, 321–329.

Amato, L., Davoli, M., Ferri, M., Gowing, L., & Perucci, C.A. (2004a). Effectiveness of interventions on opiate withdrawal treatment: an overview of systematic reviews. *Drug and Alcohol Dependence, 73*, 219–226.

Amato, L., Davoli, M., Minozzi, S., Ali, R., & Ferri, M. (2005b). Methadone at tapered doses for the management of opioid withdrawal. *Cochrane Database of Systemic Reviews, 3*, CD003409.

Amato, L., Minozzi, S. Davoli, M., Vecchi, S. Ferri, M., & Mayet, S. (2004b). Psychosocial combined with agonist maintenance treatments versus agonist maintenance treatments alone for treatment of opioid dependence. *Cochrane Database of Systematic Reviews, 4*, CD004147.

American Psychiatric Association. (2000). *Diagnostic and statistical manual of mental disorders.* Washington, DC: Author.

Anton, R. F., O'Malley, S. S., Ciraulo, D. A., Cisler, R. A., Couper, D., Donovan, D. M., et al. (2006). Combined pharmacotherapies and behavioral interventions for alcohol dependence: The COMBINE study: A randomized controlled trial. *Journal of the American Medical Association, 295*, 2003–2017.

Apelt, S., & Emrich, H.M. (1990). Sodium valproate in benzodiazepine withdrawal. *American Journal of Psychiatry, 147*, 950–951.

Baker, D. A., McFarland, K., Lake, R. W., Shen, H., Toda, S., & Kalivas, P. W. (2003). N-acetyl cysteine-induced blockade of cocaine-induced reinstatement. *Annals of the New York Academy of Science, 1003*, 349–351.

Balldin, J., Berglund, M., Borg, S., Mansson, M., Bendtsen, P., Franck, J., et al. (2003). A 6-month controlled naltrexone study: Combined effect with cognitive behavioral therapy in outpatient treatment of alcohol dependence. *Alcoholism: Clinical and Experimental Research, 27*, 1142–1149.

Barker, I., & Grant, I. S. (1982). Convulsions after abrupt withdrawal of baclofen. *Lancet, 2*, 556–557.

Batki, S., Moon, J., Bradley, M., Hersh, D., Smolar, S., Mengis, M., et al. (1999). Fluoxetine and methamphetamine dependence–A controlled trial: Preliminary analysis. *NIDA Research Mongraph, 180*, 235.

Benjamin, D., Grant, E. R., & Pohorecky, L. A. (1993). Naltrexone reverses ethanol-induced dopamine release in the nucleus accumbens in awake, freely moving rats. *Brain Research, 621*, 137–140.

Bjorkqvist, S. E., Isohanni, M., Makela, R., & Malinen, L. (1976). Ambulant treatment of alcohol withdrawal symptoms with carbamazepine: A formal multicentre double-blind comparison with placebo. *Acta Psychiatrica Scandinavica, 53*, 333–342.

Bonnet, U., Banger, M., Leweke, F. M., Maschke, M., Kowalski, T., & Gastpar, M. (1999). Treatment of alcohol withdrawal syndrome with gabapentin. *Pharmacopsychiatry, 32*, 107–109.

Bouza, C., Angeles, M., Munoz, A., & Amate, J. M. (2004). Efficacy and safety of naltrexone and acamprosate in the treatment of alcohol dependence: a systematic review. *Addiction, 99*, 811–828.

Bozikas, V., Petrikis, P., Gamvrula, K., Savvidou, I., & Karavatos, A. (2002). Treatment of alcohol withdrawal with gabapentin. *Progress in Neuro-psychopharmacology and Biological Psychiatry, 26*,197–199.

Brodie, J. D., Figueroa, E., & Dewey, S. L. (2003). Treating cocaine addiction: From preclinical to clinical trial experience with gamma-vinyl GABA. *Synapse, 50*, 261–265.

Brodie, J. D., Figueroa, E., Laska, E. M., & Dewey, S. L. (2005). Safety and efficacy of gamma-vinyl GABA (GVG) for the treatment of methamphetamine and/or cocaine addiction. *Synapse, 55*, 122–125.

Brooner, R. K., King, V. L., Kidorf, M., Schmidt, C. W., Jr., & Bigelow, G. E. (1997). Psychiatric and substance use comorbidity among treatment-seeking opioid abusers. *Archives of General Psychiatry, 54*, 71–80.

Cahill, K., Stead, L., & Lancaster, T. (2007). Nicotine receptor partial agonists for smoking cessation. *Cochrane Database of Systemic Reviews, 1*, CD006103.

Calsyn, D. A., Malcy, J. A., & Saxon, A. J. (2005). Slow tapering from methadone maintenance in a program encouraging indefinite maintenance. *Journal of Substance Abuse Treatment, 30*, 159–163.

Carpenter, K. M., Brooks, A. C., Vosburg, S. K., & Nunes, E. V. (2004). The effect of sertraline and environmental context on treating depression and illicit substance use among methadone maintained opiate dependent patients: A controlled clinical trial. *Drug and Alcohol Dependence, 74*, 123–134.

Carroll, K. M., Fenton, L. R., Ball, S. A., Nich, C., Frankforter, T. L., Shi, J., et al. (2004). Efficacy of disulfiram and cognitive behavior therapy in cocaine-dependent outpatients: A randomized placebo-controlled trial. *Archives of General Psychiatry, 61*, 264–272.

Carroll, K. M., Nich, C., Ball, S. A., McCance, E., & Rounsavile, B. J. (1998). Treatment of cocaine and alcohol dependence with psychotherapy and disulfiram. *Addiction, 93*, 713–727.

Carroll, K. M., Rounsaville, B. J., Nich, C., Gordon, L. T., Wirtz, P. W., & Gawin, F. (1994). One-year follow-up of psychotherapy and pharmacotherapy for cocaine dependence. Delayed emergence of psychotherapy effects. *Archives of General Psychiatry, 51*, 989–997.

CSAT (Center for Substance Abuse Treatment). (2006). *Detoxification and substance abuse treatment.* Treatment Improvement Protocol (TIP) Series 45. Rockville, MD: Substance Abuse and Mental Health Services Administration.

CSAT (Center for Substance Abuse Treatment). (2005). *Medication-assisted treatment for opioid addiction in opioid treatment programs.* Treatment Improvement Protocol (TIP) Series 43. Rockville, MD: Substance Abuse and Mental Health Services Administration.

CSAT (Center for Substance Abuse Treatment). (2004). *Clinical guidelines for the use of buprenorphine in the treatment of opioid addiction.* Treatment Improvement Protocol (TIP) Series 40. Rockville, MD: Substance Abuse and Mental Health Services Administration.

Chang, G., & Kosten, T. R. (2005). Detoxification. In: J. H. Lowinson, P. Ruiz, R. B. Millman, & J. G. Langrod (Eds.), *Substance abuse: A comprehensive textbook.* Philadelphia: Lippincott Williams & Wilkins. pp. 579–589.

Chatterjee, C. R., & Ringold, A. L. (1999). A case report of reduction in alcohol craving and protection against alcohol withdrawal by gabapentin. *Journal of Clinical Psychiatry, 60*, 617.

Chick, J. (1999). Safety issues concerning the use of disulfiram in treating alcohol dependence. *Drug Safety, 20*, 427–435.

Chick, J., Anton, R., Checinski, K., Croop, R., Drummond, D. C., Farmer, R., et al. (2000). A multicentre, randomized, double-blind, placebo-controlled trial of naltrexone in the treatment of alcohol dependence or abuse. *Alcohol and Alcoholism, 35*, 587–593.

Chick, J., Lehert, P., & Landron, F. (2003). Does acamprosate improve reduction of drinking as well as aiding abstinence? *Journal of Psychopharmacology, 17*, 397–402.

Clark, N., Lintzeris, N., Gijsbers, A., Whelan, G., Dunlop, A., Ritter, A., et al. (2002). LAAM maintenance vs methadone maintenance for heroin dependence. *Cochrane Database of Systemic Reviews, 2*, CD002210.

Clarke, S. F., Dargan, P. I., & Jones, A. L. (2005). Naloxone in opioid poisoning: Walking the tightrope. *Emergency Medicine Journal, 22*, 612–616.

Collins, E. D., Kleber, H. D., Whittington, R. A., & Heitler, N. E. (2005). Anesthesia-assisted vs buprenorphine- or clonidine-assisted heroin detoxification and naltrexone induction: A randomized trial. *Journal of the American Medical Association, 294*, 903–913.

Colombo, G., Addolorato, G., Agabio, R., Carai, M.A., Pibiri, F., Serra, S., et al.(2004). Role of GABA(B) receptor in alcohol dependence: Reducing effect of baclofen on alcohol intake and alcohol motivational properties in rats and amelioration of alcohol withdrawal syndrome and alcohol craving in human alcoholics. *Neurotoxicology Research, 6*, 403–414.

Colombo, G., Serra, S., Brunetti, G., Atzori, G., Pani, M., Vacca, G., et al. (2002). The GABA(B) receptor agonists baclofen and CGP 44532 prevent acquisition of alcohol drinking behaviour in alcohol-preferring rats. *Alcohol and Alcoholism, 37*, 499–503.

Cornelius, J. R., Salloum, I. M., Ehler, J. G., Jarrett, P. J., Cornelius, M. D., Perel, J. M., et al. (1997). Fluoxetine in depressed alcoholics. A double-blind, placebo-controlled trial. *Archives of General Psychiatry, 54*, 700–705.

Dackis, C. A., Kampman, K. M., Lynch, K. G., Pettinati, H. M., & O'Brien, C. P. (2005). A double-blind, placebo-controlled trial of modafinil for cocaine dependence. *Neuropsychopharmacology, 30*, 205–211.

Daeppen, J. B., Gache, P., Landry, U., Sekera, E., Schweizer, V., Gloor, S., et al. (2002). Symptom-triggered vs fixed-schedule doses of benzodiazepine for alcohol withdrawal: a randomized treatment trial. *Archives of Internal Medicine, 162,*1117–1121.

Davis, K. M., & Wu, J. Y. (2000). The role of glutaminergic and GABAergic systems in alcoholism. *Journal of Biomedical Science, 8*, 7–19.

De Waele, J. P., & Gianoulakis, C. (1994). Enhanced activity of the brain beta-endorphin system by free-choice ethanol drinking in C57BL/6 but not DBA/2 mice. *European Journal of Pharmacology, 258*, 119–129.

Dean, A. J., Saunders, J. B., Jones, R. T., Young, R. M., Connor, J. P., & Lawford, B. R. (2006). Does naltrexone treatment lead to depression? Findings from a randomized controlled trial in subjects with opioid dependence. *Journal of Psychiatry Neuroscience, 31*, 38–45.

DHHS. (2004). *The health consequences of smoking: A report of the Surgeon General.* Washington, DC: Centers for Disease and Health Promotion, Office of Smoking and Health.

Digiusto, E., Shakeshaft, A., Ritter, A., O'Brien, S., & Mattick, R. P. (2004). Serious adverse events in the Australian National Evaluation of Pharmacotherapies for Opioid Dependence (NEPOD). *Addiction, 99*, 450–460.

Dreifuss, F. E., Santilli, N., Langer, D. H., Sweeney, K. P., Moline, K. A., & Menander, K. B. (1987). Valproic acid hepatic fatalities: A retrospective review. *Neurology, 37*, 379–85.

Drummer, O. H. (2005). Recent trends in narcotic deaths. *Therapeutic Drug Monitoring, 27*, 738–740.

Erwin, W. E., Williams, D. B., & Speir, W. A. (1998). Delirium tremens. *Southern Medical Journal, 91*, 425–432.

Faggiano, F., Vigna-Taglianti, F., Versino, E., & Lemma, P. (2003). Methadone maintenance at different dosages for opioid dependence. *Cochrane Database of Systemic Reviews, 3*, CD002208.

Ferraro, L., Antonelli, T., O'Connor, W. T., Tanganelli, S., Rambert, F. A., & Fuxe, K. (1998). The effects of modafinil on striatal, pallidal and nigral GABA and glutamate release in the conscious rat: Evidence for a preferential inhibition of striato-pallidal GABA transmission. *Neuroscience Letters, 253*, 135–138.

Ferraro, L., Antonelli, T., Tanganelli, S., O'Connor, W. T., Perez de la Mora, M., Mendez-Franco, J., et al. (1999). The vigilance promoting drug modafinil increases extracellular glutamate levels in the medial preoptic area and the posterior hypothalamus of the conscious rat: Prevention by local GABAA receptor blockade. *Neuropsychopharmacology, 20*, 346–356.

Ficker, D. M., Privitera, M., Krauss, G., Kanner, A., Moore, J. L., & Glauser, T. (2005). Improved tolerability and efficacy in epilepsy patients with extended-release carbamazepine. *Neurology, 65*, 593–595.

Findlay, G. S., Wick, M. J., Mascia, M. P., Wallace, D., Miller, G. W., Harris, R. A., et al. (2002). Transgenic expression of a mutant glycine receptor decreases alcohol sensitivity of mice. *Journal of Pharmacology and Experimental Therapeutics, 300*, 526–534.

Foster, J., Brewer, C., & Steele, T. (2003). Naltrexone implants can completely prevent early (1-month) relapse after opiate detoxification: A pilot study of two cohorts totalling 101 patients with a note on naltrexone blood levels. *Addiction Biology, 8*, 211–217.

Foy, A., Kay, J., & Taylor, A. (1997). The course of alcohol withdrawal in a general hospital. *QJM, 90,* 253–261.

Fuller, R. K., Branchey, L., Brightwell, D. R., Derman, R. M., Emrick, C. D., Iber, F.L., et al. (1986). Disulfiram treatment of alcoholism. A Veterans Administration cooperative study. *Journal of the American Medical Association, 256,* 1449–1455.

Galloway, G. P., Newmeyer, J., Knapp, T., Stalcup, S. A., & Smith, D. (1996). A controlled trial of imipramine for the treatment of methamphetamine dependence. *Journal of Substance Abuse Treatment, 13,* 493–497.

Galloway, G. P., Newmeyer, J., Knapp, T., Stalcup, S. A., & Smith, D. (1994). Imipramine for the treatment of cocaine and methamphetamine dependence. *Journal of Addictive Diseases, 13,* 201–216.

Garbutt, J. C., Kranzler, H. R., O'Malley, S. S. Gastfriend, D. R., Pettinati, H. M, Silverman, B. L., et al. (2005). Efficacy and tolerability of long-acting injectable naltrexone for alcohol dependence: a randomized controlled trial. *Journal of the American Medical Association, 293,* 1617–1625.

Garcia-Borreguero, D., Bronisch, T., Apelt, S., Yassouridis, A., & Emrich, H.M. (1991). Treatment of benzodiazepine withdrawal symptoms with carbamazepine. *European Archives of Psychiatry and Clinical Neuroscience, 241,* 145–150.

Gastpar, M., Bonnet, U., Boning, J., Mann, K., Schmidt, L. G., Soyka, M., et al. (2002). Lack of efficacy of naltrexone in the prevention of alcohol relapse: Results from a German multicenter study. *Journal of Clinical Psychopharmacology, 22,* 592–598.

George, T. P., Chawarski, M. C., Pakes, J., Carroll, K. M., Kosten, T. R., & Schottenfeld, R. S. (2000). Disulfiram versus placebo for cocaine dependence in buprenorphine-maintained subjects: a preliminary trial. *Biological Psychiatry, 47,* 1080–1086.

Gonzales, D., Rennard, S. I., Nides, M., Oncken, C., Azoulay, S., Billing, C. B., et al. (2006). Varenicline, an alpha4beta2 nicotinic acetylcholine receptor partial agonist, vs sustained-release bupropion and placebo for smoking cessation: A randomized controlled trial. *Journal of the American Medical Association, 296,* 47–55.

Gonzalez, G., Desai, R., Sofuoglu, M., Poling, J., Oliveto, A., Gonsai, K., et al. (2007). Clinical efficacy of gabapentin versus tiagabine for reducing cocaine use among cocaine dependent methadone-treated patients. *Drug and Alcohol Dependence, 87,* 1–9.

Gonzalez, G., Sevarino, K., Sofuoglu, M., Poling, J., Oliveto, A., Gonsai, K., et al. (2003). Tiagabine increases cocaine-free urines in cocaine-dependent methadone-treated patients: Results of a randomized pilot study. *Addiction, 98,* 1625–1632.

Gonzalez-Sicilia, L.,Cano, A., Serrano, M., & Hernandez, J. (1998). Stevens-Johnson syndrome associated with gabapentin. *American Journal of Medicine, 105,* 455.

Gowing, L., Ali, R., & White, J. (2006). Buprenorphine for the management of opioid withdrawal. *Cochrane Database of Systemic Reviews, 2,*CD002025.

Gowing, L., Farrell, M., Ali, R., & White, J. (2004). Alpha2 adrenergic agonists for the management of opioid withdrawal. *Cochrane Database Systemic Reviews, 4,*CD002024.

Gowing, L. R., Farrell, M., Bornemann, R., Sullivan, L. E., & Ali, R.,L. (2006). Brief report: Methadone treatment of injecting opioid users for prevention of HIV infection. *Journal of General Internal Medicine, 21,* 193–195.

Grabowski, J., Rhoades, H., Elk, R., Schmitz, J., Davis, C., Creson, D., et al. (1995). Fluoxetine is ineffective for treatment of cocaine dependence or concurrent opiate and cocaine dependence: two placebo-controlled double-blind trials. *Journal of Clinical Psychopharmacology, 15,* 163–174.

Grabowski, J., Rhoades, H., Schmitz, J., Stotts, A., Daruzska, L. A., Creson, D., et al. (2001). Dextroamphetamine for cocaine-dependence treatment: A double-blind randomized clinical trial. *Journal of Clinical Psychopharmacology, 21,* 522–526.

Grabowski, J., Rhoades, H., Silverman, P., Schmitz, J. M., Stotts, A., Creson, D., et al. (2000). Risperidone for the treatment of cocaine dependence: Randomized, double-blind trial. *Journal of Clinical Psychopharmacology, 20,* 305–310.

Grabowski, J., Rhoades, H., Stotts, A., Cowan, K., Kopecky, C., Dougherty, A., et al. (2004). Agonist-like or antagonist-like treatment for cocaine dependence with methadone for heroin dependence: two double-blind randomized clinical trials. *Neuropsychopharmacology, 29,* 969–981.

Grabowski, J., Roache, J. D., Schmitz, J. M., Rhoades, H., Creson, D., & Korszun, A. (1997). Replacement medication for cocaine dependence: Methylphenidate. *Journal of Clinical Psychopharmacology, 17,* 485–488.

Green, A. I. (2006). Treatment of schizophrenia and comorbid substance abuse: Pharmacologic approaches. *Journal of Clinical Psychiatry, 67* (Suppl 7), 31–35; quiz 36–37.

Hall-Flavin, D. K., Black, J. L., Mrazek, D. A., & Sanchez-Samper, X. (2002). Screening of patients who drink on disulfiram for atypical P450 polymorphisms: A pilot study. *American Journal of Medical Genetics, 114,* 780.

Harrison, T. S., Plosker, G. L., & Keam, S. J. (2006). Extended-release intramuscular naltrexone. *Drugs, 66,* 1741–1751.

Hasin, D., Liu, X., Nunes, E., McCloud, S., Samet, S., & Endicott, J. (2002). Effects of major depression on remission and relapse of substance dependence. *Archives of General Psychiatry, 59,* 375–380.

Hobbs, W. R., Rall, T. W., & Verdoorn, T. A. (1996). Hypnotics and sedatives, alcohol. In: H. J.G. & L. L.E. (Eds.) *Goodman and Gilman's the pharmacological basis of therapeutics.* New York: McGraw-Hill.

Hubbard, R. L., Mardsen, M. E., & Rachal, J. V. (1989). *Drug abuse treatment: A national study of effectiveness.* Chapel Hill, NC: University of North Carolina Press.

Hughes, Jr., Stead, L., & Lancaster, T. (2007). Antidepressants for smoking cessation. *Cochrane Database of Systemic Reviews, 1,* CD000031.

Hughes, J.R., Stead, L. F., & Lancaster, T. (2005). Nortriptyline for smoking cessation: A review. *Nicotine and Tobacco Research, 7,* 491–499.

Hulse, G. K., Arnold-Reed, D. E., O'Neil, G., Chan, C. T., Hansson, R., & O'Neil, P. (2004). Blood naltrexone and 6-beta-naltrexol levels following naltrexone implant: Comparing two naltrexone implants. *Addiction Biology, 9,* 59–65.

Hulse, G. K., Tait, R. J., Comer, S. D., Sullivan, M. A., Jacobs, I. G., & Arnold-Reed, D. (2005). Reducing hospital presentations for opioid overdose in patients treated with sustained release naltrexone implants. *Drug and Alcohol Dependence, 79,* 351–357.

Ingersoll, K. S., & Cohen, J. (2005). Combination treatment for nicotine dependence: State of the science. *Substance Use & Misuse, 40,* 1923–1943, 2043–2048.

IVAX. (2001). Product information: Baclofen oral tablets, baclofen oral tablets. Miami, FL: IVAX Pharmaceuticals.

Johansson, B. A., Berglund, M., & Lindgren, A. (2006). Efficacy of maintenance treatment with naltrexone for opioid dependence: A meta-analytical review. *Addiction, 101,* 491–503.

Johnson, B. A., & Ait-Daoud, N. (2005). Alcohol: Clinical aspects. In: J. H. Lowinson, P. Ruiz, R. B. Millman, & J. G. Langrod (Eds.) *Substance abuse: A comprehensive textbook.* Philadelphia: Lippincott Williams & Wilkins.

Johnson, B. A., Ait-Daoud, N., Akhtar, F. Z., & Ma, J. Z. (2004). Oral topiramate reduces the consequences of drinking and improves the quality of life of alcohol-dependent individuals: a randomized controlled trial. *Archives of General Psychiatry, 61,* 905–912.

Johnson, B. A., Ait-Daoud, N., Bowden, C. L., DiClemente, C. C., Roache, J. D., Lawson, K., et al. (2003). Oral topiramate for treatment of alcohol dependence: A randomised controlled trial. *Lancet 361*(9370),1677–1685.

Jones, K. L., Lacro, R. V., Johnson, K. A., & Adams, J. (1989). Pattern of malformations in the children of women treated with carbamazepine during pregnancy. *New England Journal of Medicine, 320,* 1661–1666.

Jorenby, D. E., Hays, J. T., Rigotti, N. A., Azoulay, S., Watsky, E. J., Williams, K. E., et al. (2006). Efficacy of varenicline, an alpha4beta2 nicotinic acetylcholine receptor partial agonist, vs placebo or sustained-release bupropion for smoking cessation: a randomized controlled trial. *Journal of the American Medical Association, 296,* 56–63.

Kahn, H. D., Faguet, G. B., Agee, J. F., & Middleton, H. M., 3rd (1984). Drug-induced liver injury. In vitro demonstration of hypersensitivity to both phenytoin and phenobarbital. *Archives of Internal Medicine 144,*1677–1679.

Kalivas, P. W., McFarland, K., Bowers, S., Szumlinski, K., Xi, Z. X., & Baker, D. (2003). Glutamate transmission and addiction to cocaine. *Annals of the New York Academy of Science, 1003,* 169–175.

Kalivas, P. W., & Volkow, N. D. (2005). The neural basis of addiction: A pathology of motivation and choice. *American Journal of Psychiatry, 162,* 1403–1413.

Kampman, K. M., Dackis, C., Lynch, K. G., Pettinati, H., Tirado, C., Gariti, P., et al. (2006). A double-blind, placebo-controlled trial of amantadine, propranolol, and their combination for the treatment of cocaine dependence in patients with severe cocaine withdrawal symptoms. *Drug and Alcohol Dependence, 85,* 129–137.

Kampman, K. M., Pettinati, H., Lynch, K. G., Dackis, C., Sparkman, T., Weigley, C., et al. (2004). A pilot trial of topiramate for the treatment of cocaine dependence. *Drug and Alcohol Dependence, 75,* 233–240.

Kampman, K. M., Pettinati, H., Lynch, K. G., Sparkman, T., & O'Brien, C. P. (2003). A pilot trial of olanzapine for the treatment of cocaine dependence. *Drug and Alcohol Dependence, 70,* 265–273.

Kampman, K. M., Volpicelli, J. R., Alterman, A. I., Cornish, J., & O'Brien, C. P. (2000). Amantadine in the treatment of cocaine-dependent patients with severe withdrawal symptoms. *American Journal of Psychiatry, 157,* 2052–2054.

Kampman, K. M., Volpicelli, J. R., Mulvaney, F., Alterman, A. I., Cornish, J., Gariti, P., et al. (2001). Effectiveness of propranolol for cocaine dependence treatment may depend on cocaine withdrawal symptom severity. *Drug and Alcohol Dependence, 63,* 69–78.

Kaneko, S., Otani, K., Kondo, T., Fukushima, Y., Nakamura, Y., Ogawa, Y., et al. (1992). Malformation in infants of mothers with epilepsy receiving antiepileptic drugs. *Neurology 42*(Suppl 5), 68–74.

Karamanakos, P. N., Pappas, P., Stephanou, P., & Marselos, M. (2001). Differentiation of disulfiram effects on central catecholamines and hepatic ethanol metabolism. *Pharmacology & Toxicology, 88,* 106–110.

Kessler, R. C., Nelson, C. B., McGonagle, K. A., Edlund, M. J., Frank, R. G., & Leaf, P. J. (1996). The epidemiology of co-occurring addictive and mental disorders: Implications for prevention and service utilization. *American Journal of Orthopsychiatry, 66,* 17–31.

Kiefer, F. & Mann, K. (2006). Pharmacotherapy and behavioral intervention for alcohol dependence. *Journal of the Americal Medical Association, 296,* 1727–1728; author reply 1728–1729.

Kim, S. W., Grant, J. E., Yoon, G., Williams, K. A., & Remmel, R. P. (2006). Safety of high-dose naltrexone treatment: Hepatic transaminase profiles among outpatients. *Clinical Neuropharmacology, 29,*77–79.

King, A. C., Volpicelli, J. R., Frazer, A., & O'Brien, C. P. (1997). Effect of naltrexone on subjective alcohol response in subjects at high and low risk for future alcohol dependence. *Psychopharmacology, 129,* 15–22.

Koguchi, K., Nakatsuji, Y., Abe, K., & Sakoda, S. (2004). Wernicke's encephalopathy after glucose infusion. *Neurology, 62,* 512.

Kongsakon, R., Papadopoulos, K. I., & Saguansiritham, R. (2005). Mirtazapine in amphetamine detoxification: A placebo-controlled pilot study. *International Clinical Psychopharmacology, 20,* 253–256.

Kosten, T. R., & O'Connor, P. G. (2003). Management of drug and alcohol withdrawal. *New England Journal of Medicine, 348,* 1786–1795.

Krantz, M. J., Lewkowiez, L., Hays, H., Woodroffe, M. A., Robertson, A. D., & Mehler, P. S. (2002). Torsade de pointes associated with very-high-dose methadone. *Annals of Internal Medicine, 137,* 501–504.

Kranzler, H. R., Modesto-Lowe, V., & Van Kirk, J. (2000). Naltrexone vs. nefazodone for treatment of alcohol dependence. A placebo-controlled trial. *Neuropsychopharmacology, 22,* 493–503.

Kranzler, H. R., & Van Kirk, J. (2001). Efficacy of naltrexone and acamprosate for alcoholism treatment: A meta-analysis. *Alcoholism, Clinical and Experimental Research, 25,* 1335–13341.

Krystal, J. H., Cramer, J. A., Krol, W. F., Kirk, G. F., & Rosenheck, R. A. (2001). Naltrexone in the treatment of alcohol dependence. *New England Journal of Medicine, 345,* 1734–1739.

Lee, M. C., Wagner, H. N., Jr., Tanada, S., Frost, J. J., Bice, A. N., & Dannals, R. F. (1988). Duration of occupancy of opiate receptors by naltrexone. *Journal of Nuclear Medicine, 29,*1207–1211.

Lejoyeux, M., Solomon, J., & Ades, J. (1998). Benzodiazepine treatment for alcohol-dependent patients. *Alcohol and Alcoholism, 33,* 563–575.

Lerman, C., Kaufmann, V., Rukstalis, M., Patterson, F., Perkins, K., Audrain-McGovern, J., et al. (2004). Individualizing nicotine replacement therapy for the treatment of tobacco dependence: A randomized trial. *Annals of Internal Medicine, 140,* 426–433.

Lesscher, H. M., Bailey, A., Burbach, J. P., Van Ree, J. M., Kitchen, I., & Gerrits, M. A. (2003). Receptor-selective changes in mu-, delta- and kappa-opioid receptors after chronic naltrexone treatment in mice. *European Journal of Neuroscience, 17*, 1006–1012.

Lima, M. S., Reisser, A. A., Soares, B. G., & Farrell, M. (2003). Antidepressants for cocaine dependence. *Cochrane Database of Systemic Reviews, 2*, CD002950.

Litten, R. Z., Fertig, J., Mattson, M., & Egli, M. (2005). Development of medications for alcohol use disorders: recent advances and ongoing challenges. *Expert Opinion on Emerging Drugs, 10*, 323–343.

Maccioni, P., Serra, S., Vacca, G., Orru, A., Pes, D., Agabio, R., et al. (2005). Baclofen-induced reduction of alcohol reinforcement in alcohol-preferring rats. *Alcohol, 36*, 161–168.

Malcolm, R., Ballenger, J. C., Sturgis, E. T., & Anton, R. (1989). Double-blind controlled trial comparing carbamazepine to oxazepam treatment of alcohol withdrawal. *American Journal of Psychiatry, 146*, 617–621.

Malcolm, R., Myrick, H., Brady, K. T., & Ballenger, J. C. (2001). Update on anticonvulsants for the treatment of alcohol withdrawal. *American Journal of Addiction, 10* (Suppl), 16–23.

Mann, K. (2004). Pharmacotherapy of alcohol dependence: A review of the clinical data. *CNS Drugs, 18*, 485–504.

Mariani, J. J., Rosenthal, R. N., Tross, S., Singh, P., & Anand, O. P. (2006). A randomized, open-label, controlled trial of gabapentin and phenobarbital in the treatment of alcohol withdrawal. *American Journal of Addiction, 15*, 76–84.

Mariolis, P., Rock, V. J., Asman, K., Merritt, R., Malarcher, A. Husten, C., & Pechacek, T. (2006). Tobacco use among adults — United States. *MMWR, 55*, 1145–1148.

Mark, T. L., Woody, G. E., Juday, T., & Kleber, H. D. (2001). The economic costs of heroin addiction in the United States. *Drug and Alcohol Dependence, 61*, 195–206.

Martz, A., Deitrich, R. A., & Harris, R. A. (1983). Behavioral evidence for the involvement of gamma-aminobutyric acid in the actions of ethanol. *European Journal of Pharmacology, 89*, 53–62.

Mason, B. J., Goodman, A. M., Chabac, S., & Lehert, P. (2006). Effect of oral acamprosate on abstinence in patients with alcohol dependence in a double-blind, placebo-controlled trial: The role of patient motivation. *Journal of Psychiatric Research, 40*, 383–393.

Mattick, R. P., Breen, C., Kimber, J., & Davoli, M. (2003). Methadone maintenance therapy versus no opioid replacement therapy for opioid dependence. *Cochrane Database of Systemic Reviews, 2*, CD002209.

Mattick, R. P., Kimber, J., Breen, C., & Davoli, M. (2002). Buprenorphine maintenance versus placebo or methadone maintenance for opioid dependence. *Cochrane Database Systemic Reviews, 4*, CD002207.

Maxwell, S., Bigg, D., Stanczykiewicz, K., & Carlberg-Racich, S. (2006). Prescribing naloxone to actively injecting heroin users: A program to reduce heroin overdose deaths. *Journal of Addictive Diseases, 25*, 89–96.

Mayo-Smith, M. F. (1997). Pharmacological management of alcohol withdrawal. A meta-analysis and evidence-based practice guideline. American Society of Addiction Medicine Working Group on Pharmacological Management of Alcohol Withdrawal. *Journal of the American Medical Association, 278*, 144–151.

McCance-Katz, E. F. (2005). Treatment of opioid dependence and coinfection with HIV and hepatitis C virus in opioid-dependent patients: The importance of drug interactions between opioids and antiretroviral agents. *Clinical Infectious Diseases: an official publication of the Infectious Diseases Society of America, 41* (Supp. 1), S89–S95.

McCaul, M. E., Wand, G. S., Eissenberg, T., Rohde, C. A., & Cheskin, L. J. (2000a). Naltrexone alters subjective and psychomotor responses to alcohol in heavy drinking subjects. *Neuropsychopharmacology. 22*, 480–492.

McCaul, M. E., Wand, G. S., Rohde, C., & Lee, S. M. (2000b). Serum 6-beta-naltrexol levels are related to alcohol responses in heavy drinkers.[see comment]. *Alcoholism: Clinical & Experimental Research, 24*, 1385–1391.

McDowell, D., Nunes, E. V., Seracini, A. M., Rothenberg, J., Vosburg, S. K., Ma, G. J., et al. (2005). Desipramine treatment of cocaine-dependent patients with depression: A placebo-controlled trial. *Drug and Alcohol Dependence, 80*, 209–221.

McGrath, P. J., Nunes, E. V., Stewart, J. W., Goldman, D., Agosti, V., Ocepek-Welikson, K., et al.(1996). Imipramine treatment of alcoholics with primary depression: A placebo-controlled clinical trial. *Archives of General Psychiatry, 53*, 232–240.

Medtronic (2002a). *Product information: Lioresal(R) Intrathecal (baclofen injection)/overdose procedure, Baclofen intrathecal overdose procedure*. Minneapolis, MN: Medtronic.

Medtronic (2002b). *Medwatch: Important drug warning*. Minneapolis, MN: Medtronic, Inc.

Minozzi, S., Amato, L., Vecchi, S., Davoli, M., Kirchmayer, U., & Verster, A. (2006). Oral naltrexone maintenance treatment for opioid dependence. *Cochrane Database of Systemic Reviews, 1*, CD001333.

Miotto, K., McCann, M. J., Rawson, R. A., Frosch, D., & Ling, W. (1997). Overdose, suicide attempts and death among a cohort of naltrexone-treated opioid addicts. *Drug and Alcohol Dependence, 45*, 131–134.

Montoya, I. D., Preston, K. L., Rothman, R., & Gorelick, D. A. (2002). Open-label pilot study of bupropion plus bromocriptine for treatment of cocaine dependence. *American Journal of Drug and Alcohol Abuse, 28*, 189–196.

Munafo, M., Bradburn, M., Bowes, L., & David, S. (2004). Are there sex differences in transdermal nicotine replacement therapy patch efficacy? A meta-analysis. *Nicotine and Tobacco Research, 6*, 769–776.

Myrick, H., & Anton, R. (2004). Recent advances in the pharmacotherapy of alcoholism. *Current Psychiatry Reports, 6*, 332–338.

Neppe, V. M., & Sindorf, J. (1991). Carbamazepine for high-dose diazepam withdrawal in opiate users. *The Journal of Nervous and Mental Disease, 179*, 234–235.

Ngo, H. T. T., Tait, R. J., Arnold-Reed, D. E., & Hulse, G. K. (2007). Mental health outcomes following naltrexone implant treatment for heroin-dependence. *Progress In Neuro-Psychopharmacology & Biological Psychiatry, 31*, 605–612.

Nunes, E. V., & Levin, F. R. (2006). Treating depression in substance abusers. *Current Psychiatry Reports, 8*, 363–370.

Nunes, E. V., Liu, X., Samet, S., Matseoane, K., & Hasin, D. (2006). Independent versus substance-induced major depressive disorder in substance-dependent patients: Observational study of course during follow-up. *Journal of Clinical Psychiatry, 67*, 1561–1567.

Nunes, E. V., Quitkin, F. M., Donovan, S. J., Deliyannides, D., Ocepek-Welikson, K., Koenig, T., et al. (1998). Imipramine treatment of opiate-dependent patients with depressive disorders. A placebo-controlled trial. *Archives of General Psychiatry, 55*, 153–160.

O'Brien, C. P. (2001). Naltrexone for alcohol dependence: Compliance is a key issue. *Addiction, 96*, 1857.

Okuyemi, K. S., Nollen, N. L., & Ahluwalia, J. S. (2006). Interventions to facilitate smoking cessation. *American Family Physician, 74*, 262–271.

Olive, M. F., Koenig, H. N., Nannini, M. A., & Hodge, C. W. (2001). Stimulation of endorphin neurotransmission in the nucleus accumbens by ethanol, cocaine, and amphetamine. *Journal of Neuroscience, 21*, RC184.

O'Malley, S. S., & Froehlich, J. C. (2003). Advances in the use of naltrexone: An integration of preclinical and clinical findings. *Recent Developments in Alcoholism, 16*, 217–245.

Oreskovich, M. R., Saxon, A. J., Ellis, M. L., Malte, C. A., Reoux, J. P., & Knox, P. C. (2005). A double-blind, double-dummy, randomized, prospective pilot study of the partial mu opiate agonist, buprenorphine, for acute detoxification from heroin. *Drug and Alcohol Dependence, 77*, 71–79.

Ortho-McNeil Pharmaceutical Inc. (2004). *Product information: Topamax(R) tablets, Topamax(R) sprinkle capsules, topiramate tablets, capsules, sprinkle capsules*. Raritan.

Peles, E., Kreek, M. J., Kellogg, S., & Adelson, M. (2006). High methadone dose significantly reduces cocaine use in methadone maintenance treatment (MMT) patients. *Journal of Addictive Diseases, 25*, 43–50.

Petrakis, I. L., Carroll, K. M., Nich, C., Gordon, L. T., McCance-Katz, E. F., Frankforter, T., et al. (2000). Disulfiram treatment for cocaine dependence in methadone-maintained opioid addicts. *Addiction, 95*, 219–228.

Porter, R. J. (1987). How to initiate and maintain carbamazepine therapy in children and adults. *Epilepsia, 28* (Supp. 3), S59–S63.

Quinlan, J. J., Ferguson, C., Jester, K., Firestone, L. L., & Homanics, G. E. (2002). Mice with glycine receptor subunit mutations are both sensitive and resistant to volatile anesthetics. *Anesthesia and Analgesia, 95*, 578–582, table of contents.

Regier, D. A., Farmer, M. E., Rae, D. S., Locke, B. Z., Keith, S. J., Judd, L. L., et al. (1990). Comorbidity of mental disorders with alcohol and other drug abuse. Results from the Epidemiologic Catchment Area (ECA) Study. *Journal of the American Medical Association, 264*, 2511–2518.

Reoux, J. P., & Miller, K. (2000). Routine hospital alcohol detoxification practice compared to symptom triggered management with an Objective Withdrawal Scale (CIWA-Ar). *American Journal of Addiction, 9*, 135–144.

Reoux, J. P., Saxon, A. J., Malte, C. A., Baer, J. S., & Sloan, K. L. (2001). Divalproex sodium in alcohol withdrawal: A randomized double-blind placebo-controlled clinical trial. *Alcoholism, Clinical and Experimental Research, 25*, 1324–1329.

Rettig, R. A., & Yarmolinsky, A. (1995). Federal Regulation of Methadone Treatment. Washington DC: Institute of Medicine. National Academy Press.

Ries, R., Cullison, S., Horn, R., & Ward, N. (1991). Benzodiazepine withdrawal: Clinicians' ratings of carbamazepine treatment versus traditional taper methods. *Journal of Psychoactive Drugs, 23*, 73–76.

Ries, R. K., Roy-Byrne, P. P., Ward, N. G., Neppe, V., & Cullison, S. (1989). Carbamazepine treatment for benzodiazepine withdrawal. *American Journal of Psychiatry, 146*, 536–537.

Rosa, F. W. (1991). Spina bifida in infants of women treated with carbamazepine during pregnancy. *New England Journal of Medicine, 324*, 674–677.

Roy-Byrne, P. P., Sullivan, M. D., Cowley, D. S., & Ries, R. K. (1993). Adjunctive treatment of benzodiazepine discontinuation syndromes: a review. *Journal of Psychiatric Research, 27* (Suppl 1), 143–153.

Roy-Byrne, P. P., Ward, N. G., & Donnelly, P. J. (1989). Valproate in anxiety and withdrawal syndromes. *Journal of Clinical Psychiatry, 50* (Suppl.), 44–48.

Rzany, B., Correia, O., Kelly, J. P., Naldi, L., Auquier, A., & Stern, R. (1999). Risk of Stevens-Johnson syndrome and toxic epidermal necrolysis during first weeks of antiepileptic therapy: A case-control study. Study Group of the International Case Control Study on Severe Cutaneous Adverse Reactions. *Lancet, 353*, 2190–2194.

Saitz, R., Mayo-Smith, M. F., Roberts, M. S., Redmond, H. A., Bernard, D. R., & Calkins, D. R. (1994). Individualized treatment for alcohol withdrawal. A randomized double-blind controlled trial. *Journal of the Americal Medical Association, 272*, 519–523.

Saitz, R., & O'Malley, S. S. (1997). Pharmacotherapies for alcohol abuse. Withdrawal and treatment. *Medical Clinics of North America, 81*, 881–907.

Sass, H., Soyka, M., Mann, K., & Zieglgansberger, W. (1996). Relapse prevention by acamprosate. Results from a placebo-controlled study on alcohol dependence. *Archives of General Psychiatry, 53*, 673–680.

Schachter, S. (2007). Pharmacology of antiepileptic drug. *Up to Date Online 15.1.*

Schmitz, J. M., Averill, P., Stotts, A. L., Moeller, F. G., Rhoades, H. M., & Grabowski, J. (2001). Fluoxetine treatment of cocaine-dependent patients with major depressive disorder. *Drug and Alcohol Dependence, 63*, 207–214.

Schubiner, H., Saules, K. K., Arfken, C. L., Johanson, C. E., Schuster, C. R., Lockhart, N., et al. (2002). Double-blind placebo-controlled trial of methylphenidate in the treatment of adult ADHD patients with comorbid cocaine dependence. *Experimental and Clinical Psychopharmacology, 10*, 286–294.

Schuckit, M. A. (2006). Comorbidity between substance use disorders and psychiatric conditions. *Addiction, 101* (Suppl 1) 76–88.

Schweizer, E., Rickels, K., Case, W. G., & Greenblatt, D. J. (1991). Carbamazepine treatment in patients discontinuing long-term benzodiazepine therapy. Effects on withdrawal severity and outcome. *Archives of General Psychiatry, 48*, 448–452.

Seip, M. L. (1976). Growth retardation, dysmorphic facies and minor malformations following massive exposure to phenobarbitone in utero. *Acta Paediatrica Scandinavica, 65*, 617–621.

Shoptaw, S., Huber, A., Peck, J., Yang, X., Liu, J., Jeff, D., et al. (2006). Randomized, placebo-controlled trial of sertraline and contingency management for the treatment of methamphetamine dependence. *Drug and Alcohol Dependence, 85*, 12–18.

Shoptaw, S., Kintaudi, P. C., Charuvastra, C., & Ling, W. (2002). A screening trial of amantadine as a medication for cocaine dependence. *Drug and Alcohol Dependence, 66*, 217–224.

Shoptaw, S., Rawson, R. A., McCann, M. J., & Obert, J. L. (1994). The Matrix model of outpatient stimulant abuse treatment: evidence of efficacy. *Journal of Addictive Diseases, 13*, 129–141.

Shoptaw, S., Yang, X., Rotheram-Fuller, E. J., Hsieh, Y. C., Kintaudi, P. C., Charuvastra, V. C., et al. (2003). Randomized placebo-controlled trial of baclofen for cocaine dependence: preliminary effects for individuals with chronic patterns of cocaine use. *Journal of Clinical Psychiatry, 64*, 1440–1448.

Sieghart, W. (1995). Structure and pharmacology of gamma-aminobutyric acidA receptor subtypes. *Pharmacology Review, 47*, 181–234.

Silagy, C., Lancaster, T., Stead, L., Mant, D., & Fowler, G. (2004). Nicotine replacement therapy for smoking cessation. *Cochrane Database of Systemic Reviews, 3*, CD000146.

Simpson, D. D., Joe, G. W., Broome, K. L., Hiller, M. L., Knight, K., & Rowan-Szal, G. A. (1997). Program diversity and treatment retention rates in the Drug Abuse Treatment Outcome Study (DATOS). *Psychology of Addictive Behaviors, 11*, 279–293.

Simpson, D. D., & Sells, S. B. (1982). Effectiveness of treatment for drug abuse: An overview of the DARP research program. *Advances in Alcohol and Substance Abuse, 2*, 7–29.

Simpson, D. D., & Sells, S. B. (Eds.). (1990). *Opioid addiction and treatment: A 12-year follow up.* Malabar, FL.: Krieger.

Smith, G. B., & Olsen, R. W. (1995). Functional domains of GABAA receptors. *Trends in Pharmacological Science, 16*, 162–168.

Smyth, B., Hoffman, V., Fan, J., & Hser, Y. I. (2007). Years of potential life lost among heroin addicts 33 years after treatment. *Preventative Medicine, 44*, 369–374.

Sneddon, I. B. (1967). Steven-Johnson syndrome with eye lesions. *British Journal of Dermatology, 79*, 715.

Srisurapanont, M., & Jarusuraisin, N. (2002). Opioid antagonists for alcohol dependence. *Cochrane Database of Systemic Reviews, 2*,CD001867.

Srisurapanont, M., Kittiratanapaiboon, P., & Jarusuraisin, N. (2001). Treatment for amphetamine psychosis. *Cochrane Database of Systemic Reviews, 4*, CD003026.

Stine, S. M., Krystal, J. H., Kosten, T .R., & Charney, D. S. (1995). Mazindol treatment for cocaine dependence. *Drug and Alcohol Dependence, 39*, 245–252.

Stromberg, M. F., Sengpiel, T., Mackler, S. A., Volpicelli, J. R., O'Brien, C. P., & Vogel, W. H. (2002). Effect of naltrexone on oral consumption of concurrently available ethanol and cocaine in the rat. *Alcohol, 28*, 169–179.

Studies, O.o.A. (2006). *Results from the 2005 National Survey on Drug Use and Health: National Findings.* Rockville, MD.: Substance Abuse and Mental Health Services Administration.

Sullivan, J. T., Sykora, K., Schneiderman, J., Naranjo, C. A., & Sellers, E. M. (1989). Assessment of alcohol withdrawal: The revised clinical institute withdrawal assessment for alcohol scale (CIWA-Ar). *British Journal of Addicttion, 84*, 1353–1357.

Sullivan, L. E., Metzger, D. S., Fudala, P. J., & Fiellin, D. A. (2005). Decreasing international HIV transmission: The role of expanding access to opioid agonist therapies for injection drug users. *Addiction, 100*, 150–158.

Sullivan, M. A., Vosburg, S. K., & Comer, S. D. (2006). Depot naltrexone: Antagonism of the reinforcing, subjective, and physiological effects of heroin. *Psychopharmacology (Berl), 189*, 37–46.

Suzdak, P. D., Schwartz, R. D., Skolnick, P., & Paul, S. M. (1986). Ethanol stimulates gamma-aminobutyric acid receptor-mediated chloride transport in rat brain synaptoneurosomes. *Proceedings of the National Academy of Sciences USA, 83*, 4071–4075.

Swift, R. M., Whelihan, W., Kuznetsov, O., Buongiorno, G., & Hsuing, H. (1994). Naltrexone-induced alterations in human ethanol intoxication. *American Journal of Psychiatry, 151*, 1463–1467.

Tabakoff, B., & Hoffman, P. L. (1983). Alcohol interactions with brain opiate receptors. *Life Sciences, 32*, 197–204.

Thompson, G. H., & Hunter, D. A. (1998). Nicotine replacement therapy. *Annals of Pharmacotherapy, 32*, 1067–1075.

Thomsen Healthcare Inc. (2006). *Physician's desk reference.* Montvale, NJ: Thomsen Healthcare Inc.

Ticku, M. K., Lowrimore, P., & Lehoullier, P. (1986). Ethanol enhances GABA-induced 36Cl-influx in primary spinal cord cultured neurons. *Brain Research Bulletin, 17*, 123–126.

Tiihonen, J., Kuoppasalmi, K., Fohr, J., Tuomola, P., Kuikanmaki, O., Vorma, H., et al. (2007). A comparison of aripiprazole, methylphenidate, and placebo for amphetamine dependence. *American Journal of Psychiatry, 164*, 160–162.

Tonstad, S., Tonnesen, P., Hajek, P., Williams, K. E., Billing, C. B., & Reeves, K. R. (2006). Effect of maintenance therapy with varenicline on smoking cessation: A randomized controlled trial. *Journal of the American Medical Association 296*, 64–71.

Trafton, J. A., Minkel, J., & Humphreys, K. (2006). Determining effective methadone doses for individual opioid-dependent patients. *PLoS Medicine, 3*, e80.

Tucker, T. K., & Ritter, A. J. (2000). Naltrexone in the treatment of heroin dependence: A literature review. *Drug and Alcohol Review, 19*, 73–78.

Victor, M., Adams, R. A., & Collins, G. H. (1989). *The Wernicke-Korsakoff syndrome and related disorders due to alcoholism and malnutrition.* Philadelphia: FA Davis.

Volpicelli, J. R., Alterman, A. I., Hayashida, M., & O'Brien, C. P. (1992). Naltrexone in the treatment of alcohol dependence. *Archives of General Psychiatry, 49*, 876–880.

Volpicelli, J. R., Davis, M. A., & Olgin, J. E., (1986). Naltrexone blocks the post-shock increase of ethanol consumption. *Life Sciences, 38*, 841–847.

Volpicelli, J. R., Rhines, K. C., Rhines, J. S., Volpicelli, L. A., Alterman, A. I., & O'Brien, C. P. (1997). Naltrexone and alcohol dependence. Role of subject compliance. *Archives of General Psychiatry, 54*, 737–742.

Voris, J., Smith, N. L., Rao, S. M., Thorne, D. L., & Flowers, Q. J. (2003). Gabapentin for the treatment of ethanol withdrawal. *Substance Abuse, 24*,129–132.

Vornik, L. A., & Brown, E. S. (2006). Management of comorbid bipolar disorder and substance abuse. *Journal of Clinical Psychiatry, 67* (Suppl 7) 24–30.

Waal, H., Frogopsahl, G., Olsen, L., Christophersen, A. S., & Morland, J. (2006). Naltrexone implants — duration, tolerability and clinical usefulness. A pilot study. *European Addiction Research, 12*, 138–144.

Weinhouse, G. L., & Manaker, S. (2007). Alcohol withdrawal syndromes *Up to Date Online 15.1.*

Wesson, D. R., Smith, D. E., Ling, W., & Seymour, R. B. (2005). Sedative-Hypnotics. In: L. J. H. R. P; M. RB & L. JG (Eds.), *Substance abuse: A comprehensive textbook.* Philadelphia: Lippincott Williams & Wilkins.

Williams, K. L., Ferko, A. P., Barbieri, E. J., & DiGregorio, G. J. (1995). Glycine enhances the central depressant properties of ethanol in mice. *Pharmacology, Biochemistry and Behavior, 50*, 199–205.

Wright, C. T., Vafier, J. A., & Lake, C. R. (1988). Disulfiram-induced fulminating hepatitis: guidelines for liver-panel monitoring. *Journal of Clinical Psychiatry, 49*, 430–434.

Wuis, E. W., Dirks, M. J., Termond, E. F., Vree, T. B., & Van der Kleijn, E. (1989). Plasma and urinary excretion kinetics of oral baclofen in healthy subjects. *European Journal of Clinical Pharmacology, 37*, 181–184.

Yudkin, P. L., Jones, L., Lancaster, T., & Fowler, G. H. (1996). Which smokers are helped to give up smoking using the transdermal nicotine patches? Results from a randomized, double-blind, placebo-controlled trial. *British Journal of General Practice. 46*,145–148.

Zellweger, H. (1974). Anticonvulsants during pregnancy: A danger to the developing fetus? *Clinical Pediatrics (Phila), 13*, 338–341.

26

Motivational Interviewing

Bryan Hartzler, David B. Rosengren, and John S. Baer

University of Washington

Contents

Nearly a quarter century ago, William R. Miller published a first paper (1983) describing motivational interviewing (MI). Several years later, he and Stephen Rollnick would co-author what is now a seminal text (1991) that delineated the method, its underlying conceptual basis, and application to various treatment populations. MI evolved from observations in the research literature that brief interventions, containing specific elements, could have powerful effects. It suggested that instead of instruction, skills-training, or shaping of behavior via contingencies, what clients need most is a supportive and nonjudgmental relationship with a practitioner where ambivalence about substance use behavior could be more fully explored and effectively resolved.

As do many new approaches, MI garnered much attention and scrutiny, and was viewed in contrast to prevailing confrontational models of American substance abuse treatment. Although a handful of studies documenting efficacy were available at the time of Miller & Rollnick's (1991) first edition, the decade that followed brought with it a burgeoning scientific base in which MI was evaluated in a variety of formats, with a range of health behaviors, and in a host of clinical settings. On a broader level, this ensuing decade included a call to "bridge the research-practice gap" (Lamb, Greenlick, & McCarty, 1998), prompting national organizations to publish definitions, policies, and guidelines for evidence-based practice in substance abuse treatment. Of note was the inclusion of motivational enhancement therapy (MET), an adaptation of MI that integrates individualized assessment feedback, among a list of empirically supported treatments (NIDA, 1999).

Recent scientific inquiry has begun to explore other questions about MI. Among these are questions of its mechanisms of action (e.g., how does MI work?), measurement (e.g., how does one assess how MI is performed?), adoption (e.g., how does one learn to do MI?), and implementation (e.g., how does one integrate MI into daily practice?).

What is MI?

Miller and Rollnick (2002) define MI as, "A client-centered, directive method for enhancing intrinsic motivation to change by exploring and resolving ambivalence". As a client-centered approach MI makes use of traditional Rogerian concepts of accurate empathy, genuineness, and unconditional positive regard. Yet as a directive method, MI practitioners selectively and strategically seek to explore ambivalence about change in a manner that increases the likelihood that change will occur. MI does not advance specific skills or strategies for client behavior change. Some have suggested that all change is self-change, even that involving formal treatment (DiClemente, 2003). Presumably, MI encourages natural change processes to emerge, which clients use to alter long-standing, repetitive, and self-defeating patterns of behavior.

MI could be misinterpreted by some as a bag of tricks, used to convince clients to change who otherwise may not. Its originators emphasize *MI spirit*, differentiating the global style with which one works from specific techniques one may employ. MI spirit is governed by a collaborative, eliciting, and respectful interpersonal style thought to facilitate open and honest client discussion of hopes and concerns about the prospect of behavior change. In employing MI, one pairs this interpersonal spirit with strategic use of linguistic techniques that structure conversation so clients may articulate whether, why, when, and how change occurs. Thus, the intent of MI is not to manipulate clients, nor to demand or enforce that change occur.

Although MI was not developed based on a specific theoretical framework (Allsop, 2007), its principles are, in fact, linked to social psychology theories (Leffingwell, Neumann, Babitzke, Leedy, & Walters, 2007; Markland, Ryan, Tobin, & Rollnick, 2005), most notably Bem's (1972) self-perception theory that postulates we more readily commit to what we hear ourselves defend. This may be particularly true when our beliefs are not well-defined, as when we are ambivalent about a behavior or a change. By extension, the intent of MI is to elicit arguments for change from the client—statements of desire, ability, reason, need, and commitment to change—termed *change talk* (Miller & Rollnick, 2002). The premise is that clients hear their own discussion of change and thereby more readily commit to actions that follow. If one accepts this conceptual basis for the approach, then practicing MI is more clearly seen as a goal-directed activity—one in which we seek to elicit change talk from clients and in doing so strengthen their commitment to change.

MI Spirit

Clients come to us with a daunting task of deciphering a mixture of internal competing motivations, some that incite change, others that maintain circumstances, and all that are both personal and reasonable from at least one perspective. Should we be surprised that some omit, filter, or misrepresent information when feeling judged or perceiving pressure to change? The therapeutic process benefits from efforts to promote client trust and comfort with self-disclosure. To effectively use MI is to do just that, by exuding a collaborative, eliciting, and supportive "way of being" (Miller & Rollnick, 2002). More than simple courtesy, it requires sincere interest in, understanding of, and tolerance for people: what they believe, how they feel, and what they do. Accordingly, MI spirit has been defined as a confluence of: *collaboration, evocation, autonomy*. These qualities are further defined in Table 26.1.

TABLE 26.1
The Spirit of Motivational Interviewing

Fundamental Approach of Motivational Interviewing	*Mirror-Image Opposite Approach to Counseling*
Collaboration. Counseling involves a partnership that honors the client's expertise and perspectives. The counselor provides an atmosphere that is conducive rather than coercive to change.	*Confrontation.* Counseling involves overriding the client's impaired perspectives by imposing awareness and acceptance of "reality" that the client cannot see or will not admit.
Evocation. The resources and motivation for change are presumed to reside within the client. Intrinsic motivation for change is enhanced by drawing on the client's own perceptions, goals, and values.	*Education.* The client is presumed to lack key knowledge, insight, and/or skills that are necessary for change to occur. The counselor seeks to address these deficits by providing the requisite enlightenment.
Autonomy. The counselor affirms the client's right and capacity for self-direction and facilitates informed choice.	*Authority.* The counselor tells the client what he or she must do.

Source. Adapted from Miller and Rollnick (2002).

Rollnick & Miller (1995) offer the following as additional description of MI spirit:

1. *Motivation to change is elicited, not imposed.* Coercion, persuasion, or confrontation may provoke behavior change at times, but fails to draw on clients' intrinsic motivations.
2. *It is a client's responsibility to articulate and resolve competing motivations.* Practitioner is responsible for supporting free expression and guiding decisions about change.
3. *Direct persuasion does not effectively resolve client ambivalence.* If anything, such tactics strengthen client resistance and thereby lessen likelihood that change will occur.
4. *A quiet eliciting style promotes client comfort and trust in the therapeutic process.* This aids in generating achievable, rather than unrealistic or counterproductive, client goals.
5. *Practitioners are active in directing clients to explore and resolve ambivalence.* Once resolve is solidified, there may not be need for further intervention in many cases.
6. *Readiness to change is not static, but perpetually fluctuating.* Thus, client statements about change (whether for or against) are critical feedback to which the practitioner should be attuned.
7. *The practitioner–client bond is a partnership, not a hierarchy.* Cooperation and mutual respect support change more than assertion of practitioner expertise or empowerment.

We wish to emphasize that MI is spirit-driven, with the aim of exuding perpetual support, not confrontation nor hoodwinking of clients when it suits one's agenda. Although MI, like most innovations, may be diluted during its diffusion (Rogers, 2003), retention of its spirit is an area of particular attention for those invested in its dissemination. Indeed, a nascent research base suggests MI spirit is an important predictor of its impact (Moyers, Miller, & Hendrickson, 2005b).

Four Guiding Principles

Miller and Rollnick (1991) outline a set of four principles, derived through expert consensus and based on brief intervention research, to more directly guide practitioners' behavior during clinical encounters. If appreciation of MI spirit affords practitioners a global sense of purpose, then the principles listed in Table 26.2 offer greater clarity of the nature and timing of strategies employed by practitioners in pursuit of that purpose.

Expressing Empathy

The capacity to understand the world from another's perspective has long been considered necessary for effective therapeutic intervention. Rogers (1959) coined the term *accurate empathy*, incorporating appreciation for client thoughts, feelings, and action, but also the need to convey that understanding explicitly. Expression of empathy—or reflective listening—communicates respect, normalizes ambivalence, encourages collaborative alliance, and continually supports a client's self-exploration. An important, sometimes overlooked distinction is that expressing empathy may not necessarily mean identifying with a client's experience, let alone approving of values or beliefs. What is critical, from an

> ### TABLE 26.2
> ### Four Principles of Motivational Interviewing
>
> **Principle 1: Express Empathy**
>
> Acceptance facilitates change.
> Skillful reflective listening is fundamental.
> Ambivalence is normal.
>
> **Principle 2: Develop Discrepancy**
>
> The client rather than the counselor should present the arguments for change.
> Change is motivated by a perceived discrepancy between present behavior and important
>   personal goals or values.
>
> **Principle 3: Roll with Resistance**
>
> Avoid arguing for change.
> Resistance is not directly opposed.
> New perspectives are invited but not imposed.
> The client is a primary resource in finding answers and solutions.
> Resistance is a signal to respond differently.
>
> **Principle 4: Support Self-Efficacy**
>
> A person's belief in the possibility of change is an important motivator.
> The client, not the counselor, is responsible for choosing and carrying out change.
> The counselor's own belief in the person's ability to change becomes a self-fulfilling prophecy.
>
> *Source.*   Adapted from Miller and Rollnick (2002).

MI perspective, is that practitioners sustain efforts to understand the client's perspective. Expressing empathy has been considered a defining characteristic of MI since its inception (Miller, 1983).

Developing Discrepancy

If empathy were expressed solely in classic Rogerian terms, there would be no direction within this therapeutic approach. To the contrary, those who employ MI strategically seek to develop discrepancy by heightening client awareness of gaps between values and behavior. Recognition of such gaps is a source of intrinsic motivation among substance users (Downey, Rosengren, & Donovan, 2000; Wagner & Sanchez, 2002), whose actions may contradict values apparent in social connections they desire with family, friends, and community. In an MI session, the client first articulates aspirations and regrets, then hears a practitioner selectively repeat these back as a contrast with current behavior. This process differs from that advocated by traditional disease model concepts in which discrepancy between client behavior and societal values is highlighted, and from which clients may reasonably feel undue pressure. From an MI perspective, it is critical that discrepancies originate in client statements, and be offered back from a position of attempting to understand—not convince—the client. Thus, discrepancies are not ammunition in support of practitioner arguments, but rather reflection of the client's internal discourse, which the practitioner helps bring to the surface and assists the client in exploring.

Rolling with Resistance

Therapist may be tempted to oversimplify client resistance and reinterpret it as characterological defensiveness. An alternative view is that resistance is a transient, ever-fluctuating product of the therapeutic alliance. An MI perspective holds that practitioners use resistance to better understand the client's ambivalence. Miller and Rollnick (2002) offer strategies for responding to resistance, among them: (1) reflective listening to acknowledge, strategically overstate, or normalize ambivalence; (2) shifting conversational focus; (3) reframing statements in a supportive light; (4) offering agreement with latent reframing (e.g., "agreement with a twist"); and (5) reinforcing autonomy and perceived control. Whatever the strategy, the underlying aim is to acknowledge and show interest in the client perspective rather than to disagree or dismiss. In MI parlance, client resistance cues the practitioner to change his or her own behavior.

Supporting Self-Efficacy

A practitioner may express empathy, develop discrepancy, and defuse client resistance as described. However, this alone may only aid a client's sense of being understood and understanding of substance-related harms. Many have limited confidence that they can change behavior. Thus, it's critical that confidence is built by reinforcing optimism that change can occur. Support for client self-efficacy, or perceived ability to achieve a desired outcome, reflects practitioner expectations about change. Such expectations strongly influence treatment outcome (Leake & King, 1977). Support may involve simply conveying the belief that change is achievable. To do so, one must first allow that clients can choose whether and how change occurs, and that the necessary resources lie within the client. This runs contrary to notions that resources reside in the counselor and the client needs to learn specific skills that the counselor must teach. Support of client self-efficacy does not assume that a relapse prevention plan or drink refusal skills are unimportant, but rather notes that clients often have a great deal of wisdom already, including information about what is and is not helpful for them. Client self-efficacy is further supported by referencing the success of others facing similar challenges as well as those in the client's own past.

Taken together, these four principles guide practitioner behavior in exploring and resolving client ambivalence. Furthermore, they are intended both individually and collectively to reinforce the collaborative, eliciting, and supportive spirit of MI described previously. Application of these principles involves practitioner use of particular conversational skills and techniques described in the next section.

Core Skills and Supplemental Techniques

The set of four core skills within MI are illustrated in Table 26.3. From an MI perspective, the classical reflective listening techniques (i.e., open-ended questions, affirmations, reflections, and summary statements) that form a basis of many approaches to counseling (Rogers, 1959) are utilized to engender intrinsic motivation within the client. An important distinction is that, within MI, reflective listening is used with the explicit intention of eliciting discussion of change from clients.

**TABLE 26.3
OARS: Motivational Interviewing's Core
Tools for Moving the Session**

1. Asking Open-Ended Questions (e.g., questions that do not invite brief answers)
   Is a way of eliciting narrative from the client
   Helps establish an atmosphere of acceptance and trust
   May strategically target a useful topic for exploration

2. Affirming Client Strengths Or Efforts
   Is a way of articulating support and encouragement
   Strengthens rapport and reinforces the client's self-exploration
   Is particularly effective when salient efforts or idiosyncratic qualities are targeted

3. Listening Reflectively
   Is an active process of hypothesis-testing as to what the client's words mean
   Sustains client's focus to further explore potential ambivalence
   Can vary in form, from simple repeating to more complex paraphrasing, expanding,
      abbreviating, or underscoring of client ideas

4. Summarizing Client Statements
   Is a way of linking together and selectively reinforcing the client's statements
   Can serve to help organize the client's thoughts about an issue
   May reflect a process of collecting and recounting client change statements, of linking
      current statements to previously offered material, or of a strategic transition from
      one topic of self-exploration to another

Source.   Adapted from Miller and Rollnick (2002).

Practitioners use Open questions to elicit client narrative, as opposed to eliciting little more than one-word responses (e.g., "yes/no," "12," "Thursday"). Practitioners then listen, and identify underlying client qualities (e.g., honesty, perseverance) to reinforce with Affirmations, or statements recognizing those qualities. Practitioners may also offer reflective listening statements, or Reflections, to convey understanding of what the client has said. These take many forms: repeating a client's own words, adding meaning by paraphrasing, increasing depth by introducing affective language or a metaphor, or linking common themes among client statements. The latter example constitutes a Summary, which are offered periodically (after 4–5 reflections, although this is not a hard-and-fast rule). Summaries organize a client's thoughts, offered back by the practitioner as if flowers in a bouquet (Miller & Rollnick, 2002).

There are many purposes for *OARS*, including establishing rapport, facilitating client comfort with exploring difficult topics, and creating momentum within a clinical encounter. *OARS* are also employed to elicit arguments for behavior change from clients. Miller (1983) originally labeled such arguments *self-motivational statements* to encompass advantages of change, disadvantages of status quo, optimism for, and/or intention, to change. Terminology changed with publication of the second edition of the MI text (Miller & Rollnick, 2002), in which this broad category of speech acts was labeled "change talk." The inability to document hypothesized links between change talk and behavioral outcomes (Miller, Benefield, & Tonigan, 1993; Miller, Yahne, & Tonigan, 2003) prompted psycholinguistic analysis of client speech, the results of which (Amrhein, Miller, Yahne, Palmer, & Fulcher, 2003) led to classification into five categories reflected by the acronym *DARN-C*. The categories were as follows: (1) *Desire* (e.g., "I want to stop drinking"); (2) *Ability* (e.g., "I could stop drinking");

(3) *Reasons* (e.g., "The hangovers just kill me"); (4) *Need* (e.g., "I've got to stop drinking"); and (5) *Commitment* (e.g., "I intend to stop drinking"). Amrhein and colleagues (2003) further provided data in support of a progression within this taxonomy, wherein client statements of desire, ability, reasons, and need for change (e.g., *DARN*) predicted commitment statements (e.g., *C*) which, in turn, predicted behavior change outcomes. This has led the training community to label *DARN* statements as preparatory language (Miller et al., 2006a), in contrast to commitment language. As this work remains in its preliminary stages, there is a need for research to further address the role and nature of client's speech in behavior change

In addition to *OARS* skills, there are supplemental techniques that may also be employed to elicit and reinforce change talk (Miller & Rollnick, 2002). These include:

1. *Asking Evocative Questions:* This simply involves posing direct questions (e.g., "In what ways does your use of _____ concern you?"). Such questions can be influential, and it's important to follow them with subsequent use of *OARS*.

2. *Using Readiness Rulers:* This popular technique involves eliciting paired client ratings, on 1–10 scales, about the importance of change, and confidence in achieving it. Ratings provide segues into how client perceptions might be influenced in either direction.

3. *Exploring Decisional Balance:* This involves prompting a client to discuss positive and negative aspects of substance use, to increase self-disclosure, and clarify ambivalence. Many variants exist, from structured conversation to written pros/cons lists.

4. *Asking for Elaboration:* This asks for expansion of client comments about change or difficulties with the status quo. Through clarification, requesting an example, or simply asking "What else," the practitioner may elicit greater detail about current behavior, and perhaps about the prospect of behavior change.

5. *Querying Extremes:* This involves selectively asking a client to describe best-case and worst-case scenarios of maintaining, or changing, current behavior. Typically, one elicits worst-case scenarios for maintaining behavior, and best-case scenarios for change.

6. *Looking Back:* This perspective-taking approach prompts a client to discuss personal history when substance use was a lesser problem, as a contrast to current circumstances. This often assists in developing discrepancy between client values and behavior.

7. *Looking Forward:* The converse of *looking back*, clients are asked to envision the future in contrast to current circumstances. Picturing continued substance use may prompt client concerns, whereas visualizing change may prompt recognition of resulting benefits.

8. *Exploring Goals/Values:* Inherent in asking clients to discuss goals and values, one assumes clients are motivated by a variety of sources (e.g., aspirations, relationships). The aim is to identify what is important and valued by the individual. Once clear, discrepancies between these and current behavior may be highlighted via *OARS*.

All of the described techniques offer avenues for eliciting client change talk. *OARS* does so by promoting client narrative through effective questions, support for client self-efficacy through affirmation of client qualities, selective reinforcement of change talk through reflections, and clarification of the client perspective through summaries that strategically link client statements. The supplemental techniques may additionally facilitate aspects of client self-disclosure, develop discrepancy between values and behavior, and contribute to assessment of client readiness for change. However, MI spirit and principles should underlie the use of each described skill and/or technique. That is, although the techniques are meant to embody this spirit and these principles, the spirit and principles are not inherent in their use. For example, one might imagine a practitioner effectively eliciting values about being a good parent, but then confronting the client about how drug dependence impedes this relationship. Thus, practitioners must remain mindful that the spirit in which a technique is implemented is as or more important than the technique itself.

Efficacy of MI

As of this writing, we are aware of over 160 published randomized clinical trials (RCTs) of MI, and many more planned or underway. Although initially developed in the treatment of substance users, the crossover of MI to other healthcare domains is considerable. Surveying recent publications, we found MI trials for pregnancy and sexually transmitted disease (Petersen et al., 2007), medication adherence (Golin et al., 2006), nutrition (Ahluwalia et al., 2007), postnatal care (Wilhelm et al., 2006), self-management of chronic illness (Bennett et al., 2007b), and preparation for group psychotherapy (Westra & Dozois, 2006). Consistent with the intent of this text, this discussion focuses on the efficacy of MI in intervening with domains of substance use.

In addition to its application to a range of clinical problems, MI has also been employed in varying intervention formats. For instance, researchers often use MI as a standalone treatment for direct facilitation of behavior change. MET, as implemented in Project MATCH (1997), is an example. But MI can also serve as a prelude to other approaches (e.g., 12-step facilitation, relapse prevention) or treatment-as-usual, with the intent being to facilitate client engagement in such interventions. MI has often been employed in this adjunctive manner, including a recent large, multisite trial (Carroll et al., 2002). MI may also contribute to an integrated treatment approach, promoting greater client-centeredness and reducing resistance to clinical methods such as social skills-training (SST) or cognitive-behavioral therapy (CBT). Descriptions of strategic integration have been offered (Arkowitz & Westra, 2004; Baer et al., 1999; Carroll et al., 2006), although the fidelity of treatment hybrids that may result from such integration has not been well studied.

Differences in intervention format likely beget variability in the type and dose (e.g., number and/or length of clinical sessions) of MI that clients receive. Such variability creates challenges when evaluating efficacy reported in formal trials. In studies to date that have employed standalone or adjunctive formats, client contact is typically limited to a single, 30–60 minute interview (Brown & Miller, 1993; Carroll et al., 2001; Longabaugh et al., 2001; Martino, Carroll, O'Malley, & Rounsaville, 2000; Miller et al., 1993; Saunders, Wilkinson, & Phillips, 1995; Soria, Leguido, Escolano, Lopez-Yeste, & Montoya, 2006). Interestingly, beneficial impacts of MI have been reported at 1-year follow-up for single-session interventions as brief as 15 minutes (Senft, Polen, Freeborn, & Hollis, 1997; Smith et al., 2003). Investigations comparing MI with established, alternative treatments often employ multisession MI interventions (Project MATCH, 1997; UKATT Research Team, 2005) to better account for dose effects. Similarly, efficacy studies wherein MI is integrated with an alternative treatment (e.g., CBT/SST) report a range of 2.5–12 hours of direct client contact (Alwyn, John, Hodgson, & Phillips,

2004; Baker, Boggs, & Lewin, 2001; Baker et al., 2006; Barrowclough et al., 2001; Dennis et al., 2004; Kelly, Halford, & Young, 2000; Morganstern et al., 2007; Reid, Teesson, Sannibale, Matsuda, & Haber,2005). Additional considerations that bear on efficacy of an MI intervention include: the setting and population for whom it is offered, the behavioral target it is intended to address, interventionist(s) background and training, the procedures used to monitor intervention fidelity, the standard of care to which it is compared, the method by which its impact is assessed, and the timeframe of that assessment.

Published reviews of MI efficacy (Burke, Arkowitz, & Dunn, 2002; Burke, Arkowitz, & Menchola, 2003; Dunn et al., 2001; Hettema et al., 2005; Noonan, 1997; Vasilaki, Hosier, & Cox, 2006) have typically restricted their focus to results reported from RCTs. Considered by many a methodological gold standard for evaluating treatment efficacy, RCT designs control for alternative influences (e.g., attention, measurement reactivity, faith/hope effects) that might otherwise account for changes in client functioning. Collectively, recent reviews address the quantification of effect sizes and clinical impact, moderators of efficacy, indicators of fidelity (or lack thereof), and general methodological quality of studies. Here, we offer a summarization of these collective findings with respect to efficacy of individually administered MI interventions targeting behavior change in three domains of substance use: alcohol, illicit drugs, and tobacco.

Alcohol

A review of efficacy studies by Noonan and Moyers (1997) included nine such investigations focused on alcohol use as a behavioral target of MI interventions employed in a range of intervention formats and settings. Collective results supported efficacy of MI on change in alcohol use, albeit with variable effect sizes (0.39–1.06). Dunn and colleagues' subsequent review (2001) included 12 studies and similarly compared effect sizes, as well as other aspects of study methodology. Variable effect sizes were again reported, both proximate to interventions (0.26–0.83) and more distally at 6 months (–0.08–0.45) and 1 year (0.09–0.78) posttreatment. Of note, little attenuation of MI effects was observed over time. The authors indicate a lack of consistent evidence that MI is differentially suited to specific client attributes (e.g., readiness for change, problem severity). A later review by Burke and colleagues (2003) note reliable support for efficacy of MI on change in alcohol use and problems, and estimate its clinical impact as contributing to a 56% reduction in drinking behavior. A need for greater attention to, and reporting of, treatment fidelity among studies is also noted. Still later reviews (Hettema, Steele, & Miller, 2005; Vasilaki et al., 2006) similarly report small-to-medium effect sizes for MI, with some indication of enhanced effects with ethnic minorities. Taken together, there appears to be strong and consistent evidence for efficacy of MI in intervening with drinkers in a variety of settings, intervention formats, and client populations.

Illicit Drugs

Noonan and Moyers' (1997) initially reviewed two studies focused on illicit drug use as a behavioral target for MI interventions, with modest results reported. Dunn and colleagues'

(2001) subsequent review included 6 studies, with variable effect sizes (0.25–0.95) at three months posttreatment. Notably, MI was most effective when used as a precursor to more intensive treatment services for illicit drug users. As with MI interventions targeting alcohol use, there was no evidence of differential effects of MI related to clients' readiness for change. A later review by Burke and colleagues (2003) similarly highlights MI as optimally efficacious as an adjunctive service provided in advance of more intensive treatment, and estimate a large effect size (0.90) on measures of clinical impact (e.g., social, occupational, or physical problems). A subsequent review by Hettema and colleagues (2005) specifies a medium posttreatment effect size (0.51) that attenuates somewhat after a follow-up window of up to one year (0.29). Taken together, the evidence suggests MI is generally effective in intervening with illicit drug users, and may be particularly so when implemented as a prelude to more structured and intensive treatment services.

Tobacco

The conduct and reporting of efficacy trials on use of tobacco was slower to develop than for the alcohol and illicit drugs. Thus, early reviews of MI either omitted tobacco use from consideration (Noonan, 1997), or drew appropriately limited conclusions regarding its efficacy in this substance domain (Burke, Arkowitz, & Dunn, 2002; Dunn et al., 2001). Burke and colleagues (2003) did note that the limited available data were not encouraging, with no significant intervention effects of MI observed in efficacy trials published prior to their review. The more recent review by Hettema and colleagues (2005) indicates only one of six efficacy trials detected a significant impact of MI. Several efficacy trials targeting smoking cessation (Ahluwalia et al., 2006; Borrelli et al., 2005; Horn et al., 2007; Kelly & Lapworth, 2006; Soria et al., 2006) have recently been published, although the collective results appear equivocal. Taken together, the current evidence for MI as means of intervening with tobacco users is weak; however, this may be considered in the context of a larger smoking cessation literature in which utility of individual counseling approaches (Lancaster & Stead, 2005) is variable at best.

A few additional points bear mention. A predominant focus of MI research has been directed to external validity (e.g., can MI be adapted for a given setting/population?) rather than central issues of internal validity (e.g., how and why does MI work?). As noted above, there are now numerous studies applying MI to varied clinical problems and populations. What is notably lacking in the research literature, as indicated by Burke and colleagues (2003), are studies of the content and quality of MI interventions, and relation of these intervention components to clinical outcomes. Furthermore, extant research provides little guidance for using MI in formats that are popular and/or cost-effective in the treatment community. An example is use of group interventions—a format relied on nearly universally for some level of service provision in substance abuse treatment settings—and for which the process of adapting the dyadic style and techniques of MI is unclear. Accordingly, it may come as little surprise that a review by Walters and colleagues (2002) presents discouraging evidence for the efficacy of group-based MI. Clearly, the field would benefit from empirical studies that directly address the internal validity of MI as a behavioral intervention.

The goals of better identifying and describing the processes by which MI works are all the more attainable given treatment integrity systems designed by Moyers and colleagues (2003, 2005a) that quantify MI skill as ratings and behavior tallies. This multivariate quantification of MI has allowed some initial forays into treatment process research in MI, with findings that have contributed to a categorizing client change talk (Amrhein et al., 2003), assessing individual practitioner techniques (Catley & Harris, 2006; Moyers & Martin, 2006), and weighting of the relative value of practitioner style versus technique (Boardman et al., 2006; Moyers et al., 2005b). Although generally supportive of the basic tenants of MI, treatment process research needs to be extended via creative study designs that target, dismantle, or isolate therapeutic elements to determine and describe their impact. Paramount in this process research, in addition to creative study designs, are instruments that allow measurement of therapy process and MI skillfulness.

Measuring MI

Several features of evidenced-based practice are thought to promote better outcomes in substance abuse treatment. Beyond demonstrating treatment effectiveness, evidence can also describe treatment elements and processes. Such data are necessary for testing mechanisms of action and, perhaps more importantly, effective training and implementation in practice settings. Technology models for behavioral intervention (Bellg et al., 2004; Rounsaville et al., 2001) advocate that critical treatment elements be specified, which often occurs in the form of manuals of intervention content, standardized training procedures, assessments to ensure practitioners acquire skills, and regular monitoring of treatment provision to minimize drift over time. Clearly, training and performance-monitoring in research and clinical settings require methods of measuring practitioner skills (Baer et al., 2007; Bellg et al., 2004).

Fortunately, researchers have been active in developing methods to assess MI skills (Madson & Campbell, 2006). As described earlier in the chapter, an overall MI spirit governs the use of core communication skills and strategies for eliciting discussions about change. Notably, MI requires no specific therapeutic tasks (e.g., homework), behavioral goals, in-session exercises, or specific cognitive or emotional insights. Thus, measuring MI necessarily relies on assessing the style and conduct of clinical encounters rather than their content. Colleagues at the University of New Mexico deserve credit for their extensive and ongoing efforts to develop systems for measuring MI, including the Motivational Interviewing Skills Code, or MISC (Miller, 2000; Moyers et al., 2003).

The MISC involves sequential review of a clinical encounter involving three "passes," each designed to reveal unique data. The first MISC pass yields 7-point global ratings of MI-relevant dimensions focused on practitioner, client, and their interaction. The second pass tallies the frequency of 27 practitioner behaviors (some congruent with MI principles, others incongruent) and 4 client behaviors (e.g., statements suggesting favor for, resistance against, or neutrality toward change). The third pass specifies the proportion of time in which the practitioner speaks. Resulting data allow for comparison of practitioner skills against competency standards for a number of summary scores (Miller, 2000), such as the (1) percentage of questions that are "open" (50% or greater), (2) percentage of reflections that are "complex," (40% or greater), (3) ratio of reflections to questions (1:1 or greater), (4) rate of reflections (1/min or greater), and (5) percentage of overall behavior that is MI-consistent (80% or greater). Similar comparison to competency standards is possible for global ratings (score of 5 or greater) as well. There are limitations to the MISC. The competency standards are preliminary, based on coding of expert demonstrations and have modest empirical support (Miller & Mount, 2001). The MISC also requires considerable resources and skill for reliable coding. Moyers and colleagues (2003) report 40+ training hours for raters, after which reliability estimates between raters (e.g., inter-rater reliability) ranged from poor to excellent with more frequent behaviors rated more reliably. Thus, Moyers and colleagues (2003) conclude that a simpler rating system may be useful, and streamlined variants of the MISC have emerged.

Among these are the Motivational Interviewing Treatment Integrity scale (MITI; 2005a) and Motivational Interviewing Supervision and Training Scale (MIST; 2005). These instruments limit focus to practitioner behavior, excluding counts/ratings of client indices and calculation of practitioner talktime. Accordingly, both save time by limiting scoring to fewer passes. Based on factor analysis of a subset of sessions reviewed in MISC development, Moyers and colleagues (Moyers et al., 2005a) reduced the number of global ratings in the MITI to two, and categories of counted behavior to seven. This led to improved reliability of ratings, with 70% of ratings in the excellent range. Moyers and colleagues (2005a) demonstrated the MITI's sensitivity to practitioner training, and its strong correlation with the MISC. Independent psychometric evaluations are additionally encouraging (G. A. Bennett et al., 2007a; Pierson et al., 2007). By comparison, the MIST was developed from reviews of 50 MET sessions. It includes tallying of 9 practitioner behaviors and a more expansive set of 16 MI-relevant dimensions on which 7-point global ratings are derived. Madson and colleagues (2005) report that the MIST can be scored with good reliability among raters, and comparison with a more general rating system provides some initial though modest validity data. Thus, the MITI and MIST are both simplified, less labor-intensive alternatives to the MISC.

Most recently Martino and colleagues (Martino et al., 2008) have developed the Independent Tape Rater Scale (ITRS) adapted from the Yale Adherence Competence Scale (Carroll et al., 2000). The scale includes 30 items, each rated on a 7-point scale, that measure therapeutic dimensions that are MI-consistent, MI-inconsistent, or consistent with alternative counseling approaches. MI-consistent items tap both reflective listening skills and higher order or strategic techniques. Items are rated on two dimensions: "adherence," the extent to which an intervention was delivered, and "competence," the degree of skill with which it was delivered. Analysis of the ITRS, as used by 76 raters in two large multisite trials of MI, suggest excellent internal reliability and strong support for the a priori two-factor structure. The successful use of the ITRS by raters who work in community treatment agencies and who had little prior expertise in MI suggests that it can be used effectively when implementing MI in clinical settings.

As noted earlier in the chapter, interest in adapting MI for health care settings is strong. The brevity of many health care conversations prompted Rollnick and colleagues to adapt MI to an approach termed Behavior Change Counseling (Rollnick et al., 2002, 1999). The Behavior Change Counseling Index (BECCI) consists of 11 items designed to assess practitioner fidelity and rated on 5-point Likert scales. Based on review of simulated interviews, Lane and colleagues (2005) developed items to reflect relevant skills for brief medical consultations (e.g., inviting client to talk, encouraging discussions of change, providing information sensitively). As do prior instruments, the BECCI requires that a rater review a clinical encounter, but scoring takes little additional time to complete. Preliminary inter- and intrarater scoring reliability was adequate, and the scale demonstrated sensitivity to change based on practitioner training. Thus, the BECCI appears a viable alternative to the other coding instruments, and may be particularly useful in assessing practitioner fidelity in settings where clinical encounters are brief.

Recording clinical encounters does present real-world challenges. Fidelity monitoring via regular session recording is a desired standard for clinical practice, yet is rarely achieved. We've speculated previously (Baer et al., 2004) that performance anxiety, perceived threats to confidentiality, cherry-picking of unrepresentative sessions, and faulty equipment limit the viability of such data. For example, Miller and colleagues (2004) struggled to achieve a 50% return rate in their MI training trial. An alternative is to record interactions with standardized patients (SPs), laypersons or actors trained to consistently and realistically portray clients. Use of SPs is beneficial in many ways; they remove concerns about client confidentiality, provide a consistent stimulus, flexibly schedule appointments, and manage recording equipment. Miller and colleagues (Miller & Mount, 2001; Miller et al., 2004) first used SPs in MI training trials, to be followed by others more recently (Bennett et al., 2007a; Pierson et al., 2007). Our own studies (Baer et al., 2004; Hartzler et al., 2007a) use SPs to assess MI skills prior to and following training as well as at a predetermined follow-up point. Although we are encouraged by preliminary evidence that coding of recorded SP encounters is sensitive to change in practitioner skill in our training trials, we also believe more work is needed to document authenticity of SP responses to behavioral interventions like MI.

Although variably labor-intensive, all of the coding systems described to this point require reviews of clinical sessions. Some may reasonably seek less time-consuming alternatives. One brief, paper and pencil method is the Helpful Responses Questionnaire (HRQ) (Miller et al., 1991) which has been used in studies of learning MI (Baer et al., 2004; Rubel et al., 2000). The HRQ consists of six brief clinical scenarios in written form to which respondents are asked to write down "what they would say next." Responses are scored based on degrees of reflective listening, with lowest scores given to "roadblocks" (e.g., responses that raise client defensiveness), better scores given to basic MI techniques (e.g., simple reflections, open questions), and the highest scores given to complex reflections (e.g., accurate reflections that infer added meaning and/or affect). The HRQ should be more narrowly interpreted as a measure of reflective listening, however, it has shown sensitivity to the effects of practitioner training in MI.

In an effort to design a less costly and labor-intensive method of assessing MI skills, we recently developed the Video Assessment of Simulated Encounters (VASE; Rosengren, Baer, Hartzler, Dunn, & Wells, 2005). It consists of three videotaped vignettes of actors portraying substance users, with each vignette broken down into several video clips to which respondents provide written responses akin to the HRQ (e.g., write what you would say next). One advantage of the VASE is its provision of standardized, yet realistic stimuli to which practitioners respond. A second potential advantage is that it is structured for targeted and multivariate assessment of MI skills, with several skill-specific subscales (e.g., responding to resistance). Consequently, the VASE taps several dimensions of MI skill while avoiding the time and resources necessary for recording and review of clinical sessions. Admittedly, further data are needed to validate VASE effectiveness in measuring some dimensions of MI skillfulness. The initial instrument was piloted with a small sample of 22 practitioners (Rosengren et al., 2005), in which it evidenced good interrater reliability and association with other established measures of MI (e.g., HRQ, MISC). Based on these initial findings, we refined the items and subscales, and the resulting instrument is the VASE-Revised or VASE-R (Rosengren et al., 2008).

The described instruments provide a modest set of options. Review and scoring of recorded clinical encounters is a gold standard as means of assessing MI skill, yet is time-consuming and costly. Simpler coding systems (e.g., MITI) are a distinct improvement, and result in more reliable scoring. Video- and computer-based methods of assessment hold promise for the future. And integration of practitioner self-reports with objective assessment methods provide a fuller picture of practitioners' learning processes (Hartzler, Baer, Rosengren, Dunn, & Wells, 2007a; Miller & Mount, 2001). Despite these concerted efforts, there is clearly room to further develop measures of MI skill. For instance, empathy and reflective listening appear well represented in existing instruments; however, Moyers and colleagues (2005a) appropriately note the relatively limited focus that such instruments have in tapping intentional and strategic aspects of MI practice (Martino et al., 2008 is a recent exception). Of additional concern, evidence of instrument validity is often lacking in published efficacy and training trials and thus empirical bases for existing instruments are admittedly thin. Thus, research is needed to estimate associations among existing instruments, as well as between instruments and clinical outcomes.

Learning and Maintenance of MI Skills

Questions remain about how one learns to perform this behavioral intervention, including to what extent MI can be learned, what teaching methods best facilitate learning, and what other considerations might optimize training impact? In this section, we address these primary questions based on the results of published training trials to date, and with reference to a broader dissemination literature and our experiences as facilitators of MI training.

Can MI Skills Be Learned?

Answers to that question are influenced by the skills targeted, the assessment methods, and the timing of the assessment. A review of dissemination practices in substance abuse treatment (Miller et al., 2006b) notes that most training packages are fairly limited in scope and bear little resemblance to what research suggests is effective. A growing MI training literature suggests highly variable acquisition and maintenance of MI skills; this may be the product of many influences including the nature and format in which training occurs. An oft-used vehicle for introduction to MI to practitioners is the two-day workshop, which typically features a blend of didactic, observational, and experiential activities.

One way to evaluate training events is to assess trainee knowledge, specifically trainee familiarity with MI principles and concepts, at their conclusion. Studies often show knowledge acquisition, despite instruction methods as diverse as didactics, video demonstration (Handmaker et al., 1999, 2004), self-instruction (Miller et al., 2004), or distance education (Shafer, Rhode, & Chong, 2004). However, knowledge of MI principles and practices, as well as practitioner reports of their use, are uncorrelated with observable skills (Miller & Mount, 2001; Shafer et al., 2004). This supports Miller and colleagues' (2004) contention that self-instruction (e.g., reading MI text, watching videos) is insufficient to acquire MI skills. However, they also note it may be a precursor to developing behavioral skills. Metaphorically, this has been referred to as the "ground school for flying" (2006b), where foundational concepts are grasped but practitioners are not yet ready to fly without instruction. If the learning goal is to effectively implement MI skills in clinical practice, knowledge-based indices appear insufficient as markers of training success.

Increasingly, training trials employ behavioral tests—recorded encounters with a client or an SP—that document outcomes by requiring that practitioners demonstrate their MI skill in a sample of practice behavior. A two-day training workshop appears to result in immediate skill gains when behavioral tests are used to assess training outcomes. For instance, Miller and colleagues (2001) found probation officers increased MI-consistent behaviors, but failed to suppress MI-inconsistent behaviors after such a workshop. Baer and colleagues (2004) also found postworkshop increases in MI-consistent behaviors among highly educated addiction and mental health practitioners, but less need to eliminate MI-inconsistent behavior. Both studies included an additional assessment after a brief follow-up window (e.g., 2–3 months), and similarly reported deterioration of MI skills to near pretraining levels for many practitioners. Although the collective evidence suggests MI knowledge and skills can be acquired, concern remains about what training methods promote skill maintenance over time.

What Teaching Methods are Best for Learning MI?

Need for greater skill maintenance has led to variation and comparison of training methods. Miller and colleagues (2004) employed an RCT in which a two-day workshop was tested against self-directed methods (e.g., reading, watching videos) as well as two-day workshops with one of three added training components: written feedback on recorded practice sessions, telephone-based coaching with a trainer, or integration of written feedback and phone-based coaching. All practitioners improved over the course of the trial, but those receiving feedback or coaching showed still greater rates of MI proficiency when assessed a year after training. This finding parallels that of a large training trial for CBT (Sholomskas et al., 2005). Thus, it appears that additional training processes (e.g., feedback, coaching) may help to maintain and expand use of MI skills.

Training processes that utilize structured skills-practice and performance-based feedback are being tested. Rollnick and colleagues (2002) advocate *contextualizing* of training: adapting content to the needs of a clinical environment, with structured practice an integral component. Our own ongoing work tests this model, by way of an RCT wherein six community agencies have personnel trained via two-day workshop or Context-Tailored Training (CTT). CTT occurs over nine weeks, with five 3-hour group sessions set at two-week intervals between which personnel conduct skills-practice interviews with an SP and receive trainer and SP feedback. Preliminary data suggest similar skill acquisition and maintenance in CTT and workshop formats, and thus no added benefit from the conduct and feedback from skills-practice interviews. Interestingly, a comparison (2006) of brief training formats (one integrating SP interviews, the other role-plays between practitioners) reported no differential benefit of these skills-practice activities. Clearly, the evidence is mixed as to the added value of skills-practice with SPs and feedback as training processes, and there is much still to learn about practitioners' subjective learning experience, in particular, their receptivity to and understanding of performance-based feedback. These and other findings (Miller et al., 2004; Sholomskas et al., 2005) highlight a need to further explore other processes, such as coaching.

Coaching may take a variety of forms in a clinical setting. Coaches, presumed to have expertise in MI, provide structured guidance to practitioners, although the frequency, mode, and format of such contacts have been variously conceptualized in training trials to date. Miller and colleagues (Miller et al., 2004) defined it as one-to-one activity occurring as a series of up to six, half-hour phone conversations over a four-month period. An innovative and similarly effective extension of this model (Smith et al., 2007) allowed live coaching by teleconference (e.g., "bug in the ear" teleconnection) during clinical sessions. Schoener and colleagues (2006) note that a series of in-person, group coaching sessions after a two-day workshop contributed to broad improvements in use of MI techniques. The UK Alcohol Treatment Trial (Tober et al., 2005; UKATT, 2005), which trained community practitioners to a competence-based criterion, found postworkshop individual coaching (by phone or in person) was critical for practitioners reaching competency, and that it took longer than similar training-to-criterion procedures for an alternative therapy. Other attempts to provide coaching in conjunction with formal training processes have been less successful. Shafer and colleagues (2004) note under-utilized opportunities for coaching in a distance-learning format for training, perhaps due in part to technical and logistical challenges. Forrester and colleagues (2008) also indicate that offers of several no-cost individual coaching contacts after a workshop were met with little interest. Coaching clearly holds potential to influence learning and practice habits, but how to best harness this potential remains an open question.

Technological advances allow introduction of innovative teaching techniques. For instance, Carpenter and colleagues (2003) describe a computer-based MI tutorial that delivers targeted training (e.g., smoking cessation) via interactive multimedia teaching and simulation. Respondents show increased knowledge and more MI-consistent responses to written clinical scenarios after its administration. Others (Villaume, Berger, & Barker, 2006) describe a process for scripting a "virtual client." Learners develop branching components of practitioner–client dialogue, including the generation of both sample client statements and subsequent practitioner responses. This iterative process also resulted in increased knowledge and more MI-consistent responses among learners. Advances in computer and video-based technology will continue to enhance methods of practitioner learning.

What Other Considerations Might Effect Training Impact?

There seem to be other sources of potential influence in practitioner learning and maintenance of skills. For example, it is possible that personal characteristics of learners influence who learns and/or deploys MI more easily. Our prior work, as well as studies by Miller and colleagues (2004), has yielded little beyond the notion that those who enter training with better developed skills seem to benefit more from training (Baer et al., 2004). The relatively small sample sizes in most training trials make evaluation of individual predictors of training impact a difficult challenge. Many colleagues in the training community offer the notion that some persons seem more receptive and better equipped to learn MI than others; however, there is also strong sentiment that poor learning may reflect a mismatch between trainer and learner styles and needs.

Some of our most recent work suggests that learning and maintenance of MI skills may be influenced by whether practitioners view clients from a deficit framework (Miller & Moyers, 2007). Some may ascribe more strongly to ideas that clients are in denial, or that difficulties derive from deficient knowledge, insight, or personal skills. This manner of thinking is fairly common in substance abuse treatment in the United States, no doubt influenced by treatment models that liken misuse of substances to a disease. This view stands in contrast with the principles and spirit of MI that affirms a more strength-based view of clients. Preliminary findings of our ongoing training trial (Hartzler et al., 2006) suggest that practitioners who endorse beliefs congruent with this disease model of addiction acquire MI skills at similar rates as their counterparts, but are less apt to maintain skills over time. This finding may suggest that initial MI skill acquisition occurs at a more superficial, behavioral level, and irrespective of how the conceptual underpinnings of MI fit with personal beliefs about substance use; however, sustained use of MI in the context of daily clinical practice may more rigorously test the goodness-of-fit between these therapeutic concepts and practitioner beliefs, consequently leading some to resume alternative practices congruent with their beliefs. Indeed, practitioner beliefs about the efficacy and validity of any empirically supported intervention might well influence the quality of its implementation.

Qualities of the setting wherein practitioners work also seem a possible influence on the learning and implementation of MI. Increasing attention is now being given to the study of treatment organizations (Simpson, 2002). A recent review of dissemination practices in substance abuse treatment (Miller et al., 2006b) suggests an organization's readiness to support adoption of new practices influences their success with implementation of those practices. Our ongoing work has only just begun to explore aspects of organizations (e.g., staff perceptions of available resources/support, organizational cohesion/stress) that may influence practitioner learning. Given uneven findings reported in training trials to date, it may be fair to speculate that variability observed in training outcomes may be due in part to variance in the work contexts where MI skills are implemented. This area, like others noted previously, merits further research before conclusions are drawn.

As noted earlier, coaching and feedback may be important in maintaining MI skills. In community practice, these forms of support most often are incorporated into an ongoing process of clinical supervision. Due in part to a prevailing supervision model in substance abuse treatment (Powell & Brodsky, 2004) that blends administrative, evaluative, clinical, and support functions, practitioners may hold disparate views of the relative importance of these domains. Kerwin and colleagues (2006) note that historically substance abuse counselors are groomed via apprenticeship in which knowledge and skills are acquired literally on-the-job. This contrasts with most health disciplines, which emphasize structured learning and commitment to adopting and monitoring empirically supported practice. As the demand for effective approaches grows, substance abuse treatment settings face increasing incentives to train (or retrain) personnel and formalize supervision processes to document implementation. This may steer the field away from an apprenticeship model to which some are accustomed and toward practices ascribed by other disciplines. To that end, MI is among the psychosocial interventions that treatment directors and personnel are most ready to adopt (McGovern, Fox, Xie, & Drake, 2004).

A recent review of multisite treatment studies (Baer et al., 2007) distills an emerging set of standards that may serve as a blueprint for effective integration of supervision in community-based settings, namely the monitoring/review of therapeutic sessions, use of established fidelity measures, specification of standards for competence, and provision (and oversight) of support activities for supervisees. With the recent advent of the coding systems outlined earlier in this chapter (Moyers et al., 2003, 2005a) and other available supervision tools (Madson et al., 2005; Martino et al., 2006), MI appears well suited for achieving such aims. Furthermore, available tools have generally been designed to promote their use in monitored practice, feedback, and coaching: all recommended dissemination practices (Miller et al., 2006b). Thus, a basic set of tools appears to be available to community supervisors seeking to monitor practitioner fidelity in the practice of MI.

But formalizing a supervision process invites other challenges. A key consideration is choice of supervisor; that is, what characteristics are desirable? Most agree that proficiency in MI, and supervisory experience, are necessary precursors for effective supervision of MI (Hecht et al., 2005; Miller et al., 2006b). But not all settings have a staffperson who possesses these attributes, and the time/cost of developing them internally may be prohibitive. Furthermore, internal designees may feel ambivalent about the supervisory role, with added responsibility and change in the nature of interpersonal dealings with co-workers. An alternative is to seek fidelity monitoring and coaching externally, such as contracting with a member of the Motivational Interviewing Network of Trainers (MINT; www.motivationalinterview.org). A recent review (Baer et al., 2007) notes considerable variation in the nature of supervisors chosen for controlled trials, with studies often relying on a mix of internal and external resources. Clearly, this arena merits further study to determine optimal supervision practices, as well as consideration of cost-effectiveness for treatment settings.

Beyond choice of supervisor, additional practical challenges are noted by Carroll and colleagues (2002) in their undertaking of a multisite MI effectiveness trial. Many challenges relate to issues of practitioner diversity, in experience and education, interest or motivation, comfort with monitoring procedures, and notably insight into MI skill development and retention. A particular challenge is supervising practitioners whose sense of personal competency exceeds observable skills (e.g., "I'm already doing MI."). Issues of practitioner diversity are exacerbated by staff turnover, a salient obstacle to durable implementation of any new practice (McLellan, 2006). This list of challenges may appear daunting. However, in the spirit of the MI approach we may find a template for addressing many of these obstacles.

A salient issue in supervising practitioners learning a new approach, particularly early on, is how to manage practitioner ambivalence, mixed feelings about having work reviewed and, more generally, the prospect of changing practice behavior. From an MI perspective, supervised practitioners may in this way resemble clients, torn between the safety and security of what is familiar, and the prospect and pressure of trying something new. A suggested approach to teaching MI, and supervision by extension, is to actively model its use in the supervision session (Miller & Rollnick, 2002). So, instead of demanding MI-consistent practice, a supervisor might express empathy for supervisee ambivalence about learning MI, develop discrepancy between supervisees' MI-consistent values and less MI-consistent practice behaviors, roll with supervisee frustration with the awkwardness of trying a novel clinical method, or support supervisee self-efficacy for improving and continued use of MI techniques. Certainly, a supervisor's adherence to MI principles alone may not address all of the aforementioned challenges to effective supervision. But a supervisor guided by these principles and a collaborative, supportive spirit may positively influence the staff they supervise in a number of ways: increasing willingness to try and adopt MI, enhancing comfort with evaluation of their work, improving insight into their own competencies, and perhaps most important, strengthening their commitment to remain in their current post. If one believes a client-centered approach to therapeutic intervention facilitates behavior change in clients, might one reasonably expect a supervisee-centered approach to supervision may assist with adoption and implementation of MI as clinical practice?

Recommendations for Facilitating the Learning of MI

Miller and Moyers (2007) recently offered an intuitively derived, eight-stage model for learning MI. It suggests a sequence of skill areas that a practitioner masters, beginning with central concepts such as MI spirit and use of reflective listening and proceeding through more challenging areas like rolling with resistance, negotiating behavior change plans, and consolidating client commitment. The model provides a framework from which researchers may develop testable hypotheses to confirm, or disconfirm, this suggested sequential learning process. This model is not without some, albeit modest, empirical support. For example, research does suggest that MI spirit is an important predictor of other MI skills (2005b); thus, it may be a logical and appropriate initial focus for learning MI. There is, however, much we still do not know about this learning process. To what extent does it occur in stages, and if so, are stages linked directly to skill areas? In what order do such stages actually occur, and is the progression the same for everyone? Does one need to complete an earlier stage before starting the next? These are all open questions at present, a point Miller and Moyers (2007) readily acknowledge and which leads them to advocate for empirical validation of the proposed model.

We close this section with a brief set of recommendations for learning MI, based on the literature presented and our own collective experiences as researchers, trainers, and clinicians.

- Reading about MI and watching demonstrations of its practice can be valuable as a preliminary step. However, such "book knowledge" of MI is clearly not the same as skillfulness, and may be more useful as a precursor for some learners than others.
- To acquire a set of core MI skills, a minimum of a two-day training workshop is needed. We advocate that training include considerable opportunity for experiential practice of skills. Developing a cognitive framework to understand and direct the use of skills may be beneficial; but to learn to ride a bicycle, one needs to feel the pedals under one's feet.
- Achieving proficiency in use of MI likely requires a combination of additional skills-practice, feedback, and/or coaching for most practitioners. As noted earlier, these can take many different forms, and may be most useful when paired together.
- Skill acquisition and maintenance are related, yet distinct, learning goals. Training workshops that offer additional training processes, like those noted above, and that do so longitudinally seem likely to be more effective in maintaining skills.
- Institutional support may be a necessary condition for skill maintenance. To the extent that a treatment organization actively reminds and reinforces its personnel to use MI, the quality of its implementation should profit and thus benefit practitioners and clients alike.

Looking Forward

This chapter has described MI principles and practices, and reviewed its efficacy in substance abuse treatment, how it is measured, how it may be learned, implemented, and supervised. As an empirically supported behavioral intervention, there is strong support for application of MI in everyday practice. Yet, much is still unknown. Specification of the causal mechanisms by which MI acts remains an area in need of more definitive findings. Conclusive data regarding its mechanisms of action may certainly influence estimates of its efficacy as well as the methods by which MI is measured, learned, implemented, and monitored. We look forward with interest and optimism as the base of evidence for this behavioral intervention further unfolds, and hope to see the following areas addressed by future research.

- MI proposes use of an array of different clinical responses. Are specific clinician responses particularly beneficial or detrimental to engaging clients in change processes? If so, how do we best train clinicians to selectively use the most beneficial responses?
- MI contains both empathic and directive elements. Yet research has yet to demonstrate the relative importance of these two domains. Does MI need to be directive to be effective? If so, what directive elements, used in what ways, toward what goals, are most effective? Can we more effectively assess skills in directive aspects of MI?
- Much of the directive focus in MI involves eliciting and reinforcing change talk, yet data supporting the link between client change talk and eventual behavior change is limited. Is articulation and reinforcement of change talk causative of change, or a reflection of an internal process? Does facilitation of the use of change language alter clinical course?
- The literature on MI training methods is in its infancy, with many questions still to be answered. Does training practitioners to observe client responses lead to changes in practice behavior? If so, does this lead to changes in client behavior? Do practitioners need a "ground school" for learning, or can they simply be taught to perform specific practice behaviors? Are there specific interpersonal skills or styles that make learning MI particularly easy or challenging? Can these differences be effectively utilized in training?
- Advances in technology continue to unfold, and consequently present novel opportunities for training practitioners as well as measuring and monitoring their skills. How can such technologies be best utilized to facilitate dissemination of MI? Are there limits to the simulation or automation of the complex, human process of therapeutic intervention?
- Increasingly, health care organizations are provided incentives to train and monitor use of evidence-based practices by their staff. What motivates organizations to effectively embrace such change? What aspects of organizational climate facilitate adoption of MI? How do organizations monitor staff to ensure maintenance of evidence-based practices?

References

Ahluwalia, J. S., Nollen, N., Kaur, H., James, A. S., Mayo, M. S., & Resnicow, K. (2007). Pathway to health: Cluster-randomized trail to increase fruit and vegetable consumption among smokers in public housing. *Health Psychology, 26*, 214–221.

Ahluwalia, J. S., Okuyemi, K., Nollen, N., Choi, W. S., Kaur, H., Pulvers, K., et al. (2006). The effects of nicotine gum and counseling among African American light smokers: A 2 x 2 factorial design. *Addiction, 101*, 883–891.

Allsop, S. (2007). What is this thing called motivational interviewing? *Addiction, 102*, 343–345.

Alwyn, T., John, B., Hodgson, R. J., & Phillips, C. J. (2004). The addition of a psychological intervention to a home detoxification program. *Alcohol and Alcoholism, 39*, 536–541.

Amrhein, P. C., Miller, W. R., Yahne, C. E., Palmer, M., & Fulcher, L. (2003). Client commitment language during motivational interviewing predicts drug use outcomes. *Journal of Consulting and Clinical Psychology, 71*, 862–878.

Arkowitz, H., & Westra, H. A. (2004). Integrating motivational interviewing and cognitive-behavioral therapy in the treatment of depression and anxiety. *Journal of Cognitive Psychotherapy, 18*, 337–350.

Baer, J. S., Ball, S. A., Campbell, B. K., Miele, G. M., Schoener, E. P., & Tracy, K. (2007). Training and fidelity monitoring of behavioral interventions in multi-site addictions research. *Drug and Alcohol Dependence, 87*, 107–118.

Baer, J. S., Kivlahan, D. R., & Donovan, D. M. (1999). Integrating skills training and motivational therapies: Implications for the treatment of substance dependence. *Journal of Substance Abuse Treatment, 17*, 15–23.

Baer, J. S., Rosengren, D. R., Dunn, C., Wells, E., Ogle, R., & Hartzler, B. (2004). An evaluation of workshop training in motivational interviewing for addiction and mental health clinicians. *Drug and Alcohol Dependence, 73*, 99–106.

Baker, A., Boggs, T. G., & Lewin, T. (2001). Randomized controlled trial of brief cognitive-behavioural interventions among regular users of amphetamine. *Addiction, 96*, 1279–1287.

Baker, A., Bucci, S., Lewin, T., Kay-Lambkin, F., Constable, P. M., & Carr, V. J. (2006). Cognitive-behavioural therapy for substance use disorders in people with psychotic disorders: Randomised controlled trial. *British Journal of Psychiatry, 188*, 439–448.

Barrowclough, C., Haddock, G., Tarrier, N., Lewis, S. W., Moring, J., O'Brien, R., et al. (2001). Randomized controlled trial of motivational interviewing, cognitive behavior therapy, and family intervention for patients with comorbid schizophrenia and substance use disorders. *American Journal of Psychiatry, 158*, 1706–1713.

Bellg, A. J., Borrelli, B., Resnick, B., Hecht, J., Minicucci, D. S., Ory, M., et al. (2004). Enhancing treatment fidelity in health behavior change studies: Best practices and recommendations from the nih behavior change consortium. *Health Psychology, 23*, 443–451.

Bem, D. J. (1972). Self-perception theory. In L. Berkowitz (Ed.), *Advances in experimental social psychology* (Vol. 6, pp. 1–62). New York: Academic Press.

Bennett, G. A., Roberts, H. A., Vaughan, T. E., Gibbons, J. A., & Rouse, L. (2007a). Evaluating a method of assessing competence in motivational interviewing: A study using simulated patients in the united kingdom. *Addictive Behaviors, 32*, 69–79.

Bennett, J. A., Lyons, K. S., Winters-Stone, K., Nail, L. M., & Scherer, J. (2007b). Motivational interviewing to increase physical activity in long-term cancer survivors: A randomized controlled trial. *Nursing Research, 56*, 18–27.

Boardman, T., Catley, D., Grobe, J. E., Little, T. D., & Ahluwalia, J. S. (2006). Using motivational interviewing with smokers: Do therapist behaviors relate to engagement and therapeutic alliance? *Journal of Substance Abuse Treatment, 31*, 329–339.

Borrelli, B., Novak, S., Hecht, J., Emmons, K., Papandonatos, G., & Abrams, D. B. (2005). Home health care nurses as a new channel for smoking cessation treatment: Outcomes from project cares (community-nurse assisted research and education on smoking). *Preventive Medicine, 41*, 815–821.

Brown, J. M., & Miller, W. R. (1993). Impact of motivational interviewing on participation in residential alcoholism treatment. *Psychology of Addictive Behaviors, 7*, 211–218.

Burke, B. L., Arkowitz, H., & Dunn, C. (2002). The efficacy of motivational interviewing. In W. R. Miller & Rollnick, S. (Eds.), *Motivational interviewing: Preparing people for change* (2nd ed., pp. 217–250). New York: Guilford Press.

Burke, B. L., Arkowitz, H., & Menchola, M. (2003). The efficacy of motivational interviewing: A meta-analysis of controlled clinical trials. *Journal of Consulting and Clinical Psychology, 71*, 843–861.

Carpenter, K. M., Watson, J. M., Raffety, B., & Chabal, C. (2003). Teaching brief interventions for smoking cessation via an interactive computer-based tutorial. *Journal of Health Psychology, 8*, 149–160.

Carroll, K. M., Easton, C. J., Nich, C., Hunkele, K. A., Neavins, T. M., Sinha, R., et al. (2006). The use of contingency managment and motivational/skills-building therapy to treat young adults with marijuana dependence. *Journal of Consulting and Clinical Psychology, 74*, 955–966.

Carroll, K. M., Farentinos, C., Ball, S. A., Crits-Christoph, P., Libby, B., Morgenstern, J., et al. (2002). Met meets the real world: Design issues and clinical strategies in the clinical trials network. *Journal of Substance Abuse Treatment, 23*, 73–80.

Carroll, K. M., Libby, B., Sheehan, J., & Hyland, N. (2001). Motivational interviewing to enhance treatment initiation in substance abusers: An effectiveness study. *The American Journal on Addictions, 10*, 335–339.

Carroll, K. M., Nich, C., Sifry, R., Frankforter, T. L., Nuro, K. F., Ball, S. A., et al. (2000). A general system for evaluating therapist adherence and competence in psychotherapy research in the addictions. *Drug and Alcohol Dependence, 57*, 225–238.

Catley, D., & Harris, K. J. (2006). Adherence to principles of motivational interviewing and client within-session behavior. *Behavioural and Cognitive Psychotherapy, 34*, 43–56.

Dennis, M., Godley, S. H., Diamond, G., Tims, F. M., Babor, T., Donaldson, J., et al. (2004). The cannabis youth treatment (cyt) study: Main findings from two randomized trials. *Journal of Substance Abuse Treatment, 27*, 197–213.

DiClemente, C. C. (2003). *Addiction and change: How addictions develop and how addicted people recover.* New York: Guilford Press.

Downey, L., Rosengren, D. B., & Donovan, D. M. (2000). To thine own self be true: Self-concept and motivation for abstinence among substance abusers. *Addictive Behaviors, 25*, 743–757.

Dunn, C., Deroo, L., & Rivara, F. P. (2001). The use of brief interventions adapted from motivational interviewing accross behavioural domains: A systematic review. *Addiction, 96*, 1725–1742.

Forrester, D., McCambridge, J., Waissbein, C., & Rollnick, S. (2008). How do child and family social workers talk to parents about child welfare concerns? *Child Abuse Review, 17*, 23–35.

Golin, C. E., Earp, J., Tien, H. C., Stewart, P., Porter, C., & Howie, L. (2006). A 2-arm, randomized, controlled trial of a motivational interviewing-based intervention to improve adherence to antiretroviral therapy (art) among patients failing or initiating art. *Journal of Acquired Immune Deficiency Syndromes, 42*, 42–51.

Handmaker, N. S., Hester, R. K., & Delaney, H. D. (1999). Videotape training in alcohol counseling for obstetric care practitioners: A randomized control trial. *Obstetrics & Gynecology, 93*, 213–218.

Hartzler, B., Slade, A., Todd, A., Peterson, D. G., Rosengren, D., & Baer, J. S. (2006). Predictors of training impact: The role of disease model beliefs in retention of MI skills among substance abuse treatment staff. *Motivational Interviewing Network of Trainers Bulletin, 13*, 37–38.

Hartzler, B., Baer, J. S., Rosengren, D. B., Dunn, C., & Wells, E. A. (2007a). What is seen through the looking glass: The impact of training on practitioner self-rating of motivational interviewing skills. *Behavioural and Cognitive Psychotherapy, 35*, 431–445.

Hecht, J., Borrelli, B., Breger, R. K. R., DeFrancesco, C., Ernst, D., & Resnicow, K. (2005). Motivational interviewing in community-based research: Experiences from the field. *Annals of Behavioral Medicine, 29*(Special Supplement), 29–34.

Hettema, J., Steele, J., & Miller, W. R. (2005). Motivational interviewing. *Annual Review of Clinical Psychology, 1*, 91–111.

Horn, K., Dino, G., Hamilton, C., & Noerachmanto, N. (2007). Efficacy of an emergency department-based motivational teenage smoking intervention. *Preventing Chronic Disease, 4*, A08.

Kelly, A. B., Halford, W. K., & Young, R. M. (2000). Maritally distressed women with alcohol problems: The impact of a short-term alcohol focused intervention on drinking behavior and marital satisfaction. *Addiction, 95*, 1537–1549.

Kelly, A. B., & Lapworth, K. (2006). The hyp program-targeted motivational interviewing for adolescent violations of school tobacco policy. *Preventive Medicine, 43*, 466–471.

Kerwin, M. E., Walker-Smith, K., & Kirby, K. C. (2006). Comparative analysis of state requirements for the training of substance abuse and mental health counselors. *Journal of Substance Abuse Treatment, 30*, 173–181.

Lamb, S., Greenlick, M. R., & McCarty, D. (1998). *Bridging the gap between practice and research: Forging partnerships with community-based drug and alcohol treatment.* Washington, DC: National Academy Press.

Lancaster, T., & Stead, L. F. (2005). Individual behavioural counselling for smoking cessation. In *Cochrane database of systematic reviews* (Vol. 2, CD001292): John Wiley & Sons.

Lane, C., Huws-Thomas, M., Hood, K., Rollnick, S., Edwards, K., & Robling, M. (2005). Measuring adaptations of motivational interviewing: The development and validation of the behavior change counseling index (becci). *Patient Education and Counseling, 56*, 166–173.

Leake, G. J., & King, A. S. (1977). Effect of counselor expectations on alcoholic recovery. *Alcohol, Health, and Research World, 11*, 16–22.

Leffingwell, T. R., Neumann, C. A., Babitzke, A. C., Leedy, M. J., & Walters, S. T. (2007). Social psychology and motivational interviewing: A review of relevant principles and recommendations for research and practice. *Behavioral and Cognitive Psychotherapy, 35*, 31–45.

Longabaugh, R., Woolard, R. F., Nirenberg, T. D. Minugh, A. P., Becker, B., Clifford, P. R., & et al. (2001). Evaluating the effects of a brief motivational intervention for injured drinkers in the emergency department. *Journal of Studies on Alcohol, 62*, 806–816.

Madson, M. B., & Campbell, T. C. (2006). Measures of fidelity in motivational enhancement: A systematic review. *Journal of Substance Abuse Treatment, 31*, 67–73.

Madson, M. B., Campbell, T. C., Barrett, D. E., Brondino, M. J., & Melchert, T. P. (2005). Development of the motivational interviewing supervision and training scale. *Psychology of Addictive Behaviors, 19*, 303–310.

Markland, D. A., Ryan, R. M., Tobin, V. J., & Rollnick, S. (2005). Motivational interviewing and self-determination theory. *Journal of Social and Clinical Psychology, 24*, 811–831.

Martino, S., Ball, S. A., Gallon, S. L., Hall, D., Garcia, M., Ceperich, S., et al. (2006). *Motivational interviewing assessment: Supervisory tools for enhancing proficiency (mia:Step)*. Salem, OR: Northwest Frontier Addiction Technology Transfer Center, Oregon Health Sciences University.

Martino, S., Ball, S. A., Nich, C., Frankforter, T. L., & Carroll, K. M. (2008). Community program therapist adherence and competence in motivational enhancement therapy. *Drug and Alcohol Dependence, 96*, 37–48.

Martino, S., Carroll, K. M., O'Malley, S. S., & Rounsaville, B. J. (2000). Motivational interviewing with psychiatrically ill substance abusing patients. *American Journal of Addictions, 9*, 88–91.

McGovern, M. P., Fox, T. S., Xie, H., & Drake, R. E. (2004). A survey of clinical practices and readiness to adopt evidence-based practicies: Dissemination research in an addiction treatment system. *Journal of Substance Abuse Treatment, 26*, 305–312.

McLellan, A. T. (2006). What we need is a system: Creating a responsive and effective substance abuse treatment system. In W. R. Miller & K. Carroll (Eds.), *Re-thinking substance abuse: What the science shows, and what we should do about it* (pp. 275–292). New York: Guilford Press.

Miller, W. R. (1983). Motivational interviewing with problem drinkers. *Behavioral Psychotherapy, 11*, 147–172.

Miller, W. R. (2000). *Motivational interviewing skill code: Coders manual*. University of New Mexico Center on Alcoholism Substance Abuse, and Addictions website: http://casaa-0031.unm/edu/.

Miller, W. R., Benefield, R. G., & Tonigan, J. S. (1993). Enhancing motivation for change in problem drinking: A controlled comparison of two therapist styles. *Journal of Consulting and Clinical Psychology, 61*, 455–461.

Miller, W. R., Hedrick, K. E., & Orlofsky, D. (1991). The helpful responses questionnaire: A procedure for measuring therapeutic empathy. *Journal of Clinical Psychology, 47*, 444–448.

Miller, W. R., & Mount, K. A. (2001). A small study of training in motivational interviewing: Does one workshop change clinician and client behavior? *Behavioural and Cognitive Psychotherapy, 29*, 457–471.

Miller, W. R., & Moyers, T. (2007). Eight stages in learning motivational interviewing. *Journal of Teaching the Addictions, 5*, 3–17.

Miller, W. R., Moyers, T., Amrhein, P. C., & Rollnick, S. (2006a). A consensus statement on defining change talk. *MINT Bulletin, 13*, 6–8.

Miller, W. R., & Rollnick, S. (1991). *Motivational interviewing: Preparing people to change addictive behavior*. New York: Guilford Press.

Miller, W. R., & Rollnick, S. (2002). *Motivational interviewing: Preparing people for change* (2nd ed.). New York: Guilford Press.

Miller, W. R., Sorensen, J. L., Selzer, J. A., & Brigham, G. S. (2006b). Disseminating evidence-based practices in substance abuse treatment: A review with suggestions. *Journal of Substance Abuse Treatment, 31*, 25–39.

Miller, W. R., Yahne, C., & Tonigan, J. S. (2003). Motivational interviewing in drug abuse services: A randomized trial. *Journal of Consulting and Clinical Psychology, 71*, 754–763.

Miller, W. R., Yahne, C. E., Moyers, T. B., Martinez, J., & Pirritano, M. (2004). A randomized trial of methods to help clinicians learn motivational interviewing. *Journal of Counseling and Clinical Psychology, 72*, 1050–1062.

Morganstern, J., Irwin, T. W., Wainberg, M. L., Parsons, J. T., Muench, F., Bux, D. A., et al. (2007). A randomized controlled trial of goal choice interventions for alcohol use disorders among mena who have sex with men. *Journal of Consulting and Clinical Psychology, 75*, 72–84.

Mounsey, A. L., Bovbjerg, V., White, L., & Gazewood, J. (2006). Do students develop better motivational interviewing skills through role-play with standardised patients or with student colleagues? *Medical Education, 40*, 775–780.

Moyers, T. B., & Martin, T. (2006). Therapist influence on client language during motivational interviewing sessions. *Journal of Substance Abuse Treatment, 30*, 245–251.

Moyers, T. B., Martin, T., Catley, D., Harris, K. J., & Ahluwalia, J. S. (2003). Assessing the integrity of motivational interviewing interventions: Reliability of the motivational interviewing skills code. *Behavioural and Cognitive Psychotherapy, 31*, 177–184.

Moyers, T. B., Martin, T., Manuel, J. K., Hendrickson, S. M. L., & Miller, W. R. (2005a). Assessing competence in the use of motivational interviewing. *Journal of Substance Abuse Treatment, 28*, 19–26.

Moyers, T. B., Miller, W. R., & Hendrickson, S. M. L. (2005b). How does motivational interviewing work? Therapist interpersonal skill predicts client involvement within motivational interviewing sessions. *Journal of Consulting and Clinical Psychology of Addictive Behaviors, 73*, 590–598.

NIDA. (1999). Principles of drug addiction treatment: A research-based guide. *#99–4180.*

Noonan, W., & Moyers, T. (1997). Motivational interviewing: A review. *Journal of Substance Misuse, 2*, 8–16.

Petersen, R., Albright, J., Garrett, J. M., & Curtis, K. M. (2007). Pregnancy and std prevention counseling using an adaptation of motivational interviewing: A randomized controlled trial. *Perspective on Sex and Reproductive Health, 39*, 21–28.

Pierson, H. M., Hayes, S. C., Gifford, E. V., Roget, N., Padilla, M., Bissett, R., et al. (2007). An examination of the motivational interviewing treatment integrity code. *Journal of Substance Abuse Treatment, 32*, 11–17.

Powell, D. J., & Brodsky, A. (2004). *Clinical supervision in alcohol and drug abuse counseling.* San Francisco, CA: Jossey-Bass.

Project MATCH. (1997). Matching alcoholism treatments to client heterogeneity: Project match post-treatment drinking outcomes. *Journal of Studies on Alcohol, 58*, 7–29.

Reid, S. C., Teesson, M., Sannibale, C., Matsuda, M., & Haber, P. S. (2005). The efficacy of compliance therapy in pharmacotherapy for alcohol dependence: A randomized controlled trial. *Journal of Studies on Alcohol, 66*, 833–841.

Rogers, C. R. (1959). A theory of therapy, personality, and interpersonal relationships as developed in a client-centered framework. In P. Koch (Ed.), *The study of a science* (Vol. 3, pp. 184–256). New York: McGraw-Hill.

Rogers, E. M. (2003). *Diffusion of innovations.* (Vol. 5). New York: Free Press.

Rollnick, S., Kinnersley, P., & Butler, C. (2002). Context-bound communication skills training: Development of a new method. *Medical Education, 36*, 377–383.

Rollnick, S., Mason, P., & Butler, C. (1999). *Health behavior change: A guide for practitioners.* London: Churchill Livingstone.

Rollnick, S., & Miller, W. R. (1995). What is motivational interviewing? *Behavioral and Cognitive Psychotherapy, 23*, 325–334.

Rosengren, D. B., Baer, J. S., Hartzler, B., Dunn, C., & Wells, E. (2005). The video assessment of simulated encounters (vase): Development and validation of a group-administered method for evaluating clinician skills in motivational interviewing. *Drug and Alcohol Dependence, 79*, 321–330.

Rosengren, D. B., Hartzler, B., Baer, J. S., Wells, E. A., & Dunn, C. W. (2008). The video assessment of simulated encounters-revised (vase-r): Reliability and validity of a revised measure of motivational interviewing skills. *Drug and Alcohol Dependence, 97*, 130–138.

Rounsaville, B. J., Carroll, K. M., & Onken, L. S. (2001). A stage model of behavioral therapies research: Getting started and moving on from stage i. *Clinical Psychology: Science and Practice, 8*, 133–142.

Rubel, E., Shepell, W., Sobell, L., & Miller, W. (2000). Do continuing education workshops improve participants' skills? Effects of a motivational interviewing workshop on substance-abuse counselor's skills and knowledge. *Behavior Therapist, 23,* 73–77.

Saunders, B., Wilkinson, C., & Phillips, M. (1995). The impact of a brief motivational intervention with opiate users attending a methadone programme. *Addiction, 90,* 415–424.

Schoener, E. P., Madeja, C. L., Henderson, M. J., Ondersma, S. J., & Janisse, J. J. (2006). Effects of motivational interviewing training on mental health therapist behavior. *Drug and Alcohol Dependence, 82,* 269–275.

Senft, R. A., Polen, M. R., Freeborn, D. K., & Hollis, J. F. (1997). Brief intervention in a primary care setting for hazardous drinkers. *American Journal of Preventive Medicine, 13,* 464–470.

Shafer, M. S., Rhode, R., & Chong, J. (2004). Using distance education to promote the transfer of motivational interviewing skills among behavioral health professionals. *Journal of Substance Abuse Treatment, 26,* 141–148.

Sholomskas, D. E., Syracuse-Siewert, G., Rounsaville, B. J., Ball, S. A., Nuro, K. F., & Carroll, K. M. (2005). We don't train in vain: A dissemination trial of three strategies of training clinicians in cognitive-behavioral therapy. *Journal of Consulting and Clinical Psychology, 73,* 106–115.

Simpson, D. D. (2002). A conceptual framework for transferring research to practice. *Journal of Substance Abuse Treatment, 22,* 171–182.

Smith, A. J., Hodgson, R. J., Bridgeman, K., & et.al. (2003). A randomized controlled trial of a brief intervention after alcohol-related facial injury. *Addiction, 98,* 43–52.

Smith, J. L., Amrhein, P. C., Brooks, A. C., Carpenter, K. M., Levin, D., Schreiber, E. A., et al. (2007). Providing live supervision via teleconferencing improves acquisition of motivational interviewing skills after workshop attendance. *The American Journal of Drug and Alcohol Abuse, 33,* 163–168.

Soria, R., Leguido, A., Escolano, C., Lopez-Yeste, A., & Montoya, J. (2006). A randomized controlled trial of motivational interviewing for smoking cessation. *British Journal of General Practice, 56,* 768–774.

Tober, G., Godfrey, C., Parrott, S., & et al. (2005). Setting standards for training and competence: The UK alcohol treatment trial. *Alcohol and Alcoholism, 40,* 413–418.

UK Alcohol Treatment Trial (UKATT) Research Team. (2005). Effectiveness of treatment for alcohol problems: Findings of the randomized UK alcohol treatment trial (UKATT). *British Medical Journal, 331,* 541.

Vasilaki, E. I., Hosier, S. G., & Cox, W. M. (2006). The efficacy of motivational interviewing as a brief intervention for excessive drinking: A meta-analytic review. *Alcohol & Alcoholism, 41,* 328–335.

Villaume, W. A., Berger, B. A., & Barker, B. N. (2006). Learning motivational interviewing: Scripting a virtual patient. *American Journal of Pharmacy Education, 70,* 33.

Voss, J. D., & Wolf, A. M. (2004). Teaching motivational interviewing in chronic care: A workshop approach. *Journal of General Internal Medicine, 19,* 213.

Wagner, C. C., & Sanchez, F. P. (2002). The role of values in motivational interviewing. In W. R. Miller & S. Rollnick (Eds.), *Motivational interviewing: Preparing people for change* (2nd ed., pp. 284–298). New York: Guilford Press.

Walters, S. T., Ogle, R., & Martin, J. E. (2002). Perils and possibilities of group-based motivational interviewing. In W. R. Miller & S. Rollnick (Eds.), *Motivational interviewing: Preparing people for change.* (2nd ed., pp. 377–390). New York: Guilford Press.

Westra, H. A., & Dozois, D. J. A. (2006). Preparing clients for cognitive behavioral therapy: A randomized pilot study of motivational interviewing for anxiety. *Cognitive Therapy and Research., 30,* 481–498.

Wilhelm, S. L., Stepans, M. B., Hertzog, M., Rodehorst, T. K., & Gardner, P. (2006). Motivational interviewing to promote sustained breastfeeding. *Journal of Obstetric, Gynecological, & Neonatal Nursing, 35,* 340–348.

27

Faith-Based Approaches

Thomas J. Johnson and Patrick R. Bennett
Indiana State University

Contents

Religion & Spirituality

Definitions

Religion is often thought of as an organized social system of beliefs and practices, whereas spirituality refers to individuals' unique, subjective existential concerns, sense of meaning, and/ or transcendent or mystical experiences (Miller, 1998; Pargament, 1997). Both religion and spirituality involve a connection with the transcendent, something larger and more important than the individual and potentially considered sacred or divine. R/S are multidimensional phenomena including public and private practices, experiences (e.g., mystical experiences, connection to God and others, inner peace, etc.), beliefs (e.g., specific creeds, belief in angels or demons, concepts of God as loving or punitive, etc.), R/S coping and support, R/S struggles or distress, and other concepts (Hill, 2005).

Positive and Negative Religious Coping

Religious coping practices have both positive and negative effects. Positive religious coping includes forgiveness, seeking support from clergy or congregation members, active surrender, and benevolent religious reappraisal (e.g., viewing negative events as a lesson from God, etc.; Pargament, Ano, & Wachholtz, 2005). Negative religious coping includes passive deferral to God, pleading for direct intercession, and appraising negative events as demonic action or punishment from God (Pargament et al., 2005). Ano and Vasconcelles' (2005) meta-analysis confirmed that use of positive religious coping strategies was significantly related to better psychological outcomes when dealing with stressful situations, whereas negative religious coping strategies were significantly related to increased negative outcomes. Reviewing the religion and coping research, Pargament (2002) concluded: "a religion that is internalized, intrinsically motivated, and built on a belief in a great meaning in life, a secure relationship with God, and a sense of spiritual connectedness with others has positive implications for well-being. Conversely, a religion that is imposed, unexamined, and reflective of a tenuous relationship with God and the world bodes poorly for well-being" (p. 177).

American Religious Landscape

The most common faith groups in the United States are Christianity (approximately 80% of the U.S. population), Judaism (1%), Islam (.5%), and Buddhism (.5%). Atheists and agnostics make up around 3% of the population and 10% give no specific religious preference (source for all statistics: Adherents.com). The largest Christian denomination is the Roman Catholic Church, followed by the Southern Baptist Convention, United Methodist Church, and the Church of Jesus Christ of Latter Day Saints (Mormon).

"Main-Line" protestant denominations generally arose between the Reformation and the early nineteenth century. Examples include the Episcopal Church, Evangelical Lutheran Church in America, Presbyterian Church (USA), and the United Methodist Church (Wuthnow & Evans, 2002). Members tend to view the Bible as inspired, but not literally true, and to see other faiths as containing at least some religious truths (Wuthnow & Evans, 2002). Several different, but overlapping conservative Protestant groups can also be identified, most stressing the importance of a "born again" experience. Fundamentalist Christians claim that the Bible is free from factual errors. Evangelicals are not as focused on doctrine as fundamentalists and place more emphasis on winning converts (Wolfe, 2003). Pentecostals emphasize emotional worship that may involve participants speaking in tongues or believing they have healing powers (Wolfe, 2003).

In the United States, different faith traditions have different norms and values regarding alcohol and other drugs, as well as different rates of abstinence and dependence (Booth & Martin, 1998). Jewish Americans often report lower rates of alcohol dependence than the general population (Vex & Blume, 2001). Among Jews, the cultural stereotype that only non-Jews have drinking problems has been perceived as a barrier to recovery (Spiegel & Kravitz, 2001). Similar stigmas may be present among Muslims (Suliman, 1983) and Evangelical Christians (Stoltzfus, 2006) and also interfere with members of these groups seeking help. Relative to the general population, both rates of abstinence from alcohol and rates of problematic alcohol use are higher among members of some faiths that ban all alcohol use (Booth & Martin, 1998). This could be due to guilt over drinking, lack of social norms for moderate drinking (Rivers, 1994), or punishing reactions to drinking from members of the denomination (Booth & Martin).

Defining Faith-Based (FB) Approaches

We distinguish between faith-based organizations (FBOs) and FB treatments or interventions. Both concepts are helpful to understand the full spectrum of FB approaches to addiction.

FBOs

Several recent books on FBOs devote entire chapters to the topic of definition (Kennedy & Bielefeld, 2006; Unruh & Sider, 2005). Their reviews suggest great diversity among FBOs in the degree to which their organizational structure (e.g., whether staff assignments are based on religious criteria, use of prayer or religious literature to guide organizational decisions, etc.)

and the services they offer are guided by religion, as well as the degree of visible (e.g., clients required to participate in religious activities or make religious commitments, etc.) and implicit (e.g., presence of religious symbols in the facility, etc.) religiousness present in the organization. Wuthnow (2004) noted that some organizations, such as the YMCA, originally included strong religious components, but have become largely secular in their activities. Other groups, such as Catholic Charities, Lutheran Social Services, and Jewish Family Services, are "separately incorporated non-profit charitable organizations" (Kennedy & Bielefeld, 2003, p. 14). Such diversity in organizational structure, services offered, and the degree to which R/S are integrated into FBOs makes it difficult to conduct research on FB programs and/or to make general statements about FBOs and faith-based treatment (FBT). Wuthnow (2004) estimated that there are about 6,500 FB nonprofit human services organizations in the United States. This figure would not include for-profit providers that self-identify as FB, nor would it include programs offered by local congregations. There are more than 330,000 congregations in the United States (Hadaway & Marler, 2005), including approximately 75,000 local congregations in the six largest "main-line" Protestant denominations (Wuthnow, 2002). Cnaan (2002) surveyed nearly 300 congregations in the United States and Canada, and reported that 90% offered some form of social or human service program.

Between FB human service providers and congregations, there are literally thousands of FB groups offering social services. However, there is little information on the number of programs addressing addiction issues. Dominguez, Ip, Hoover, Oleari, McMinn, Lee et al., (2005) reported that only 10% of 141 Christian clergy they surveyed had some form of addiction support program within their church.

FBTs

The most obvious definition of a FB treatment would be one provided by a FBO. However, given the variation in how much R/S inform the activities of FBOs, this is too simple a solution. Studies of FB nonprofits typically find that one fourth or less of such organizations indicate that religion is a primary element in all their activities and services (Wuthnow, 2004). Neff, Shorkey, and Windsor (2006) noted that identifying a treatment as FB may be more complicated in the addiction field than in other areas due to the pervasiveness of spiritually based 12-step approaches in the United States. We define FB treatments as approaches where both the conceptual model underlying treatment and at least some of the specific interventions employed derive from a particular religious or spiritual tradition. By our definition, 12-step-based programs are FBTs. Various forms of meditation have been studied as treatments for addiction, but the conceptual model used to explain their effects is typically psychological or physiological rather than religious or spiritual.

Most studies of FBT for addiction identify programs as FB based on self-identification by the provider. FBT programs are diverse in their balance between R/S and secular elements, sources of funding, and additional programs offered. For example, Dominguez and colleagues (2006) conducted interviews with staff from 15 (out of an initial pool of 97) FB addiction treatment centers in northern Illinois. They identified three categories of programs: those emphasizing faith as the primary element of treatment ($N = 3$), those following a mental health model ($N = 6$), and those that had a mixed emphasis on faith and mental health interventions ($N = 6$). Most of the programs in all three categories also emphasized helping clients meet basic needs (e.g., education, job placement, housing, etc.). The programs that included a faith emphasis were Christian in their orientation and faith development was a major goal of treatment. Those with a mental health orientation included both Christian programs that disavowed evangelism as a goal and programs based on a more generic spiritual model such as that found in 12-step programs. Dominguez et al. also noted that some programs with a faith emphasis are opposed to clients using psychotropic drugs to treat co-morbid mental health problems.

Neff et al. (2006) found that the FB and traditional addiction treatment programs they studied shared common features, such as an empathic climate, elements to promote engagement with treatment, and role modeling and support. However, FB programs were also more likely to emphasize spiritual activities and beliefs, structure and discipline, and readiness for work.

Why Practitioners should know about FB Approaches

Surveys typically show that 90% or more of the U.S. population believe in God and over 60% belong to a church and consider religion important in their lives, but only 30–50% of psychotherapists belong to a theistic religion (Richards & Bergin, 2005). Despite this gap, codes of ethics for health professionals in various specialties require respect for and sensitivity to clients' R/S beliefs and practices (Richards & Bergin). This might include helping a client locate a treatment program, social support system, or social services consistent with his or her faith. However, ethical principles preclude attempting to convert a client into a particular faith. Given the emphasis on conversion in many FB programs, knowledge about a range of FB and non-FB options for treatment, aftercare, and support is crucial for ethical practice. For example, some Evangelical Christian or Jewish clients may be uncomfortable with traditional 12-step groups. In both cases, religiously sensitive programs may be available.

Although 94% of Christian, Jewish, and Muslim clergy surveyed by the National Center on Addiction and Substance Abuse felt that addiction issues were important in their congregations, only 12.5% had any training on addictions while studying to be a member of the clergy (CASA, 2001). Thus, addiction professionals could potentially play a valuable role in consulting with and being a resource for clergy, congregations, and FB programs.

The past two decades have also seen a growing emphasis on evidence-based practice. Professionals need to be aware of the current status of the evidence regarding FB approaches and relationships between R/S and addiction. In addition, aspects of a client's beliefs or practices may at times be self-defeating or dangerous (Johnson, Ridley, & Nielsen, 2000; Richards & Bergin, 2005). In such cases the professional's task is to attempt to address the "toxic" portions of the client's R/S system without dismantling the entire structure. Although a full discussion of such issues is beyond the scope for this chapter (see Miller, 2003; Pargament, 2007; Richards & Bergin, 2005, etc.), the information presented here may help addiction professionals be better prepared to address these complex ethical and practice issues.

Examples of a Spectrum of FB Approaches to Addiction Treatment

It is impossible to offer a comprehensive list of all FBTs. However, we briefly describe several FBTs and list additional examples.

Twelve-step-based Mutual Help Groups and Treatments

Alcoholics Anonymous (AA) and other 12-step group programs are considered to be mutual help programs rather than formal treatment, in that members share experiences, aid, and support with other members. However, the Minnesota Model (MM) and Twelve-Step Facilitation therapy (TSF) utilize 12-step principles and could thus be considered FBTs that could be offered by either FB or secular organizations.

AA had its origins in the conservative Evangelical Christian Oxford Group movement of the early twentieth century (Mercadante, 1996; Kurtz, 1979). The original AA members kept the Oxford Group emphasis on conversion and group support, but rejected what they felt was perfectionism and absolutism in that movement in favor of a more personal spirituality, "God as we understood him" (Nelson, 2004). Many of AA's founders criticized organized religion as divisive, rigid, perfectionistic, moralistic, and judgmental (Nelson, 2004). Nonetheless, both Christian (Baker, 2004) and non-Christian (Imani, 1992; Olitzky & Copans, 1991) groups have adopted and adapted the 12-step approach by putting religious elements back into their programs (e.g., some Christians refer to Jesus Christ instead of a higher power). Christian groups derived from the 12-step approach include Celebrate Recovery, Overcomers Outreach, and Alcoholics Victorious. Jewish Alcoholics, Chemically Dependent Persons, and Significant Others (JACS), a program of the Jewish Board of Family and Child Services, provides resources for Jewish addicts and their families, supports Jews in recovery, and promotes understanding of addiction within the Jewish community. Millati Islami has adapted the 12-steps for Muslims. The Faces and Voices of Recovery website maintains a list of secular and FB mutual help programs (http://www.facesandvoicesofrecovery.org/resources/support_groups.php#mi) with descriptions of each, recommendations for whom to refer to which program, and web addresses when available.

Members of 12-step programs, "work the steps," which include admitting powerlessness over their addiction, seeking help from a higher power, reflecting on their moral failures and attempting to make amends, and carrying the message to others in need. Step work is intended to produce a gradual or sudden spiritual awakening, essentially a conversion experience.

The core literature on AA does not identify addiction as a disease (Miller, 1998), but the MM does endorse the disease concept. The MM developed in the 1940s and 1950s and is thought to be the model used at most addiction treatment facilities in the United States. According to Cook (1988a), the key concepts underlying the MM are: (1) change is possible; (2) addiction is a disease; (3) treatment goals are abstinence and "improvement of lifestyle" (p. 626); and (4) 12-step principles form the core of treatment. Treatment includes various forms of group therapy and discussion, educational lectures and activities about

12-step and disease model concepts, 12-step group participation, and step work (Cook, 1988a; Stinchfield & Owen, 1998).

TSF, one of the manualized treatment approaches evaluated in Project MATCH, includes activities and interventions designed to help a client get involved in a 12-step program and begin to work the steps (Nowinski, Baker, & Carroll, 1992). Clients do 12-step readings and homework and are expected to attend 12-step group meetings. The client is instructed that addiction is a chronic and progressive disease, characterized by denial. A full discussion of the controversy regarding the validity of the disease model of addiction is not possible here, but see Thombs (1999) and Nelson (2004) for two different views.

Salvation Army Programs

William Booth founded the Salvation Army in England during the 1880s out of his concern for the poor. Historically, the Salvation Army has offered a number of programs that address addiction and other social problems. Katz (1964) estimated that by 1961, it is likely that more individuals were being treated annually for alcoholism in Salvation Army Men's Social Service Centers than in all of the outpatient clinics in the United States.

Salvation Army programs attempted to provide comprehensive services from an early date. Treatment at the 119 centers reported on by Katz (1964) always included spiritual counseling, religious services, recreational and work opportunities, and usually regular medical treatment. In addition, many centers offered group and/or individual psychotherapy, A.A. meetings, bible study, and educational lectures or films. Facilities usually had physicians on staff, and some also included psychologists, psychiatrists, and/or social workers. By the 1970s centers had begun to provide detoxification services and to employ a larger number of professional staff (Judge, 1971). Currently Salvation Army Adult Recovery Centers across the United States are residential programs providing Christian worship services and education, individual and group therapy, 12-step group participation and self-study, medical services, recreational and work activities, G.E.D. classes, and various other educational programs.

Teen Challenge

Teen Challenge was started in 1958 by David Wilkerson, a Pentecostal minister who wanted to provide a safe loving home for the gang members he was ministering to in New York City. The first treatment center opened in 1960, and the program now includes nearly 200 centers in the United States and more than 500 worldwide. The original treatment program consisted of several months at an Induction Center (Phase 1), typically located in an urban area, followed by 6–9 months at a Training Center located in a rural area (Phase 2). The full program was approximately one year long and involved bible study, religious education and activities, and involvement in work. The original Training Center in Pennsylvania was in fact a working farm, run by the "students," as program participants were called. More information about the origins and program can be found in Glasscote et al. (1972), Wilkerson (1986), and from the Teen Challenge website (www.teenchallengeusa.com). Curricula currently used in the residential program include workbooks for group study that focus on aspects of Evangelical and Pentecostal Christian faith (with titles such as: "How Can I Know I'm a Christian?," "Obedience to God," "Obedience to Man," "Christian Practices," and "Spiritual Power and the Supernatural") and more general life skills (also from a Christian perspective) such as developing relationships with others, dealing with anger, forgiveness, dealing with boredom, and self-acceptance.

Although the name Teen Challenge has been retained and some residential programs for youth still exist (Youth Challenge & Teen Challenge Christian Academy), the residential programs now primarily house adults. Most are for men, but there are also programs for women. In addition to the residential treatment facilities, Teen Challenge Centers may offer additional programs such as outpatient and prevention services, crisis hotlines, support groups, programs for at-risk children, GED training, and vocational and job skills training. Teen Challenge does not directly receive federal funds, but residents may get food stamps and some Teen Challenge centers are accepting vouchers as part of the Access to Recovery program (see below).

Other Programs

Spiritual Self-Schema therapy (3-S; Avants & Margolin, 2004) is based on both social cognitive theory and Buddhist concepts, and thus only partially meets our definition of a FBT. A manualized treatment suitable for persons of all faiths, 3-S attempts deactivate clients' view of self as an addict and activate their view of self as a spiritual being.

FB programs are seen as significant resources within minority communities (Irwin, 2002; Wolfe, 2003). Black churches have historically been a source of support and a place where African Americans could exercise power and control denied them in the larger society (Poole, 1990). The Abyssinian Baptist Church in Harlem has offered social programs since its inception in 1923, and in 1993 began a FB community mentoring program aimed at reducing delinquency and drug use in youth by providing positive mentoring, role modeling, and Afro-centric rites of passage (Irwin). A variety of FB addiction programs continue to be available in African-American communities nationwide, including programs that also include services aimed at reducing HIV risk (Collins, Whiters, & Braithwaite, 2007; MacMaster et al., 2007). In addition, despite the lack of training in addictions common to many clergy, Black pastors are sought out for help with addiction problems by members of their congregations and communities (Sexton, Carlson, Siegal, Leukefeld, & Booth, 2006). McNeese and DiNitto (2005) provide descriptions of a number of prevention and treatment programs that attempt to integrate Native American spirituality to better address needs of Native Americans and Alaska Natives. FB programs have also developed in many Hispanic communities (Ringwald, 2002; Wolfe, 2003).

In addition to treatment facilities sponsored by specific denominations, in many communities congregations or local coalitions have various programs that address addiction. We are not aware of any firm estimate of the number of these programs that exist. To use our own region as an example, in West Central Indiana where we live there are chapters of national groups such as Celebrate Recovery, modifications of Celebrate Recovery, ministries that provide support to addicts, residential programs including various degrees of R/S emphasis, and youth prevention programs with strictly secular content delivered at FB community centers. The Rush Center of the Johnson Institute has developed a nondenominational, multifaith program to help local congregations develop "Faith Partners teams" in an effort to decrease stigma associated with addiction and increase the likelihood of congregation members with addiction problems seeking and obtaining help (Allem & Merrill, 2004). Ringwald (2002) provides descriptions of a large number of FB approaches to addiction, including some of those mentioned in this chapter. The Substance Abuse and Mental Health Services Administration also has published a list of FB and recovery-related programs affiliated with various U.S. faith groups (SAMHSA, 2006).

Yet another FB support program is the "recovery church," originating among individuals with current or past addiction problems who did not feel welcomed in a traditional house of worship. Most attendees at a recovery church identify themselves as "in recovery" or relatives of individuals in recovery. One example is Central Park United Methodist in St. Paul, Minnesota (Francis, 2005), but recovery churches exist in a number of large cities.

History and Controversies Regarding Faith-Based Services

Brief History of Faith-Based Approaches

Ideas of charity for the poor and aid to those in need have been a part of Judaism, Christianity, and Islam from their beginnings. Religious groups in the United States began offering social services well before the federal government became involved during the Great Depression (Kennedy & Bielefeld, 2006). Blumburg (1978) described nineteenth century residential programs for alcoholics that resemble many contemporary FB programs in their emphasis on mutual help and total abstinence, reliance on God, and focus on moral persuasion. A major barrier to keeping such institutions open was lack of funding, although some money seems to have come from municipal or state governments (Blumburg, 1978). White and Whiters (1992) provide a brief but thorough history of FB recovery programs in the United States. They identified several common elements of such programs, including transcendence of self, reconstruction of identity and values, various rituals to facilitate transformation or conversion, and the role of a community of shared belief.

Public awareness of FBOs began to increase with the passage of the House Personal Responsibility and Work Opportunity Reconciliation Act of 1996 (HR 3734). Section 104 of this bill, the Charitable Choice provision, allowed states to make contracts with both secular and sectarian (FB) groups for selected types of social services (Formicola et al., 2003). Other approaches to funding FBOs proposed at around the same time included offering income tax credits for charitable contributions to FBOs, even for those who do not itemize, and programs to offer vouchers that could be redeemed for services at secular or FB organizations. The White House Office of Faith Based and Community Initiatives was created in 2001 by executive order. Later executive orders expanded the range of services eligible for Charitable Choice funding.

Access to Recovery

The Access to Recovery (ATR) program was proposed in 2003 as a voucher program with goals of expanding consumer choice, measuring results of treatment, and increasing treatment capacity. Funds were allocated to support both treatment and recovery support services (e.g., case management, family support, child care, transportation services, employment services, housing assistance, "spiritual support," etc.) by FB and traditional providers. An RFA was issued and 44 states and 22 tribes and territories submitted proposals in June 2004. In August 2004, 14 states (CA, CT, FL, ID, IL, LA, MO, NJ, NM, TN, TX, WA, WI, WY) and one tribal organization (CA Rural Indiana Health Board) were announced as recipients of three-year grants. The original program served 190,144 individuals, 75,000 more than had originally been hoped (Clay, 2007). In 2007, a new set of three-year grants was awarded to 18 states, the District of Columbia, and five tribal organizations.

Clients are assessed and eligibility and need for ATR services determined. Clients in need of services are referred to at least two providers and select one. Vouchers are then issued to obtain the services. All providers participating in ATR are required to collect outcome data, including abstinence from drugs or alcohol, retention in treatment, and other indicators such as education, employment, and criminal activity. However, outcome data are based only on client self-report. The initial ATR announcement left certification and standards of care requirements for providers up to individual states. Some groups were concerned that FB providers would not have adequate training or credentials to effectively work with addicted populations (Hughes & Farris, 2005; NAADAC, 2007), but currently all ATR providers are supposed to follow the same standards of care and certification requirements.

Criticisms and Controversies Surrounding FBOs

Program Effectiveness   Relatively little data exist on effectiveness of faith-based social service programs (Kennedy & Bielefeld, 2006). Arguments in support for FBOs typically stated that such programs are more effective and efficient (e.g., they cost less because they rely on volunteer staff) than similar secular programs (Hodge, 2000; Kuo, 2006). However, even some supporters of FB programs pointed out the lack of research evidence for this alleged effectiveness (Johnson, Tompkins, & Webb, 2002; Kuo, 2006). Kennedy & Bielefeld (2006) conducted what is probably the largest scale study of a FB social service, a three-year study of over 5,000 cases of individuals in welfare to work programs in two Indiana counties. When controlling for county, gender, race, education, and year, they found no differences between FB and non-FB providers in percentage of clients placed in jobs or in hourly wages when placed. However, FB providers were less likely to place clients in full-time work and clients placed by FB providers were less likely to have health insurance. Several studies of FB prison programs suggest that such programs may have positive outcomes, but there are a number of methodological limitations with these studies (Johnson et al., 2002). The current status of evidence regarding FBTs for addiction is discussed in a later section.

Violation of Separation of Church and State   Perhaps the most contentious issue in recent debate surrounding FB programs is the question of whether government funding for FBOs violates the First Amendment to the Constitution (Formicola et al., 2003; Kennedy & Bielefeld, 2006). Thus far, the ability of FBOs to hire and fire based on religious grounds and to display religious materials and symbols has been upheld, and charitable choice regulations have stipulated that federal money cannot be utilized to pay for religious services of prosetylizing, that

FBOs may not discriminate against clients on the basis of faith, and that secular alternatives must be made available for clients who request them. However, at the time of this writing, lawsuits are in progress in several states questioning use of public funds for various FB programs, typically those where the goal of the program is conversion to Christianity.

Government Involvement may Hinder Activities of FBOs   The flip side of the separation of church and state argument is the fear that government involvement would hamper the provision of services. For example, paperwork requirements that accompany government funds might consume resources and actually impede service delivery. Smaller congregations might lack the resources to even apply for funds, which is one proposed explanation for why few African American churches have obtained funds from FB grants (Bullock, 2006). Religiously conservative and evangelical FBOs are typically less interested in obtaining government funding than other FBOs (Ebaugh, Chafetz, & Pipes, 2006a, 2006b; Hodge, 2000).

Christian and other religious leaders sometimes refer to the "prophetic role" of the church in society (Formicola et al., 2003). Examples from history include the abolitionist and civil rights movements. Some critics expressed the fear that accepting government money could compromise religious groups' role as social critics and forces for justice (Formicola et al., 2003).

Lack of Credentialing and Regulation   Several proposed Charitable Choice programs in the 1990s attempted to prohibit states from requiring specific training or credentials for individuals providing addiction services. These proposals were opposed by the National Association of State Alcohol and Drug Abuse Directors and the National Association of Alcohol and Drug Abuse Counselors and did not pass. The lack of clergy training in addictions identified by CASA (2001) and the heavy reliance on nonprofessional staff in many FBOs are still concerns. Although some FBOs view reliance on nonprofessional staff as a limitation (Dominguez et al., 2006), others have defended it as consistent with their evangelizing mission (Hodge, 2000). Nonetheless, at a December 2006 conference on FB programs sponsored by the Roundtable on Religion & Social Welfare Policy, there was general agreement by both supporters and detractors that FB programs should be subject to the same forms of guidance and oversight required for secular programs (Hughes & Farris, 2006). The Clergy Training Project, initiated by the National Association for Children of Alcoholics and the Johnson Institute, in collaboration with SAMHSA and the NIAAA is an attempt to address the lack of clergy training in substance abuse issues. Initially an expert consensus panel produced a list of Core Competencies for Clergy (Core Competencies, 2003), and subsequent efforts are developing curricula to provide training in the competency areas.

Other Concerns   Some critics accused backers of FBOs of having political rather than humanitarian motivations (Formicola et al., 2003; Kennedy & Bielfeld, 2006; Kuo, 2006). Following passage of the initial Charitable Choice legislation, several conservative Christian leaders and politicians publicly stated that certain religious groups, including Muslims, Wiccans, Hare Krishnas, and Scientologists should not receive funding, raising concerns that funding might be biased toward Evangelical Christian programs (Formicola, et al., 2003; Kuo, 2006). Finally, the FBT programs studied by Hodge (2000) expressed that finding and retaining staff was difficult. Hodge therefore expressed doubt that increasing funds for FBOs could have a measurable impact on availability of services.

Arguments in Support of FBOs

Who Else will do this Kind of Work?   Many FBOs operate in contexts where there are few other options for people in need. Whether in the poverty-stricken rural south (Bartkowski & Regis, 2003) or the equally poor regions of the inner city (Wolfe, 2003), many people in need, particularly minorities, are argued to be beyond the reach of traditional social services, either because of geographic isolation, lack of culturally appropriate services, mistrust of government, cultural barriers that inhibit access to and/or utilization of services, marginalization, and/or other factors. FBOs are argued to be well integrated into a community, whereas the market sector is thought to have no significant financial incentive to work with individuals who have no insurance and in some cases may not even qualify for or have accessed Medicaid or Medicare. Even in less destitute areas, FBOs are seen as important community resources.

Development of Social Capital   Religious communities are thought to promote "social capital" by establishing stable social networks that work for social change and engage in actions aimed at the collective good, rather than pursuing self-interest and profit as in the market sector (Bartkowski & Regis, 2003; Bicknese, 1999). Several studies suggest that social capital predicts lower alcohol use at the community level (Weitzman & Chen, 2005; Weitzman and Kawachi, 2000). If FBTs produce better citizens and enhance social capital, this could have a positive effect not only on the individuals treated, but other members of the local community.

Consumer Options   Services offered by FBOs might increase consumer options (Kuo, 2006). Cooney et al. (2003) suggested that the treatments studied in Project MATCH may all have been effective because they mobilized client resources, enhanced motivation for change and expectancy of success, and provided access to social support for recovery. They noted that perhaps "the real value of having an array of treatments available is to promote healthy competition for the wide variety of people who benefit from any treatment, but who would be more attracted to one because of reputation, convenience, or personal preference" (p. 225). This argument would apply to FBTs only if they have uniformly positive results comparable to other effective treatments (as was the case with the approaches studied in Project MATCH).

Conceptual Basis of FB Addiction Treatment

Hypotheses and Claims

A full discussion of theological and ethical issues related to alcohol and addiction is beyond the scope of this chapter, but we do provide an overview of some of the major positions. In-depth discussions from the perspective of various faith traditions are available (Baker, 2004; Cook, 2006; Groves and Farmer, 1994; Marlatt, 2002; Mercadante, 1996; Plantinga, 2003; Spiegel

& Kravitz, 2001; etc.). Miller (1998) claimed that it is possible to separate spiritual models of addiction from moralistic views "that [blame] . . . alcoholics or addicts for being morally deficient" (p. 982). Published R/S conceptualizations of addiction often propose that use (or heavy use) of alcohol or other drugs represents attempts to cope with lack of meaning and purpose in life (Bicknese, 1999; Doweiko, 1999; Piedmont, 2004) or (in theistic religions) lack of perceived connection to God (May, 1988; Mercadante, 1996; Plantinga, 2003). A related R/S conceptualization of addiction is as idolatry, with the addictive substance (or behavior) taking the place of God in one's life (Miller, 1998).

Some R/S groups equate addiction or substance use with sin, a view that may or may not be detrimental to the individual depending on how a group defines and responds to behaviors labeled as sinful (Mercadante, 1996; Nelson, 2004). There is some evidence that the belief that alcohol use is morally wrong at least partially explains the lower rates of drinking among individuals who belong to faith groups stressing abstinence (see below). However, if communities shun or reject members who use alcohol or drugs, or if they refuse to recognize that such problems exist among their members, users or addicts may experience guilt and/or be less likely to obtain treatment (Stoltzfus, 2006; Suliman, 1983).

As noted above, belief that God is punitive and harsh is associated with increased risk for mental health problems, whereas belief in a loving God who functions as a collaborative partner is associated with positive mental health (Koenig et al., 2001; Pargament, 1997). It is possible that believing that substance use or addiction is a sin would be more detrimental among individuals or groups who hold a punishing concept of God. Belief that health or mental health problems are the result of demonic forces has also been associated with poorer mental health (Koenig et al., 2001). Mariz (1991) claimed that, at least in Brazil, Pentecostal Christians view "addiction as the action of the devil" and that this provides "an important element in the motivation to stop drinking" (p. 78). Research on the interaction of beliefs about sin and beliefs about demonic forces could help clarify how these might be related to addiction. Stoltzfus (2006) recommended that professionals working with religious individuals or congregations attempt to avoid getting into debates about whether addiction is best seen as a disease or as sin. However, the first of the Core Competencies (2004) listed by the NCOA Expert Consensus Panel was that clergy "be aware of the generally accepted definition of alcohol and drug dependence."

Pentecostal Christians and members of some other religions believe to varying extents in divine or magical healing. Such beliefs could be potential barriers to utilizing health care services or lead to guilt if healing does not occur (Koenig et al., 2001). Stoltzfus (2006) noted that the founder of Teen Challenge initially expected that conversion would immediately cure addiction problems, but later concluded from experience that a long period of immersion in a positive supportive environment was also necessary for abstinence to be maintained.

Studies of FBOs

Several studies have surveyed staff at FB addiction treatment centers regarding the conceptual models they use to understand addiction (Dominguez et al., 2005; Hodge, 2000; McCoy et al., 2004). Although a minority of programs relied exclusively on religious methods (prayer, bible study, etc.) and viewed addiction only as a spiritual problem, most programs in these studies took a broader view. Although most viewed addiction as a spiritual problem (e.g., "attempts to fill a spiritual void through the use of substances" McCoy et al., pp. 5–6; etc.), staff also often admitted that biological, social/environmental, and psychological factors could be involved and/or indicated that they utilized not only R/S practices, but techniques drawn from cognitive, behavioral, existential, or psychodynamic approaches and even biomedical treatments. It is not clear whether these diverse conceptual models are integrated into a unified bio-psycho-social-spiritual model, or if they merely serve as a source for deriving interventions that are applied eclectically or in an atheoretical fashion.

Proposed Integrative Model: Conversion, Transformation, and Conservation

Most of the FBTs we reviewed, including 12-step programs, aim to produce some form of conversion. This should probably not be surprising, given that prior to the twentieth century most individuals probably understood personal change primarily in religious terms, with examples such as Siddhartha, St. Paul, St. Augustine, or Mohammed. There is an extensive research literature on conversion, although much of it involves descriptive studies conducted from a Protestant perspective (Spilka et al., 2003). Spilka et al. defined conversion as a transformation of self within a religious context, and noted that conversions can be sudden or more gradual. Core personality traits show little change as a result of a conversion experience. However, considerable changes may occur in attitudes, goals, and behaviors and perhaps profound changes in sense of meaning, purpose, and identity (Paloutzian, Richardson, & Rambo, 1999).

Paloutzian (2005) proposed that conversion is a subset of the broader phenomenon of spiritual transformation (Hill, 2002). Spiritual transformation applies not only to conversion from one faith to another or from no faith to having faith, but to intensifications of existing faith (such as "born again" experiences) and even to losses of faith. According to Paloutizian, the essential prerequisite for a spiritual transformation is "*discrepancy* between the *ought* and the *is* of a person's life" (p. 337, italics original). For a spiritual transformation to occur, some event or experience, often doubts or "crises (not necessarily catastrophic) of purpose, value, efficacy, or self-worth" (p. 336), has called into question a person's current way of understanding and making meaning in the world. Spiritual transformation is the reconstruction of a framework of meaning (or loss of faith or meaning). R/S may help create meaning through both relations with the transcendent (e.g., God, sacred goals or values, etc.) and with others. Conversions occurring in supportive social environments seem to produce longer-lasting changes than when the social context involves pressure or coercion (Spilka et al., 2003).

R/S models tracing addiction to a lack of meaning or lack of connection with God fit well within Paloutzian's framework. Both of these situations reflect a discrepancy between what is and what ought to be. A crisis of meaning could trigger drug or alcohol use as an attempt to cope. In the project MATCH sample, Tonigan, Miller, and Schermer (2002) found that individuals who were unsure about their belief in God, and thus potentially experiencing R/S struggle, drank more often than atheists and those who were certain that God exists.

Alternatively, some aspects of addiction could themselves trigger a crisis of meaning. Users who have developed symptoms of physiological dependence or experience cravings may feel they have no control over their own behavior. A person who has been detoxified may look back over his or her behavior while using and be shocked by actions such as neglect of children or other responsibilities. Such experiences could easily create crises of worth, meaning, or efficacy or reveal discrepancies between one's behavior and important values or goals.

However, a crisis also sets the stage for reconstruction of meaning. Twelve-step programs often refer to the necessity of hitting bottom before change can occur. One Teen Challenge staff member interviewed by Glascotte et al. (1972) indicated that the program preferred to admit individuals who were desperate. However, an intense crisis might not be necessary. Miller (2006) wrote: "change occurs when a person perceives significant discrepancy between his or her present state and his or her desired goals or values" (p 149). Saunders, Lucas, and Kuras (2007) explicitly linked motivational models to R/S. They proposed that Spiritual or Religious Functioning (SRF) is a subjective judgment and that all individuals experience some degree of discrepancy between their current and ideal levels of SRF. Their hypothesis that such a discrepancy might be a causal factor in addiction is consistent with Paloutzian's broader framework.

Pargament (1997) noted that people do not always experience transformation. If stresses are not overwhelming, they may instead focus on maintaining or conserving their current ways of making meaning and/or their existing goals and values. The concepts of transformation and conservation bear further study in the specific context of addiction treatment, but they may provide heuristic constructs that clinicians can use in attempting to understand R/S functioning. FBTs may be helpful when individuals are experiencing a crisis of meaning, because such individuals have the necessary pre-requisite for a spiritual transformation.

Research on FBT for Addiction

Outcome Studies on FBT

With the exception of research on AA and related programs, most published studies of FB treatments are from the 1960s and 1970s. Methodologically, they are weak by contemporary standards (usually no control group, small sample size, low percentages of participants available for follow-up, no means to verify self-reports of outcome, often relatively short follow-up periods, outcomes assessed only in terms of abstinence, etc.). In addition it is possible that the types of individuals seen or treatments offered could have changed over the past 40 years.

Success rates reported for FB treatment could depend to a great extent on how FBT is defined. Desmond and Maddux (1981) reported outcomes for a sample of 248 predominantly Hispanic heroin addicts treated in "religious programs" (including Teen Challenge) and a variety of secular programs. They obtained urine screens to verify abstinence from heroin one year or more after completing treatment. They reported that 45% (15 out of 33) of patients who entered a religious program were abstinent at one year versus 2–5% for hospital-based or methadone maintenance programs and 18% for residential or therapeutic community treatment.

These results seem to favor FBT over secular treatments. However, Desmond and Maddux (1981) included among the 33 patients in religious programs 9 individuals "abstinent for 3 years or more" (p. 74) who "did not join a formal program, but attributed prolonged abstinence to religious conversion or to involvement in church activities" (p. 74). If these patients are excluded, which seems permissible given that they did not in fact receive formal FBT, the success rate for FBT becomes 24% (6/24). Desmond and Maddux also reported data on 38 individuals who entered a methadone maintenance program that included a religious component and noted that this program worked "no better than conventional methadone programs without a religious component" (pp. 75–76.). If these 38 are added to the original 33, then the success rate for FBT is around 24%, but if they are added to the 24 who actually received FBT, then the overall success rate for formal programs including a religious component goes down to 13% (8/62). Desmond and Maddux concluded that "religious programs" may be attractive to and effective for some individuals, but added that they "would not expect to bring about marked increases in abstinence in an addict population by coercing more into religious programs" (p. 77). They suggested FBT may have been beneficial to some Mexican-American men due to cultural familiarity with and acceptance of healing rituals or supernatural healing. In reference to the small proportion of the sample that entered FBT (11% of participants), Desmond and Maddux (1981) noted that "from the standpoint of attractiveness or acceptability to opioid users, religious programs do not appear especially effective" (p. 75).

Studies of AA and 12-step-based Treatments   Although the drop-out rate in AA is high, involvement in AA (e.g., working the steps rather than simply attending meetings) predicts better outcomes across a variety of treatment modalities (Tonigan, Connors, & Miller, 2003). Tonigan, Toscova, and Miller (1996) performed a meta-analysis of AA studies, most of which involved 12-step-inspired treatments or the relationship between AA involvement and outcome while receiving formal treatment rather than focusing on AA alone. AA involvement was generally positively related to drinking outcomes, especially abstinence. The mean weighted rs were around .20 across different outcomes, on the border between a small and medium effect size. Reviews of studies of court-ordered AA clearly indicate that mandated AA attendance is not generally effective (Miller, Wilbourne, & Hettema, 2003). Thus, although there is evidence that AA appears to be beneficial in individuals who voluntarily attend while undergoing formal addiction treatment, we know relatively little about the effect of AA in individuals who attend without also being in treatment (Tonigan et al., 1996). In Project MATCH, TSF did at least as well as Cognitive Behavioral Therapy (CBT) and Motivational Enhancement Therapy (MET). TSF was somewhat better than MET and CBT in producing continuous abstinence in outpatients. AA involvement was an independent predictor of treatment success, regardless of which type of treatments clients received (Miller & Longabough, 2003).

Abstinence rates of 40–60% at 12-month follow-up have been reported in studies of MM programs (Cook, 1988b; Winters, Stinchfield, Opland, Weller, & Latimer, 2000). Winters et al. (2000) reported abstinence rates of 53% for adolescents who completed a MM program, compared to 15% for dropouts and 28% for a waiting list control group. However, Miller et al. (2003) reported that the only controlled trial of the MM they could locate showed MM no better than the control condition. They also noted that educational interventions, as often used in MM programs, are the least effective of the nearly 50 interventions they reviewed.

Studies of Salvation Army Programs   Katz (1966) reported on outcomes of men treated at two Salvation Army Men's Service Centers in California. Follow-up (f/u) data regarding abstinence was obtained on 26% of the 293 men treated in 1962. Twenty-five percent reported total abstinence during the f/u period, and 56% reported being abstinent for more than one half of the f/u period. Sixty-eight percent of men reported increased proportion of time abstinent in the 6 month f/u period compared to the six months prior to admission. Utilizing a larger dataset, Katz suggested that length of time spent in treatment was positively related to outcome. Katz also added that "The role of religion can be a major and very dramatic one in certain cases; when a religious conversion is experienced rehabilitation seems to follow almost 'automatically'" (p. 645). Unfortunately he gave no information on the prevalence of conversions.

Moos, Mehren, and Moos (1978) obtained self-report data at intake ($N = 121$) and 6 months posttreatment ($N = 97$) from a sample of alcohol-dependent individuals treated at a Salvation Army facility. At f/u, participants reported fewer drinking problems, less physical and behavioral impairment, and greater well-being, occupational functioning, and likelihood of abstinence. The 26% of participants who dropped out of treatment were less likely than completers to be abstinent and more likely to report a serious drinking problem at f/u. Greater involvement in program activities predicted statistically significant improvement in physical impairment, self-rating of drinking problems, past month abstinence, and social functioning.

Studies of Teen Challenge   The most frequently cited outcome study of a FBT is the federally funded study of Teen Challenge conducted by Hess in 1975. The study attempted to follow up 369 men who entered Teen challenge programs 7 years earlier in 1968. Sixty-six percent dropped out during the induction phase, leaving 144 to enter the Training Center phase. Fifty-three percent dropped out of the Training Center, leaving only 18% completing the program (Hess, 1978). This is similar to Glasscote et al.'s (1972) report that 20% of those entering a Teen Challenge Center they studied stayed in the program beyond the first two weeks.

Hess' (1978) sample consisted of "3 populations" (p. 273), P1 = 44 of the 222 men who dropped out of the Brooklyn Induction Center, P2 = 77 men who dropped out of the Training Center, and P3 = 67 men who graduated from the Training Center. Hess (1978) stated that "70% *of all three populations* were not using drugs at the time of the interview (March through August, 1975). This is confirmed by urinalysis report." (p. 273, italics added). That the majority of both treatment completers and noncompleters were drug-free suggests that maturation may have accounted for the observed changes in drug use. However, a larger percentage of graduates were employed at f/u (75%) than of the P1 (50%) or P2 (56%) samples (Hess, 1978).

Gruner (1984) administered the Purpose in Life (PIL) test at intake, ($N = 160$), and after 6 months ($N = 138$) and 12 months ($N = 128$) of treatment at Teen Challenge programs in India, Holland, Germany, France, Guam, and Hawaii. He found that PIL increased significantly over the course of treatment, but did not attempt to relate changes in PIL score to treatment outcome.

An unpublished Political Science dissertation by Bicknese (1999) included 59 Teen Challenge participants and a matched control group of 118 patients from a variety of public Short Term Inpatient (STI) treatment facilities. Bicknese characterized the study as a test of the "AA 'disease model' of drug treatment against the Teen Challenge 'character building model'" (p. 128). Ignoring the issue of whether these models accurately characterize either the Teen Challenge or AA programs, the study would be better described as a comparison between 2–4 weeks of treatment (in STI) and 12–14 months of treatment (in Teen Challenge). A Therapeutic Community would probably have been a more appropriate control group.

Not surprisingly, Bicknese (1999) found that the Teen Challenge "students" performed better on a variety of outcome measures than the STI patients. Although his study is an impressive undertaking for a dissertation and he attempted to be rigorous in his treatment of the data he had available, the low response rate (less than 40%) in both groups limits the generalizability of the findings (which he acknowledges). What is probably most notable about the study is not that it proves anything either way about the effectiveness of Teen Challenge, but that it suggests that, as with studies of Salvation Army programs, FB providers are willing to cooperate in evaluation studies. The results summarized here suggest that more extensive studies with rigorous methodologies conducted by experienced outcome researchers may be worth government funding, particularly given that FBTs currently receive funds through the ATR program.

Other Studies   In an uncontrolled study, clients who completed 8 weeks of Spiritual Self-Schema (3-S) Therapy showed decreases in drug use and other HIV risk behaviors, increased self-identification as spiritual, and increases in spiritual experiences and practices (Avants, Beitel, & Margolin, 2005). In a controlled trial, 3-S therapy clients showed greater increases in spirituality and fewer HIV risk behaviors than controls (Margolin, Beitel, Schuman-Olivier, & Avants, 2006). Case studies are available for 3-S therapy (Marcotte, Margolin, & Avants, 2003) as well as for various integrations of R/S into addiction treatment (Richards & Bergin, 2004).

Patient Characteristics and Treatment Matching

Attitudes Towards FBT   Two studies of Midwestern Christian clergy found that these clergy were more likely to refer clients to FBT rather than secular treatment (Collet, Guidry, Martin, and Sager, 2006; Dominguez et al., 2006). However, these results may not generalize to other regions or faiths. Goldfarb, Galanter, McDowell, Lifshutz, & Dermatis (1996) reported that medical students had more negative attitudes toward inclusion of spirituality in dual diagnosis treatment programs than did patients in those programs. Arnold, Avants, Margolin, and Marcote (2002) reported that the majority of opioid-dependent patients they surveyed expressed interest in spiritually focused addiction treatment, with African-American women being more interested than African-American men. Aromin, Galanter, Solhkhah, Dermatis, and Bunt (2006) reported that adolescents were more likely than adults to express interest in 12-step and spiritual components in Therapeutic Community Treatment.

Who Benefits from FBT?   With the exception of the Hess (1978) study, most of the studies we located suggested that success in FBT was unrelated to faith background or pretreatment levels of religiousness. Hess (1978) found that individuals who were not religious before entering Teen Challenge were more likely to complete the program than those who were religious. Neither prior evangelical affiliation nor knowledge of evangelical concepts/church referral predicted outcome among the Teen Challenge participants studied by Bicknese (1999). Tonigan, Miller, and Schermer (2002) reported that, although atheists and agnostics attended AA less often than religious clients, greater AA attendance predicted greater abstinence regardless of participants' belief in God. In Project MATCH, religious clients did no better in TSF than in MET or CBT. Similarly, Winzelberg and Humphries (1999) found that religious background did not alter the ability of referrals to 12-step programs to predict meeting attendance or the fact that 12-step attendance predicted better outcomes. In contrast to these studies that did not find R/S to be predictive of attitudes toward FB treatment, Aromin et al. (2006) found that perceived connectedness to others, frequency of prayer, and level of intrinsic spirituality predicted greater interest among adolescents in 12-step and spiritually focused treatment.

In Project MATCH, TSF was more effective than MET for outpatient clients whose social networks supported their drinking. Much of this effect appeared to be due to the success of TSF in getting clients involved in AA (Cooney et al., 2003). In outpatients, TSF was also superior to CBT for clients low in comorbid psychopathology. In the aftercare arm CBT surpassed TSF in effectiveness for clients low in dependence symptoms, whereas TSF was superior to CBT for clients with higher levels of dependence. Clearly more research is needed to clarify what types of individuals are likely to be interested in and benefit from FBT.

Other Relevant Research

Given the paucity of outcome studies, it may be useful to consider additional sources of information to help clarify the potential efficacy of FBT. We present information regarding potential mediators of the relationship between R/S and substance use, R/S factors that might increase risk of addiction, changes in R/S variables in response to treatment, and mediators of treatment outcome. A mediating variable is a variable that could be part of a causal chain linking other variables, for example, explaining how R/S might cause lower levels of substance use. Hypothetically, variations in the level of R/S cause changes in the level of the mediator, which in turn causes lower levels of substance use or problems.

Religious Involvement and Alcohol and Other Drug Use

In studies of the general population, higher levels of R/S are consistently associated with lower levels of substance use and problems (Booth and Martin, 1998), but there is currently no published meta-analysis on the strength of these effects. We examined a dozen recent studies. They tended to report small effect sizes for the relationship between R/S and alcohol use, and low to medium effect sizes for the relationship between R/S and use of other drugs.

R/S has been proposed to cause lower levels of substance use by affecting social influences, beliefs or values, and well-being (Gorsuch, 1995; Koenig et al., 2001). Path analytic and other multivariate studies in adolescents (Burkett, 1980, 1993; Mason & Windle, 2002), college students (Johnson, Sheets, & Kristeller, 2008), and adults (Drerup, 2005) are consistent with the hypothesis that highly religious individuals tend to have friends and associates that also show low levels of substance use. Thus, their exposure to social influences on use (e.g., modeling of drinking behavior, being offered alcohol or other drugs, etc.) is less than individuals who are not religious. Reduced exposure in turn leads to lower use. R/S also may impact use via parental or family influences (Mason & Windle, 2002; Stewart & Bolland, 2002).

Religious individuals often hold negative attitudes toward use of alcohol and other drugs (Francis, 1992, 1997; Stylianou, 2004), and religious objections are commonly listed as reasons for not drinking (Johnson & Cohen, 2004). Path analytic studies suggest that the relationship between R/S and substance use may be mediated by disapproval of use (Bachman et al., 2002) or negative beliefs, but the effect of beliefs on drinking is not as strong as the effect of social influences (Drerup, 2005; Johnson et al., 2008).

Johnson et al. (2008) and Drerup (2005) found that individuals higher in R/S had higher levels of meaning in life and inner peace. This in turn was associated with lower use of alcohol as a coping mechanism and fewer alcohol-related problems. Religiosity (Jang & Johnson, 2001; Wills, Yaeger, & Sandy, 2003) and positive religious coping (Johnson, Aten, Madson, & Bennett, 2006) have been shown to reduce the effect of various life stressors on substance use.

R/S Variables that Might Increase Risk

Several authors have reported the clinical observation that punitive religious experiences or belief in a punitive God are associated with alcohol problems (Doweiko, 1999; Gorsuch, 1995). Drerup (2005) reported that belief in a punitive God, life stress, and negative interactions with members of one's faith community predicted higher levels of religious struggle (Pargament, 2002). Johnson et al. (2008) and Drerup found that individuals who reported higher levels of religious struggle reported lower levels of meaning and peace. This in turn appeared to increase the motive to use alcohol as a coping mechanism and thereby increase alcohol related problems.

R/S Variables in Response to Addiction Treatment

A number of studies have reported that purpose in life increases over the course of treatment or recovery (Bammer & Weeks, 1994; Carroll, 1993; Waisberg & Porter, 1994) or that meaning-seeking decreases (Walitzer & Barrick, 2003). Piedmont (2004) reported that experiences of spiritual transcendence in a treatment sample increased over the course of eight weeks of treatment, but did not report whether the increase predicted treatment outcome.

Robinson et al. (2007) examined changes in multiple dimensions of R/S from intake to six months later in a sample of 157 clients with alcohol problems (92% dependence, 8% abuse). Measures reflecting religious beliefs (e.g., belief in God, concept of God) did not change significantly, whereas religious practices, Positive Religious Coping, and several types of R/S experiences (Daily Spiritual Experiences, Purpose in Life, & Forgiveness) did increase significantly from baseline to six months. Furthermore, increases in Purpose in Life and Daily Spiritual Experiences were predictive of positive treatment outcomes.

In Project MATCH, the effect of AA attendance on outcome was mediated not by having had a spiritual awakening or by decreases in meaning-seeking, but by establishing non-drinking social networks (Cooney et al., 2003; Tonigan, in Owen et al., 2003). However, Tonigan noted that the lack of findings could reflect inadequate measurement of complex constructs.

Effects of Religious or Spiritual Practices and Behaviors

Given that FBTs often employ a number of R/S practices such as prayer, it is worth examining what is known about the effects of such practices on health and well-being. A comprehensive review is beyond the scope of this chapter, so we limit our focus.

Prayer

Several types of prayer appear to have positive effects on health and well-being, including contemplative/meditative prayer and colloquial prayer (e.g., conversations with God; McCullough & Larson, 1999). Ritual prayer (e.g., rote recitation) and petitionary prayer (pleading for God's help) are associated with poorer well-being, although the direction of causation cannot be established. Carroll (1993) reported that frequency of prayer was positively associated with PIL scores among alcoholics in treatment. Walker, Tonigan, Miller, Comer, and Kahlich (1997) conducted a randomized trial of intercessory prayer for alcoholics in treatment, but found no differences in outcome between controls and alcoholics who were being prayed for.

Pennebaker (1997) proposed that prayer may function as self-disclosure to God and therefore enhance R/S coping. The process of self-disclosure by writing narratives about difficult life events has been shown to promote a number of positive health outcomes including lower levels of distress, perhaps by providing an opportunity for meaning-making (Greenberg, Wortman, & Stone, 1996; Rimé, 1995). A prospective experimental study by Bennett (2005) found that the content of prayer narratives is structurally similar to more traditional forms of self-disclosure and that writing prayers about previously nondisclosed traumatic events was associated with improvements in physical and emotional health.

Forgiveness

Thoresen, Harris, and Luskin (2000) define forgiveness as, ". . . the decision to reduce negative thoughts, affect, and behavior, such as blame and anger, toward an offender or hurtful situation, and to begin to gain a better understanding of the offence and the offender" (p. 255). Although forgiveness can be a secular value, it is also a central tenet of many faith traditions.

In relation to addiction recovery, Wuthnow (2000) found that those who were part of groups that helped them forgive were more likely to overcome an addiction. Lin, Mack, Enright, Krahn, and Baskin (2004), found that inpatient substance abuse clients who participated in forgiveness therapy experienced greater self-esteem, less anger, anxiety, depression, and less vulnerability to drug use than those receiving an alternative treatment. Recent evidence suggests that forgiveness could benefit psychological adjustment to life stress by allowing individuals to satisfy their need for control (Witvliet, Ludwig, and Vander Laan, 2001).

Meditation

Transcendental meditation (TM) is a technique used to attain a state of restful alertness with the goal of experiencing "transcendental consciousness." A meta-analysis of TM used in alcohol treatment suggested that TM was superior to a number of other relaxation and prevention interventions (Alexander, Robinson, & Rainforth, 1994). Mindfulness meditation is a practice that pairs relaxation and focus with the nonjudgmental examination of one's thoughts and feelings. Witkiewitz, Marlatt, and Walker (2005), suggest that the process of mindfulness meditation can be beneficial because it "reduce[s] an individual's susceptibility to act in response to a drug cue or cue stimulus, and decrease[s] an individual's inclination to behave impulsively." Bowen et al. (2006) showed that practice of mindfulness meditation in an incarcerated population was associated with reduced substance abuse after release.

Summary & Recommendations

There is substantial evidence that 12-step program attendance by individuals in treatment improves treatment outcome. This may be due to providing a nonusing social support network and/or promoting spiritual transformation. Future research should examine the effect of matching clients with mutual help groups that reflect their specific faith background. It may be reasonable for clinicians to attempt to do such matching with their clients when alternative programs are available, but this would require knowledge of and familiarity with local resources.

There is reasonable, but not conclusive evidence to suggest that TSF and MM programs are as helpful as some other treatment modalities. Additional randomized clinical trials of MM programs would be helpful. Data from the 1960s and 1970s indicate some improvement in alcohol use and employment after participation in Salvation Army programs.

The current evidence for FB programs that rely almost exclusively on R/S interventions is suggestive enough to justify spending time and money on additional research. However, ethical and legal issues aside, one could question whether the existing data justify directing public funds toward all such programs. Given the possibility of negative effects associated with R/S, research is needed to help clarify what types of FB programs and what types of clients are least likely to produce negative outcomes. Data from the Access to Recovery program may be useful in addressing such issues, but will be limited by reliance on self-report outcome data and the diversity of FB programs participating (e.g., some offering treatment, others offering specific types of recovery support services).

A plausible case can be made that in the general population R/S may causally affect substance use and problems by influencing attitudes and values, affecting social influence variables, and increasing well-being and sense of meaning in life. Even in secular treatment programs, R/S variables might mediate treatment outcome and are worthy of further study. Some specific techniques utilized in FBTs might be beneficial components of FB or secular treatment, including prayer, meditation, and facilitating forgiveness. In addition, it is possible that FBTs promote changes in self-concept and belief systems, support development of new goals and meaning in life, and provide positive social support systems that can facilitate recovery.

Based on the above findings, we offer the following recommendations for practitioners:

1. Knowledge of local FB resources and clergy will help the addiction professional or clinician make informed decisions regarding patient care issues.

2. Collaborative efforts with FB programs, clergy, and congregations may have mutual benefits to both these groups and to clinicians.

3. Understanding clients' R/S background and beliefs may allow clinicians to establish a better working alliance, make better use of clients' R/S coping resources, integrate clients' R/S practices into even secular treatments, identify discrepancies between ideal and actual level of R/S functioning, make appropriate referrals, and help clients transform or conserve meaning.

4. Knowledge, collaboration, and understanding are necessary for making informed and appropriate referrals to FB (and/or secular) mutual help groups or other programs.

5. R/S groups and FB programs may offer valuable sources of social support or other kinds of human services (e.g., child care, job training, transportation, etc.) that could help support treatment and recovery.

6. Clinicians should be aware of the potential negative effects of R/S involvement, including R/S struggle. Richards and Bergin (2005) suggested that many clients perceive these issues as too threatening or dangerous to bring up at their place of worship and may therefore be more likely to bring them up in the more secular setting of counseling or psychotherapy.

References

Allem, J., & Merrill, T. (2004). *Healing places: How faith institutions can effectively address chemical dependency.* Washington, DC: The Rush Center of the Johnson Institute.

Alexander, C. N., Robinson, P., & Rainforth, M. (1994). Treating and preventing alcohol, nicotine, and drug abuse through transcendental meditation: A review and statistical meta-analysis. *Alcohol Treatment Quarterly, 11,* 13–87.

Ano, G. G., & Vasconcelles, E. B. (2005). Religious coping and psychological adjustment to stress: A meta-analysis. *Journal of Clinical Psychology, 61,* 461–480.

Arnold, R. M., Avants, S. K., Margolin, A., & Marcotte, D. (2002). Patient attitudes concerning the inclusion of spirituality into addiction treatment. *Journal of Substance Abuse Treatment, 23,* 319–326.

Aromin, R. A., Jr., Galanter, M., Solhkhah, R., Dermatis, H., & Bunt, G. (2006). Preference for spirituality and twelve-step oriented approaches among adolescents in a residential therapeutic community. *Journal of Addictive Diseases, 25,* 89–96.

Avants, S. K., Beitel, M., & Margolin, A. (2005). Making the shift from 'addict self' to 'spiritual self': results from a stage I study of spiritual self-schema (3-S0 therapy for the treatment of addiction and HIV risk behavior. *Mental Health, Religion, & Culture, 8,* 167–177.

Avants, S. K., & Margolin, A. (2004). Development of spiritual self-schema (3-S) therapy for the treatment of addictive and HIV risk behavior: A convergence of cognitive and Buddhist psychology. *Journal of Psychotherapy Integration, 14,* 253–289.

Bachman, J. G., O'Malley, P. M., Schulenberg, J. E., Johnston, L. D., Bryant, A. L., & Merline, A. C. (2002). *The decline of substance use in young adulthood: Changes in social activities, roles, and beliefs.* Mahwah, NJ: Erlbaum.

Baker, M. O. (2004). *Understanding alcohol and drug addiction: An LDS perspective.* Springville, UT: Cedar Fort.

Bammer, G., & Weekes, S. (1994). Becoming an ex-user: Insights into the process and implications for treatment and policy. *Drug & Alcohol Review, 13,* 285–292.

Bartkowski, J. P., & Regis, H. A. (2003). *Charitable choices: Religion, race, and poverty in the post-welfare era*. New York: New York University Press.

Bennett, P. R. (2005). Prayers about traumatic experiences as self-disclosure to God: Implications for health and well-being. Unpublished doctoral dissertation, University of Nevada, Reno, Nevada.

Bicknese, A. T. (1999). *The Teen Challenge program in comparative perspective*. Unpublished Doctoral Dissertation, Northwestern University, Evanston, IL.

Blumburg, L. U. (1978). The institutional phase of the Washingtonian total abstinence movement: A research note. *Journal of Studies on Alcohol, 39*, 1591–1606.

Booth, J., & Martin, J. E. (1998). Spiritual and religious factors in substance use, dependence, and recovery. In H. G. Koenig (Ed.), *Handbook of religion and mental health* (pp. 175–200). San Diego: Academic Press.

Bowen, S., Witkiewitz, K., Dillworth, T. M., Chawla, N., Simpson, T. L., Ostafin, B. D., et al. (2006). Mindfulness meditation and substance use in an incarcerated population. *Psychology of Addictive Behaviors, 20*, 343–347.

Bullock, L. M. (October 1, 2006). Few black churches take part in faith based initiative program. *The Louisiana Weekly*. Retrieved January 31, 2007, from www.socialpolicyandreligion.org/news/article.cfm?id = 5120.

Burkett, S. R. (1980). Religiosity, beliefs, normative standards, and adolescent drinking. *Journal of Studies on Alcohol, 41*, 662–671.

Burkett, S. R. (1993). Perceived parents' religiosity, friends' drinking, and hellfire: A panel study of adolescent drinking. *Review of Religious Research, 35*, 134–154.

Carroll, S. (1993). Spirituality and purpose in life in alcoholism recovery. *Journal of Studies on Alcohol, 54*, 297–301.

CASA - National Center on Addiction and Substance Abuse at Columbia University (2001). *So help me God: Substance abuse, religion and spirituality. A CASA white paper*. New York: National Center on Addiction and Substance Abuse at Columbia University.

Chamberlain, K., & Zika, S. (1992). Religiosity, meaning in life, and psychological well-being. In J. F. Schumaker (Ed.), *Religion and mental health* (pp. 138–148). New York: Oxford University Press.

Clay, R. A. (2007, November/December). Access to recovery: Enhancing consumer choice. *SAMHSA News, 15(6)*. Retrieved June 25, 2008, from http://www.samhsa.gov/SAMHSA_News/VolumeXV_6?article8.htm.

Cnaan, R. (2002). *The invisible caring hand: American congregations and the provision of welfare*. New York: New York University Press.

Cochran, J. K., Beeghley, L., & Bock, E. W. (1992). The influence of religious stability and homogamy on the relationship between religiosity and alcohol use among Protestants. *Journal of Scientific Study of Religion, 31*, 441–456.

Collett, J. L., Guidry, T. E., Martin, N. J., & Sager, R. (2006). Faith-based decisions? The consequences of heightened religious salience in social service referral decisions. *Journal for the Scientific Study of Religion, 45*, 119–127.

Collins, C. E., Whiters, D. L., & Braithwaite, R. (2007). The Saved Sista Project: A faith-based HIV prevention program for black women in addiction recovery. *American Journal of Health Studies, 22*, 76–82.

Cook, C. C. H (1988a). The Minnesota Model in the management of drug and alcohol dependency: Miracle, method, or myth? Part I. The philosophy and the programme. *British Journal of Addiction, 83*, 625–634.

Cook, C. C. H (1988b). The Minnesota Model in the management of drug and alcohol dependency: Miracle, method, or myth? Part II. Evidence and conclusions. *British Journal of Addiction, 83*, 735–748.

Cook, C. C. H. (2006). *Alcohol, addiction and Christian ethics*. New York: Cambridge University Press.

Cooney, N. L., Babor, T. F., DiClemente, C. C., & Del Boca, F. K. (2003). Clinical and scientific implications of Project MATCH. In T. F. Babor & F. K. Del Boca (Eds.), *Treatment matching in alcoholism* (pp. 222–237). Cambridge: Cambridge University Press.

Core competencies for clergy and other pastoral ministers in addressing alcohol and drug dependence and the impact on family members (2004). DHHS Pub. No. (SMA) 04-3900. Rockville, MD: Center for Substance Abuse Treatment, Substance Abuse and Mental Health Services Administration.

Desmond, D. P., & Maddux, J. F. (1981). Religious programs and careers of chronic heroin users. *American Journal of Drug and Alcohol Abuse, 8*, 71–83.

Dominguez, A. W., Ip, C.-C., Hoover, D., Oleari, A., McMinn, M. R., Lee, T. W. et al. (2006). Faith-based substance abuse treatment programs. In M. R. McMinn & A. W. Dominguez (Eds.), *Psychology and the church* (pp. 19–30). New York: Nova Science.

Doweiko, H. E. (1999). Substance use disorders as a symptom of a spiritual disease. In O. J. Morgan & M. Jordan (Eds.), *Addiction and spirituality: A multidisciplinary approach* (pp. 33–53). St Louis: Chalice Press.

Drerup, M. L. (2005). Religion, spirituality and motives for drinking in an adult community sample. (Doctoral dissertation, Indiana State University). *Dissertation Abstracts International, 66*(12) Jun 2006. (UMI No. 3199426).

Ebaugh, H. R., Chafetz, J. S., & Pipes, P. E. (2006a). The influence of evangelicalism on government funding of faith-based social service organizations. *Review of Religious Research, 47*, 380–392.

Ebaugh, H. R., Chafetz, J. S., & Pipes, P. E. (2006b). Where's the faith in faith-based organizations? Measures and correlates of religiosity in faith-based social service coalitions. *Social Forces, 84*, 2259–2272.

Formicola, J. R., Segers, M. C., & Weber, P. (2003). *Faith-based initiatives and the Bush administration: The good, the bad, and the ugly.* Lanham, MD: Rowman & Littlefield.

Francis, D. J. (June 4, 2005). Faith & values: Recovery church. *Chicago Star Tribune*. Retrieved February 15, 2007, from: http://www.facesandvoicesofrecovery.org/in_the_news/2005-06-04_recovery_church.php.

Francis, L. J. (1992). Attitude towards alcohol, church attendance, and denominational identity, *Drug and Alcohol Dependence, 31*, 45–50.

Francis, L. J. (1997). The impact of personality and religion on attitude towards substance use among 13–15 year olds. *Drug and Alcohol Dependence, 44*, 95–103.

Glasscotte, R. M., Sussex, J. N., Jaffe, J. H., Ball, J., & Brill, L. (1972). *The treatment of drug abuse: Programs, problems, prospects.* Washington, DC: The Joint Information Service of the American Psychiatric Association and the National Association for Mental Health.

Goldfarb, L. M., Galanter, M., McDowell, D., Lifshutz, H., & Dermatis, H. (1996). Medical student and patient attitudes toward religion and spirituality in the recovery process. *American Journal of Drug & Alcohol Abuse, 22*, 549–561.

Gorsuch, R. L. (1995). Religious aspects of substance abuse and recovery. *Journal of Social Issues, 51*, 65–83.

Greenberg, M. A., Wortman, C. B., & Stone, A. A. (1996). Emotional expression and physical health: Revising traumatic memories or fostering self-regulation. *Journal of Personality and Social Psychology, 71*, 588–602.

Groves, P., & Farmer, R. (1994). Buddhism and addictions. *Addiction Research, 2*, 183–194.

Hadaway, C. K., & Marler, P. L. (2005). How many Americans attend worship each week? An alternative approach to measurement. *Journal for the Scientific Study of Religion, 44*, 307–322.

Hess, C. B. (1978). A seven-year follow-up of 186 males in a religious therapeutic community indicates by personal interview and urinalysis that 70% are drug free. 57% never used an illegal drug following graduation from the program. In A. Schecter, H. Alksne, & E. Kaufman (Eds.), Critical concerns in the field of drug abuse: *Proceedings of the Third National Drug Abuse Conference, Inc., New York* (pp. 270–274). New York: Marcel Dekker.

Hill, P. C. (2002). Spiritual transformation: Forming the habitual center of personal energy. *Research in the Social Scientific Study of Religion, 13*, 87–108.

Hill, P. C. (2005). Measurement in the psychology of religion and spirituality: Current status and evaluation. In R. F. Paloutzian & C. L. Park (Eds.), *Handbook of the psychology of religion and spirituality* (pp. 43–61). New York: Guilford.

Hodge, D. R. (2000). The spiritually committed: An examination of the staff at faith-based substance abuse providers. *Social Work & Christianity, 27*, 150–167.

Hughes, C., & Farris, A. (December 12, 2006). *Faith-based organizations serve important role, but need guidance.* Roundtable on Religion and Social Welfare Policy News Release. Retrieved January 31, 2007, from www.socialpolicyandreligion.org/news/article.cfm?id = 5704.

Imani, Z. (1992). *Millati Islami (The Path of Peace): Islamic Treatment for Addiction.* Baltimore: Millati Islami Program, 1997.

Irwin, D. D. (2002). Alternatives to delinquency in Harlem: A study of faith-based community mentoring. *The Justice Professional, 15,* 29–36.

Jang, S. J., & Johnson, S. J. (2001). Neighborhood disorders, individual religiosity, and adolescent use of illicit drugs: A test of multilevel hypotheses. *Criminology, 39,* 109–143.

Johnson, B. R., Tompkins, R. B., & Webb, D. (2002). *Objective hope: Assessing the effectiveness of faith-based organizations: A review of the literature.* Philadelphia: Center for Research on Religion and Urban Civil Society.

Johnson, T. J., Aten, J., Madsen, M., & Bennett, P. (2006, July). *Alcohol use and meaning in life among survivors of hurricane Katrina.* Paper presented at the International Network on Personal Meaning Conference: Meaning and Addiction, Vancouver, British Columbia.

Johnson, T. J., & Cohen, E. A. (2004). College students' reasons for not drinking and not playing drinking games. *Substance Use and Misuse, 39,* 1137–1160.

Johnson, T. J., Sheets, V. L., & Kristeller, J. (2008). Identifying mediators of the relationship between religiousness/spirituality and alcohol use. *Journal of Studies on Alcohol and Drugs, 69,* 160–170.

Johnson, W. B., Ridley, C. R., & Nielsen, S. L. (2000). Religiously sensitive rational emotive behavior therapy: Elegant solutions and ethical risks. *Professional Psychology: Research and Practice, 31,* 14–20.

Judge, J. J. (1971). Alcoholism treatment at the Salvation Army: A new men's social service center. *Quarterly Journal of Studies on Alcohol, 32,* 462–467.

Katz, L. (1964). The Salvation Army men's social service center: I. Program. *Quarterly Journal of Studies on Alcohol, 25,* 324–332.

Katz, L. (1966). The Salvation Army men's social service center: II. Results. *Quarterly Journal of Studies on Alcohol, 27,* 636-647.

Kennedy, S. S., & Bielefeld, W. (2006). *Charitable choice at work: Evaluating faith-based job programs in the states.* Washington, DC: Georgetown University Press.

Koenig, H. G., McCollough, M. E., & Larson, D. B. (2001). *Handbook of religion and health.* NewYork: Oxford University Press.

Kurtz, E. (1979). *Not-God: A history of Alcoholics Anonymous.* Center City, MN: Hazelden.

Lin, W., Mack, D., Enright, R. D., Krahn, D., & Baskin, T.W. (2004). Effects of forgiveness therapy on anger, mood, and vulnerability to substance use among inpatient substance-dependent clients. *Journal of Consulting and Clinical Psychology, 72,* 1114–1121.

MacMaster, S. A., Crawford, S. L., Jones, J. L., Rasch, R. F. R., Thompson, S. J., & Sanders, E. C. (2007). Metropolitan community AIDS network: Faith-based culturally relevant services for African American substance users at risk of HIV. *Health & Social Work, 52,* 151–154.

Marcotte, D., Margolin, A., & Avants, S. K. (2003). Addressing the spiritual needs of a drug user living with human immunodeficiency virus: A case study. *The Journal of Alternative and Complementary Medicine, 9,* 169–175.

Margolin, A., Beitel, M., Schuman-Oliver, Z., & Avants, S.K. (2006). A controlled study of a spirituality-focused intervention for HIV prevention among drug users. *AIDS Education and Prevention, 18,* 311–322.

Mariz, C. L. (1991). Pentecostalism and alcoholism among the Brazilian poor. *Alcoholism Treatment Quarterly, 8,* 75–82.

Mason, W. A., & Windle, M. (2002). A longitudinal study of the effects of religiosity on adolescent alcohol use and alcohol-related problems. *Journal of Adolescent Research, 17,* 346–363.

May, G. G. (1988). *Addiction & grace: Love and spirituality in the healing of addictions.* San Francisco: Harper.

McCoy, L. K., Hermos, J. A., Bokhour, B. G., & Frayne, S. M. (2004). Conceptual bases of Christian, faith-based substance abuse rehabilitation programs qualitative analysis of staff interviews. *Substance Abuse, 25,* 1–11.

McCrady, B. S., Horvath, A. T., & Delany, S. I. (2003). Self-help groups. In R. K. Hester & W. R. Miller (Eds.), *Handbook of alcoholism treatment approaches: Effective alternatives* (3rd ed., pp. 165–187). Boston: Allyn & Bacon.

McCullough, M. E., & Larson, D. B. (1999). Prayer. In W.R. Miller (Ed.), *Integrating spirituality into treatment: Resources for practitioners*, (pp. 85–110). Washington, DC: American Psychological Association.

McNeese, C. A., & DiNitto, D. M. (2005). *Chemical dependency: A systems approach* (3rd ed.). Boston: Allyn & Bacon.

Mercadante, L. (1996). *Victims & sinners: Spiritual roots of addiction and recovery*. Louisville, KY: Westminster John Knox Press.

Miller, G. (2003). *Incorporating spirituality in counseling and psychotherapy: Theory and Technique*. Hoboken, NJ: Wiley.

Miller, W. R. (1998). Researching the spiritual dimensions of alcohol and other drug problems. *Addiction, 93*, 979–990.

Miller W. R., & Hester, R. K. (2003). Treating alcohol problems: Toward an informed eclecticism. In R. K. Hester & W. R. Miller (Eds.), *Handbook of alcoholism treatment approaches: Effective alternatives* (3rd ed., pp. 1–12). Boston: Allyn and Bacon.

Miller, W. R., & Longabough, R. (2003). Summary and conclusions. In T. F. Babor & F. K. Del Boca (Eds.), *Treatment matching in alcoholism* (pp. 207–221). Cambridge, UK: Cambridge University Press.

Miller, W. R., Wilbourne, P. L., & Hettema, J. E. (2003). What works? A summry of alcohol treatment outcome research. In R. K. Hester & W. R. Miller (Eds.), *Handbook of alcoholism treatment approaches: Effective alternatives* (3rd ed., pp. 13–63). Boston: Allyn & Bacon.

Minehan, J. A., Newcomb, M. D., & Galaif, E. R. (2000). Predictors of adolescent drug use: Cognitive abilities, coping strategies and purpose in life. *Journal of Child & Adolescent Substance Abuse, 10*, 33–52.

Moos, R. H., Mehren, B., & Moos, B. S. (1978). Evaluation of a Salvation Army alcoholism treatment program, *Journal of Studies on Alcohol, 39*, 1267–1275.

Murphy, T. S., Pagano, R. R., & Marlatt, G. A. (1986). Lifestyle modification with heavy alcohol drinkers: Effects of aerobic exercise and meditation. *Addictive Behaviors, 11,* 175–186.

NAADAC – National Association of Alcohol and Drug Abuse Counselors (2007). *Issue brief: Access to recovery*. Retrieved January 25, 2007, from http://naadac.org/documents/print.php?DocumentID=100.

Neff, J. A., Shorkey, C. T., & Windsor, L. C. (2006). Contrasting faith-based and traditional substance abuse treatment programs. *Journal of Substance Abuse Treatment, 30*, 49–61.

Nelson, J. B. (2004). *Thirst: God and the alcoholic experience*. Louisville: Westminster John Knox.

Nicholson, T., Higgins, W., Turner, P., James, S., Stickle, F., & Pruitt, T. (1994). The relation between meaning in life and the occurrence of drug abuse: A retrospective study. *Psychology of Addictive Behavior, 1*, 24–28.

Nowinski, J., Baker, S., & Carroll, K. (1992). *Twelve step facilitation manual: A clinical research guide for therapists treating individuals with alcohol abuse and dependence*. Rockville, MD: National Institute on Alcohol Abuse and Alcoholism.

Olitzky, K. M., & Copans, S. A. (1991). *Twelve Jewish steps to recovery: A personal guide to turning from alcoholism and other addictions*. Woodstock, VT: Jewish Lights.

Owen, P. L., Slaymaker, V., Tonigan, J. S., McCrady, B. S., Epstein, E. E., Kaskutas, L. A., et al. (2003). Participation in Alcoholics Anonymous: Intended and unintended change mechanisms. *Alcoholism: Clinical and Experimental Research, 27*, 524–532.

Padelford, B. L. (1974). Relationships between drug involvement and purpose in life, *Journal of Clinical Psychology, 30*, 303–305.

Paloutzian, R. F. (2005). Religious conversion and spiritual transformation: A meaning-system analysis. In R. F. Paloutzian & C. L. Park (Eds.), *Handbook of the psychology of religion and spirituality* (pp. 331–347). New York: Guilford.

Paloutzian, R. F., Richardson, J. R., & Rambo, L. R. (1999). Religious conversion and personality change. *Journal of Personality, 67*, 1047–1079.

Pargament, K. I. (1997). *The psychology of religion and coping: Theory, research, practice*. New York: Guilford.

Pargament, K. I. (2002). The bitter and the sweet: An evaluation of the costs and benefits of religious-ness. *Psychological Inquiry, 13*, 168–181.

Pargament, K. I. (2007). *Spiritually intergrated psychotherapy: Understanding and addressing the sacred.* New York: Guilford.

Pargament, K. I., Ano, G. G., & Wachholtz, A. B. (2005). The religious dimension of coping: Advances in theory, research, and practice. In R. F. Paloutzian & C. L. Park (Eds.) *Handbook of the psychology of religion and spirituality* (pp. 479–495). New York: Guilford.

Park, C. L., & Blumberg, C. J. (2002). Disclosing trauma through writing: Testing the meaning-making hypothesis. *Cognitive Therapy & Research, 26*, 597–616.

Pennebaker, J. W. (1997). *Opening up: The healing power of expressing emotions* (rev. ed.). New York: Guilford Press.

Piedmont, R. L. (2004). Spiritual transcendence as a predictor of psychosocial outcome from an outpa-tient substance abuse program. *Psychology of Addictive Behaviors, 18*, 213–222.

Platinga, C., Jr. (2003). Sin and addiction. In R. C. Roberts & M. R. Talbot (Eds.), *Limning the psyche: Explorations in Christian psychology*. Eugene, OR: Wipf and Stock.

Poole, T. G. (1990). Black families and the black church: A sociohistorical perspective. In Cheatham, H. E., & Stewart, J. B. (Eds), *Black families* (pp. 33–48). New Brunswick, NJ: Transaction.

Richards, P. S., & Bergin, A. E. (2004). *Casebook for a spiritual strategy in counseling and psychotherapy.* Washington, DC: American Psychological Association.

Richards, P. S., & Bergin, A. E. (2005). *A spiritual strategy for counseling and psychotherapy* (2nd ed.). Washington, DC: American Psychological Association.

Rimé, B. (1995). Mental rumination, social sharing, and the recovery from emotional exposure. In Pennebaker, J. W. (Ed.), *Emotion, disclosure, and health* (pp. 271–291). Washington, DC: American Psychological Association.

Ringwald, C. D. (2002). *The soul of recovery: Uncovering the spiritual dimension in the treatment of addic-tions.* New York: Oxford University Press.

Rivers, P. C. (1994). *Alcohol and human behavior: Theory, research and practice.* Englewood Cliffs, NJ: Prentice Hall.

Robinson, E. A. R., Cranford, J. A., Webb, J. R., & Brower, K. J. (2007). Six-month changes in spiritu-ality, religiousness, and heavy drinking in a treatment-seeking sample. *Journal of Studies on Alcohol and Drugs, 68*, 282–290.

SAMHSA (2006). *Targeted outreach: Clergy and faith based groups.* Retrieved February 15, 2007, from download.ncadi.samhsa.gov/recoverymonth/2006/kit/Targeted_Outreach_Pdfs/Clergy.pdf.

Saunders, S. M., Lucas, V., & Kuras, L. (2007). Measuring the discrepancy between current and ideal spiritual and religious functioning in problem drinkers. *Psychology of Addictive Behaviors, 21*, 404–408.

Sexton, R. L., Carlson, R. G., Siegal, H. A., Leukefeld, C. G., & Booth, B. M. (2006). The role of African-American clergy in providing informal services to drug users in the rural south: Preliminary ethnographic findings. *Journal of Ethnicity in Substance Abuse, 5*, 1–21.

Smith, T. B., McCullough, M. E., & Poll, J. (2003). Religiousness and depression: Evidence for a main effect and the moderating influence of stressful life events. *Psychological Bulletin, 129*, 614–636.

Smith, S. R., & Sosin, M. R. (2001). The varieties of faith-related agencies. *Public Administration Review, 61*, 125–141.

Spiegel, M.C., & Kravitz, Y. (2001). Confronting addiction. In D. A. Friedman (Ed.), *Jewish pastoral care: A practical handbook from traditional and contemporary sources* (pp. 264–285).Woodstock, VT: Jewish Lights.

Spilka, B., Hood, R. W., Hunsberger, B., & Gorsuch, R. (2003). *The psychology of religion.* New York: Guilford Press.

Stewart, C., & Bolland, J. M. (2002). Parental style as a possible mediator of the relationship between religiosity and substance use in African-American adolescents. *Journal of Ethnicity in Substance Abuse, 1*, 63–81.

Stoltzfus, K. M. (2006). An elephant in the sanctuary: Denial and resistance in addicted Christians and their churches. *Social Work & Christianity, 33*, 141–163.

Stylianou, S. (2004). The role of religiosity in the opposition to drug use. *International Journal of Offender Therapy and Comparative Criminology, 48*, 429–448.

Suliman, H. (1983). Alcohol and Islamic faith. *Drug and Alcohol Dependence, 11*, 63–65.

Tangenberg, K. (2004). Spirituality and faith-based social services: Exploring provider values, beliefs, and practices. *Journal of Religion & Spirituality in Social Work, 23*, 3–23.

Thombs, D. L. (1999). *Introduction to addictive behaviors* (2nd ed.). New York: Guilford.

Thoresen, C. E., Harris, A. H. S., & Luskin, F. (2000). Forgiveness and health: An unanswered question. In McCullough, M. E., Pargament, K. I., & Thoresen, C. E. (Eds.), *Forgiveness: Theory, research, and practice* (pp. 254–280). New York: Guilford Press.

Tonigan, J. S., Connors, G. J., & Miller, W. R. (2003). Participation and involvement in Alcoholics Anonymous. In T. F. Babor & F. K. Del Boca (Eds.), *Treatment matching in alcoholism* (pp. 184–204). Cambridge, UK: Cambridge University Press.

Tonigan, J. S., Miller, W. R., & Shermer, C. (2002). Atheists, agnostics and Alcoholics Anonymous. *Journal of Studies on Alcohol, 63*, 534–541.

Tonigan, J. S., Toscova, R., & Miller, W. R. (1996). Meta-analysis of the literature on Alcoholics Anonymous: Sample and study characteristics moderate findings. *Journal of Studies on Alcohol, 57*, 65–72.

Unruh, H. R., & Sider, R. J. (2005). *Saving souls, serving society: Understading the faith factor in church-based social ministry.* New York: Oxford University Press.

VandeCreek, L., Janus, M. D., Pennebaker, J. W., & Binau, B. (2002). Praying about difficult experiences as self-disclosure to God. *The International Journal for the Psychology of Religion, 12*, 29–39.

Vex, S. L., & Blume, S. B. (2001). The JACS Study I: Characteristics of a population of chemically dependent Jewish men and women. *Journal of Addictive Diseases, 20*, 75–94.

Waisberg, J. L., & Porter, J. E. (1994). Purpose in life and outcome of treatment for alcohol dependence. *British Journal of Clinical Psychology, 33*, 49–63.

Weitzman, E. R., & Chen, Y.-Y. (2005). Risk modifying effect of social capital on measures of heavy alcohol consumption, alcohol abuse, and secondhand effects: National survey findings. *Journal of Epidemiology & Community Health, 59*, 303–309.

Weitzman, E. R., & Kawachi, I. (2000). Giving means receiving: The protective effect of social capital on binge drinking on college campuses. *American Journal of Public Health, 90*, 1936–1939.

White, W. L., & Whiters, D. (October, 2005). Faith-based recovery: Its historical roots. *Counselor, The Magazine for Addiction Professionals, 6*, 58–62.

Witkiewitz, K., Marlatt, G. A., & Walker, D. (2005). Mindfulness-based relapse prevention for alcohol and substance use disorders. *Journal of Cognitive Psychotherapy: An International Quarterly, 19*, 211–228.

Wilkerson, D., Sherrill, J., & Sherrill, E. (1986). *The cross and the switchblade* (reissue edition). New York: Jove Books.

Wills, T. A., Yaeger, A. M., & Sandy, J. M. (2003). Bufffering effect of religiosity for adolescent substance abuse. *Psychology of Addictive Behaviors, 17*, 24–31.

Winters, K. C., Stinchfield, R. D., Opland, E., Weller, C., & Latimer, W. W. (2000). The effectiveness of the Minnesota Model approach in the treatment of adolescent drug abusers. *Addiction, 95*, 601–612.

Winzelberg, A., & Humphreys, K. (1999). Should patients' religiosity influence clinicians' referral to 12-step self-help groups? Evidence from a study of 3,018 male substance abuse patients. *Journal of Consulting and Clinical Psychology, 67*, 790–794.

Witvliet, C. V., Ludwig, T. E., & Vander Laan, K. L. (2001). Granting forgiveness or harboring grudges: Implications for emotion, physiology, and health. *Psychological Science, 12*, 117–123.

Wolfe, A. (2003). *The transformation of American religion: How we actually live our faith.* New York: Free Press.

Wuthnow, R. (2000). How religious groups promote forgiving: A national study. *Journal for the Scientific Study of Religion, 39*, 125–139.

Wuthnow, R. (2004). *Saving America: Faith-based services and the future of civil society.* Princeton, NJ; Princeton University Press.

Wuthnow, R., & Evans, J. H. (2002). Introduction. In R. Wuthnow & J. H. Evans (Eds.) *The quiet hand of God: Faith-based activism and the public role of mainline Protestantism* (pp. 1–24). Berkeley: University of California Press.

28

Future of Treatment for Substance Use: A View from 2009

Kenneth J. Sher and Julia A. Martinez

University of Missouri

Contents

There have never been more evidence-based treatments for substance dependence and substance use as there are at present. Although this statement may seem tautological (because, presumably, the number of evidence-based treatments can only grow over time), the issue of note is that recent years have witnessed an explosion of new treatment options that did not exist until recently. Some of these new treatments appear to have considerably greater efficacy than prior treatments (e.g., varenicline for tobacco dependence; Jorenby et al., 2006), some appear to work in ways entirely differently than previously available treatments (e.g., topiramate for alcohol dependence; Johnson, 2005), and some represent new compounds developed for treating one or more forms of substance dependence or represent new indications for established compounds (e.g., buprenorphine to treat concurrent opiate and cocaine dependence; Montoya et al., 2004). Clearly, the trends that led to these innovations should be expected to continue.

Attempting to predict future developments in any area of science is always hazardous and the history of the treatment of substance dependence is littered with numerous trends, fads, and disappointments (White, 1998). Although often based upon our best science and compelling in principle, objective assessment of efficacy and/or tolerability often dashes the hopes of both the developers of new approaches and those supporting their efforts (e.g., drug companies, funding agencies). We do not have to look far to see disappointing findings associated with initially promising psychological treatments (e.g., cue exposure; Conklin & Tiffany, 2002) or pharmacological treatments (e.g., cannabinoid receptor antagonists; Soyka et al., 2008) that fail to live up to our initial hopes.

Thus, in attempting to preview the future, we can at best point to what types of novel treatments or improved treatments might be explored and why it would be worthwhile to explore them. This is still important because substance use disorders represent some of the most prevalent mental disorders in the United States (e.g., Kessler, Chiu, Demler, & Walters, 2005), imposing tremendous suffering to afflicted individuals, their friends, and families (Room, Graham, Rehm, Jernigan, & Monteiro, 2003), as well as considerable economic costs to society (e.g., Cartwright, 2008). For example, it was estimated that in one year alone, the United States shouldered approximately $98.5 billion in losses attributable to substance use (i.e., deaths, incarcerations; Cartwright, 2008).

In conceptualizing where new treatments are likely to come from, it is important to consider evolving concepts of the etiology and course of substance use and dependence because basic etiological research can suggest new approaches or "targets" for the development of novel interventions. It is also important to recognize that treatments can work independently of etiology if enough is known concerning the systems that can influence the expression of substance-related behavior.

Impelling Versus Restraining Tendencies and the Implications for Treatment Interventions

As noted by Orford (2001), we can view addictive behavior as the product of competing restraining and impelling forces that manifests itself when the balance of these forces tips in favor of expression. From this perspective, treatments can be developed to either: (1) strengthen restraint or (2) reduce underlying substance-seeking tendencies. In addition, we can add that (3) the availability of the addictive substance is a necessary precondition for the expression of addiction, suggesting that the battle between impelling forces can only meaningfully occur if the addictive substance is available. Although traditionally alcohol and drug availability have been conceptualized as physical availability and controlled through social policies such as prohibition in the form of illegal substances or various restrictions on sales (e.g., price, limiting the number and types of vendors, age restrictions on purchases) on legal substances, some types of pharmacological strategies block availability of a consumed substance to key neural circuits either through pharmacological blockage of critical neural receptors (e.g., naltrexone;

Littleton & Zieglagänsberger, 2003) or by preventing the drug from crossing the blood–brain barrier (e.g., drug vaccines; Haney & Kosten, 2005). Although in prosecuting a crime we must establish that a suspect has the means, motive, and opportunity to have committed that crime, in identifying promising treatments, any of the three components might lead to a potentially useful therapeutic approach.

Historically, most treatments have focused on supporting restraining forces (e.g., self-help groups, contingency management) although a number of pharmacological approaches target the incentive value of drugs with agonist (Cousins, Roberts, & de Wit, 2002) and partial agonist (e.g., varenicline; Keating & Siddiqui, 2006) approaches. The issue of whether aversion treatments, when effective, primarily strengthen restraint or reduce incentive value is complex and it seems likely that these forms of treatment can affect both aspects of restraint and approach.

New Targets for Drug Development

Neuropharmacologists are attempting to identify new targets for drug development and test compounds that may work on these targets that can be thought of as directly affecting impelling and restraining tendencies. The range of systems that are being studied is extremely broad and encompasses systems involved in drug reward, attentional processing, withdrawal symptomatology, general inhibitory and excitatory systems, and chronic stress reactions, employing compounds directly interacting with systems involving dopamine, serotonin, GABA, glutamate, (nicotinic and muscarinic) cholinergic systems, and the HPA axis (Heidbreder & Hagan, 2005; Please also see Koob in this volume), as well as immunotherapeutic approaches that prevent drugs such as nicotine, cocaine, and methamphetamine from crossing the blood–brain barrier (e.g., Kantak, 2003; Kosten & Owens, 2005). The range of potentially useful targets increases proportionally as the basic neurobiology of addiction continues to be characterized more fully.

For those drugs that are already FDA-approved but with indications for conditions other than substance dependence (e.g., topiramate for alcohol dependence; Johnson, 2005), it is not clear if drug companies will pursue substance-related indications and the effect of this on dissemination is not clear. Also, as discussed below, there remains a gap between what is known to be effective from efficacy trials and what is practiced in the clinic and community. It is important that barriers to dissemination of effective treatments do not unduly affect drug discovery and development efforts. That is, the basic science of addiction is providing numerous opportunities to develop novel treatments but for these efforts to continue it is important that pharmacological interventions are viewed favorably by providers and payers. If they are not, the stream of innovation may be narrowed.

Specific Versus General Disorder and Implications for Treatment

Substance use disorders are not only among the most common mental disorders (Kessler et al., 2005) catalogued in the *Diagnostic and Statistical Manual of Mental Disorders–IV* (DSM; American Psychiatric Association, 2000), they are also among the most comorbid with other

Axis I (Grant et al., 2004; Kessler, Chiu, Demler, & Walters, 2005) and Axis II (Grant et al., 2004; Trull, Sher, Minks-Brown, Durbin, & Burr, 2000) disorders. This high comorbidity has important implications for both conceptualizing the nature of disorder and the range of potential interventions.

Substance Use Disorders and the Externalizing Spectrum

Investigations into the dimensional and hierarchical structure of mental disorders consistently show that substance use disorders (specifically, alcohol use disorders and drug use disorders) are strongly related to other externalizing pathology such as conduct disorder and adult anti-social behavior leading some theorists to view these disorders as specific manifestations of a general externalizing problem (Krueger, 1999; Krueger, Markon, Patrick, & Iacono, 2005). From this perspective, alcohol and drug use disorders represent a general form of behavior disorder characterized by underlying vulnerabilities common to a range of other externalizing disorders (Iacono, 1998; Krueger et al., 2002; Sher & Slutske, 2003), perhaps most notably, specific forms of impulsivity (Smith et al., 2007; Whiteside & Lynam, 2003). This view of alcohol and drug use disorders as somewhat nonspecific manifestations of general external-izing behavior has its roots in psychometric studies of childhood and adolescent psychopathol-ogy (Achenbach & Edelbrock, 1978) and adolescent problem behavior (Donovan & Jessor, 1985; Jessor, Donovan, & Costa, 1991) but is gaining increasing currency as problems with current diagnostic systems come to the fore and there is accumulating evidence for many com-mon etiological factors across ostensibly distinct forms of psychopathology.

If we take the viewpoint that much of the underlying pathology of substance use dis-orders is attributable to externalizing psychopathology, an important target for treatment becomes strengthening self-regulation or self-control. Although traditionally self-regulation has been viewed as a relatively stable individual trait and measured by traditional personality traits measures such as "constraint" (Tellegen, 1994) and "conscientiousness" (e.g., Costa & McCrae, 1992), recent research suggests that there are highly mutable aspects of self-con-trol. Indeed, Muraven and Baumeister (2000) argue that self-control is "like a muscle" and, analogously, can be strengthened through regular use, decrease with lack of use, and exhibit short-term fatigue after recent use. This somewhat optimistic view of self-control provides novel approaches for training or rehabilitating self-control in persons suffering from substance use disorders and holds out the promise for highly generalized treatments across a range of externalizing problems and impediments to healthy functioning in school, the labor market, interpersonal relationships, and the more general pursuit of long-term goals. Some examples of self-control "exercises" which have led to improvements in other self-regulatory behaviors, such as smoking fewer cigarettes and drinking less alcohol, include regular physical exercise, dietary monitoring, money management planning and working on improving study habits (Baumeister, Gailliot, DeWall, & Oaten, 2006). Additionally, it has been shown that self-control behaviors, including smoking cessation, are improved by restoring individuals' blood glucose to a sufficient level (Gailliot & Baumeister, 2007). It seems likely that we will con-tinue to see the development of a wide range of approaches that target self-control as a general treatment strategy for successful and healthy living. These interventions could span the range of current treatments including behavioral approaches, cognitive-behavioral approaches, mindfulness training (Baer, 2003), and pharmacological interventions that target neural circuitry involved in self-regulation (Baumeister & Vohs, 2004).

Treatments for Individuals at Various Stages of Dependence

It has now been approximately 20 years since two Institute of Medicine (IOM) reports (IOM, 1989, 1990) attempted to identify new avenues for addressing alcohol problems in our society. The IOM recognized the need to broaden the base of treatment (IOM, 1990), move away from a near exclusive focus on the small subpopulation of the most severe cases, and recommended the development and testing of treatments for the entire population affected by alcohol. Looking back at the range of substance use and related problems and at the diversity of substance-using populations that have been targeted in recent years, these reports do seem prescient. Moreover, the changing definitions of substance use disorders over successive revisions of the DSM (American Psychiatric Association, 1980, 1987, 1994) highlights the limitations of only treating those who meet formal diagnostic criteria for a given substance use disorder.

Extending treatment to "less severe" cases requires not only developing new treatment approaches such as brief intervention and motivational interviewing (Dunn, Deroo, & Rivara, 2002; Moyer, Finney, Swearingen, & Vergun, 2002) but also suggests the utility of innovative modifications of existing treatments. For example, naltrexone which was originally approved for treatment for alcohol dependence (O'Malley et al., 1992) has been reformulated in a long-acting, injectable form (Garbutt et al., 2005) that might be useful for treating severe levels of dependence characterized by poor compliance. At the other end of the scale, there have been studies documenting the viability of using "targeted" (i.e., situational) dosing of naltrexone for "early problem drinkers" (Kranzler et al., 2003). Thus, with respect to broadening the base of treatment to a wider spectrum of the substance-using population, we can think of innovations that are both wider (i.e., bringing in new approaches) and deeper (i.e., tailoring existing approaches to a more diverse range of clients).

Patient–Treatment Matching Revisited

Although empirical evidence in support of patient–treatment matching has been equivocal (e.g., Project MATCH Research Group, 1997), this does not mean the general strategy is flawed and further efforts should be abandoned. A potential limitation of major efforts such as Project Match (Project MATCH Research Group, 1997) is that the designers of these studies examined previously established treatments and then hypothesized individual differences in treatment responsiveness conditional upon treatment strategy. Although a reasonable strategy to explore, other, more etiologically relevant approaches to patient–treatment matching may be more useful. For example, rather than taking previously established treatments as a starting point and then assessing relevant individual differences that may moderate treatment effects, the reverse strategy could be employed. For example, one could look at important individual differences (e.g., personality, motives for substance use) and develop treatments targeted at predominant substance use motivations. Such an approach has been explored by Conrod, Stewart, and their colleagues (2000) who have suggested that classifying individuals by differences in factors such as anxiety, sensitivity, and sensation-seeking tends to reveal groups who are also different in terms of addictive psychopathology and coping skills deficits, and that these differences may be used as specific targets for intervention. That is, interventions that target individuals' particular underlying motivations for use are more effective than interventions which do not target such underlying motivations (Conrod, Castellanos, & Mackie, 2008; Conrod et al., 2000).

Perhaps nowhere is the promise of patient–treatment matching more exciting than in the area of pharmacogenomics. A vision of the NIH is personalized medicine where preventive and treatment efforts are tailored to an individual's unique health profile informed by genomics, proteomics, and other relevant fields (Culliton, 2006; Zerhouni, 2006). Pharmacogenomics represents one facet of personalized medicine and is the field that addresses how specific pharmacological treatments interact in unique ways with an individual's genotype (please see Ray & Hutchison in this volume).

Because substance use disorders arise from the use of specific drugs and there is genetic variation in susceptibility to different drugs of abuse, pharmacogenomics play an increasingly important part in our understanding of substance use disorder etiology, holding out hope that we will be able to profile risk based on an individual's genomic profile and that a long-term goal of modern health care research is not only health care in the future to be more personalized but also to make it predictive (i.e., anticipating the health risks before manifest disorder based on individual characteristics) and pre-emptive (i.e., intervening to prevent the development of specific diseases; Zerhouni, 2006). At present, such models for medicine are aspirational but as we know more about how specific genes work to promote the development of dependence, we will have a rational guide for devising pharmacological strategies to pre-emptively intervene early in the course of the disorder (e.g., Edenberg & Kranzler, 2005). However, given the relatively small effect sizes associated with vulnerability genes for most mental disorders (including substance use disorders; Kendler, Myers, & Prescott, 2007), it is not clear how effective pre-emptive interventions based on genotype alone are likely to be.

However, data are beginning to accrue which indicate that there are important, genetically based individual differences in response to medications used to treat substance dependence. Among the most discussed of these is a report by Oslin et al. (2003; see also Oslin, Berttini, & O'Brien, 2006) which found that allelic variation in the μ-opioid receptor moderated treatment response to naltrexone in alcohol-dependent individuals. In this study, the treatment effect for naltrexone varied as a function of genotype which, in turn, was unrelated to outcome in the placebo arm of the study. Given the range of neuronal systems targeted by existing treatments and rapidly increasing knowledge concerning functional polymorphisms associated with these systems, we can expect rapid accumulation of findings concerning the extent to which relevant genotypes are important etiologically with respect to moderating reinforcing effects of psychoactive substances and with respect to moderating treatment effects (e.g., Edenberg & Kranzler, 2005; Kenna, McGeary, & Swift, 2004a, 2004b; Lichtermann, Franke, Maier, & Rao, 2000).

Reexamining Existing Treatments in Light of Evolving Science

As science progresses, theories are revised in light of new data and new insights. Even some of the most basic notions of behavioral science are revised in light of continuing research. For example, principles of learning (especially operant and Pavolovian conditioning) have guided the development of treatments for substance dependence for many years including aversion therapies (e.g., emetic and covert conditioning for alcohol dependence; Howard, 2001) and extinction-based procedures such as cue-exposure treatments (Heather & Bradley, 1990).

However, in recent years, our views of what takes place in both acquiring and retrieving conditioned associations and during extinction has changed considerably. For example, the great importance of context on learning (especially for later learning which would be important in changing problematic behaviors) is being increasingly recognized (Bouton, 2000, 2002). Perhaps more important, the notion that extinction and counterconditioning procedures "destroy" prior learning is most likely incorrect and, extinction, rather than causing "unlearning" most likely lays down alternative learning that competes with what was learned previously (Bouton, 2002). Conklin and Tiffany (2002) describe a number of ways we can use new knowledge regarding the nature of conditioning to develop more effective exposure-based treatments that have greater potential to be durable and show clinically necessary generalization.

Additionally, as the neurobiology of learning continues to unfold, we can hope to develop various pharmacological interventions to facilitate the degree of learning that occurs. For example, recent research has shown promising effects of D-cycloserine (a partial NMDA receptor agonist) on facilitating extinction learning in the treatment of phobias in humans (Ressler et al., 2004) and preclinical work suggests that certain compounds can modulate the nature of drug-related associations in rodents (Feltenstein & See, 2007; Schroeder & Packard, 2004). Thus it seems likely that treatment approaches that have been found to be of limited effectiveness can be revisited and tweaked to improve the likelihood of obtaining clinically meaningful behavior change.

Are there Secular Changes in the Nature of Substance Dependence and its Responsiveness to Treatment?

Just as the Red Queen in *Through the Looking Glass* (Carroll, 1871) noted "it takes all the running you can do, to keep in the same place," cultural changes in norms surrounding substance use and related problems and effective prevention programs could result in the need to constantly upgrade the efficacy of treatments just to maintain the success rates of treatments today. Breslau, Johnson, Hiripi, and Kessler (2001) found that individuals from more recent birth cohorts were less likely to use tobacco products than those from earlier birth cohorts but the risk of tobacco dependence among smokers was substantially higher in the more recent cohorts. In attempting to explain this phenomenon, the authors speculated that "the growing awareness of the addictive potential of smoking and its adverse health effects has resulted in declining numbers who take up smoking. Those in recent cohorts who do take up smoking might be more deviant than smokers in earlier cohorts with respect to personality traits that influence smoking and the progression to nicotine dependence (e.g., risk taking, impulsivity)" (p. 815). Based on this type of explanation, it is a reasonable hypothesis that the average severity of dependence among those using is likely to be higher when public health efforts or cultural change alter the distribution of severity (or comorbid psychopathology, or interest in behavior change) so that there is relatively little "low hanging fruit" with respect to treatment. Although it is not clear if cessation rates among treatment-seeking individuals have gone down overall in recent years, some subpopulations of tobacco-dependent individuals (e.g., chronically mentally ill) may represent "hardened" populations that are less treatment responsive and represent a growing percentage of the population (see also Hughes & Brandon 2003; Warner & Burns, 2003). The major point here is that substance-dependent individuals in the future may differ from those who are being treated today. As we increase our ability to prevent and successfully treat an increasing proportion of affected individuals, the remaining population of treatment-resistant individuals can present new challenges and highlight the need for continuing innovation.

If you Build it will they Come? Disseminating and Paying for New Treatments

Regardless of the efficacy of new and existing treatments, their effectiveness in dealing with the burden of substance-related disorder and disability will be limited if they are not employed by "real-world" providers with treatment-seeking populations. Unfortunately, the area of substance abuse treatment has been slow to adopt evidence-based treatments and, at least with respect to alcohol use disorders, it's been claimed that "the most effective treatments … are least often used … whereas the least effective treatments are most often used" (Gotham, 2004, p. 160). Barriers to successful diffusion of substance use disorder treatments from research settings to community settings occur at each step of the dissemination process; including the level of patients, counselors, supervisors, administrators, and the treatment delivery system (Fals-Stewart, Logsdon, & Birchler, 2004). Developing and evaluating strategies for successful implementation of evidence-based practices should be a major focus of treatment-related research in the future. Models of technology transfer (e.g., Rogers, 2003) may represent one useful approach to conceptualizing diffusion of innovation and actively seeding new treatments in appropriate settings (see Gotham, 2004) but until there are major changes in our ability to successfully diffuse new treatments into the clinic, our ability to improve real-world treatment outcomes will be severely limited.

It is somewhat dismaying that, at present, there has been relatively poor diffusion of efficacious pharmacotherapies for substance dependence into clinical practice. Although changes in mental health and substance abuse parity laws may alter the landscape in the near future, pharmacological interventions appear to be utilized at a very low rate. For example, in 2001, costs associated with medications for treatment of substance abuse in the United States represented less than 1% of the total costs of treatments (Mark et al., 2005). Moreover, access to pharmacological treatments for substance dependence is often highly restricted by private insurers. For example, buprenorphine is often excluded entirely from the formularies of private insures and when it is included, is included only in the highest cost-sharing tier (Horgan, Reif, Hodgkin, Garnick, & Merrick, 2008). Horgan et al. found that of three medications surveyed (naltrexone, disulfiram, and burprenorphine), only generic naltrexone was invariably included in the formulary and placed in a less expensive tier. Systematic data on insurance coverage of other expensive medications that either have FDA indications for substance dependence (e.g., depot naltrexone, and varenicline) or used off-label but with reasonable empirical support (e.g., topiramate) are not readily available but given existing practice would appear to receive only limited coverage by insurers at present.

Clearly, the future of substance dependence treatment requires not only the continued development of efficacious treatments but concerted efforts by treatment developers, treatment providers, and other stakeholders to disseminate these into practice. Thoughtful implementation plans, perhaps coordinated by government agencies (e.g., Saxon & McCarty, 2005) are probably necessary when the nature of treatments and how they are delivered pose systemic changes to provider networks and treatment systems. Implementation of costly treatments, especially to drug abusers who are often dependent upon public treatment systems, will require careful cost-benefit analyses if public and private payers of treatment will be persuaded of the value of providing and paying for expensive new treatments (Cartwright, 2000; Cartwright & Solano, 2003).

Innovations in Assessment

At present, there is an abundance of useful tools for the clinician and the researcher interested in assessing substance use and dependence. These include: structured diagnostic interviews for assessing substance use disorders and related psychopathology (Cottler et al., 1997), clinician and patient rating scales for assessing various aspects of dependence (Heatherton, Kozlowski, Frecker, & Fagerstrom, 2006; McLellan, Luborsky, Woody, & O'Brien, 1980; Wanberg, Horn, & Foster, 1985), timeline follow-back interviews (Sobell & Sobell, 1992) for taking detailed retrospective assessments of substance use, measures of constructs related to substance use motivations such as explicit outcome expectancies (Fromme & D'Amico, 2000; Wetter et al., 1994) for different substances and "reasons" for use (Cooper, Russell, Skinner, & Windle, 1992), specialized measures of dependence-related concepts such as "restraint" (Collins & Lapp, 2006) and craving (Sayette et al., 2000), and many more. Most of these assessments are based on traditional approaches to test/measure development via self-report or observation.

In attempting to identify new assessment approaches that are likely candidates for wider use in the future, three emerging technologies that represent a break with tradition stand out. These include the use of electronic diaries for assessing individuals in their natural environments in real time, the use of implicit measures of cognition to capture substance-relevant motivation that is automatic and possibly outside of one's awareness, and transdermal real-time monitoring of substance use.

The use of electronic diaries (usually palmtop computers) to assess substance use and relevant covariates in real-time and in their natural environments is referred to by a number of terms including ecological momentary assessment (EMA), electronic diaries, experience sampling, and real-time data capture (see Piasecki, Hufford, Solhan, & Trull, 2007; Shiffman, Stone, & Hufford, 2008). Although this technology has been increasingly applied to studying a range of psychological phenomena and health-related behaviors, it has shown particular promise for the study of substance use and its correlates. Using these techniques, individuals can record their substance use as it occurs in their day-to-day life along with the contexts surrounding use, stressors, moods, reasons for use, and activities engaged in throughout the day. These electronic diaries can be flexibly programmed to correspond to the needs of an assessment protocol and have been useful in the study of the situational determinants of use and consequences. Because they can provide exquisitely sensitive data on the patterning of substance use, these techniques can provide useful baseline, process, and outcome data in formal clinical trials as well as "real-life" treatment. Although their primary application has been within the context of formal research studies of substance use and substance abuse treatment, the proliferation of smart phones with graphical interfaces and wireless connectivity suggests that this type of assessment can be ported to individuals' own personal communication devices and flexibly incorporated into ongoing treatment.

Another emerging trend is the application of various implicit cognitive measures of substance use motivation and related constructs. Traditionally, most substance use and dependence assessments have been "explicit," meaning that patients are asked to provide voluntary self-reports on their substance use and related variables. In contrast, implicit measurement approaches refer to a range of indirect measures that assess automatic cognitive processes that might be outside of ones awareness. As noted by Wiers and Stacy (2006), these approaches have great potential for supplementing traditional approaches because they "assess cognitive processes that are unavailable to introspection, ... are less sensitive to self-justification and social desirability, ... explain unique variance or different aspects of behavior [than explicit measures ... and provide] ... a new important bridge between diverse disciplines as well as human and animal research on addiction" (p. 1). Indeed, implicit measures can be used to assess what are possibly core features of dependence such as incentive salience (Robinson & Berridge, 1993) by objectively assessing the extent that substance-related stimuli can "grab" one's attention or are positively or negatively valenced. Indeed, as we have argued elsewhere (Sher, Wolf, & Martinez, in press), these measures might be particularly useful for tracking the course of dependence, even in individuals who are abstinent and "recovering" from substance dependence.

Although the implicit measurement approach is compelling on a theoretical level, at present these measures have not met the psychometric standards that are expected in clinical assessment instruments (Buchner & Wippich, 2000; Cunningham, Preacher, & Banaji, 2002) and most practicing substance abuse clinicians and counselors are not accustomed to employing cognitive measures in their practice (neuropsychologists being an obvious exception to this generalization). However, if the promise of implicit measurement is fulfilled, then it seems likely that clinicians will find supplementation of explicit measures with implicit ones to be clinically highly useful.

There is a long history of using biomarkers from urine, blood, expired air for assessing baseline levels of substance use and treatment compliance (Allen, Litten, Strid, & Sillanauke, 2001; Lakshman & Tsutsumi, 2001; McClure, 2002), and biomarker research remains an active area of clinical research. However, traditionally, biomarker assessments are conducted at the clinic during patient visits and are therefore not useful for characterizing the timing patterning of substance use. Indeed, because most biomarkers are used for screening and assessing compliance or abstinence, they ideally have a fairly long half-life so that recent use can be detected over a period of days. Similar to EMA approaches described above, the ability to objectively assess drug exposure in real-time and in the natural environment is of great potential clinically and holds the potential for both improving the validity of EMA reports of use (i.e., patients know that objective measurements of substances are being taken and should be extra-motivated to be accurate) and capturing substance use with patients noncompliant with EMA.

Although still in its infancy, real-time objective assessment of substance use has proven to be feasible. For example, Swift (2000) and Sakai, Mikulich-Gilbertson, Long, and Crowley (2006) have shown that transdermal ethanol sensors (i.e., wearable electrochemical devices that sample the concentration of alcohol in sweat) are a valid means of measuring blood alcohol concentrations (BAC), aligning well with breath measures of BAC; additionally, they can easily be worn in drinking environments and can continuously sample the BAC over time. Further development of this technique to make it robust enough for clinical practice and extension of real-time, objective, in vivo, assessment of substance use or exposure to other substances could represent an extraordinary leap forward for the assessment of substance use.

Delivering Addiction Services over the Internet

The development of the Internet, especially over the past 10 years, has changed the way a number of human activities are conducted ranging from delivery of news and entertainment, shopping, information retrieval, and forming and maintaining interpersonal relations to name just a few. The Internet's ability to engage individuals who are widely dispersed geographically, at low cost and efficiently, and with a degree of anonymity represents just a few features that make it attractive as a means for delivering services to persons with substance use disorders. Internet interventions for nicotine and alcohol use disorders have been proliferating for several years and, although varying in form and content, often include screening tools, informational resources and links, online journals, and discussion forums (Copeland & Martin, 2004). Those interventions can be easily disseminated, are conveniently available at all hours of the day (making them particularly useful for some subpopulations such as college students, Escoffery et al., 2005), are readily accessible to a large proportion of substance users at present (Cunningham, Peter, Kypri, & Hymphreys, 2006), can provide rapid questionnaire feedback, and may be less expensive than traditional therapy involving face-to-face contact, on site, with a therapist or even telephone-based treatments (Walker, Roffman, Picciano, & Stephens, 2007).

The potential reach of the Internet for various forms of social networking is almost limitless and online affiliation with a wide range of different substance recovery groups (e.g., Alcoholics

Anonymous, Narcotics Anonymous, and Smart Recovery) has gained popularity among recovering substance users throughout the world (Hall & Tidwell, 2003). It seems likely that the Internet's ability to foster virtual communities of individuals with common interests could provide new opportunities for various social support and recovery groups.

To date, little is known concerning the relative effectiveness of Internet-based interventions compared to more traditionally administered interventions. The few existing studies examining the efficacy of these types of interventions produce inconsistent results, perhaps because so little is known at present about the precise mechanisms that would make these types of interventions work most effectively (Bewick et al., 2008). Consequently, we do not yet know how to optimize Internet-based services, for whom they are most appropriate (Copeland & Martin, 2004), and how best to integrate these services into the broader health care system.

In predicting the future of treatment for substance use disorders, one prediction seems almost certain; the Internet will become an increasing presence in our lives and come to serve increasing functions including those related to substance use treatment. As the portability of the web continues to increase (i.e., the "mobile Web") with smartphones on high-speed data networks, each individual has increased opportunity to access some forms of services at a time and place that is convenient for them.

Along with these opportunities come new challenges such as insuring the quality of services provided, confidentiality of "patient" data, continuum of care, licensing of providers, and legal and administrative issues related to the geographic location of service delivery. It is anticipated that, over time, the market and cultural forces coupled with provider concerns will likely goad integration of the Internet into the larger health care delivery system.

Concluding Comments

At present, research on substance abuse treatment is proceeding at an exciting pace and along numerous fronts. Advances in basic biomedical and behavioral research provide an ever-flowing source of knowledge for refining current interventions and developing new ones. The technological revolution that has led to the penetration of the Internet into many facets of our daily lives presents new opportunities for both assessing and treating substance use and dependence. Although all of these new opportunities present challenges, perhaps the biggest challenges are those that have plagued the area of substance abuse treatment for many years, the all-too-frequent failure for evidence-based practices to be incorporated into standard care. Although some highly efficacious treatments have been around for many years (e.g., community reinforcement and contingency management approaches; Gianini, Lundy, & Smith in this volume; Hunt & Azrin, 1973) and are repeatedly shown to have some of the highest effect sizes in the substance abuse treatment literature, they are often not provided in the community (Dutra et al., 2008). If past is prologue to the future, we might expect the future to show a dramatically improved state-of-the-art and a disappointing level of standard care.

References

Achenbach, T. M., & Edelbrock, C. S. (1978). The classification of child psychopathology: A review and analysis of empirical efforts. *Psychological Bulletin, 85,* 1275–1301.

Allen, J. P., Litten, R. Z., Strid, N., & Sillanauke, P. (2001). The role of biomarkers in alcoholism medication trials. *Alcoholism: Clinical and Experimental Research, 25,* 1119–1125.

American Psychiatric Association. (1980). *Diagnostic and statistical manual of mental disorders* (3rd ed.). Washington, DC: Author.

American Psychiatric Association. (1987). *Diagnostic and statistical manual of mental disorders* (3rd ed., revised). Washington, DC: Author.

American Psychiatric Association. (1994). *Diagnostic and statistical manual of mental disorders* (4th ed.). Washington, DC: Author.

American Psychiatric Association. (2000). *Diagnostic and statistical manual of mental disorders* (4th ed., Text Revision). Washington, DC: Author.

Baer, R. A. (2003). Mindfulness training as a clinical intervention: A conceptual and empirical review. *Clinical Psychology: Science and Practice, 10,* 125–143.

Baumeister, R. F., Gailliot, M., DeWall, C. N., & Oaten, M. (2006). Self-regulation and personality: How interventions increase regulatory success, and how depletion moderates the effects of traits on behavior. *Journal of Personality, 74,* 1173–1802.

Baumeister, R. F., &Vohs, K. D. (Eds.). (2004). *Handbook of self-regulation: Research, theory and applications.* New York: Guilford.

Bewick, B. M., Trusler, K., Barkham, M., Hill, A. J., Cahill, J., & Mulhern, B. (2008). The effectiveness of web-based interventions designed to decrease alcohol consumption—a systematic review. *Preventive Medicine, 47,* 17–26.

Bouton, M. E. (2000). A learning theory perspective on lapse, relapse, and the maintenance of behavior change. *Health Psychology, 19*(Suppl. 1), 57–63.

Bouton, M. E. (2002). Context, ambiguity, and unlearning: Sources of relapse after behavioral extinction. *Biological Psychiatry, 52,* 976–986.

Breslau, N., Johnson, E. O., Hiripi, E., & Kessler, R. (2001). Nicotine dependence in the United States: Prevalence, trends and smoking persistence. *Archives of General Psychiatry, 58,* 810–816.

Buchner, A., & Wippich, W. (2000). On the reliability of implicit and explicit memory measures. *Cognitive Psychology, 40,* 227–259.

Carroll, L. (1871). *Through the looking-glass: And what Alice found there.* London: Macmillan.

Cartwright, W. S. (2000). Cost-benefit analysis of drug treatment services: Review of the literature. *The Journal of Mental Health Policy and Economics, 3,* 11–26.

Cartwright, W. S. (2008). Economic costs of drug abuse: Financial, cost of illness, and services. *Journal of Substance Abuse Treatment, 34,* 224–233.

Cartwright, W. S., & Solano, P. L. (2003). The economics of public health: Financing drug abuse treatment services. *Health Policy, 66,* 247–260.

Collins, R. L., & Lapp, W. M. (2006). The temptation and restraint inventory for measuring drinking restraint. *Addiction, 87,* 625–633.

Conklin, C. A., & Tiffany, S. T. (2002). Applying extinction research and theory to cue-exposure addiction treatments. *Addiction, 97,* 155–167.

Conrod, P. J., Castellanos, N., & Mackie, C. (2008). Personality-targeted interventions delay the growth of adolescent drinking and binge drinking. *Journal of Child Psychology and Psychiatry, 49,* 181–190.

Conrod, P. J., Stewart, S. H., Pihl, R. O., Côté, S., Fontaine, V., & Dongier, M. (2000). Efficacy of brief coping skills interventions that match different personality profiles of female substance abusers. *Psychology of Addictive Behaviors, 14,* 231–242.

Cooper, M. L., Russell, M., Skinner, J. B., & Windle, M. (1992). Development and validation of a three-dimensional measure of drinking motives. *Psychological Assessment, 4,* 123–132.

Copeland, J., & Martin, G. (2004). Web-based interventions for substance use disorders: A qualitative review. *Journal of Substance Abuse Treatment, 26,* 109–116.

Costa, P. T., & McCrae, R. R. (1992). Normal personality assessment in clinical practice: The NEO personality Inventory. *Psychological Assessment, 4*, 5–13.

Cottler, L. B., Grant, B. F., Blaine, J., Mavreas, V., Pull, C., Hasin, D., et al. (1997). Concordance of *DSM–IV* alcohol and drug use disorder criteria and diagnoses as measured by AUDADIS-ADR, CIDI and SCAN. *Drug and Alcohol Dependence, 47*, 195–205.

Cousins, M. S., Roberts, D. C. S., & de Wit, H. (2002). GABAB receptor agonists for the treatment of drug addiction: A review of recent findings. *Drug and Alcohol Dependence, 65*, 209–220.

Culliton, B. J. (2006). Extracting knowledge from science: A conversation with Elias Zerhouni. *Health Affairs, 25*, w94–w103.

Cunningham, J., Peter, S., Kypri, K., & Hymphreys, K. (2006). Access to the internet among drinkers, smokers and illicit drug users: Is it a barrier to the provision of interventions on the world wide web? *Medical Informatics and the Internet in Medicine, 31*, 53–58.

Cunningham, W. A., Preacher, K. J., & Banaji, M. R. (2002). Implicit attitude measures: Consistency, stability and convergent validity. *Psychological Science, 12*, 163–170.

Donovan, J. E., & Jessor, R. (1985). Structure of problem behavior in adolescence and young adulthood. *Journal of Consulting & Clinical Psychology, 53*, 890–904.

Dunn, C., Deroo, L., & Rivara, F. P. (2002). The use of brief interventions adapted from motivational interviewing across behavioral domains: A systematic review. *Addiction, 96*, 1725–1742.

Dutra, L., Stathopoulou, G., Basden, S. L., Leyro, T. M., Powers, M. B., & Otto, M. W. (2008). A meta-analytic review of psychosocial interventions for substance use disorders. *American Journal of Psychiatry, 165*, 179–187.

Edenberg, H. J., & Kranzler, H. R. (2005). The contribution of genetics to addiction therapy approaches. *Pharmacology & Therapeutics, 108*, 86–93.

Escoffery, C., Miner, K. R., Adame, D. D., Butler, S., McCormick, L., & Mendell, E. (2005). Internet use for health information among college students. *Journal of American College Health, 53*, 183–188.

Fals-Stewart, W., Logsdon, T., & Birchler, G. R. (2004). Diffusion of an empirically supported treatment for substance abuse: An organizational autopsy of technology transfer success and failure. *Clinical Psychology: Science and Practice, 11*, 177–182.

Feltenstein, M. W., & See, R. E. (2007). NMDA receptor blockade in the basolateral amygdala disrupts consolidation of stimulus-reward memory and extinction learning during reinstatement of cocaine-seeking in an animal model of relapse. *Neurobiology of Learning and Memory, 88*, 423–444.

Fromme, K., & D'Amico, E. J. (2000). Measuring adolescent alcohol outcome expectancies. *Psychology of Addictive Behaviors, 14*, 206–212.

Gailliot, M. T., & Baumeister, R. F. (2007). The physiology of willpower: Linking blood glucose to self-control. *Personality and Social Psychology Review, 11*, 303–327.

Garbutt, J. C., Kranzler, H. R., O'Malley, S. S., Gastfriend, D. R., Pettinati, H. M., Silverman, B. L., et al. (2005). Efficacy and tolerability of long-acting injectable naltrexone for alcohol dependence: A randomized controlled trial. *Journal of the American Medical Association, 293*, 1617–1625.

Gotham, H. J. (2004). Diffusion of mental health and substance abuse treatments: Development, dissemination, and implementation. *Clinical Psychology: Science and Practice, 11*, 160–176.

Grant, B. F., Stinson, F. S., Dawson, D. A., Chou, S. P., Dufour, M. C., Compton, W., et al. (2004). Prevalence and co-occurrence of substance use disorders and independent mood and anxiety disorders: Results from the national epidemiologic survey on alcohol and related conditions. *Archives of General Psychiatry, 61*, 807–816.

Grant, B. F., Stinson, F. S., Dawson, D. A., Chou, S. P., Ruan, W. J., & Pickering, R. P. (2004). Co-occurrence of 12-month alcohol and drug use disorders and personality disorders in the United States: Results from the National Epidemiologic Survey on Alcohol and Related Conditions. *Archives of General Psychiatry, 61*, 361–368.

Hall, M. J., & Tidwell, W. C. (2003). Internet recovery for substance abuse and alcoholism: An exploratory study of service users. *Journal of Substance Abuse Treatment, 24*, 161–167.

Haney, M., & Kosten, T. R. (2005). Therapeutic vaccines for substance dependence. *Drug Discovery Today: Therapeutic Strategies, 2*, 65–69.

Heather, N., & Bradley, B. P. (1990). Cue exposure as a practical treatment for addictive disorders: Why are we waiting? *Addictive Behaviors, 15,* 335–337.

Heatherton, T. F., Kozlowski, L. T., Frecker, R. C., & Fagerstrom, K. O. (2006). The Fagerström test for Nicotine dependence: A revision of the Fagerstrom tolerance questionnaire. *Addiction, 86,* 1119–1127.

Heidbreder, C. A., & Hagan, J. J. (2005). Novel pharmacotherapeutic approaches for the treatment of drug addiction and craving. *Current Opinion in Pharmacology, 5,* 107–118.

Horgan, C. M., Reif, S., Hodgkin, D., Garnick, D. W., & Merrick, E. L. (2008). Availability of addiction medications in private health plans. *Journal of Substance Abuse Treatment, 34,* 147–156.

Howard, M. O. (2001). Pharmacological aversion treatment of alcohol dependence. I. Production and prediction of conditioned alcohol aversion. *American Journal of Drug and Alcohol Abuse, 27,* 561–585.

Hughes, J. R., & Brandon, T. H. (2003). A softer view of hardening. *Nicotine and Tobacco Research, 5,* 961–962.

Hunt, G. M., & Azrin, N. H. (1973). The community-reinforcement approach to alcoholism. *Behaviour Research and Therapy, 11,* 91–104.

Iacono, W. G. (1998). Identifying psychophysiological risk for psychopathology: Examples from substance abuse and schizophrenia research. *Psychophysiology, 35,* 621–637.

Institute of Medicine. (1989). *Prevention and treatment of alcohol problems: Research Opportunities.* Washington, DC: National Academy Press.

Institute of Medicine. (1990). *Broadening the base of treatment for alcohol problems.* Washington, DC: National Academy Press.

Jessor, R., Donovan, J. E., & Costa, F. M. (1991). *Beyond adolescence: Problem behavior and young adult development.* New York: Cambridge University Press.

Johnson, B. A. (2005). Recent advances in the development of treatments for alcohol and cocaine dependence: Focus on topiramate and other modulators of GABA or glutamate function. *CNS Drugs, 19,* 873–896.

Jorenby, D. E., Hays, J. T., Rigotti, N. A., Azoulay, S., Watsky, E. J., Williams, K. E., et al., (2006). Efficacy of varenicline, an α4β2 nicotinic acetylcholine receptor partial agonist, vs. placebo or sustained-release bupropion for smoking cessation: A randomized controlled trial. *Journal of the American Medical Association, 296,* 56–63.

Kantak, K. M. (2003). Vaccines against drugs of abuse: A viable treatment option? *Drugs, 63,* 341–352.

Keating, G. M., & Siddiqui, A. A. (2006). Varenicline: A review of its use as an aid to smoking cessation therapy. *CNS Drugs, 20,* 945–960.

Kendler, K. S., Myers, J., & Prescott, C. A. (2007). Specificity of genetic and environmental risk factors for symptoms of cannabis, cocaine, alcohol, caffeine, and nicotine dependence. *Archives of General Psychiatry, 64,* 1313–1320.

Kenna, G. A. (2005). Pharmacotherapy of alcohol dependence: Targeting a complex disorder. *Drug Discovery Today: Therapeutic Strategies, 2,* 71–78.

Kenna, G. A., McGeary, J. E., & Swift, R. M. (2004a). Pharmacotherapy, pharmacogenomics, and the future of alcohol dependence treatment, part 1. *American Journal of Health-System Pharmacy, 61,* 2272–2279.

Kenna, G. A., McGeary, J. E., & Swift, R. M. (2004b). Pharmacotherapy, pharmacogenomics, and the future of alcohol dependence treatment, part 2. *American Journal of Health-System Pharmacy, 61,* 2380–2388.

Kessler, R. C., Chiu, W. T., Demler, O., & Walters, E. E. (2005). Prevalence, severity, and comorbidity in the national comorbidity survey replication. *Archives of General Psychiatry, 62,* 617–627.

Kosten, T., & Owens, S. M. (2005). Immunotherapy for the treatment of drug abuse. *Pharmacology & Therapeutics, 108,* 76–85.

Kranzler, H. R., Armeli, S., Tennen, H., Blomqvist, O., Oncken, C., Petry, N., et al., (2003). Targeted naltrexone for early problem drinkers. *Journal of Clinical Psychopharmacology, 23,* 294–304.

Krueger, R. F. (1999). The structure of common mental disorders. *Archives of General Psychiatry, 56,* 921–926.

Krueger, R. F., Hicks, B. M., Patrick, C. J., Carlson, S. R., Iacono, W. G., & McGue, M. (2002). Etiologic connections among substance dependence, antisocial behavior, and personality: Modeling the externalizing spectrum. *Journal of Abnormal Psychology, 111,* 411–424.

Krueger, R. F., Markon, K. E., Patrick, C. J., & Iacono, W. G. (2005). Externalizing psychopathology in adulthood: A dimensional-spectrum conceptualization and its implications for *DSM–V. Journal of Abnormal Psychology, 114,* 537–550.

Lakshman, M. R., & Tsutsumi, M. (2001). Alcohol biomarkers: Clinical significance and biochemical basis. *Alcohol, 25,* 171–172.

Lichtermann, D., Franke, P., Maier, W., & Rao, M. L. (2000). Pharmacogenomics and addiction to opiates. *European Journal of Pharmacology, 410,* 269–279.

Littleton, J., & Zieglagänsberger, W. (2003). Pharmacological mechanisms of naltrexone and acamprosate in the prevention of relapse in alcohol dependence. *American Journal on Addictions, 12,* S3–S11.

Mark, T. L., Coffey, R. M., Vandivort-Warren, R., Harwood, H. J., King, E. C., & MHSA Spending Estimates Team (2005). U.S. spending for mental health and substance abuse treatment, 1991–2001. *Health Affairs (Millwood), W5,* 133–142.

McClure, J. B. (2002). Are biomarkers useful treatment aids for promoting health behavior change? An empirical review. *American Journal of Preventive Medicine, 22,* 200–207.

McCollister, K. E., & French, M. T. (2003). The relative contribution of outcome domains in the total economic benefit of addiction interventions: A review of first findings. *Addiction, 98,* 1647–1659.

McLellan, A. T., Luborsky, L., Woody, G. E., & O'Brien, C. P. (1980). An improved diagnostic evaluation instrument for substance abuse patients: The addiction severity index. *Journal of Nervous and Mental Disease, 168,* 26–33.

Montoya, I. D., Gorelick, D. A., Preston, K. L., Schroeder, J. R., Umbricht, A., Cheskin, L. J., et al. (2004). Randomized trial of buprenorphine for treatment of concurrent opiate and cocaine dependence. *Clinical Pharmacology & Therapeutics, 75,* 34–48.

Moyer, A., Finney, J. W., Swearingen, C. E., & Vergun, P. (2002). Brief interventions for alcohol problems: A meta-analytic review of controlled investigations in treatment-seeking and non-treatment seeking populations. *Addiction, 97,* 279–292.

Muraven, M., & Baumeister, R. F. (2000). Self-regulation and depletion of limited resources: Does self-control resemble a muscle? *Psychological Bulletin, 126,* 247–259.

O'Malley, S. S., Jaffe, A. J., Chang, G., Schottenfeld, R. S., Meyer, R. E., & Rounsaville, B. (1992). Naltrexone and coping skills therapy for alcohol dependence. *Archives of General Psychiatry, 49,* 881–887.

Orford, J. (2001). *Excessive appetites: A psychological view of addictions* (2nd ed.). New York: Wiley.

Oslin, D. W., Berrettini, W. H., Kranzler, H. R., Pettinati, H., Gelernter, J., Volpicelli, J. R., et al. (2003). A functional polymorphism of the mu-opioid receptor gene is associated with naltrexone response in alcohol-dependent patients. *Neuropsychopharmacology, 28,* 1546–1552.

Oslin, D. W., Berrettini, W. H., & O'Brien, C. P. (2006). Targeting treatments for alcohol dependence: The pharmacogenetics of naltrexone. *Addiction Biology, 11,* 397–403.

Piasecki, T. M., Hufford, M. R., Solhan, M., & Trull, T. J. (2007). Assessing clients in their natural environments with electronic diaries: Rationale, benefits, limitations, and barriers. *Psychological Assessment, 19,* 25–43.

Project MATCH Research Group. (1997). Matching alcoholism treatments to client heterogeneity: Project MATCH posttreatment drinking outcomes. *Journal of Studies on Alcohol, 58,* 7–29.

Ressler, K. J., Rothbaum, B. O., Tannenbaum, L., Anderson, P., Graap, K., Zimand, E., et al.(2004). Cognitive enhancers as adjuncts to psychotherapy: Use of d-cycloserine in phobic individuals to facilitate extinction of fear. *Archives of General Psychiatry, 61,* 1136–1144.

Robinson, T. E., & Berridge, K. C. (1993). The neural basis of drug craving: An incentive-sensitization theory of addiction. *Brain Research Reviews, 18,* 247–291.

Rogers, E. M. (2003). *Diffusion of innovations* (5th ed.). New York: Free Press.

Room, R., Graham, K., Rehm, J., Jernigan, D., & Monteiro, M. (2003). Drinking and its burden in a global perspective: Policy considerations and options. *European Addiction Research, 9,* 165–175.

Sakai, J. T., Mikulich-Gilbertson, S. K., Long, R. J., & Crowley, T. J. (2006) Validity of transdermal alcohol monitoring: Fixed and self-regulated dosing. *Alcoholism: Clinical and Experimental Research, 30,* 26–33.

Saxon, A. J., & McCarty, D. (2005). Challenges in the adoption of new pharmacotherapeutics for addiction to alcohol and other drugs. *Pharmacology & Therapeutics, 108,* 119–128.

Sayette, M. A., Shiffman, S., Tiffany, S. T., Niaura, R. S., Martin, C. S., & Shadel, W.G. (2000). The measurement of drug craving. *Addiction, 95*(Suppl. 2), S189–S210.

Schroeder, J. P., & Packard, M. G. (2004). Facilitation of memory for extinction of drug-induced conditioned reward: Role of amygdala and acetylcholine. *Learning and Memory, 11,* 641–647.

Sher, K. J., & Slutske, W. (2003). Disorders of impulse control. In G. Stricker, T. A. Widiger, & I. B. Weiner (Eds.), *Comprehensive handbook of psychology, Vol. 8: Clinical Psychology* (pp. 195–228). New York: John Wiley & Sons.

Sher, K. J., Wolf, S. T., & Martinez, J. A., (in press). How can etiological research inform the distinction between normal drinking and disordered drinking? In L. M. Scheier (Ed.), *Handbook of drug use etiology.* Washington, DC: American Psychological Association.

Shiffman, S., Stone, A. A., & Hufford, M. R. (2008). Ecological momentary assessment. *Annual Review of Clinical Psychology, 4,* 1–32.

Smith, G. T., Fischer, S., Cyders, M. A., Annus, A. M., Spillane, N. S., & McCarthy, D. M. (2007). On the validity and utility of discriminating among impulsivity-like traits. *Assessment, 14,* 155–170.

Sobell, L. C., & Sobell, M. B. (1992). Timeline follow-back: A technique for assessing self-reported alcohol consumption. In R. Z. Litten & J. P. Allen (Eds.), *Measuring alcohol consumption: Psychosocial and biochemical methods* (pp. 41–72). Totowa: Humana Press.

Soyka, M., Koller, G., Schmidt, P., Lesch, O., Leweke, F., Fehr, C., et al. (2008). Cannabinoid receptor 1 blocker rimonabant (SR 141716) for treatment of alcohol dependence: Results from a placebo-controlled, double-blind trial. *Journal of Clinical Psychopharmacology, 28,* 317–324.

Swift, R. (2000). Transdermal alcohol measurement for estimation of blood alcohol concentration. *Alcoholism: Clinical and Experimental Research, 24,* 422–423.

Tellegen, A. (1994). *The multidimensional personality questionnaire*: Minneapolis: University of Minnesota Press.

Trull, T. J., Sher, K. J., Minks-Brown, C., Durbin, J., & Burr, R. (2000). Borderline personality disorder and substance use disorders: A review and integration. *Clinical Psychology Review, 20,* 235–253.

Walker, D. D., Roffman, R. A., Picciano, J. F., & Stephens, R. S. (2007). The check-up: In person, computerized, and telephone adaptations of motivational enhancement treatment to elicit voluntary participation by the contemplator. *Substance Abuse Treatment, Prevention, and Policy, 8,* 22.

Wanberg, K. W., Horn, J. L., & Foster, F. M. (1985). *Manual for the alcohol use inventory.* Denver: Multivariate Measurement Consultants.

Warner, K. E., & Burns, D. M. (2003). Hardening and the hard-core smoker: Concepts, evidence, and implications. *Nicotine and Tobacco Research, 5,* 37–48.

Wetter, D. W., Smith, S. S., Kenford, S. L., Jorenby, D. E., Fiore, M. C., Hurt, R. D., et al. (1994). Smoking outcome expectancies: Factor structure, predictive validity, and discriminant validity. *Journal of Abnormal Psychology, 103,* 801–811.

White, W. L. (1998). *Slaying the dragon: The history of addiction treatment and recovery in America.* Bloomington, IL: Chestnut Health Systems/Lighthouse Institute.

Whiteside, S. P., & Lynam, D. R. (2003). Understanding the role of impulsivity and externalizing psychopathology in alcohol abuse: Application of the UPPS Impulsive Behavior Scale. *Experimental & Clinical Psychopharmacology 11,* 210–217.

Wiers, R. W., & Stacy, A. W. (Eds.). (2006). *Handbook of implicit cognition and addiction.* Thousand Oaks: Sage.

Zerhouni, E. A. (2006). Clinical research at a crossroads: The NIH roadmap. *Journal of Investigative Medicine, 54,* 171–173.

About the Editors

Lee M. Cohen, PhD, is an associate professor and director of clinical training in the Department of Psychology at Texas Tech University. Dr. Cohen also holds adjunct status in the Departments of Psychiatry and Pediatrics at the Texas Tech University Health Sciences Center. Dr. Cohen completed his predoctoral clinical internship and a postdoctoral fellowship funded by the National Institute of Drug Abuse (NIDA) at the University of California, San Diego, specializing in behavioral medicine. He completed his graduate training in clinical psychology at Oklahoma State University. Dr. Cohen's research interests involve systematically exploring the behavioral and physiological mechanisms that contribute to nicotine use and dependence. Dr. Cohen may be contacted at Department of Psychology, Texas Tech University, Lubbock, Texas.

Frank L. Collins, Jr, PhD, is a professor of psychology and director of clinical training for the Clinical Health Psychology and Behavioral Medicine Program at the University of North Texas. He received his PhD from Auburn University in 1980 and has served on the faculties of West Virginia University, Rush Medical College, and Oklahoma State University, before moving to the University of North Texas in the fall of 2007. Dr. Collins' research interests focus on the behavioral pharmacology of nicotine and health behavior choices. Dr. Collins may be contacted at Department of Psychology, Oklahoma State University, Stillwater, Oklahoma.

Katrina L. Cook, BA, is a doctoral student in clinical psychology at Texas Tech University. She earned her undergraduate degrees from Baylor University in biology and Texas Tech University in psychology where she also served as an undergraduate research assistant for Dr. Lee Cohen. Her research interests include risk factors associated with adolescents and their families, particularly in underserved populations. Ms Cook may be contacted at Department of Psychology, Texas Tech University, Lubbock, Texas.

Thad R. Leffingwell, PhD, is an associate professor and director of clinical training in the Department of Psychology at Oklahoma State University. He completed his graduate training at the University of Washington. His research interests include brief motivational interventions for health behavior change, including smoking cessation and harm-reduction for high-risk alcohol use. Dr. Leffingwell may be contacted at Department of Psychology, Oklahoma State University, Stillwater, Oklahoma.

Dennis E. McChargue, PhD, is an assistant professor and associate director of clinical training in the Clinical Psychology Training Program of the Department of Psychology at the University of Nebraska-Lincoln. He completed his predoctoral clinical internship at Boston University/Boston Veterans Affairs Medical Center Consortium and completed his postdoctoral training at the University of Illinois at Chicago. He completed his graduate training in clinical psychology at Oklahoma State University. His research interest focuses on examining biobehavioral mechanisms that contribute to the development, maintenance, and eventual treatment of addictive and health behaviors, especially among those vulnerable to psychopathology. Dr. McChargue may be contacted at Department of Psychology, University of Nebraska-Lincoln, Lincoln, Nebraska.

Alice M. Young PhD, is a professor of psychology at Texas Tech University and of pharmacology and neuroscience at Texas Tech University Health Sciences Center. Her current research and teaching focus on behavioral and pharmacological processes that modulate tolerance to and dependence on psychoactive drugs, with particular attention to learning and memory processes and the roles of efficacy and receptor activity in drug dependence and withdrawal. Before joining the Texas Tech University System in 2004, Dr. Young was professor of psychology and of psychiatry and behavioral neurosciences at Wayne State University. Dr. Young is a fellow of the American Psychological Association, the Association for Psychological Science, and the College on Problems of Drug Dependence. She is past president of the Behavioral Pharmacology Society and currently serves as associate editor for *The Journal of Pharmacology and Experimental Psychology*. She received a PhD in psychology from the University of Minnesota and postdoctoral training in pharmacology at the University of Michigan. Dr. Young may be contacted at Department of Psychology, Texas Tech University, Lubbock, Texas.

About the Contributors

Mustafa al'Absi, PhD, is a professor of behavioral medicine and the holder of the Max & Mary LaDue Pickworth Research Chair at University of Minnesota School of Medicine, Duluth, MN. He is the founding director of the Duluth Medical Research Institute (DMRI). Professor. al'Absi's research programs focus on psychobiology of stress, pain perception, and tobacco addiction. His research has been funded by grants from the National Institute on Drug Abuse, the National Cancer Institute, the National Health, Lung, and Blood Institute, and the American Heart Association. Prof. al'Absi completed his biological psychology training at the University of Oklahoma. He has received several honorary awards, including the Neal E. Miller Young Investigator Award from the Academy for Behavioral Medicine Research and the Herbert Weiner Early Career Award from the American Psychosomatic Society. He may be contacted at University of Minnesota Medical School, University Drive, Duluth, Minnesota.

Sheila M. Alessi, PhD, earned her doctorate in psychology from Wayne State University in 2000 after which she completed a National Institute on Drug Abuse Post-Doctoral Research Fellowship in the human behavioral pharmacology laboratory at the University of Vermont. Dr. Alessi is currently an Assistant Professor in the Department of Medicine at the University of Connecticut Health Center and a member of the Alcohol Research Center at the same institution. She conducts research on substance use disorders with an emphasis on treatment. Dr. Alessi can be contacted at Calhoun Cardiovascular Center-Behavioral Health, Farmington, Connecticut.

Richard M. Allen, PhD, is an associate professor of psychology at the University of Colorado Denver. Dr. Allen earned his PhD in neurobiology from the University of North Carolina at Chapel Hill. Dr. Allen's research program investigates glutamatergic mechanisms of drug tolerance and dependence, most recently studying the escalation of cocaine consumption using a rodent self-administration procedure. Dr. Allen may be contacted at Department of Psychology, University of Colorado Denver, Denver, Colorado.

John S. Baer, PhD, is a research professor in the Department of Psychology at the University of Washington in Seattle, and is currently associate director for training and education and director of the Interdisciplinary Fellowship in Substance Abuse Treatment at the Center of Excellence for Substance Abuse Treatment and Education at the Veterans Affairs Puget Sound Health Care System. Dr. Baer received his doctoral degree in clinical psychology from the University of Oregon in 1986 after a clinical internship in the department of psychiatry and behavioral sciences at the University of Washington. Dr. Baer's research and clinical interests focus on the assessment, prevention, treatment, and relapse of substance use and abuse. He has specialized in the study of brief interventions for both prevention and treatment of substance use problems, and has studied adult, young adult, and adolescent populations. Dr. Baer can be reached at S-116-ATC, VA Medical Center, Seattle.

Danielle Barry, PhD, is an assistant professor in the Department of Medicine at the University of Connecticut Health Center. She received her PhD in clinical psychology from Rutgers, The State University of New Jersey, in 2004. Dr. Barry may be contacted at Calhoun Cardiovascular Center-Behavioral Health, University of Connecticut Health Center, Farmington, Connecticut.

Patrick R. Bennett, PhD, is an assistant professor and associate director of the Center for the Study of Health, Religion, and Spirituality at Indiana State University. He completed his graduate training in social psychology at the University of Nevada, Reno. His research focuses primarily on the interface between religion and health, with an emphasis on the utilization of religious practice to cope with difficult life experiences and its impact on physical and emotional health outcomes. Dr. Bennett may be contacted at Department of Psychology, Indiana State University, Terre Haute, Indiana.

Warren K. Bickel, PhD, is professor at the University of Arkansas for Medical Sciences (UAMS) in the College of Medicine and College of Public Health (COPH) and holds the Wilbur D. Mills Chair of Alcoholism and Drug Abuse Prevention. He serves as director of the UAMS Center for Addiction Research and as director of COPH's Center for the Study of Tobacco Addiction at UAMS. In these roles, he oversees the development of research addressing addiction and tobacco dependence. Dr. Bickel received his PhD in developmental and child psychology in 1983 from the University of Kansas, completed postdoctoral training at Johns Hopkins University School of Medicine in 1985, and then joined the faculty of the Albert Einstein College of Medicine. In 1987, he relocated to the University of Vermont where he became a professor in the departments of psychiatry and psychology and interim-chair of the department of psychiatry. He serves as principal investigator on several NIDA grants. His recent research includes the application of behavioral economics to drug dependence with an emphasis on the discounting of the future and the use of information technologies to deliver science-based prevention and treatment. Dr. Bickel is the recipient of numerous awards and honors including the Joseph Cochin Young Investigator Award from the College on Problems of Drug Dependence (CPDD), the Young Psychopharmacologist Award from the Division of Psychopharmacology and Substance Abuse of the American Psychological Association, a NIH Merit Award from NIDA, and Researcher of the Year from the Arkansas Psychological Association (ArPA) Honors for Outstanding Contribution. He served as president of the Division of Psychopharmacology and Substance Abuse, American Psychological Association and as president of CPDD. Dr. Bickel was editor of the journal, *Experimental and Clinical Psychopharmacology*, has co-edited five books, and published over 250 papers. Dr. Bickel may be contacted at Department of Psychiatry, University of Arkansas for Medical Sciences, Little Rock, Arkansas.

Arthur W. Blume, PhD, is associate professor and director of the Health Psychology PhD Program at the University of North Carolina at Charlotte. Dr. Blume was a National Institute of Alcohol Abuse and Alcoholism predoctoral fellow in the Addictive Behaviors Research Center. He graduated with his PhD in clinical psychology from the University of Washington and was assistant professor at the University of Texas at El Paso before moving to Charlotte. Dr. Blume investigates cognitive and behavioral factors associated with changes in substance abuse among high-risk and traditionally underserved populations, such as young adults, ethnic minority groups, and people with co-occurring disorders. Dr. Blume can be contacted at Department of Psychology, University of North Carolina at Charlotte, Charlotte, North Carolina.

Leslie D. Braddy, BA, graduated with her degree in psychology from UNC Charlotte. She served as an undergraduate research assistant in the laboratory of Dr. Arthur Blume before her graduation. Ms Braddy may be contacted at Department of Psychology, University of North Carolina at Charlotte, Charlotte, North Carolina.

Thomas H. Brandon, PhD, is professor of psychology at the University of South Florida, in Tampa, and he holds a secondary appointment in the Department of Oncologic Sciences in the College of Medicine. He also directs the Tobacco Research and Intervention Program at the H. Lee Moffitt Cancer Center & Research Institute. He received his doctorate from the University of Wisconsin-Madison, and served his clinical psychology internship at the Indiana University Medical Center. Prior to his current appointments, he was on the psychology faculty at the State University of New York at Binghamton. Dr. Brandon's research ranges from basic human behavioral studies of factors influencing tobacco dependence, through the development of theory-based interventions, with a focus on relapse-prevention. He may be contacted at Tobacco Research and Intervention Program, H. Lee Moffitt Cancer Center, Tampa, Florida.

Robert Kevin Brooner, PhD, is professor of medical psychology and psychiatry in the Johns Hopkins University School of Medicine and Director of the Addiction Treatment Services program at Johns Hopkins Bayview Medical Center. Dr. Brooner completed his internship and postdoctoral supervision at the Johns Hopkins University School of Medicine, where he trained in medical psychology, biological bases of behavior and motivated disorders, and both dimensional and categorical assessment of psychological and psychiatric problems and disorders. Dr. Brooner earned a doctorate in clinical psychology from the California School of Professional Psychology. His current research interests focus on the assessment of substance use disorder with and without other psychiatric comorbidity; development of interventions for substance-dependent patients with specific types of psychiatric comorbidity; testing of combination treatments that incorporate behavioral reinforcement to motivate patient adherence; and the development of adaptive treatment models to improve treatment participation and response in substance dependent patients with and without other psychiatric problems. Dr. Brooner's contact information is The Johns Hopkins Bayview Campus, Behavioral Biology Research Center, Addiction Treatment Services, Baltimore, Maryland.

Ryan M. Caldeiro, MD, is an addiction psychiatry fellow at the University of Washington Department of Psychiatry and the Puget Sound Veterans Administration Healthcare System in Seattle, Washington. He completed his psychiatry residency and internship training at the University of Washington. He completed his graduate training in medicine at Case Western Reserve University School of Medicine. His research interests focus on the interrelation of chronic pain and addictions and developing treatments to enhance substance use outcomes for patients with co-occurring chronic pain and addictive disorders. He may be contacted at Department of Psychiatry and Behavioral Sciences, University of Washington School of Medicine, Seattle.

Jennifer L. Callahan, PhD, ABPP, is an assistant professor in the Department of Psychology at the University of North Texas. Dr. Callahan also holds a visiting appointment in the department of psychiatry at Yale University School of Medicine. Dr. Callahan completed her predoctoral clinical internship and a postdoctoral fellowship in the department of psychiatry at Yale University School of Medicine. She completed her graduate training in clinical psychology at the University of Wisconsin-Milwaukee. Dr. Callahan's research interests involve exploring the role of clinical competencies in the provision of psychological services for the purpose of improving training and enhancing client outcomes. Dr. Callahan may be reached at Department of Psychology, University of North Texas, Denton, Texas.

Donald A. Calsyn, PhD, is a professor in the Department of Psychiatry and Behavioral Sciences, School of Medicine, and a research affiliate with the Alcohol and Drug Abuse Institute at the University of Washington. He previously served as the director of outpatient services, Addiction Treatment Center, Veterans Affairs Puget Sound Health Care System-Seattle Division where for 30 years he provided treatment services to veterans with substance abuse disorders. He completed his graduate training in counseling at University of Washington. He completed his predoctoral clinical internship at Seattle Veterans Affairs Medical Center. His research interest focuses on substance treatment outcomes and HIV/STI prevention among substance abusers. Dr. Calsyn may be contacted at University of Washington, Seattle, Washington.

Sandra D. Comer, PhD, is an associate professor of clinical neuroscience in the Department of Psychiatry at the College of Physicians and Surgeons of Columbia University, and a Research Scientist at the New York State Psychiatric Institute. Dr. Comer received her undergraduate degree at Vanderbilt University, and completed her graduate training at the University of Michigan, Ann Arbor, where she studied the analgesic and discriminative stimulus effects of opioid drugs using preclinical models. Following graduate school, Dr. Comer completed a two-year postdoctoral fellowship at the University of Minnesota, Minneapolis. There she received further training in preclinical models of drug self-administration. Dr. Comer subsequently joined the faculty in the division on substance abuse at Columbia University. Her research focus has been on the development and testing of novel approaches to the treatment of opioid dependence in human research volunteers, and the influences of sex, gonadal hormones, and drug use history on responses to pain and opioid medications. Dr. Comer may be contacted at Department of Psychiatry, Columbia University, New York.

Ziva D. Cooper, PhD, is a postdoctoral fellow in the Division on Substance Abuse at the New York State Psychiatric Institute, Department of Psychiatry of the College of Physicians and Surgeons of Columbia University. Dr. Cooper completed her undergraduate (2001) and graduate (2007) training in the area of biopsychology in the Department of Psychology at the University of Michigan where she studied behavioral pharmacology in rats in the laboratory of Dr. James Woods. As a graduate student, her research focused on the effects of opiate dependence on operant responding maintained by various stimuli. She also investigated the effects of a naturally occurring cocaine esterase on cocaine-induced toxicity. Dr. Cooper is currently receiving training in human preclinical studies under the mentorship of Drs. Sandra Comer and Margaret Haney focusing on potential pharmacotherapies for opiate and marijuana dependence. Dr. Cooper can be contacted at the Division on Substance Abuse, Department of Psychiatry, College of Physicians and Surgeons of Columbia University, New York.

Christopher J. Correia, PhD, is an associate professor in the Department of Psychology at Auburn University. He is a faculty member in the Clinical Psychology Training Program. He is also the primary clinical supervisor for the Health Behavior Assessment Center, which provides brief motivational alcohol interventions to college students. Dr. Correia completed his graduate training in clinical psychology at Syracuse University. He completed his predoctoral clinical internship at the Syracuse Veterans Affairs Medical Center, and he completed his postdoctoral training at the Johns Hopkins School of Medicine's Behavioral Pharmacology Research Unit. His research interests focus on examining a range of factors that influence the use and abuse of substances, with a special emphasis on behaviorally based laboratory and treatment studies. Dr. Correia may be contacted at Department of Psychology, Auburn University, Auburn, Alabama.

William D. Crano, PhD, is the Oskamp Professor of Psychology in the Department of Psychology at Claremont Graduate University. He was educated at Princeton and Northwestern University. His specialty is social psychology. In addition to serving on the faculties of Michigan State University, Texas A&M University, the University of Arizona, and Claremont Graduate University, he has served as Director of the NSF Program in Social Psychology, as a liaison scientist for the U.S. Office of Naval Research-London, and as a Fulbright Senior Scientist at the Universidade Federal do Rio Grande do Sul in Porto Alegre, Brazil. His research interests involve the application of principles of persuasion to preventive behaviors, especially behaviors involving youth and drug abuse, and in the novel application of established methodological designs to complex research issues. He may be contacted at Department of Psychology, Claremont Graduate University, Claremont, California.

Gayle A. Dakof, PhD, is research associate professor of epidemiology and public health at the University of Miami Miller School of Medicine's Center for Treatment Research on Adolescent Drug Abuse (CTRADA; H. Liddle, Director). She has been central to the design and implementation of all of CTRADA's controlled trials and process studies examining MDFT efficacy and therapeutic mechanisms, serving as Co-PI on both of Liddle's NIDA-funded multisite centers. She has over 20 years of experience conducting clinical trials research. She is PI of a NIDA-funded randomized clinical trial comparing home-based family drug services with standard services within the juvenile drug court context. In addition to her expertise and experience with juvenile justice involved drug-abusing youth, Dakof has designed and implemented intervention research with adult drug abusers. As PI, Dr. Dakof developed a specialized drug abuse treatment enrollment and retention intervention for drug-abusing mothers of young children called the Engaging Moms Program (Dakof et al., 2003), and currently is PI of a NIDA-funded randomized clinical trial of the Engaging Moms intervention with adult women in dependency drug court. Dr. Dakof may be contacted at the University of Miami Miller School of Medicine, Miami, Florida.

Joseph W. Ditre, MA, is a doctoral student in clinical psychology at the University of South Florida. He received his undergraduate training at the State University of New York at Binghamton. His particular research interest is in the comorbidity of tobacco dependence and chronic pain, and their causal relationships. He may be contacted at the Tobacco Research and Intervention Program, Moffitt Cancer Center, Tampa, Florida.

David J. Drobes, PhD, is professor of oncologic sciences and psychology at the University of South Florida, and Associate Director of the Tobacco Research and Intervention Program at the H. Lee Moffitt Cancer Center & Research Institute. He received his doctorate in clinical psychology from Purdue University, and served his clinical internship at the University of Florida Health Science Center. He was previously on the faculty of the Center for Drug and Alcohol Programs at the Medical University of South Carolina. Dr. Drobes' research interests include biobehavioral studies of drug craving, affective and cognitive effects of nicotine and withdrawal, and development of brief and intensive interventions for smoking cessation. He may be contacted at Tobacco Research and Intervention Program, Moffitt Cancer Center, Tampa, Florida.

Mitch Earleywine, PhD, is associate professor of clinical psychology at the University at Albany, State University of New York, where he teaches drugs and human behavior, substance abuse treatment and clinical research methods. He has received 11 teaching commendations, including the coveted General Education Teaching Award from the University of Southern California. His research funding has come from the National Institute on Alcohol Abuse and Alcoholism, the Alcoholic Beverage Medical Research Foundation, and the Marijuana Policy Project. He serves on the editorial boards of four psychology journals, reviews for over a dozen, and has more than 90 publications on drug use and abuse, including *Understanding Marijuana* (Oxford University Press, 2002). Dr. Earleywine may be contacted at Department of Psychology, University of Albany, Albany, New York.

John J. Echeverry, PhD, was a clinical/community psychologist who received his doctorate from the University of Maryland at College Park in 1991. His postdoctoral career included a combination of clinical work and research. His clinical work focused on adults with anxiety and mood disorders, HIV/AIDS, substance abuse, and issues of adaptation to a new culture. His research focused on issues related to HIV/AIDS as well as the supervision of students in clinical psychology and social work. At the time of his passing, he was on the faculty in the Departments of Psychology, and Psychiatry and Behavioral Sciences at The George Washington University in Washington, DC At that time he was funded by the National Institute on Drug Abuse (NIDA) to conduct a study on the use of club drugs among Latino young men. Dr. Echeverry published in the areas of Latino access to mental health care, and the psychosocial aspects of HIV-positive status among Latino gay and bisexual men.

Andrea Elibero, MA, is a doctoral student in clinical psychology at the University of South Florida. She received her undergraduate training at George Washington University. Her particular research interest is in the effects of exercise on smoking motivation, and the incorporation of exercise-based interventions within smoking cessation treatment. She may be contacted at the Tobacco Research and Intervention Program, Moffitt Cancer Center, Tampa, Florida.

Loren Gianini, MS, is a doctoral student in the clinical psychology program at the University of New Mexico. She has worked as a research assistant on a CSAT grant which employs the Community Reinforcement Approach with alcohol and substance-using adolescents. Ms Gianini may be contacted at Department of Psychology, University of New Mexico, Albuquerque, New Mexico.

Jeremy T. Goldbach, LMSW, is a doctoral student at the University of Texas at Austin, and project director in prevention at the Texas Department of State Health Services. Jeremy completed his Masters degree at UT-Austin and has been been funded through fellowship under the Substance Abuse and Mental Health Services Administration's (SAMHSA) Center for Substance Abuse Prevention (CSAP), specializing in prevention science. Jeremy's research interests involve cultural competence in prevention practice, with a special focus on minority youth. Jeremy may be contacted at University of Texas at Austin, School of Social Work, Austin, Texas.

Mark S. Goldman, PhD, is distinguished research professor and director of the Alcohol and Substance Use Research Institute at University of South Florida (USF). He also served as associate director of the National Institute on Alcohol Abuse and Alcoholism from June, 2003, until May, 2006, and as director of clinical psychology training at USF from 1985 to 1995. He received his PhD in January, 1972, from Rutgers University and has been on the faculty at Wayne State University (1973–1985) and USF (since 1985). He is a fellow of Divisions 3, 6, 12, 28, and 50, a member of 40 of the American Psychological Association (APA), and is board certified (ABPP) in clinical psychology. In addition to research and clinical work in the addictions field since 1969, Dr. Goldman has served as psychology field editor for the *Journal of Studies on Alcohol*, consulting editor (masthead) of a number of APA journals, member and then chair of the psychosocial research review committee of the National Institute on Alcohol Abuse and Alcoholism (NIAAA), member of NIAAA's National Advisory Council on Alcohol Abuse and Alcoholism, chair or member of a number of NIAAA portfolio review committees, member of the NIAAA research priority committee, co-chair (with Father Edward A. Malloy, president of the University of Notre Dame) of the NIAAA subcommittee on college drinking, member of the board of professional affairs of the APA, member of the task force on psychological intervention guidelines (APA), president of the division on addictions for APA, and member and then chair of the psychosocial advisory review group for the Alcoholic Beverage Medical Research Foundation. In 1992, Dr. Goldman received a MERIT Award from the NIAAA. Dr. Goldman's major research interest is in alcohol expectancies and cognitive mediators of alcoholism risk, and the development of drinking and risk for drinking in children, adolescents, and young adults (over 260 articles and presentations). Dr. Goldman may be contacted at Department of Psychology, University of South Florida, Tampa, Florida.

John H. Halpern, MD, is an assistant professor of psychiatry, Harvard Medical School, Associate Psychiatrist of McLean Hospital, and is the director of McLean Hospital's Laboratory for Integrative Psychiatry as well as associate director of Substance Abuse Research of the Biological Psychiatry Laboratory. Dr. Halpern completed his residency in psychiatry at the Harvard Longwood Psychiatry Residency Training Program and a three-year National Institute on Drug Abuse (NIDA) supported postdoctoral fellowship at McLean Hospital's Alcohol and Drug Abuse Research Training Program. Dr. Halpern also was awarded by NIDA a Mentored Patient-Oriented Research Career Development Award (K23) for his research of "Cognitive Effects of Substance Use in Native Americans" (use of peyote or alcohol) and "Neurocognitive Consequences of Long-Term Ecstasy Use," with this latter investigation receiving further federal grant support. Dr. Halpern's research interests primarily focus on basic and clinical research of hallucinogens, including the study of neurocognitive consequences, treatment potential (study of MDMA-assisted psychotherapy for anxious cancer patients; study of LSD and psilocybin for cluster headache), religions with "hallucinogenic" sacraments (Native American Church, Santo Daime Church), emerging drugs of abuse and social trends, psychoactive botanicals (ethnography, basic pharmacology, medical application), and psychiatric comorbidity. Dr. Halpern may be contacted at the Laboratory for Integrative Psychiatry, Division of Alcohol and Drug Abuse, McLean Hospital, Belmont, Massachusetts.

Bryan Hartzler, PhD, is a research scientist in the Alcohol and Drug Abuse Institute at the University of Washington. Dr. Hartzler received a doctoral degree in clinical psychology in 2003 from the University of Texas at Austin after completing a clinical internship at the Veterans Affairs Puget Sound Healthcare System (VA PSHCS). He subsequently completed an interdisciplinary clinical fellowship at the VA PSHCS Center of Excellence for Substance

Abuse Treatment and Education. Dr. Hartzler's research and clinical interests include the design, evaluation, and dissemination of behavioral interventions for substance users. He is a member of the Motivational Interviewing Network of Trainers (MINT) and trained in use of Motivational Interviewing Assessment: Supervisory Tools for Enhanced Proficiency (MIA-STEP). Dr. Hartzler may be contacted at the University of Washington, Alcohol & Drug Abuse Institute, Seattle, Washington.

Vanessa Hemovich, MA, is a fifth-year doctoral student in social psychology at Claremont Graduate University. In addition to her current work studying drug use trends among adolescent populations, she also holds adjunct status in the psychology department at Crafton Hills College. Her most recent research exploring anti-drug media campaigns is funded by the National Institute of Drug Abuse (NIDA) and focuses both on distinguishing resolute from vulnerable adolescent marijuana nonusers as well as identifying factors linked with risk variations associated with later usage. Her additional research interests include the role of family structure on adolescent problem behavior, parental attachment as a factor for drug use among youth, and relapse prevention among current drug users. She can be contacted at Department of Psychology, Claremont Graduate University, Claremont, California.

Craig E. Henderson, PhD, is assistant professor of psychology at Sam Houston State University (SHSU) and an adjunct research assistant professor of Epidemiology and Public Health at the University of Miami Center for Treatment Research on Adolescent Drug Abuse (CTRADA; H. Liddle, Director). Dr. Henderson was a psychology intern, postdoctoral research fellow, and faculty member at the CTRADA between 2000 and 2005 before joining the faculty of SHSU. In addition to his work on clinical trials of juvenile justice involved adolescent drug abusers and surveys in the juvenile justice system, Dr. Henderson has considerable expertise in a range of state-of-the-art methodological approaches for analyzing change over time, including latent growth curve modeling. Dr. Henderson may be contacted at Department of Psychology & Philosophy, Sam Houston State University, Huntsville, Texas.

Lori K. Holleran Steiker, PhD, CISW, ACSW, was an addictions therapist for over a dozen years and during her doctoral program at ASU, she transitioned to research on adolescent substance abuse and prevention. She helped design and evaluate the model Drug Resistance Strategies Project's "Keepin' It REAL" curriculum and is presently working on a study of culturally grounded adaptations of that curriculum for high-risk youth in community settings. She is an associate professor at the University of Texas at Austin School of Social Work and her present research on substance abuse prevention is a K01 Mentored Research Scientist Development Award from the National Institute on Drug Abuse. She is the recent recipient of the Deborah K. Padgett Early Career Achievement Award given by the Society for Social Work and Research. She is co-editor of a book entitled *Substance Abusing Latinos*. Dr. Holleran Steiker can be contacted at the University of Texas School of Social Work, Austin, Texas.

Laura M. Hopson, PhD, is an assistant professor at the University at Albany School of Social Welfare. Dr. Hopson completed her doctoral degree at the University of Texas at Austin School of Social Work, specializing in school-based substance abuse prevention. She is interested in dissemination of evidence-based interventions that prevent risk behavior for youth, especially in school settings. Her current research examines risk and protective factors during the transition from middle to high school. Dr. Hopson may be contacted at the University at Albany School of Social Welfare, Albany, New York.

Pedro E. Huertas, MD, PhD, MBA, is an Instructor in Medicine, Harvard Medical School and Scientist, Massachusetts Institute of Technology (MIT), and is the associate director of the Laboratory for Integrative Psychiatry, Division of Alcohol and Drug Abuse, McLean Hospital. Dr. Huertas completed his Internal Medicine Residency, Rheumatology Fellowship, and Palliative Care Medicine Fellowship at the Massachusetts General Hospital (MGH). He completed his PhD in Cell and Developmental Biology at Harvard University and also holds an MBA from MIT's Sloan School of Management. Dr. Huertas has an extensive career in drug development. He is chief medical officer of ExSAR, and was the chief development and strategy officer at Amicus Therapeutics, Inc., chief medical officer (Acting) at StemCells, Inc., chief medical officer at Novazyme, Inc., and director of strategic development and medical director at Genzyme, Inc. In addition, Dr. Huertas has served as an expert advisor to venture capital firms and governmental and non-governmental agencies on issues related to biotechnology and uses of biological resources as means of sustainable economic development. Dr. Huertas sits on the Sloan Fellows' Board of Governors at the Sloan School of Management, Advisory Board of the Division of Health Sciences and Technology at Harvard Medical School and MIT, Advisory Board of the Biomedical Entrepreneurship Program (BEP) at the Sloan School of Management, and the Advisory Board of the Program on Depression of MGH and Harvard Medical School. Dr. Huertas may be contacted at the Laboratory for Integrative Psychiatry, Division of Alcohol and Drug Abuse, McLean Hospital, Belmont, Massachusetts.

Kent E. Hutchison, PhD, is a professor of psychology and neurosciences at the University of New Mexico and the Director of the Neurogenetics Core at the Mind Research Network. Dr. Hutchison completed his graduate degree at Oklahoma State University in 1996, his internship at Brown University in 1995, and a postdoctoral fellowship in addiction at Brown University in 1998. He served as an assistant, associate, and full professor at the University of Colorado from 1998 to 2007 before moving to New Mexico. He has received funding from NIAAA and NIDA during that time. He can be reached at The Mind Research Network, Albuquerque, New Mexico.

Thomas J. Johnson, PhD, is professor of psychology and co-director of the Center for the Study of Health, Religion, and Spirituality at Indiana State University. He completed his doctorate in clinical psychology at the University of Missouri-Columbia and his clinical psychology internship at the Indiana University Medical School in Indianapolis, Indiana. His research focuses on college student drinking, addiction and spirituality (funded by NIAAA), and measurement of religiousness and spirituality. Dr. Johnson may be contacted at Department of Psychology, Indiana State University, Terre Haute, Indiana.

Van L. King, MD, is an associate professor of psychiatry and behavioral sciences at The Johns Hopkins University School of Medicine. He received a BS at the University of Wisconsin-Madison and an MD at the University of Rochester School of Medicine. He completed postdoctoral psychiatry residency training at the Massachusetts General Hospital and is board certified by the American Board of Psychiatry and Neurology. He has been the medical director of addiction treatment services at Johns Hopkins Bayview Medical Center since 1993. His research interests have focused on co-occurring psychiatric disorders in patients with substance use disorders and integration of co-occurring psychiatric disorder treatment with substance use disorder treatment. More recently, he has developed adaptive treatment strategies to extend the continuum of care for patients requiring long-term substance use treatment to minimize the intrusiveness of treatment while ensuring adequate monitoring and treatment response. Dr. King may be contacted at The Johns Hopkins University School of Medicine, Addiction Treatment Services, Baltimore, Maryland.

Hannah K. Knudsen, PhD, is assistant professor of behavioral sciences in the College of Medicine, University of Kentucky, Lexington. She earned her Bachelor's degree at the University of Puget Sound, and her Master's and PhD in sociology at the University of Georgia. She served as assistant research scientist in the Institute for Behavioral Research at the University of Georgia for three years prior to her current appointment. Dr. Knudsen was appointed to a two-year fellowship as deputy editor of the *Journal of Substance Abuse Treatment*. She has had independent grant awards from the National Institute on Drug Abuse and the Robert Wood Johnson Foundation. Her publication record focuses primarily on the adoption of treatment innovations by substance abuse service providers, and includes examination of drinking behaviors about young adults outside the collegiate environment, the impact of 9/11 on drinking behavior, and the job-related impacts of sleep problems. Dr. Knudsen may be contacted at the Department of Behavioral Science, College of Medicine, University of Kentucky, Lexington, KY.

George F. Koob, PhD, is a professor and chair of the Committee on the Neurobiology of Addictive Disorders at The Scripps Research Institute and adjunct professor in the Departments of Psychology and Psychiatry, and Adjunct Professor in the Skaggs School of Pharmacy and Pharmaceutical Sciences at the University of California, San Diego. Dr. Koob received his BS from Pennsylvania State University and his PhD in behavioral physiology from The Johns Hopkins University. He is director of the National Institute on Alcohol Abuse and Alcoholism (NIAAA) Alcohol Research Center at The Scripps Research Institute, consortium coordinator for NIAAA's multicenter Integrative Neuroscience Initiative on Alcoholism, and co-director of the Pearson Center for Alcoholism and Addiction Research. He is editor-in-chief USA for the journal *Pharmacology Biochemistry and Behavior* and senior editor for *Journal of Addiction Medicine*. His research interests have been directed at the neurobiology of addiction, with a focus on the theoretical constructs of reward and stress. Dr. Koob may be contacted at The Scripps Research Institute, Committee on the Neurobiology of Addictive Disorders, La Jolla, California.

Justin M. Laird, PhD, is a senior health educator for the Alice! Health Promotion Program at Columbia University. In his role, he manages several projects, including the coordination of health promotion efforts related to fitness, nutrition, and sexual and reproductive health. Justin also leads several initiatives related to the prevention of high-risk drinking. Prior to joining health services at Columbia, he was an assistant professor of health science at SUNY-Brockport. Justin has also been an instructor at the University of Texas, the University of Oklahoma, and Baylor University. He worked for several years at 3M in their corporate wellness department. His research interests focus on health and development in the emerging adult population. Justin may be contacted at Health Services at Columbia, New York.

Howard A. Liddle, EdD, is director of the Center for Treatment Research on Adolescent Drug Abuse (CTRADA) and Professor in the Departments of Epidemiology and Public Health, Psychology and Counseling Psychology at the University of Miami. The developer of Multidimensional Family Therapy (MDFT), Dr. Liddle has conducted treatment research with drug abusing adolescents since 1985. MDFT has been recognized as a promising or best practice by several organizations, including: NIDA, CSAT, CSAP, OJJDP, USDHHS, and Drug Strategies. Dr. Liddle has been recognized with national awards from NIDA, APA, AAMFT, and AFTA, as well as the Dan Anderson Research Award from the Hazelden Foundation, and the 2007 award for bridging research and practice from the Joint Meeting on Adolescent Treatment Effectiveness (JMATE). Dr. Liddle led the establishment of the first NIDA-funded clinical research center focusing on adolescents, the Center for Treatment Research on Adolescent Drug Abuse at Temple University, and University of Miami Miller School of Medicine. He has conducted a series of NIDA-funded clinical trials for over 20 years testing the effectiveness of MDFT in community treatment settings and the juvenile justice system. He has also been PI of several recent NIDA-funded studies designed to study implementation challenges inherent in bringing evidence-based interventions into practice settings. Dr. Liddle may be contacted at the University of Miami Miller School of Medicine, Miami, Florida.

Joshua A. Lile, PhD, is an assistant professor in the Department of Behavioral Science in the College of Medicine of the University of Kentucky. Dr. Lile received a doctorate in pharmacology from Wake Forest University School of Medicine and then completed postdoctoral training in human behavioral pharmacology at the University of Kentucky. His research has incorporated laboratory models of drug use in animals and humans in an effort to understand the neurobiology of drug addiction and to develop pharmacological treatments. Dr. Lile can be contacted at Department of Behavioral Science, University of Kentucky, Lexington, Kentucky.

Alison Looby, MA, is a doctoral student in clinical psychology at the University at Albany. She is the recipient of a National Research Service Award (NRSA) funded by the National Institute of Drug Abuse (NIDA). Ms Looby's research interests include examination of cognitive deficits among cannabis users, and identifying factors associated with the initiation and maintenance of prescription stimulant misuse. Ms Looby may be contacted at Department of Psychology, University at Albany, Albany, New York.

S. Laura Lundy, MS, is a graduate student in the Clinical Psychology Doctoral Program at the University of New Mexico. Currently, she is completing her predoctoral internship at the University of New Mexico, department of psychiatry, with an emphasis in adult neuropsychology. Her clinical and research interests involve eating disorders and neuropsychology. Laura may be contacted at Department of Psychology, University of New Mexico, Albuquerque, New Mexico.

Lisa A. Marsch, PhD, is the director of the Center for Technology and Health (CTH) at National Development and Research Institutes (NDRI) in New York City, which is an interdisciplinary research and development group focused on the creative and systematic application of cutting-edge technologies to the health sciences and health care. She is also a research scientist in the department of psychiatry at St. Luke's-Roosevelt Hospital Center. Dr. Marsch completed her PhD training in experimental psychology and behavioral pharmacology at the University of Vermont. Dr. Marsch has conducted novel and internationally recognized research on effective treatments for opioid-dependent adolescents. She also has considerable experience developing and evaluating interactive, computer-based interventions focused on substance abuse treatment, substance abuse prevention, HIV prevention, as well as prevention of HIV, hepatitis and Sexually Transmitted Infections (STIs). Dr. Marsch may be contacted at NDRI, Center for Technology and Health, New York.

Julia A. Martinez, MA, is a doctoral student at the University of Missouri, working under the direction of Dr. Kenneth J. Sher. She completed her undergraduate work at Dartmouth College. Her research interests involve the course and consequences of heavy alcohol use, underage drinking and public policy, and alcohol consumption in special and underrepresented populations. She may be contacted at Department of Psychological Sciences, University of Missouri, Columbia, Missouri.

Charles Meredith, MD, graduated from the University of Wisconsin School of Medicine and Public Health in 2001 and completed his general psychiatry residency at the University of Washington in 2005, where he served as the chief resident in psychiatry at VA Puget Sound from 2004 to 2005. He completed his addiction psychiatry residency at the University of Washington in 2006 and is board certified by the ABPN in general psychiatry as well as addiction psychiatry. His current research pursuits involve the study of subjective and objective markers of craving in cocaine and alcohol dependence, as well as the development of pharmacological treatments for alcohol, cocaine, and methamphetamine dependence. He has several publications in these areas of interest. Dr. Meredith may be contacted at Department of Psychiatry and Behavioral Sciences, University of Washington School of Medicine, VAPSHCS, Seattle, Washington.

Miriam Z. Mintzer, PhD, is an associate professor in the Department of Psychiatry and Behavioral Sciences at Johns Hopkins University School of Medicine. Dr. Mintzer completed a postdoctoral fellowship in human behavioral pharmacology funded by the National Institute on Drug Abuse (NIDA) at Johns Hopkins University School of Medicine. She received her doctorate in experimental psychology from New York University, specializing in human memory and cognition. Dr. Mintzer's research interests include the acute and chronic effects of drugs on memory and cognitive processes, neuroimaging of drug-induced amnesia, and cognitive functioning in drug abusers. Dr. Mintzer can be contacted at Behavioral Pharmacology Research Unit, Johns Hopkins University, Baltimore, Maryland.

Holly E. R. Morrell, PhD, is a postdoctoral fellow in the Center for Tobacco Control Research and Education at the University of California, San Francisco. Dr. Morrell completed her predoctoral clinical internship at the University of California, San Diego and the VA San Diego Medical Center, with an emphasis on the treatment of substance abuse and dependence. She completed her graduate training in clinical psychology at Texas Tech University. Dr. Morrell's research interests lie in elucidating the relationship between negative affect and cigarette smoking, with the ultimate goals of understanding the influence of negative affect on smoking initiation and improving the effectiveness of smoking cessation programs. Dr. Morrell may be contacted at University of California, Center for Tobacco Control Research and Education, San Francisco, California.

James G. Murphy, PhD, is an assistant professor of psychology at the University of Memphis and an adjunct assistant professor of psychiatry and human behavior at Brown University.

Dr. Murphy completed his graduate training in clinical psychology at Auburn University. He then completed a clinical internship and postdoctoral research fellowship at the Brown University Center for Alcohol and Addiction Studies. Although Dr. Murphy is interested in addictive behaviors across the lifespan, he is particularly interested in drinking and drug use among college students and other young adults. This research is informed by behavioral economic and choice theories and focuses on the role of decision making, developmental, genetic, and social/contextual variables. His research has been supported by the National Institute of Alcoholism and Alcohol Abuse, the Alcoholic Beverage Medical Research Foundation, and the U.S. Department of Education. Dr. Murphy can be contacted at Department of Psychology, University of Memphis, Memphis, Tennessee.

Mark G. Myers, PhD, is a professor in the Department of Psychiatry, at the University of California, San Diego. He received his PhD in clinical psychology from the San Diego State University/UC San Diego joint doctoral program in clinical psychology and obtained his postdoctoral training in substance abuse treatment outcome research at the Brown University Center for Alcohol and Addiction studies. Dr. Myers has conducted research on the course of addictive behavior in youth for the past 20 years. His research focuses on the study of youth tobacco use, including tobacco intervention research with substance abusing youth, investigating youth smoking cessation self-change efforts, and examining initiation and progression of smoking among college students. Dr. Myers may be contacted at Pyshcology 116B, VASDHS, San Diego, California.

Christopher D. Nettles, MA, is a doctoral student in clinical psychology at The George Washington University. Mr. Nettles completed his Master of Arts in clinical psychology at the University of Colorado at Denver and Health Sciences Center. His research interests include understanding the psychosocial characteristics that lead individuals to engage in high-risk behaviors, including substance use and high-risk sexual behaviors. Mr Nettles may be contacted at Department of Psychology, The George Washington University, Washington.

Carol A. Paronis, PhD, is an assistant professor of pharmacology at Northeastern University. Dr. Paronis received her degree in Pharmacology from Emory University and completed postdoctoral fellowships in behavioral pharmacology at the University of Michigan and Harvard University. Dr. Paronis is interested in understanding mechanisms of tolerance to the behavioral effects of opioids benzodiazepines, and cannabinoids. Her reseach has been supported by the National Institute on Drug Abuse (NIDA). Dr. Paronis may be contacted at the Department of Pharmaceutical Sciences, Northeastern University, Boston, Massachusetts.

Torsten Passie, MD, PhD, is assistant professor for clinical psychiatry and consciousness studies at Hannover Medical School, a major research institution in Germany. He studied philosophy and sociology (PhD) at Hannover University and medicine at Hannover Medical School. His medical dissertation was on existential psychiatry. For more than 20 years now, Dr. Passie has worked in the area of altered states of consciousness. He worked at the Psychiatric University Clinic in Zürich (Switzerland) with the leading European psychopathologist, Professor Christian Scharfetter, on the conceptualization of states of consciousness. During the 1990s he worked with Professor Hanscarl Leuner (Göttingen), the leading European authority on hallucinogens. Due to his specific interest in unconventional healing practices, Dr. Passie has extensively traveled through Mexico and Guatemala. He has done extensive research on the psychophysiology and neuropsychology of altered states of consciousness, their conceptualization and healing potentials, clinical research with different induction procedures including hallucinogenic drugs (cannabis, ketamine, nitrous oxide, and psilocybin). Dr. Passie is one of the very few European experts on the pharmacology and clinical/therapeutic use of hallucinogenic drugs. Other areas of interest include: consciousness, psychotherapy research, addiction medicine, phenomenological psychology, and shamanism. Dr. Passie is on the board of directors of the Swiss Physicans Society for Psycholytic Therapy. Dr. Passie may be contacted at Department of Psychiatry, Social Psychiatry and Psychotherapy, Hannover Medical School, Hannover, Germany.

Jessica M. Peirce, PhD, is assistant professor of psychiatry in the Johns Hopkins University School of Medicine and associate director of the Addiction Treatment Services program at Johns Hopkins Bayview Medical Center. Dr. Peirce completed her internship and postdoctoral fellowship at the Boston VA Medical Center, where she trained in assessment and treatment of posttraumatic stress disorder (PTSD). Dr. Peirce earned a doctorate in biological psychology from the University of Oklahoma Health Sciences Center and a clinical psychology respecialization from Oklahoma State University. Dr. Peirce's research interests focus on psychiatric comorbidity with substance use disorders, especially traumatic event exposure and PTSD. Dr. Peirce's contact information is Johns Hopkins University School of Medicine, Baltimore, Maryland.

Nancy M. Petry, PhD, earned a PhD in psychology from Harvard University in 1994, and she is presently a professor in the Department of Medicine at University of Connecticut Health Center. Dr. Petry conducts research on the treatment of addictive disorders, ranging from substance use disorders to pathological gambling, and has published over 130 peer-reviewed articles. Her work is funded by the National Institute on Drug Abuse, the National Institute of Mental Health, and the National Institute on Alcohol Abuse and Alcoholism. Dr. Petry serves as a consultant and advisor for the National Institute of Health and is on the editorial boards of six academic journals. She received the American Psychological Association Distinguished Scientific Award for Early Career Contributions to Psychology in 2003. Dr. Petry may be contacted at Calhoun Cardiovascular Center-Behavioral Health, University of Connecticut Health Center, Farmington, Connecticut.

Lara A. Ray, PhD, is an assistant professor in the Department of Psychology at the University of California, Los Angeles (UCLA). Dr. Ray also holds adjunct status in the departments of psychiatry and biobehavioral sciences at the UCLA Medical School. Dr. Ray completed her predoctoral clinical internship and a postdoctoral fellowship at Brown University, specializing in addictions. She completed her graduate training in clinical psychology at the University of Colorado at Boulder where she also received interdisciplinary graduate training at the Institute for Behavioral Genetics. Dr. Ray's research interests involve human laboratory studies, behavioral genetics of addiction, and pharmacogenetics. Dr. Ray may be contacted at Department of Psychology, University of California Los Angeles, Los Angeles, California.

Michelle R. Resor, BA, is a doctoral student in the Clinical Health Psychology PhD program at the University of North Carolina at Charlotte. She has collaborated with researchers on several federally funded research projects investigating topics including alcohol-related beliefs and behaviors of Hispanic individuals living on the United States–Mexico border, effectiveness of interventions for heavy drinking Hispanic college students, smoking and physical activity among veterans, trauma and sexual risk among patients receiving treatment for comorbid substance use and mental health disorders, evaluation of systems of caring for youths with severe emotional disturbances, and adjustment of youths and families affected by Hurricane Katrina. Michelle Resor can be contacted at Department of Psychology, University of North Carolina at Charlotte, Charlotte, North Carolina.

Paul M. Roman, PhD, has been director of the Center for Research on Behavioral Health and Human Services Delivery at the Institute for Behavioral Research, University of Georgia, since 1986 where he is also distinguished research professor of Sociology. Previously he was the Charles A. and Leo M. Favrot Professor of Human Relations and professor of sociology and epidemiology at Tulane University where he served on the faculty from 1969 to 1986. His BS and PhD degrees are from Cornell University. His research for the past 20 years has focused on the organization and management of treatment systems. Earlier in his career he originated program designs for intervention with employees with substance abuse problems and is known for deriving the Core Technology of Employee Assistance Programs (EAPs) that persists as a quality standard into the 21st century. He has served on many panels and review committees for the National Institutes of the Health, the Institute of Medicine, and the National Academy of Sciences over the past 40 years. Dr. Roman may be contacted at the University of Georgia, Institute for Behavioral Research, Athens, Georgia.

David B. Rosengren, PhD, is a clinical psychologist who splits his time between working as a research scientist at the University of Washington's Alcohol and Drug Abuse Institute, as a MI consultant and trainer, and private practice provider. The consistent themes in his work are motivation and the process of change. Presently, his treatment focus is adolescents, and his research evaluates methods of training practitioners. He completed the initial Training for Trainer's of MI course offered by Miller and Rollnick in 1993 and has provided regular training in MI since. He is a principal in 2 Steps Forward Training and Consultation (www.2sft. com) and is engaged in a state-wide MI training effort for child welfare professionals in Washington State. He is former editor of a newsletter for MI trainers and one of the founders of the Motivational Interviewing Network of Trainers (an international association representing 500+ MI trainers spread across 30+ countries and six continents and former steering committee member. Dr. Rosengren completed his graduate work at the University of Montana, his clinical internship at the Seattle Veteran's Affairs Medical Center, and a postdoctoral residency at Western State Hospital in Ft. Steilacoom, WA. Dr. Rosengren may be contacted at University of Washington, Alcohol and Drug Abuse Institute, Seattle, Washington.

Cynthia L. Rowe, PhD, is associate professor of epidemiology and Public Health, University of Miami Miller School of Medicine's Center for Treatment Research on Adolescent Drug Abuse (CTRADA; H. Liddle, Director). Dr. Rowe has been part of the CTRADA since 1994 and has extensive experience in community-based clinical research. She has trained and supervised therapists in Multidimensional Family Therapy (MDFT) in controlled trials and in community implementation projects in diverse practice settings. Dr. Rowe has particular expertise in evaluating and monitoring therapist adherence and competence. She has been project director of several MDFT clinical trials, including two multisite studies and a multi-national randomized trial of adolescent substance abuse treatment in Europe. She is also PI of a NIDA-funded randomized clinical trial that compares MDFT and group CBT with youth and families in the New Orleans area who were affected by Hurricane Katrina. Dr. Rowe may be contacted at University of Miami Miller School of Medicine, Miami, Florida.

Craig R. Rush, PhD, is a professor in the Department of Behavioral Science in College of Medicine at University of Kentucky. Dr. Rush also has appointments in the departments of psychiatry (College of Medicine) and psychology (College of Arts and Science) at the University of Kentucky. Dr. Rush completed predoctoral training at the University of Vermont (Human Behavioral Pharmacology Laboratory) and postdoctoral training at Johns Hopkins University (Behavioral Pharmacology Research Unit) both of which were funded by training grants from the National Institute of Drug Abuse (NIDA). Dr. Rush specialized in human behavioral pharmacology during both his predoctoral and postdoctoral training. Dr. Rush's research interests are focused on the conduct of human behavioral pharmacology aimed at identifying pharmacotherapies for amphetamine and cocaine abuse. Dr. Rush may be contacted at Department of Behavioral Science, University of Kentucky, Lexington, Kentucky.

Dean Sagun, BA, is a research assistant in the Center for Social Work Research at the University of Texas at Austin. Mr Sagun's research interests involve adolescent substance abuse prevention.

Andrew J. Saxon, MD, is a professor in the Department of Psychiatry and Behavioral Sciences at the University of Washington and the Director of both the Addictions Treatment Center, VA Puget Sound Health Care System and the Addiction Psychiatry Residency Program, University of Washington. Preceding his entry into psychiatry, Dr. Saxon completed an internal medicine internship and worked for four years as an emergency room physician. Subsequent to his general psychiatry residency at the University of Washington, Dr. Saxon has had 22 years of experience as a clinical and research addiction psychiatrist. Dr. Saxon is board certified with added qualifications in addiction psychiatry by the American Board of Psychiatry and Neurology. Dr. Saxon serves as one of five National Clinical Experts on office-based treatment of opioid dependence with buprenorphine for the Physician Clinical Suppport System, a national mentoring network for physicians. He is a corresponding member of the Council on Addiction Psychiatry of the American Psychiatric Association. He is a member of the Consensus Panel for the development of the Treatment Improvement Protocol, "Medication Treatment for Alcohol Dependence," as part of the Center for Substance Abuse Treatment's Knowledge Application Program. He sits on the editorial boards of the journals, *Drug and Alcohol Dependence* and *General Hospital Psychiatry*. Dr. Saxon's current research work involves pharmacotherapies and psychotherapies for alcohol, cocaine, methamphetamine, nicotine, and opioid dependence as well work in co-occurence of substance dependence and posttraumatic stress disorder. Dr. Saxon may be contacted at Department of Psychiatry and Behavioral Sciences, University of Washington School of Medicine, VAPSHCS, Seattle, Washington.

Kenneth J. Sher, PhD, is Curators' Professor of Psychological Sciences at the University of Missouri where he is associate chair for research enhancement and a pre- and post-doctoral training program in alcohol studies. His primary research interests are in the areas of the etiology of alcohol dependence, research methodology (especially longitudinal research), and the relation between personality and psychopathology. He may be contacted at University of Missouri, Columbia, Missouri.

Jane Ellen Smith, PhD, is a professor in the Psychology Department at the University of New Mexico. She received her PhD in clinical psychology from the State University of New York at Binghamton. She is currently the chair of the Psychology Department and has served as the director of clinical training for the doctoral program in Clinical Phychology at the University of New Mexico. Dr. Smith specializes in both substance abuse and eating disorders. Within the substance abuse arena she primarily has explored applications of the Community Reinforcement Approach (CRA). She has co-authored books on CRA and received grants from the National Institute on Alcohol Abuse and Alcoholism (NIAAA) to test CRA with homeless populations. Dr. Smith was just awarded the University of New Mexico's highest teaching award: the Presidential Teaching Fellowship (2007–2009). Dr. Smith may be contacted at Department of Psychology, University of New Mexico, Albuquerque, New Mexico.

William W. Stoops, PhD, is an assistant professor in the Department of Behavioral Science in the College of Medicine at the University of Kentucky. Dr. Stoops completed graduate training in the department of psychology and postdoctoral training in the department of behavioral science at the University of Kentucky. Dr. Stoops specialized in human behavioral pharmacology during both his graduate and postdoctoral training. Dr. Stoops's current research interests are focused on the conduct of human behavioral pharmacology aimed at understanding the effects of drugs that contribute to abuse and identifying pharmacotherapies for stimulant dependence. Dr. Stoops may be contacted at Department of Behavioral Science, University of Kentucky, Lexington, Kentucky.

Joji Suzuki, MD, is an instructor in psychiatry at Harvard Medical School and the Medical Director of the Addiction Psychiatry Service in the department of psychiatry at Brigham and Women's Hospital. Dr. Suzuki completed his residency in general Psychiatry at Maine Medical Center, Portland, Maine and his addition psychiatry fellowship at Boston University's Boston Medical Center, Boston, Massachusetts. Dr. Suzuki may be contacted at the Brigham and Women's Hospital, Boston, Massachusetts.

Sarah A. Ting, MA, is a doctoral candidate in Social Psychology at Claremont Graduate University. Sarah completed her master's training at Claremont Graduate University with a focus on identifying client characteristics that lead to recidivism in substance abuse treatment programs. She holds an adjunct position in the psychology department at Mt. San Antonio College. Her research involves exploration of various prevention, education, and treatment programs to identify situational, dispositional, and psychological factors that lead to initiation and continuation of risky health behaviors, such as substance use. Sarah may be contacted at Department of Psychology, Claremont Graduate University, Claremont, California.

Ryan G. Vandrey, PhD, is an assistant professor in the Department of Psychiatry and Behavioral Science at Johns Hopkins University School of Medicine. Dr. Vandrey completed his postdoctoral research fellowship at Johns Hopkins University School of Medicine. He received his doctorate in experimental psychology from the University of Vermont. Both his predoctoral and postdoctoral training were funded by institutional training grants awarded by the National Institute on Drug Abuse (NIDA). Dr. Vandrey's research includes study of the consequences of stopping heavy cannabis and tobacco use and the investigation of medications that can help people trying to quit. He also conducts research investigating novel ways to apply behavioral modification techniques such as contingency management (CM) to the treatment of drug abuse problems. Dr. Vandrey can be contacted at Behavioral Pharmacology Research Unit, Johns Hopkins University, Baltimore, Maryland.

Andrea R. Vansickel, MA, is a predoctoral student in the Department of Psychology in the College of Arts and Sciences at the University of Kentucky. Ms. Vansickel is currently a National Institute of Drug Abuse (NIDA) predoctoral trainee and also serves as the student representative to Division 28 of the American Psychological Association (APA). Ms. Vansickel completed her Bachelor of Arts at the Massachusetts College of Liberal Arts (MCLA) and completed her Master of Arts at the University of Kentucky under the supervision of Dr. Craig R. Rush. As an undergraduate, Ms. Vansickel's research focus was in the experimental analysis of behavior. Her current research focus is in human behavioral pharmacology. Ms. Vansickel's research interests are focused on the conduct of human behavioral pharmacology aimed at identifying pharmacotherapies for amphetamine and cocaine abuse as well as characterizing the effects of stimulants on tobacco smoking behavior. Ms. Vansickel may be contacted at Department of Behavioral Science, University of Kentucky, Lexington, Kentucky.

Michael R. Villanueva, BS, is a doctoral student in the Clinical Health Psychology PhD program at the University of North Carolina Charlotte. Mr Villanueva completed his undergraduate study in biology at the University of Texas at San Antonio, and was in his third year of medical school training at the Texas Tech University Health Sciences Center before changing course and pursuing his degree in clinical psychology. Mr Villanueva's research interests include investigating psychological correlates of gambling and neuropsychological correlates of addictive processes. Mr Villanueva can be contacted at Department of Psychology, University of North Carolina at Charlotte, Charlotte, North Carolina.

Rudy E. Vuchinich, PhD, did his graduate and internship training at Vanderbilt University and Brown University, respectively. Currently he is a professor and associate director of medical (clinical) psychology in the department of psychology at the University of Alabama at Birmingham. He also is affiliated with the department of health behavior in the School of Public Health and with the Center for Health Promotion and the Lister Hill Center for Health Policy. He is a fellow in four divisions of the American Psychological Association, and is past president of the APA's division on addictions. Dr. Vuchinich has published several scientific articles, books, and book chapters on substance abuse, behavioral economics, and self-control. Currently he is working on projects investigating clinical treatments for cocaine dependence, marijuana use among college students, and the behavioral economics and neuroeconomics of disordered gambling. Dr. Vuchinich may be contacted at Department of Psychology, University of Alabama at Birmingham, Birmingham, Alabama.

Index

DATE DUE

MAY 0 8 2011		

Demco, Inc. 38-293